Harborview Illustrated Tips and Tricks in Fracture Surgery

SECOND EDITION

M. Bradford Henley, MD, MBA
Professor of Orthopaedic Surgery and Sports Medicine
Department of Orthopaedics and Sports Medicine
Harborview Medical Center
University of Washington
Seattle, Washington

Michael F. Githens, MD
Assistant Professor of Orthopaedic Surgery and Sports Medicine
Harborview Medical Center
University of Washington
Seattle, Washington

Michael J. Gardner, MD
Professor and Vice Chair
Chief, Orthopaedic Trauma
Stanford University School of Medicine
Palo Alto, California

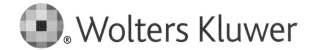

Philadelphia • Baltimore • New York • London
Buenos Aires • Hong Kong • Sydney • Tokyo

Acquisitions Editor: Brian Brown
Editorial Coordinator: Tim Rinehart
Editorial Assistant: Amy Masgay
Marketing Manager: Dan Dressler
Production Project Manager: Marian Bellus
Design Coordinator: Stephen Druding
Illustrator: Scott Bodell
Manufacturing Coordinator: Beth Welsh
Prepress Vendor: SPi Global

2nd edition

Copyright © 2019 Wolters Kluwer

9 8 7 6 5 4 3 2

Printed in China

Library of Congress Cataloging-in-Publication Data
Names: Gardner, Michael J., editor. | Henley, M. Bradford, editor. |Harborview Medical Center (Seattle, Wash.)
Title: Harborview illustrated tips and tricks in fracture surgery / [edited by] Michael J. Gardner, M. Bradford Henley.
Other titles: Illustrated tips and tricks in fracture surgery
Description: 2nd edition. | Philadelphia : Wolters Kluwer, [2018] | Includes bibliographical references and index.
Identifiers: LCCN 2017054316 | ISBN 9781496355980
Subjects: | MESH: Fractures, Bone—surgery | Orthopedic Procedures | Atlases
Classification: LCC RD101 | NLM WE 17 | DDC 617.1/5—dc23 LC record available at https://lccn.loc.gov/2017054316

LWW.com

Contributors

Mark R. Adams, MD

Assistant Professor
Orthopaedic Trauma Fellowship Director
Department of Orthopaedics
Rutgers, New Jersey Medical School
Newark, New Jersey

David P. Barei, MD, FRCSC

Professor
Department of Orthopaedic Surgery
Fellowship Director, Orthopaedic Traumatology
Harborview Medical Center
University of Washington
Seattle, Washington

Daphne M. Beingessner, BMath, BSc, MSc, MD, FRCSC

Associate Professor
Department of Orthopaedics and Sports Medicine
University of Washington
Seattle, Washington

Stephen K. Benirschke, MD

Professor of Orthopaedic Surgery and Sports Medicine
Department of Orthopaedics and Sports Medicine
Harborview Medical Center
University of Washington
Seattle, Washington

Mitchell Bernstein, MD, FRCSC

Assistant Professor
Departments of Surgery & Pediatric Surgery
McGill University
Head, Pediatric Orthopaedic Trauma
Montreal Children's Hospital
Co-Director, Limb Deformity Unit
Shriners Hospital for Children—Canada
Orthopaedic Trauma & Limb Deformity Surgery
Montreal General Hospital
Montreal, Quebec, Canada

Julius Bishop, MD

Assistant Professor and Associate Residency Director
Department of Orthopaedic Surgery
Stanford University School of Medicine
Palo Alto, California

Michael L. Brennan, MD

Vice Chairman and Director of Orthopaedic Trauma
Department of Orthopaedic Surgery
Baylor Scott and White Health
Temple, Texas

Dave Brokaw, MD

Orthopedic Trauma Surgeon
Indiana Orthopedic Hospital
Indianapolis, Indiana

Steven M. Cherney, MD

Assistant Professor
Department of Orthopaedic Surgery
University of Arkansas for Medical Sciences
Little Rock, Arkansas

Joseph Cohen, MD

Assistant Professor of Orthopedic Trauma
Department of Orthopedic Surgery
Loyola University Medical Center
Maywood, Illinois

Peter A. Cole, MD

Division Medical Director, HealthPartners Medical Group
Chair, Orthopaedic Department, Regions Hospital
Professor, University of Minnesota
Minneapolis, Minnesota

William W. Cross III, MD

Assistant Professor
Vice Chair, Department of Orthopedic Surgery
Chair, Division of Community Orthopedic Surgery
Division of Orthopedic Trauma
Department of Orthopedic Surgery
Mayo Clinic
Rochester, Minnesota

Bryce A. Cunningham, MD

Orthopedic Trauma Surgeon
Department of Orthopaedic Surgery
University of Tennessee College of Medicine—Chattanooga/Erlanger Hospital
Chattanooga, Tennessee

iii

Christopher Domes, MD

Resident
University of Washington Department of Orthopaedics and
  Sports Medicine
Harborview Medical Center
Seattle, Washington

Anthony J. Dugarte, MD

Research Fellow
Department of Orthopaedic Surgery
Regions Hospital
University of Minnesota
Minneapolis, Minnesota

Jonathan Eastman, MD

Associate Professor
Department of Orthopaedic Surgery
University of California, Davis Medical Center
Sacramento, California

Andrew R. Evans, MD, FACS

Assistant Professor of Orthopedic Surgery
Co-Director, Orthopedic Trauma, Brown University
Rhode Island Hospital
Providence, Rhode Island

Jason M. Evans, MD

Orthopaedic Trauma Surgery and Complex Fracture Care
Department of Surgery
TriStar Skyline Medical Center
Nashville, Tennessee

Eric D. Farrell, MD

Assistant Clinical Professor
Department of Orthopaedic Surgery
David Geffen School of Medicine at UCLA
Los Angeles, California

Michael J. Gardner, MD

Professor and Vice Chair
Chief, Orthopaedic Trauma
Stanford University School of Medicine
Palo Alto, California

Matthew R. Garner, MD

Assistant Professor of Orthopaedics and Rehabilitation
Division of Orthopaedic Trauma
Milton S. Hershey Medical Center
Penn State College of Medicine
Hershey, Pennsylvania

Reza Firoozabadi, MD, MA

Assistant Professor of Orthopaedic Surgery and Sports
  Medicine
Department of Orthopaedics and Sports Medicine
Harborview Medical Center
University of Washington
Seattle, Washington

Michael F. Githens, MD

Assistant Professor of Orthopaedic Surgery and Sports
  Medicine
Department of Orthopaedics and Sports Medicine
Harborview Medical Center
University of Washington
Seattle, Washington

Douglas P. Hanel, MD

Professor
Director of Orthopaedic Education
Section of Hand and Microvascular Surgery
Department of Orthopaedics and Sports Medicine
University of Washington
Seattle, Washington

Edward J. Harvey, MD, MSc, FRCSC

Professor of Surgery
McGill University
Michal and Renata Hornstein Chair in Surgical
  Excellence
Montreal General Hospital
Montreal, Quebec, Canada

Jonah Hébert-Davies, MD, FRCSC

Assistant Professor
Harborview Medical Center
University of Washington
Seattle, Washington

Garin G. Hecht, MD

Instructor
Department of Orthopaedic Surgery and Sports Medicine
Harborview Medical Center
University of Washington
Seattle, Washington

M. Bradford Henley, MD, MBA

Professor of Orthopaedic Surgery and Sports Medicine
Department of Orthopaedics and Sports Medicine
Harborview Medical Center
University of Washington
Seattle, Washington

Jessica Hooper, MD

Resident Physician
Department of Orthopaedic Surgery
NYU Langone Orthopaedic Hospital
New York, New York

Robert A. Hymes, MD

Associate Professor, Section Chief Orthopaedic Trauma,
  Director of Clinical Research
Orthopaedic Surgery
Inova Fairfax Medical Campus, VCU School of Medicine
Fairfax, Virginia

Stephen A. Kennedy, MD, FRCSC

Assistant Professor
Department of Orthopaedics and Sports Medicine
University of Washington
Seattle, Washington

Conor Kleweno, MD

Assistant Professor
Department of Orthopaedic Surgery
Harborview Medical Center
Seattle, Washington

Stephen A. Kottmeier, MD

Chief of Orthopaedic Trauma Service
Professor of Clinical Orthopaedics
Department of Orthopaedic Surgery
State University of New York—Health Sciences Center at
   Stony Brook
Stony Brook, New York

Thomas M. Large, MD

Orthopaedic Trauma Surgeon
Mission Orthopaedic Trauma Services
Mission Hospital
Asheville, North Carolina

James Learned, MD

Assistant Clinical Professor of Orthopaedic Surgery
UC Irvine Medical Center
Orange, California

Justin F. Lucas, MS, MD

Orthopedic Trauma Fellow
Department of Orthopedics and Sports Medicine
Harborview Medical Center
University of Washington
Seattle, Washington

Randall Drew Madison, MD

Clinical Instructor
Department of Orthopaedic Surgery
State University of New York—Stony Brook University Hospital
Stony Brook, New York

Aden N. Malik, MD

Resident
Department of Orthopaedic Surgery
State University of New York—Stony Brook University
Stony Brook, New York

Randall E. Marcus, MD

Charles H. Herndon Professor and Chairman
Department of Orthopedics
Case Western Reserve University
University Hospitals Cleveland Medical Center
Cleveland, Ohio

Anna N. Miller, MD

Associate Professor
Chief, Orthopaedic Trauma
Department of Orthopaedic Surgery
Washington University School of Medicine
St. Louis, Missouri

Matthew A. Mormino, MD

Professor
Department of Orthopaedic Surgery
University of Nebraska Medical Center
Omaha, Nebraska

Sean E. Nork, MD

Professor of Orthopaedic Surgery and Sports
   Medicine
Department of Orthopaedics and Sports
   Medicine
Harborview Medical Center
University of Washington
Seattle, Washington

Sarah C. Pettrone, MD (deceased)

Hand Fellow
Department of Orthopaedics
University of Washington
Commonwealth Orthopaedics
Reston, Virginia

Eric G. Puttler, MD

Orthopedic Surgeon
Rainier Orthopedic Institute
Puyallup, Washington

Motasem Refaat, MD

Clinical Instructor
Orthopaedic Surgery and Orthopaedic Trauma
University of California, San Francisco
San Francisco, California

Zachary V. Roberts, MD

Orthopedic Surgeon
DFP Orthopedics
Research Medical Center
Centerpoint Medical Center
North Kansas City Hospital
Kansas City, Missouri

Nicholas M. Romeo, DO

Assistant Professor
Department of Orthopaedic Surgery
Case Western Reserve University School of
   Medicine
MetroHealth Medical Center
Cleveland, Ohio

Milton Lee (Chip) Routt Jr, MD

The Andrew R. Burgess M.D. Professor and
  Endowed Chair
Department of Orthopedic Surgery
McGovern Medical School
University of Texas Health Science Center
Houston, Texas

John A. Scolaro, MD, MA

Associate Clinical Professor
Department of Orthopaedic Surgery
University of California, Irvine
Orange, California

Daniel N. Segina, MD

Director of Orthopaedic Trauma
Vice Chairman, Department of Orthopaedic Surgery
Holmes Regional Medical Center
Melbourne, Florida

Justin C. Siebler, MD

Associate Professor
Chief Orthopaedic Trauma
Department of Orthopaedic Surgery and Rehabilitation
University of Nebraska Medical Center
Omaha, Nebraska

Michael S. Sirkin, MD

Vice Chairman and Professor
Department of Orthopedics
Rutgers, New Jersey Medical School
Newark, New Jersey

Clay A. Spitler, MD

Assistant Professor
Department of Orthopaedic Surgery
University of Mississippi Medical Center
Jackson, Mississippi

Matthew P. Sullivan, MD

Assistant Professor of Orthopaedic Surgery
Department of Orthopaedic Surgery
State University of New York—Upstate Orthopedics
Upstate University Hospital
Syracuse, New York

Hobie Summers, MD

Associate Professor, Chief of Orthopaedic Trauma
Department of Orthopaedic Surgery and
  Rehabilitation
Loyola University Medical Center
Maywood, Illinois

Lisa A. Taitsman, MD, MPH

Associate Professor of Orthopaedic Surgery and Sports
  Medicine
Department of Orthopaedics and Sports Medicine
Harborview Medical Center
University of Washington
Seattle, Washington

Nirmal C. Tejwani, MD

Professor, NYU Langone Orthopedics
Chief of Trauma, Bellevue Hospital
New York, New York

Edward R. Westrick, MD

Assistant Professor
Drexel University College of Medicine
Orthopaedic Trauma Surgeon
Allegheny General Hospital of Allegheny Health Network
Pittsburgh, Pennsylvania

Raymond D. Wright Jr, MD

Associate Professor, Orthopaedic Surgery
Orthopaedic Trauma Fellowship Director
Department of Orthopaedic Surgery and Sports Medicine
University of Kentucky Chandler Medical Center
Lexington, Kentucky

Brad J. Yoo, MD

Associate Professor
Department of Orthopaedics and Rehabilitation
Yale University
New Haven, Connecticut

Brandon J. Yuan, MD

Assistant Professor of Orthopedics
Orthopedic Trauma Service
Mayo Clinic College of Medicine
Rochester, Minnesota

Foreword to the First Edition

When I was a resident during the mid-1970s, fracture management revolved around the use of plaster casts and traction. Young men with femur fractures remained hospitalized for weeks, lying in beds inclined on wooded boxes to counteract the pull of heavy weights. They were then placed in plaster spica casts for several months. Open fractures were treated with pins in plaster and the Orr method. Osteomyelitis and amputations were common. Some fractures were opened and fixed with straight nails or plates, but the indications were inconsistent and unclear. Custom-molded plastic bracing and functional treatment were introduced by Sarmiento, and his fracture courses in Miami were very popular. The faculty at the one I attended as a senior resident included a little-known surgeon from Seattle named Sigvard "Ted" Hansen. He reported on the initial results from Harborview Hospital with the closed nailing technique they had learned when Gerhard Kuntscher visited. To support his case for the superiority of the technique, he argued that animals with endoskeletons were more advanced than those with exoskeletons. Ted later noted that this presentation I witnessed was the launching for closed nailing and the beginning of the transition to a new era of treatment for long bone fractures.

I traveled to Davos for the annual AO course as a chief resident. There was a small zealous group of mostly European surgeons who were developing a system of internal fixation that was not yet embraced by American orthopaedic surgeons. The precisely designed Swiss implants and equipment and highly organized approach to operative fracture care were very appealing. When this system was introduced in the United States, the emphasis on early rigid fixation and rapid mobilization caused a major shift in fracture care. During this period, external fixation had a revival in the United States and was used extensively for open fractures, which were prevalent as the United States reached the peak of road traffic deaths and injuries.

Working at the Maryland Shock Trauma Center, housed then in an old wing of the hospital, I was a participant in and a witness to the birth of a new field called orthopaedic trauma. The focus became optimal care of seriously injured patients and treatment of complex musculoskeletal injuries. We incorporated the new techniques and moved away from the old methods. A pivotal moment occurred at the 1983 AAOS meeting in Las Vegas when Bob Winquist presented the highly positive Harborview experience with the closed nailing of 504 femoral fractures. Because of its significance, the presentation was scheduled in the slot before the first vice presidential address and was heard by an audience of thousands in a massive rotunda ballroom. Gus Sarmiento the leading apostle of functional bracing, who was the discussant, acknowledged that the technique offered unprecedented advantages and would change the standard of care.

Over the subsequent 27 years, the field of orthopaedic trauma has evolved constantly, and modern fracture management has spread throughout the world. The orthopaedic faculty at Harborview has been among the leading groups in the subspecialty. Serving as the trauma referral center for surrounding states, they have consistently been receiving large volume of patients, which allowed them to develop a large group of orthopaedic trauma faculty. They have amassed a large collective experience and completed many important clinical studies. Their emphasis on excellence and constant pursuit of improved methods of care has enabled them to establish and refine a series of protocols for operative management. Surgeons from all over the world visit the center to observe their approach to trauma care. Their orthopaedic trauma fellowship is considered the premier experience in the country.

Brad Henley, MD, MBA, a veteran member of the Harborview Orthopaedic Trauma group, has used his clinical expertise and business leadership skills to organize an outstanding surgical technique atlas. Members of the Harborview Orthopaedic Trauma faculty and current and former orthopaedic trauma fellows created the various chapters. A consistent approach was used combining very high-quality intraoperative photos and beautiful halftone line drawings. Details of surgical technique are conveyed in brief notes, which form legends for each illustration.

This treatise will provide valuable supplementation on surgical management and technique to the information contained in major fracture texts. There is a growing need for this type of detailed "how to do it" guidance. Successive global burden of disease and injury analyses document a growing prevalence of road traffic injuries, particularly in the developing world. The problem stems from vulnerable road travelers sharing the roads with heavy vehicles and public transportation that are overcrowded and dangerous. Increasing numbers of deaths and injuries result and disabling musculoskeletal disabilities are causing major social and economic impact. Rapid motorization in populous, economically powerful countries such as India and China is causing a surge in injuries to occupants of cars. Airbags, seat belts, and improved car design have decreased the fatality rate in developed countries, but severe lower extremity injuries are not prevented by current measures. Medical systems in many countries are evolving to levels where surgeons will be able to employ modern methods of internal and external fixation to avoid disabilities. This Harborview book will be an extremely useful resource that will assist them with the quest for optimal patient care.

Bruce Douglas Browner, MD, MS, FACS

Preface to the Alumni (Second) Edition

The genesis for this second alumni edition of *Harborview Illustrated Tips and Tricks in Fracture Surgery* came from discussions with several of our ACE graduates, many of whom are trauma surgeons at other trauma hospitals in the United States, Canada, and internationally. These surgeons found the first edition to be useful and well received by their colleagues, residents, and their orthopaedic trauma fellows. Many volunteered that they learned other "tips and tricks" during their fellowship from their Harborview faculty mentors and that these hadn't been included in the first edition. Alternatively, our graduates also either had improved on what they had learned or had their own tip(s) that they wanted to share with a wider audience in hopes of improving patient care. They encouraged me to reach out to all of graduates from Harborview's Ortho Trauma program asking for volunteers who might want to contribute one or more tips and tricks to this second "Alumni Edition." We received contributions from past trauma fellows spanning nearly 40 years of our program. The most "senior" graduate to submit a tip is Randy Marcus (Class of 1980), and we also received many tips from the most recent graduating class (2015, see Table 1 below). While most submitted just one tip, a few submitted in excess of five manuscripts.

Though these tip chapters are authored by our alumni, this doesn't mean that they are claiming ownership of any specific technique or procedure nor does authorship imply that the technique is necessarily their "invention." Some of these tips have been published previously by the same or different authors. We want to emphasize that the idea behind the first edition and now this second "Alumni Edition" of *Harborview Illustrated Tips and Tricks in Fracture Surgery* has been to further the care of trauma patients by disseminating novel or helpful ideas that hopefully will increase quality of orthopaedic trauma care. It is not to give attribution to the author for the tip but instead to credit the author for the work involved in writing and illustrating the tip for the benefit of other surgeons. Though it may have been ideal if the author could give attribution to the tip's creator, should it not be his/her own, this was not an expectation.

Mike Gardner and I have enlisted the editorial assistance of Mike Githens (class of 2016) in reviewing and revising many of the chapters from the first edition. Mike joined the Harborview Trauma faculty after completing his fellowship, and his "fresh eyes" and ideas have contributed to the breadth and depth of this second Alumni Edition. We thank him for his painstaking attention to detail and have added him as the third editor to this publication.

Mike Gardner and I also went through each of the new tip and trick submissions at least three times and took editorial license, so as to embellish, clarify, and make the text consistent with the style of the first edition. While enlarging the text significantly, we have maintained the organization of the first edition. The names of all authors contributing to a specific chapter are listed in alphabetic order at the beginning of each chapter. Some of the new alumni tips have been integrated into the text of each chapter while others are called out and featured separately. When featured as a separate tip or trick within a chapter, the name(s) of the contributor(s) submitting the specific tip is/are also associated with that feature. We should note too that we were unable to use every tip submitted though we thank the authors none the less.

As in the first edition, I would like to dedicate this book again to all of my colleagues (orthopaedic surgeons and nonorthopaedists) who provide emergency medical services to humankind. Should family or friends need emergency trauma care, I am glad to know that I can depend on the many trauma surgeons and physicians who have trained at Harborview Medical Center and at the other excellent trauma centers in the United States. I also want to acknowledge again, all of my past and present teachers and mentors but especially three of my role models, Professor Dr. med. Bernd Claudi, Dr. Kenneth D. Johnson, and Dr. Richard E. "Dickey" Jones (all former UTHSCD/Parkland physicians). Throughout their careers as orthopaedic surgeons, Bernd, Ken, and Dickey were committed to lifelong learning, teaching, and sharing their knowledge, ideas, and insights with fellows, residents, and medical students. All were incredibly generous individuals and gave their time and services freely to their patients and to their hospital's staff. They were always respectful to all members of the health care team, and both willing served the less fortunate by putting their patients' needs first and by always "doing the right thing" irrespective of reimbursement and the time of day.

I hope that the trauma faculty at Harborview, which has continued to change and expand since the first edition (Table 1), has instilled the same sense of purpose, and this service ethic in our ACEs. Since the first edition was written in 2009–2010, 36 more ACEs have been added to list found in the Preface to the first edition. Those who have completed the trauma fellowship and those currently enrolled are listed below (Table 2):

Table 1 ‖ Harborview-based UW Orthopaedic Faculty from 1988–2017

Last Name, First Name	Hire Date	Current or Departure Date
Hansen, Sigvard T.	7/1/1968	7/1/2011, now emeritus
Winquist, Robert A.	7/1/1974	5/25/1980
Veith, Robert G.	7/1/1980	3/31/1984
Mayo, Keith A.	6/25/1984 and 12/26/2012	11/12/1990 and 10/25/2015
Sack, John T.	7/1/1984	7/1/2014
Anderson, Paul A.	7/1/1985	Current
Benirschke, Stephen K.	1/1/1986	Current
Sangeorzan, Bruce J.	4/1/1987	Current
Henley, M. Bradford	2/1/1988	Current
Swiontkowski, Marc	5/1/1988	9/1/1997
Routt, M. L. Chip	7/1/1989	12/3/2012
Trumble, Thomas E.	7/1/1989	1/7/2010
Smith, Douglas G.	7/1/1990	12/31/2016, now emeritus
Chapman, Jens R.	8/1/1991	11/1/2014
Hanel, Douglas P.	6/1/1992	Current
Mirza, Sohail	9/1/1995	8/31/2008
Nork, Sean E.	8/1/1998	Current
Allan, Christopher H.	9/1/1998	current (now UWMC based)
Mills, William J.	9/10/1998	7/2/2004
Bellabarba, Carlo	10/1/1999	Current
Barei, David P.	8/1/2000	Current
Taitsman, Lisa A.	8/1/2002	Current
Bransford, Richard J.	10/6/2003	Current
Beingessner, Daphne M.	8/1/2004	Current
Dunbar, Robert P.	9/15/2005	Current
Krieg, James C.	7/1/2007	5/31/2013
Huang, Jerry I.	9/1/2008	Current (now UWMC based)
Firoozabadi, Reza	9/17/2012	Current
Kennedy, Stephen	3/5/2013	Current
Sagi, H. Claude	9/1/2015	Current
Hébert-Davies, Jonah	12/1/2016	Current
Githens, Michael	8/1/2016	Current

Table 2 I Chronology of HMC Orthopaedic Trauma ACEs from 2010–2018 (see Table 2 in the Preface to the first edition for those ACEs from 1978–2010)

Name	Begin Date	End Date	Length (mo)
Barber, Richard	8/1/2010	7/31/2011	12
Miller, Anna	8/1/2010	7/31/2011	12
Munz, John	8/1/2010	7/31/2011	12
Olson, Soren	8/1/2010	7/31/2011	12
Sharp, Lorra	8/1/2010	7/31/2011	12
Steeves, Mark	8/1/2010	7/31/2011	12
Adam, mark	8/1/2011	7/31/2012	12
Eastman, Jonathan	8/1/2011	7/31/2012	12
Frioozabadi, Reza	8/1/2011	7/31/2012	12
Large, Thomas	8/1/2011	7/31/2012	12
Schneidkraut, Jason	8/1/2011	7/31/2012	12
Bernstein, Mitchell	8/1/2012	7/31/2013	12
Maracek, Geoffrey	8/1/2012	7/31/2013	12
Scolaro, John	8/1/2012	7/31/2013	12
Shatsky, Joshua	8/1/2012	7/31/2013	12
Westrick, Edward	8/1/2012	7/31/2013	12
Fishler, Thomas	8/1/2013	7/31/2014	12
Hébert-Davies, Jonah	8/1/2013	7/31/2014	12
Learned, James	8/1/2013	7/31/2014	12
Little, Milton	8/1/2013	7/31/2014	12
Spittler, Clay	8/1/2013	7/31/2014	12
Lee, John	8/1/2014	7/31/2015	12
Schenker, Mara	8/1/2014	7/31/2015	12
Shearer, David	8/1/2014	7/31/2015	12
Toogood, Paul	8/1/2014	7/31/2015	12
Yuan, Brandon	8/1/2014	7/31/2015	12
Alton, Timothy	8/1/2015	7/31/2016	12
Garner, Matthew	8/1/2015	7/31/2016	12
Githens, Michael	8/1/2015	7/31/2016	12
Haller, Justin	8/1/2015	7/31/2016	12
Sullivan, Matthew	8/1/2015	7/31/2016	12
Cohen, Joseph	8/1/2016	7/31/2017	12
Hirschfeld, Adam	8/1/2016	7/31/2017	12
Murr, Kevin	8/1/2016	7/31/2017	12
Refaat, Motasem	8/1/2016	7/31/2017	12
Romeo, Nicholas	8/1/2016	7/31/2017	12
Donohue, David	8/1/2017	7/31/2018	12
Hecht, Garin	8/1/2017	7/31/2018	12
Lucas, Justin	8/1/2017	7/31/2018	12
Putnam, Sara	8/1/2017	7/31/2018	12
Talerico, Michael	8/1/2017	7/31/2018	12

Disclaimer

The material presented in the *Harborview Illustrated Tips and Tricks in Fracture Surgery* is for educational purposes only. This material is not intended to represent the only, nor necessarily best method or procedure appropriate for the medical situations discussed, but rather is intended to present an approach, view, statement, or opinion of the author(s), which may be helpful to others who face similar situations. The publisher, editors, and author(s) disclaim any and all liability for injury or other damages resulting to any individual for all claims that may arise out of the use of the techniques demonstrated therein by such individuals, whether these claims shall be asserted by a physician or any other person. No reproductions of any kind, including audio and video, may be made of the material presented in this publication.

FDA Statement

Some of the techniques, medical devices, and/or drugs described in the Illustrated Tips and Tricks in Fracture Surgery have been cleared by the FDA for specific purposes only, and some of the techniques, medical devices, and/or drugs may have not been cleared by the FDA. The FDA has stated that it is the responsibility of the physician to determine the FDA clearance status of each drug or medical device he or she wishes to use in clinical practice. It is the responsibility of the treating physician to disclose and discuss the "off-label" use of a drug or medical device with the patient (i.e., it must be disclosed that the FDA has not cleared the drug or device for the described purpose). Any drug or medical device is being used "off label" if the described use is not set forth on the product's approval label.

I also want to thank my wife, Ann Rutledge; my parents, Ernest and Elaine; my daughters, Taryn and Cailin; and my colleagues and friends for their support and help during this project.

Thank you very much
Brad Henley

Preface to the First Edition

I developed the idea for this book nearly 15 years ago. Like most orthopaedic surgeons, I learned surgical operations by reading about a specific or preferred technique. This was followed by observing the procedure as performed by a mentor. At some point in my training, I began performing these operations as the operating "surgeon," usually with the assistance of a senior physician. After I was awarded my first academic position at University of Texas Southwestern Health Science Center at Dallas (UTHSCD) and Parkland Hospital, I performed them independently. Also similar to most orthopaedic surgeons, after "reading one, doing one, and teaching one," I would frequently modify certain aspects of the operation to make it "better" and to improve my surgical efficiency. Throughout my career, I have continued to "refine" procedures, using what I believe are more effective and efficient methods of accomplishing the task of obtaining an anatomical reduction (an "ORIF" instead of an "OIF"[1]).

After leaving UTHSCD, I joined the University of Washington (UW) faculty at Harborview Medical Center (HMC). When I arrived in February 1988, the full-time faculty at HMC numbered only five: Sigvard "Ted" Hansen, Keith Mayo, Paul A. Anderson, Stephen K. Benirschke, and Bruce J. Sangeorzan. Steve and Bruce had recently completed fellowships in Trauma and Foot & Ankle, respectively. Later in 1988, Marc Swiontkowski joined our team expanding our number to seven. Ted, Bruce, and Paul had a nontrauma orthopaedic specialty as their primary clinical interest, though all took trauma call and cared for patients with musculoskeletal injuries. Over the next decades, the Harborview's Orthopaedic faculty contracted and expanded. Currently, we have eight full-time faculty trauma surgeons and Ted Hansen with more than 179 years of postfellowship trauma experience. Supplementing these core trauma surgeons are the other faculty based at HMC who share in covering trauma call, hand call, or spine call; I believe that the orthopaedic group at Harborview is the largest trauma group with the greatest accumulated experience treating musculoskeletal injuries in the nation (~280 physician years). Table 1 summarizes the orthopaedic faculty appointments and departures since my arrival at HMC.

The faculty at Harborview have a long history dedicated to graduate and postgraduate medical education. Beginning in the 1970s, they offered an opportunity for physicians desiring a greater trauma experience to spend time at the institution dedicated to the care of patients with musculoskeletal injuries. Both academic and community orthopaedists availed themselves of this experience and would spend either 3 or 6 months working with the residents and faculty. It was not until the mid-1980s that a few surgeons would stay for a year at a time. With the formation of the Orthopaedic Trauma Hospital Association (OTHA, the organization preceding the Orthopaedic Trauma Association [OTA; www.ota.org]), two 1-year long orthopaedic trauma fellowship positions were offered. By the late 1980s, after Marc Swiontkowski's and my arrival at HMC, three Advanced Clinical Experience (ACE) positions were offered per year. Over the next two decades, the number of positions expanded gradually from the initial three, to four, then five, and finally to the six trauma ACE positions we offer today. (Table 2 summarizes the chronology of HMC Orthopaedic Trauma ACEs.)

Being an orthopaedic trauma attending at Harborview Medical Center in Seattle allowed me to establish a practice devoted full time to musculoskeletal trauma. Performing operations, repetitively, provided many opportunities to devise my own set of tips and tricks. However, working at Harborview has also allowed me to work with some of the world's foremost thought leaders and best technical orthopaedic trauma surgeons. This environment has been conducive to collaboration and refinement of patient care. Our weekly fracture conference is renowned as it allows discourse and debate of the treatments for acute ortho trauma by six-twelve orthopaedic trauma surgeons. Additionally, my colleagues

---

[1]I ascribe this vernacular to the insights and surgical perfectionism of my partner and friend "Stevie B" (Stephen. K. Benirschke MD): ORIF — open reduction with internal fixation; OIF — open….with internal fixation.

Table 1 ▌ Harborview-Based UW Orthopaedic Faculty from 1988 to 2009

Last name, First name	Hire Date	Current or Depart Date
Hansen, Sigvard T.	7/1/1968	current
Winquist, Robert A.	7/1/1974	5/25/1980
Veith, Robert G.	7/1/1980	3/31/1984
Mayo, Keith A.	6/25/1984	11/12/1990
Sack, John T.	7/1/1984	current
Anderson, Paul A.	7/1/1985	4/30/1994
Benirschke, Stephen K.	1/1/1986	current
Sangeorzan, Bruce J.	4/1/1987	current
Henley, M. Bradford	2/1/1988	current
Swiontkowski, Marc	5/1/1988	9/1/1997
Routt, M. L. Chip	7/1/1989	current
Trumble, Thomas E.	7/1/1989	current
Smith, Douglas G.	7/1/1990	current
Chapman, Jens R.	8/1/1991	current
Hanel, Douglas P.	6/1/1992	current
Mirza, Sohail	9/1/1995	8/31/2008
Nork, Sean E.	8/1/1998	current
Allan, Christopher H.	9/1/1998	current
Mills, William J.	9/10/1998	7/2/2004
Bellabarba, Carlo	10/1/1999	current
Barei, David P.	8/1/2000	current
Taitsman, Lisa A.	8/1/2002	current
Bransford, Richard J.	10/6/2003	current
Beingessner, Daphne M.	8/1/2004	current
Dunbar, Robert P.	9/15/2005	current
Krieg, James C.	7/1/2007	current
Huang, Jerry I.	9/1/2008	current

and I can often "visit" with each other in between cases to observe each other's techniques and technical tips.

This has allowed us to disseminate our own ideas and those of our colleagues by incorporating each other's tricks, tips, and treatment philosophies into the care of our own patients and our educational philosophy.

Over the past 15 years, I have often thought of codifying these tips and tricks in journal articles or book form. Some tips and tricks have been published by HMC ACEs in orthopaedic journals but many ideas of the HMC trauma faculty are unpublished. It has been a habit of the ACEs to keep a diary or record of their cases noting surgical tips, tricks, and techniques. In September of the 2007–2008 ACE year, I pitched my idea to our six trauma fellows (Mike Brennan, Andy Evans, Jason Evans, Mike Gardner, Zach Roberts, and Ray Wright). I was greeted with enthusiastic support. Each of the ACEs digitally recorded their observations and lessons learned after each case or at the end of the day. They illustrated their notes with digital images saved from the image intensifier and planar radiographs during their 1-year experience. Their hand drawings were converted to medical illustrations by Scott Bodell, a superb medical illustrator whom I met while at UTHSCD (1985–1988). These image files were appended to their recorded observations and serve to illustrate many of the tips and tricks. This book is therefore the result of a single year's observations of select cases made by six orthopaedic trauma ACEs (8/2007–7/2008), each of whom was assigned authorship of one or more chapters.

Over the course of the year, Mike Gardner demonstrated an affinity for this book concept. He used his leadership skills to help me organize the project and served as the liaison with his peers. Based on his academic interest and his early and sustained contributions to the manuscript, I suggested that he serve as coeditor with me. Each ACE was assigned authorship of one or more chapters.

Mike and I understand that HMC is an orthopaedic center for the germination and coalescence of ideas and techniques. This is facilitated by a continuing stream of scholars, visitors, and physicians who seek education and advanced training. Together with the faculty, these individuals help catalyze the refinement of ideas and techniques, which lead to new techniques and improved patient care. We know that musculoskeletal trauma care will continue to evolve in the future. It is our hope that HMC and our ACE disciples will continue to maintain leadership roles through research and collaboration.

The editors and authors make no claim to many of the techniques, "tips," and "tricks" described in this publication. Instead, we view it as a compilation of those techniques that were used by the HMC

Table 2 ∥ Chronology of HMC Orthopaedic Trauma ACEs

Name	Begin Date	End Date	Length (mo)
Stuyck, Jos	10/13/1978	9/17/1979	11
Weber, Michael	10/1/1979	12/31/1979	3
Jackson, Robert	1/1/1980	6/30/1980	6
Marcus, Randall	4/1/1980	6/30/1980	3
Johnson, Kenneth D.	12/1/1980	6/15/1981	6
Shammas, Sameer	7/1/1980	12/31/1980	6
Jacobson, Wells	1/1/1981	3/31/1981	3
Kellam, James	4/1/1981	6/30/1981	3
Burney III, Dwight	7/1/1981	9/30/1981	3
Burman, William	10/1/1981	12/31/1981	3
Ratcliffe, Steven	1/1/1982	3/31/1982	3
Gerhart, Tobin	4/1/1982	6/30/1982	3
Webb, Lawrence	7/1/1983	12/31/1983	6
Moody,Wayne	1/3/1984	2/29/1984	2
LaMont, Justin	7/1/1984	6/30/1985	12
Wilber, John	7/1/1984	6/30/1985	12
Cotler, Howard	1/1/1985	6/30/1985	6
Lhowe, David	7/1/1985	12/31/1985	6
Moye, Daniel	7/1/1985	6/1/1986	11
Carr, James	8/1/1985	7/31/1986	12
Cornell, Charles	1/1/1986	6/30/1986	6
Jonassen, E. Andrew	7/1/1986	6/30/1987	12
Keeve, Jonathan	7/1/1986	12/31/1986	6
Donovan, Thomas	1/1/1987	4/30/1987	4
Benca, Paul	7/1/1987	6/30/1988	12
Carr, Charles	7/1/1987	12/31/1987	6
Kaehr, David	7/1/1987	6/30/1988	12
Verdin, Peter	7/1/1987	6/30/1988	12
Mirels, Hilton	7/1/1988	1/31/1989	7
Routt, Chip	7/1/1988	6/30/1989	12
Gruen, Gary	1/1/1989	6/30/1989	6
Agnew, Samuel	7/1/1989	7/31/1990	13
Santoro, Vincent	7/1/1989	7/15/1990	12
Peter, Robin	7/16/1990	7/15/1991	12
West, Gregory	7/16/1990	7/15/1991	12
Chapman, Jens	8/1/1990	1/31/1991	6
Kottmeier, Stephen	1/1/1991	7/31/1991	7
Cramer, Kathryn	8/1/1991	7/31/1992	12
Meier, Mark	8/1/1991	7/31/1992	12
Patterson, Brendan	8/1/1991	7/31/1992	12
Grujic, Les	8/1/1992	7/31/1993	12
Ott, Judson	8/1/1992	7/31/1993	12
Selznick, Hugh	8/1/1992	7/31/1993	12
Brokaw, David	8/1/1993	7/31/1994	12
Handley, Robert	8/1/1993	7/31/1994	12
Teague, David	8/1/1993	7/31/1994	12
McNamara, Kevin	4/1/1994	7/31/1994	4
Hubbard, David	8/1/1994	7/31/1995	12
Schwappach, John	8/1/1994	7/31/1995	12
Twaddle, Bruce	8/1/1994	7/31/1995	12
Weber, Tim	8/1/1994	7/31/1995	12
Clark III, Carey	8/1/1995	7/31/1996	12
Desai, Bharat	8/1/1995	7/31/1996	12
Krieg, James	8/1/1995	7/31/1996	12
Thomson, Gregory	8/1/1995	7/31/1996	12
Harding, Susan	8/1/1996	7/31/1997	12
Harvey, Edward	8/1/1996	7/31/1997	12
Mormino, Matt	8/1/1996	7/31/1997	12
O'Byrne, John	8/1/1996	7/31/1997	12
Cole, Peter	8/1/1997	7/31/1998	12
Jones, Cliff	8/1/1997	7/31/1998	12
Nork, Sean	8/1/1997	7/31/1998	12
Russell, George	8/1/1997	7/31/1998	12
Kuo, Roderick	8/1/1998	7/31/1999	12

(Continued)

Table 2 ▌ Chronology of HMC Orthopaedic Trauma ACEs (*Continued*)

Name	Begin Date	End Date	Length (mo)
Sanzone, Anthony	8/1/1998	7/31/1999	12
Segina, Daniel	8/1/1998	7/31/1999	12
Tejwani, Nirmal	8/1/1998	7/31/1999	12
Barei, David	8/1/1999	7/31/2000	12
Hymes, Robert	8/1/1999	7/31/2000	12
Schildhauer, Thomas	8/1/1999	7/31/2000	12
Schwartz, Alexandra	8/1/1999	7/31/2000	12
Ertl, William	8/1/2000	7/31/2001	12
Fowble, Coleman	8/1/2000	7/31/2001	12
Ringler, James	8/1/2000	7/31/2001	12
Vallier, Heather	8/1/2000	7/31/2001	12
Camuso, Matthew	7/1/2001	8/31/2002	14
McNair, Patrick	7/1/2001	8/31/2002	14
Taitsman, Lisa	8/1/2001	7/31/2002	12
Wagshul, Adam	8/1/2001	7/31/2002	12
Wiater, Patrick	8/1/2001	7/31/2002	12
Coles, Chad	8/1/2002	7/31/2003	12
Dunbar, Robert	8/1/2002	7/31/2003	12
Hammerberg, Eric Mark	8/1/2002	7/31/2003	12
Polonet, David	8/1/2002	7/31/2003	12
Smith, Carla	8/1/2002	7/31/2003	12
Beingessner, Daphne	8/1/2003	7/31/2004	12
Farrell, Eric	8/1/2003	7/31/2004	12
Howlett, Andrew	8/1/2003	7/31/2004	12
Molnar, Rob	8/1/2003	7/31/2004	12
Stafford, Paul	8/1/2003	7/31/2004	12
Confl itti, Joseph	8/1/2004	7/31/2005	12
Della Rocca, Gregory	8/1/2004	7/31/2005	12
Gomez, Arturo	8/1/2004	7/31/2005	12
Osgood, Gregory	8/1/2004	7/31/2005	12
Weiss, David	8/1/2004	7/31/2005	12
Bryant, Ginger	8/1/2005	7/31/2006	12
Graves, Matthew	8/1/2005	7/31/2006	12
Greene, Craig	8/1/2005	7/31/2006	12
Howard, James	8/1/2005	7/31/2006	12
O'Mara, Timothy	8/1/2005	7/31/2006	12
Yoo, Brad	8/1/2005	7/31/2006	12
Kubiak, Erik	8/1/2006	7/31/2007	12
Mehta, Samir	8/1/2006	7/31/2007	12
Mirza, Amer	8/1/2006	7/31/2007	12
Puttler, Eric	8/1/2006	7/31/2007	12
Summers, Hobie	8/1/2006	7/31/2007	12
Viskontas, Darius	8/1/2006	7/31/2007	12
Brennan, Michael	8/1/2007	7/31/2008	12
Evans, Andrew	8/1/2007	7/31/2008	12
Evans, Jason	8/1/2007	7/31/2008	12
Gardner, Michael	8/1/2007	7/31/2008	12
Roberts, Zachary	8/1/2007	7/31/2008	12
Wright, Raymond	8/1/2007	7/31/2008	12
Calafi , Leo	8/1/2008	7/31/2009	12
Maroto, Medardo	8/1/2008	7/31/2009	12
Morshed, Saam	8/1/2008	7/31/2009	12
Nwosa, Chinedu	8/1/2008	7/31/2009	12
Oldenburg, Frederick	8/1/2008	7/31/2009	12
Orec, Robert	8/1/2008	7/31/2009	12
Bishop, Julius	8/1/2009	7/31/2010	12
Cross, W. Woodie	8/1/2009	7/31/2010	12
Dikos, Greogry	8/1/2009	7/31/2010	12
Glasgow, Don	8/1/2009	7/31/2010	12
Maples, Allan	8/1/2009	7/31/2010	12
McAndrew, Christopher	8/1/2009	7/31/2010	12

faculty and observed and chronicled in a 1-year period by our six orthopaedic trauma ACEs. Some of these techniques were learned from interactions with our national and international colleagues while others may be accurately ascribed to a specific HMC faculty member. Some of these ideas may have been published previously by other authors and this is referenced only if we were aware of the prior publication.

I would like to dedicate this book to all of my colleagues (orthopaedists and nonorthopaedists) who provide emergency medical services to humankind. Should family or friends need emergency trauma care, I am glad to know that I can depend on the many trauma surgeons and physicians who have trained at Harborview and at the other excellent trauma centers in the United States. I want to acknowledge, especially, all of my past and present teachers and mentors (especially Professor Dr. med. Bernd Claudi and Dr. Kenneth D. Johnson), current and former (UTHSCD and UW/HMC) faculty colleagues, OTA colleagues and members, and HMC ACEs [see Tables 1 and 2]. It is these individuals and their disciples who have dedicated their careers to providing the emergency trauma services and are continuing graduate and postgraduate education needed by our nation. Most importantly, I want to thank my domestic partner Ann Rutledge; my parents, Ernest and Elaine; my daughters, Taryn and Cailin; and my colleagues and friends for their support and help during this project.

Thank you very much
Brad Henley

When I first visited Harborview during my residency, I attended the weekly fracture conference. After witnessing the postoperative fracture conference and X-ray presentations, I knew immediately I wanted to learn and emulate the quality, techniques, and style of fracture fixation that seemed to be consistent among all faculty. During my fellowship at Harborview, this conference was among the many highlights. The postoperative review of many fluoroscopic images in succession, often 15 or 20, made it possible to follow along the progression of the procedure, step by step. The subtleties of clamp placements for specific fracture fragments, reduction sequences for common fracture patterns, and the rationale for particular implant choices and positions were often discussed. This was an extremely effective way to teach and learn the technical aspects of fracture surgery. My co-fellows and I began to jot down names of interesting patients during the conference, and would later review and save the images. A critical mass of particularly demonstrative cases was obtained, and formed the basis of the present text. I have subsequently revisited these chapters countless times prior to operations, and hope it can similarly provide other young fracture surgeons with useful techniques. Participating in this "extra-curricular" activity during my fellowship and early career would not have been possible without the endless support and understanding from my wife, Katie, and daughter, Kelsey.

I hope that you will enjoy this compilation of tips, tricks and surgical cases that my colleagues and I have compiled.

Thank you
Mike Gardner

Tribute

On December 10, 2017, the orthopaedic trauma community was shocked and heartbroken to learn of the untimely passing of Dean G. Lorich, MD. As those who worked with Dean can attest, he was the epitome of a master surgeon. His attention to detail, relentless pursuit of perfection, and technical expertise were a few of the reasons nearly all of his trainees put him on an untouchable pedestal. He had a knack for innovative thinking that was unparalleled, and his refusal to concede that the standard was the best way to do something led him to push the envelope; his patients had better outcomes because of it. But perhaps more impressive and memorable than his personal dexterity and stamina was the energy and passion he had toward making his trainees better surgeons. He embodied "tough love," and the way he transformed and matured us as young surgeons was visible and unprecedented.

Now almost 10 years into practice, as my circle of colleagues and experience has expanded, it gets difficult to remember where I learned certain techniques or surgical approach nuances. But one never forgets where the basic principles and foundation of orthopaedic surgery were established. Dean gave that to me, and I am forever grateful. He was a mentor and friend to myself and countless residents, fellows, and others and will be deeply missed for a long time. Although he never would have wanted this much praise and gratitude, I'd like to dedicate this book to Dean, with a heartfelt "thank you," and may he rest in peace.

Mike Gardner

Contents

Section 1
Patient Positioning and Operative Principles

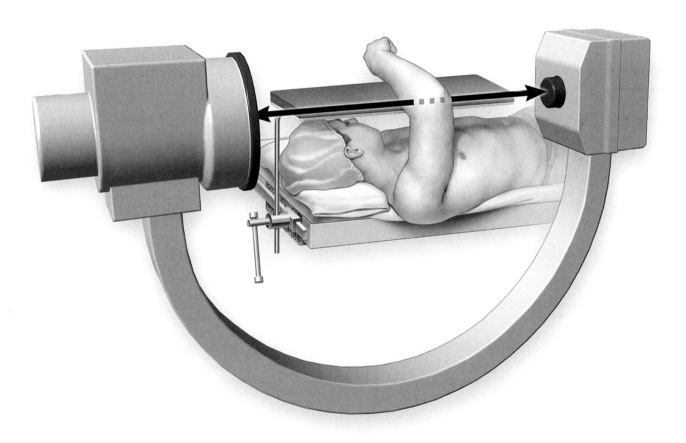

Chapter 1
Patient Positioning

MICHAEL L. BRENNAN

ERIC D. FARRELL

CONOR KLEWENO

LISA A. TAITSMAN

- The goal of positioning a patient for surgery is to allow the surgeon unrestricted access to the extremity (surgical site) for the surgical procedure and for imaging.
- Prolonged soft tissue pressure and shear forces from improper positioning may compromise quality of care and patient safety, resulting in tissue injuries such as circulatory embarrassment, perioperative pressure ulcers, and neurological injury, even in routine surgical procedures.

Upper Extremity

ORIF Clavicle, Proximal Humerus, Humeral Shaft

- Supine on reversed radiolucent cantilever table.
  - Standard beach chair positioning is an alternative.
- Patient brought as proximal and lateral on the table as possible, with head at the top corner of the table, ipsilateral to operative extremity (Figs. 1-1 and 1-2).
  - Neck should be slightly extended and head turned slightly away from operative extremity and secured with tape over a forehead towel.
- Small folded towel may be placed beneath the ipsilateral scapula if needed.
- C-arm from the top of the table, parallel to the long axis of the bed, permits axillary lateral image of the humerus in addition to standard imaging of the shoulder girdle.
- Radiolucent (e.g., Plexiglas) arm board is placed under the mattress pad with sufficient board protruding to support the arm.
  - Add height to radiolucent Plexiglas arm support with blankets (secure with tape) to match the table pad height.

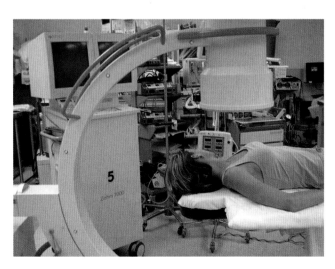

Figure 1-1 ▌ Supine positioning for upper extremity procedure, C-arm from the head of the bed.

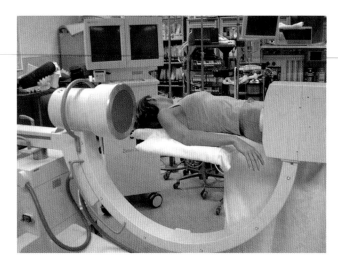

Figure 1-2 I C-arm position for axillary lateral imaging.

- Upper extremity is draped free.
- Wide prep and drape to contralateral side of midline (Figs. 1-3 and 1-4).
  - Include the sternal notch in field.

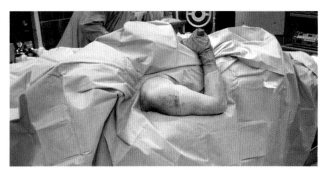

Figure 1-3 I Supine positioning for upper extremity procedure after prepping and draping.

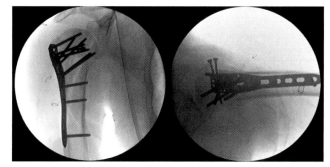

Figure 1-4 I AP and axillary fluoroscopic imaging in supine position.

IM Nail Humerus (Supine)

- Radiolucent reversed cantilever or fully radiolucent table such that the patient's head/upper extremities are placed at the cantilevered end.
- Small bump (folded towel) beneath the scapula.
- C-arm from the opposite side of the table (use fluoroscope that goes 45 degrees beyond vertical ["over the top"] and 90 degrees in the other direction).
- Uninjured arm adducted alongside the body, so that it does not impede the C-arm moving parallel to the long axis of the table/arm.
- Plexiglas arm board with stacked blankets to match the table pad height.
  - Plexiglas board is placed on the table, under the mattress pad and the patient with its long axis parallel to the table.
  - It needs only to protrude from the side of the OR table by 4 to 6 inches to support the adducted operative extremity (Figs. 1-5–1-9).

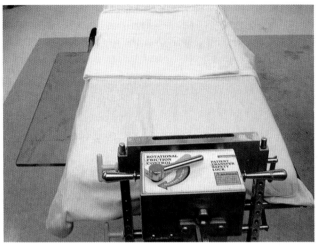

Figure 1-5 I Radiolucent flat top table with Plexiglas arm support.

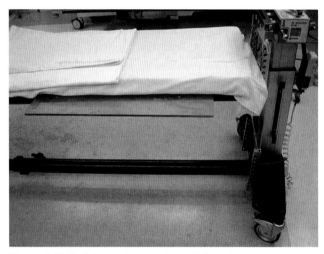

Figure 1-6 I Radiolucent flat top table with Plexiglas arm support.

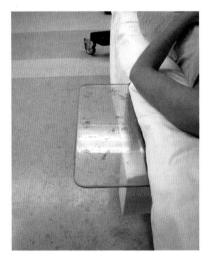

Figure 1-7 I Plexiglas board to support injured upper extremity.

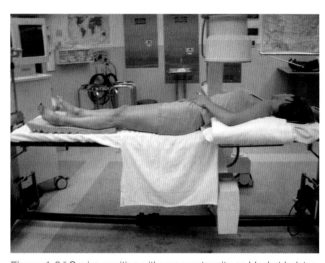

Figure 1-8 I Supine position with upper extremity on blanket bolster and Plexiglas arm support.

Figure 1-9 I Supine position with upper extremity on blanket bolster and Plexiglas arm support; view from patient's head.

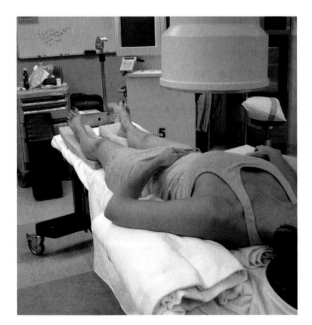

- With arm adducted, internally rotated 40 to 60 degrees, and C-arm rolled back 30 to 60 degrees—AP of the proximal humerus—a Grashey's AP image is preferred (Figs. 1-10 and 1-11).
- With arm adducted, internally rotated 40 to 60 degrees, and C-arm over the top 30 to 60 degrees, scapular "Y" lateral of the proximal humerus is obtained (Figs. 1-10 and 1-12).

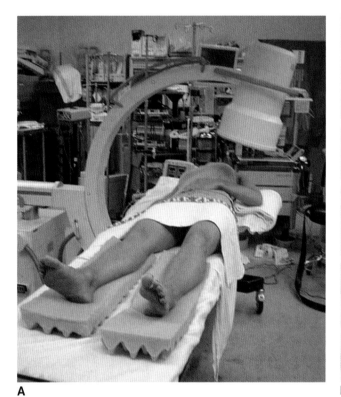 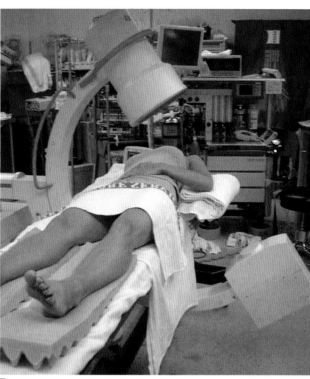

A   B

Figure 1-10 ▌ Position of C-arm for lateral **(A)** and AP **(B)** images (less than orthogonal planes are shown).

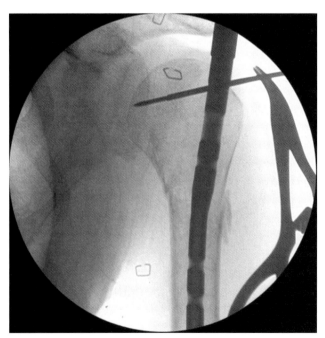 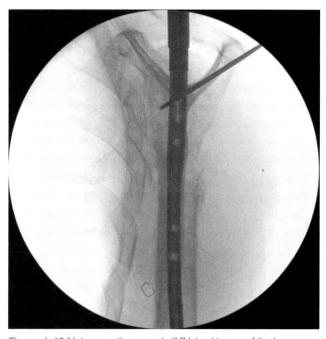

Figure 1-11 ▌ Intraoperative AP image of the humerus.   **Figure 1-12** ▌ Intraoperative scapula "Y" lateral image of the humerus.

- The C-arm should rotate in an arc of 90 degrees between the AP image and scapula "Y" lateral image to confirm orthogonal views.

ORIF Humeral Shaft: Anterolateral or Lateral Approach

- Supine.
- Radiolucent OR table.
- Small bump (folded hand towel) beneath the ipsilateral scapula.
- C-arm from the opposite side (use C-arm fluoroscope that goes 45 degrees "over the top").
- Uninjured arm adducted to the side of the body.
- Radiolucent arm table or Plexiglas arm board with blankets to match the table pad height.
- Arm internally rotated 40 to 60 degrees and C-arm over the top 30 to 60 degrees for lateral view.
- Arm internally rotated 40 to 60 degrees and C-arm back 30 to 60 degrees for AP view.
- The C-arm should rotate in an arc of 90 degrees between the AP image and scapula "Y" lateral image to confirm orthogonal views.

ORIF Humeral Shaft (Posterior Approach), Elbow Fractures (Lateral Decubitus Position)

- Radiolucent cantilever table reversed.
  - C-arm from the head (parallel to the long axis of the table).
  - Bean bag that stops at the axilla (so the down arm is free from the bean bag).
  - Rolled blankets may be used as torso supports in the front and back instead of a bean bag.
  - Plexiglas arm board for the down arm, protruding only approximately 6 inches (Fig. 1-13).

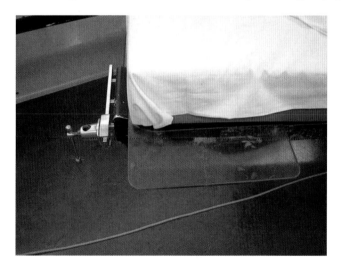

Figure 1-13 I Plexiglas arm board for the uninjured arm, attachment to the bed for radiolucent arm board for the injured arm.

- Down arm should be at maximum 90-degree shoulder abduction and 90-degree elbow flexion.
- Place a towel bolster or support to prevent excessive humeral external rotation (~70 to 80 degrees).
- Radiolucent arm board on long post (used for prone positioning) attached to rail at the top of the table, in line with the table axis for the injured arm (Figs. 1-14–1-20).

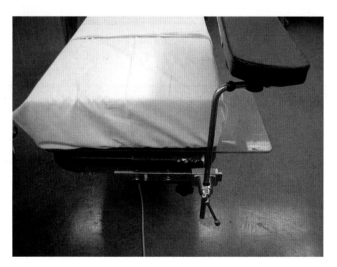

Figure 1-14 I Elevated radiolucent arm board attached to rail for an operative arm and Plexiglas arm board for an uninjured arm, viewed from the head of the bed.

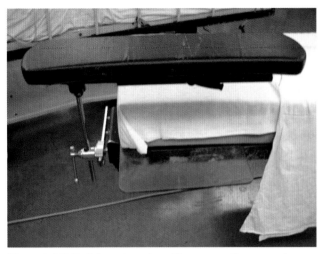

Figure 1-15 Radiolucent arm board for an operative arm and Plexiglas arm board for an uninjured arm, viewed from the side.

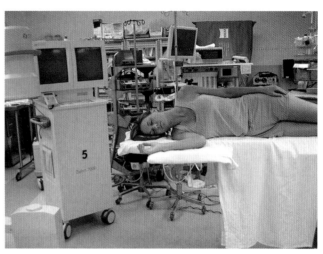

Figure 1-16 Lateral position (bean bag absent).

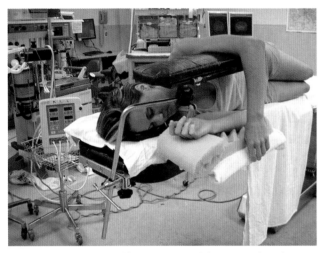

Figure 1-17 Lateral position, arms on radiolucent arm boards (bean bag absent).

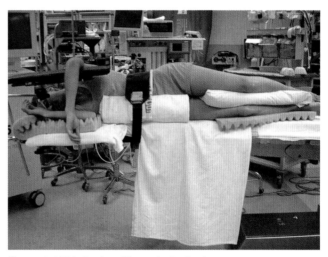

Figure 1-18 Lateral position, prior to draping.

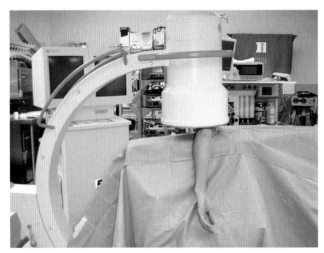

Figure 1-19 Lateral positioning and C-arm placement for intraoperative AP imaging.

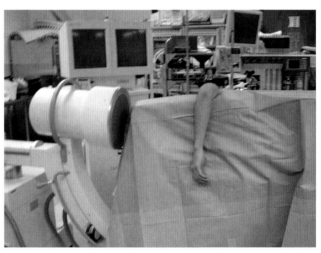

Figure 1-20 Lateral positioning and C-arm placement for intraoperative lateral imaging.

ORIF Humeral Shaft (Posterior Approach), Retrograde Nailing or Elbow Fractures with the Patient in a Prone Position

- Chest rolls (single rolled blankets) or Wilson's frame (Fig. 1-21).
- Additional cross roll at iliac crests if on rolled blankets.
- Contralateral arm adducted to lie on arm board parallel to the table or abducted <90 degrees on a "prone" positioning arm board to prevent excessive external rotation.

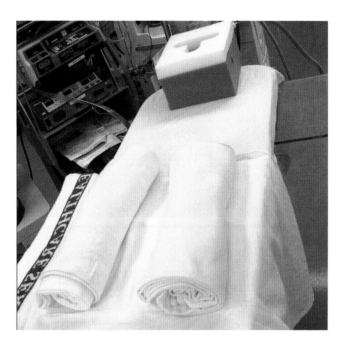

Figure 1-21 ‖ Radiolucent table with Plexiglas arm support at the upper right edge of the table.

- Operative arm abducted 90 degrees over the Plexiglas arm board padded with blankets taped on to match height of the table pad or shoulder level of Wilson's frame (Figs. 1-22 and 1-23).

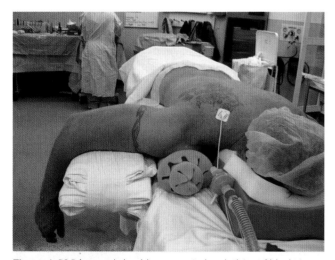

Figure 1-22 ‖ Arm and shoulder supported on bolster of blankets supported by radiolucent Plexiglas board. Elbow at 90 degrees.

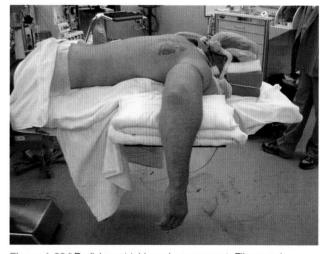

Figure 1-23 ‖ Radiolucent table and arm support. Elbow and shoulder at 90 degrees.

- Place the Plexiglas board perpendicular to the table so that only approximately 5 to 8 inches of board are exposed to allow for >90 degrees of elbow flexion.
- Contralateral arm should be <90 degrees of shoulder abduction and externally rotated <70 degrees.
- C-arm from the head of the table (parallel to the long axis of the table) (Figs. 1-24 and 1-25).

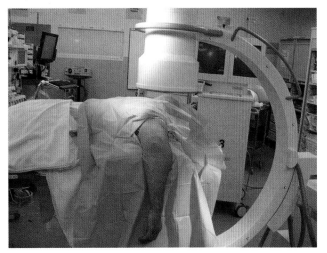

Figure 1-24 I C-arm positioning for AP imaging.

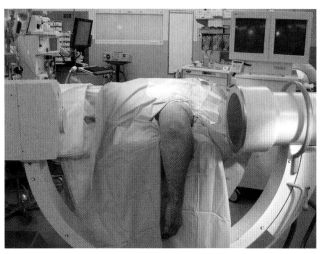

Figure 1-25 I C-arm positioning for lateral imaging.

Pelvis and Acetabulum: Anterior Approaches, Percutaneous Procedures

- Supine.
- Radiolucent table.
- C-arm from the opposite side.
- Two folded blankets centrally placed as lumbosacral support.
- Arms abducted 60 to 90 degrees on arm boards.
- Traction attachment as needed.
- Prep the ipsilateral leg in the field and both lateral flanks if iliosacral screws are needed (Figs. 1-26–1-30).

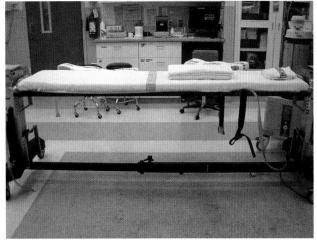

Figure 1-26 I Radiolucent flat top table with folded blankets as central (lumbosacral) support.

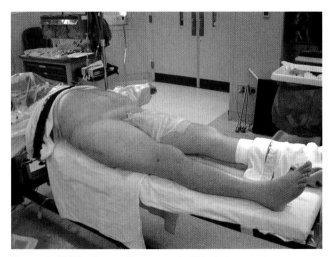

Figure 1-27 I Supine position on central blanket support.

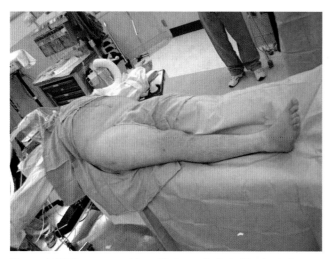

Figure 1-28 I Leg prepped free. Abdomen included to nipple line.

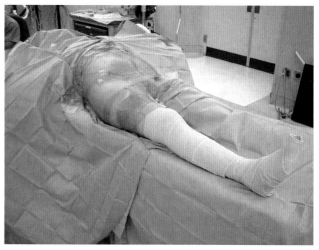

Figure 1-29 I Supine position, leg included and wrapped sterile in stockinette and elastic bandage wrap.

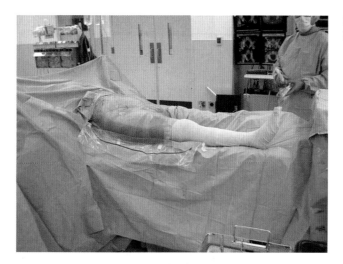

Figure 1-30 I Final supine positioning for pelvic and/or acetabular procedure.

- Prep low enough to allow iliosacral screws from both sides, even if anticipating unilateral procedure.
- Drape just above the base of the penis or labia for retrograde superior rami screws.
- Include the scrotum/penis if combined urological procedure.

Pelvis and Acetabulum: Kocher-Langenbeck

- Prone
- Radiolucent table
- C-arm from the opposite side
- Chest rolls (single rolled blankets)
- Additional cross roll at iliac crests
- Arms abducted 90 degrees, elbows flexed 90 degrees, on arm boards parallel to OR table
- Prep in the ipsilateral leg; both lateral flanks (Figs. 1-31–1-36)

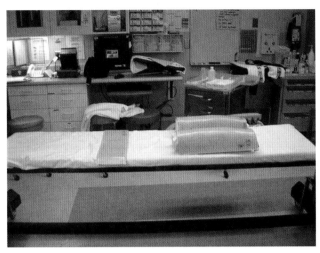

Figure 1-31 | Flat top radiolucent table with chest bolsters for prone positioning.

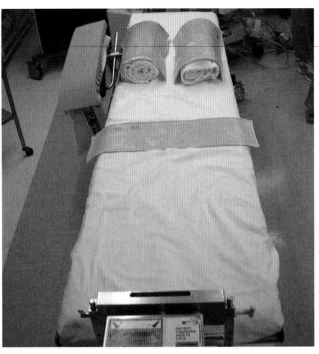

Figure 1-32 | Flat top radiolucent table with bolsters and padding for prone positioning.

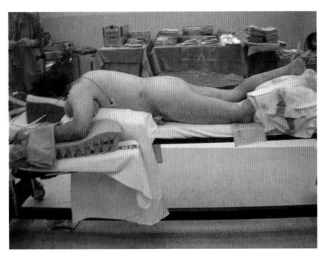

Figure 1-33 | Patient in prone position on bolsters. To avoid excessive shoulder external rotation, special arm boards are available for prone positioning.

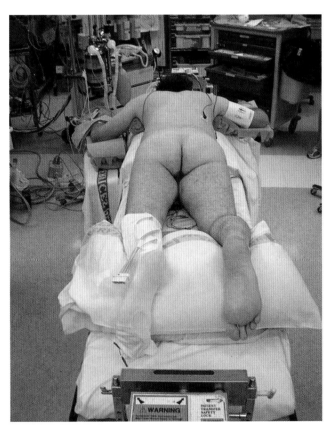

Figure 1-34 | Prone position, legs supported on pillows.

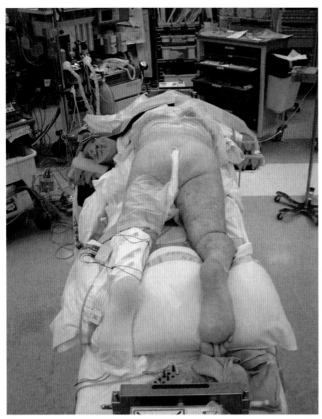

Figure 1-35 I Posterior pelvis and operative extremity isolated prior to sterile preparation.

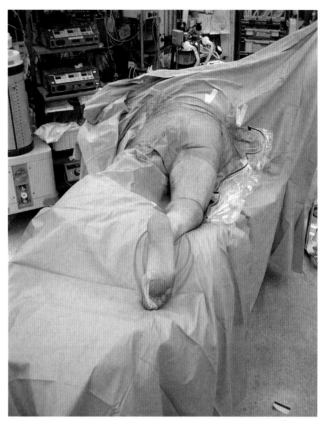

Figure 1-36 I Prone position after prepping and draping.

Lower Extremity

Antegrade Femoral Nailing, Supine Position, Hip Fractures, Subtrochanteric Fractures

- Radiolucent table to allow proximal imaging.
- Bump under the hip.
  - Single rolled blanket usually sufficient.
  - Ipsilateral buttock should hang free; that is, bump should be centrally placed.
  - Patient should be at the lateral edge of the table or just beyond the table's edge.
- Ramp pillow under the ipsilateral leg.
- C-arm from the opposite side of the table.
- Traction attachment to the end of the table on the side of the table opposite the injured limb to allow for operative lower limb adduction and ease of access to piriformis fossa or trochanter (Figs. 1-37–1-40).
- Drape traction attachment with sterile impervious stockinette.

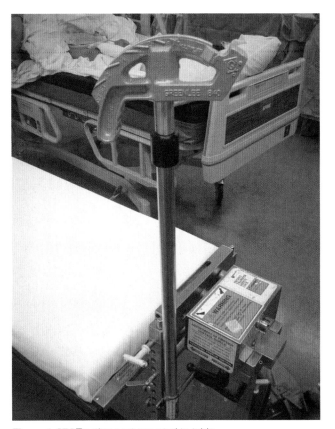

Figure 1-37 I Traction post mounted to table.

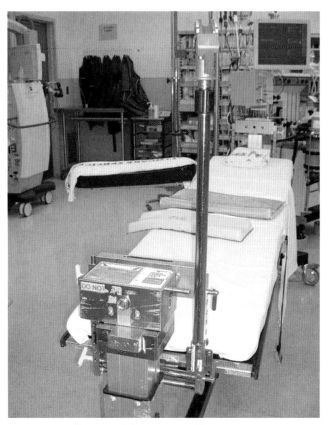

Figure 1-38 I Flat top radiolucent table with traction post mounted to the foot of the table.

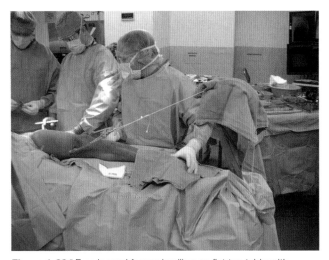

Figure 1-39 I Free legged femoral nailing on flat top table with traction attached to the Kirschner's wire bow, sterile rope over post draped with impervious stockinette. Nonsterile weights and weight pan are attached to the other end of the rope.

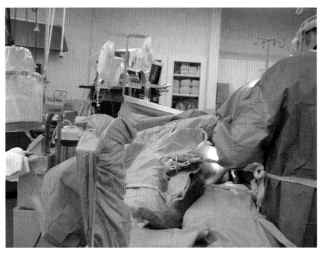

Figure 1-40 I Free legged femoral nailing on flat top table with traction post.

- Arm over the chest, not over the abdomen, to allow unencumbered access to the hip and buttock for entry portal (Figs. 1-41–1-45).
- Remove all nonradiolucent table attachments on rails on the ipsilateral side.
- Place calf compression device tubing for contralateral leg and urinary drainage tubing under the table's mattress under uninjured extremity to permit C-arm access.
- Prep and drape as posteriorly as possible on the flank and buttock to allow unencumbered access to starting point for C-arm imaging, instruments, and implants.

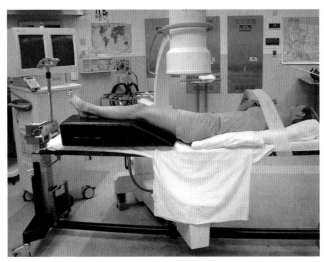

Figure 1-41 I Supine position with central flank roll. The patient is moved to the edge of the table so that the buttock hangs free. Ipsilateral arm is secured over the chest.

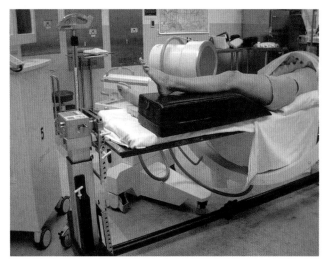

Figure 1-42 I C-arm positioning for the lateral image.

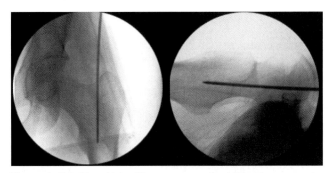

Figure 1-43 I AP and lateral images are easily obtained.

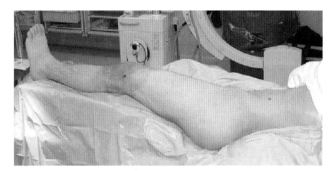

Figure 1-44 I Patient positioned with the buttock free.

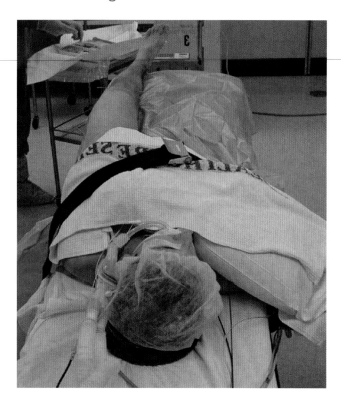

Figure 1-45 I Patient positioned, view from the head noting the elevation and rotation of the pelvis and torso as provided by the central bolster and shoulder support.

Antegrade Femoral Nail, Lateral Position, Subtrochanteric Fractures

- Lateral decubitus position.
- Flat top radiolucent table (Fig. 1-46).
- Up arm in "airplane" sling positioned with foam padding underneath the arm to protect ulnar nerve and bony prominences.
- Foam padding underneath down arm.

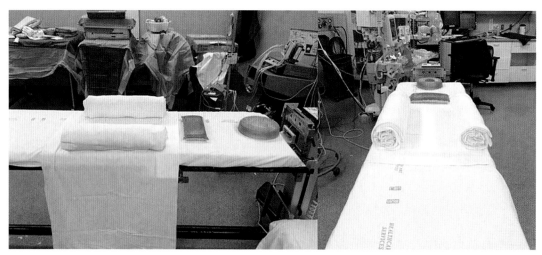

Figure 1-46 I Side and end views of flat top radiolucent OR table with high chest (axillary) gel roll and two rolled bolsters.

- Axillary roll.
  - Use rolled blankets wedged against the abdomen and spine to maintain lateral position (Fig. 1-47).
  - Create a stable platform for the operative leg by stacking folded blankets around the down leg. Secure with tape (Fig. 1-48).
- C-arm from the patient's anterior side (Fig. 1-49).

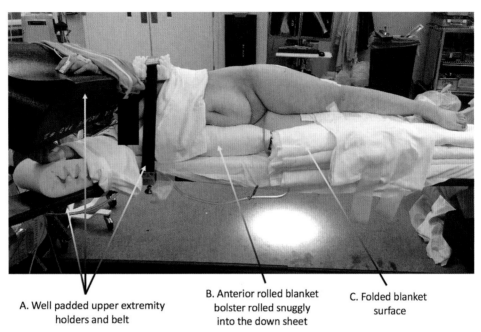

A. Well padded upper extremity holders and belt

B. Anterior rolled blanket bolster rolled snuggly into the down sheet

C. Folded blanket surface

Figure 1-47 I Anterior view of the patient in lateral position with padded upper extremity supports and blanket rolls. Lower extremities supported by folded blankets.

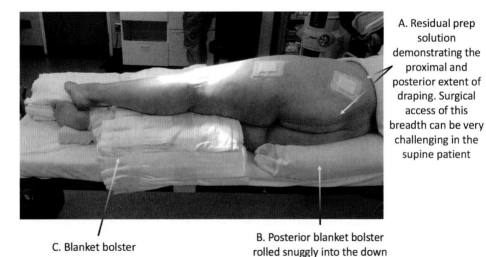

A. Residual prep solution demonstrating the proximal and posterior extent of draping. Surgical access of this breadth can be very challenging in the supine patient

C. Blanket bolster

B. Posterior blanket bolster rolled snuggly into the down sheet

Figure 1-48 I Posterior view of patient in lateral position with posterior rolled blanket bolster and lower extremity blanket support.

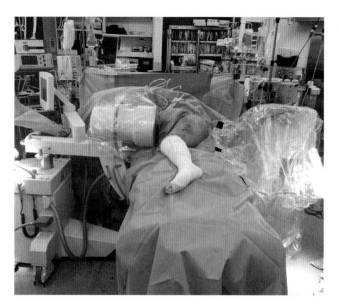

Figure 1-49 I C-arm positioning for an AP image with the patient in the lateral position.

Retrograde Femoral Nail

- Radiolucent table.
- Bump under the hip.
- C-arm from the opposite side.
- Knee flexion with wedge pillow or supporting radiolucent triangle.
  - Should permit 30 to 60 degrees of knee flexion to prevent reaming anterior tibial plateau or inferior patella.
- If traction is needed, a distal femoral or proximal tibial traction pin with traction attachment on table ipsilateral to the injured femur to facilitate reduction (Fig. 1-50).

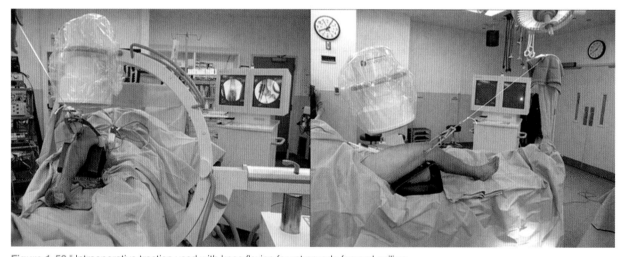

Figure 1-50 I Intraoperative traction used with knee flexion for retrograde femoral nailing.

Distal Femur, Tibial Plateau, Patella, Ankle, Foot Fractures

- Radiolucent cantilever-type table.
- Bump under the flank (rolled towels, wedge, IV bag).
- C-arm from the opposite side.
- Ramp style foam pillow to elevate the affected limb (Fig. 1-51).
- Patient at the end of the table.

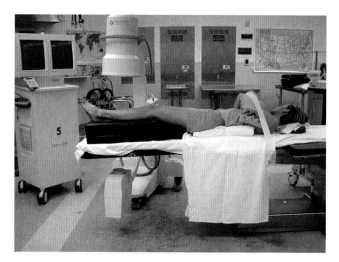

Figure 1-51 | Supine position for majority of lower extremity fractures. A flank bump is used such that leg is in neutral rotation (patella straight up).

- Consider lateral positioning for posterolateral approach to the tibia (open reduction internal fixation [ORIF] of posterior malleolus); externally rotate the limb if access to medial malleolus is needed.
  - Check for sufficient external rotation of the hip prior to positioning for trimalleolar/pilon fractures.
- Prone position, if sole approach is either posterolateral or posteromedial tibia.
  - Feet and ankle should protrude over the distal end of the table, permitting ankle dorsiflexion.
  - Protect patellae with gelfoam pads.
- Triangular pillow/ramp for metatarsal fractures to assist imaging. Consider positioning as with tibial nailing (Figs. 1-52 and 1-53).

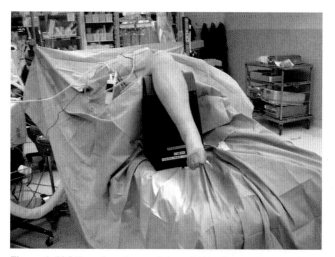

Figure 1-52 | Knee flexed on radiolucent triangle.

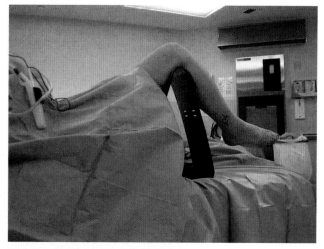

Figure 1-53 | Knee flexed on radiolucent triangle.

TIP
Lower Extremity Sequential Medial and Lateral Approaches
Eric D. Farrell

Pathoanatomy

Patient positioning can be a critical portion of many orthopaedic procedures. Bilateral lower extremity and/or "dual incision" cases can pose a positioning dilemma. Elevating one side of the pelvis with a bolster may facilitate exposure for one procedure but compromise the other approach or procedure.

Solution

Blankets and sheets may be used to elevate ("bump up") both hemipelves.

Technique

Equipment

- OR blankets and sheets, folded
- Silk tape—3-inch

Example: A 57-year-old male sustained a left bicondylar tibial plateau fracture. Two weeks post injury, he was taken to the OR for an ORIF (Fig. 1-54). A decision was made to perform a dual approach to address the fractures.

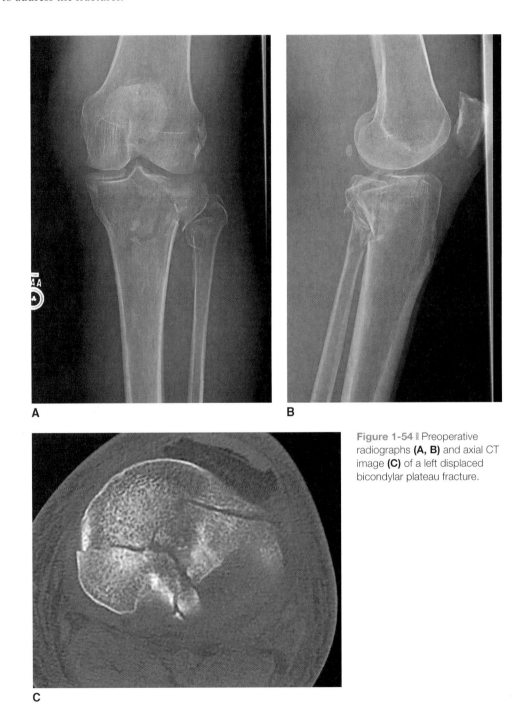

Figure 1-54 | Preoperative radiographs **(A, B)** and axial CT image **(C)** of a left displaced bicondylar plateau fracture.

- The patient is positioned on a radiolucent table, and while general anesthesia is administered, two bolsters (aka "bumps") are made.
- Since the medial approach/fixation will be addressed first, the right hemipelvis receives a larger bolster than the left. After the medial plateau ORIF is completed, the right bolster will be removed. A blanket and one sheet are combined to make this bolster. The left hemipelvis receives a one blanket bolster. The linen is rolled tightly and secured with silk tape (Fig. 1-55).
  - Depending on the habitus of the patient, different combinations of blankets/sheets may be needed. In this case, the patient was of "average" size.

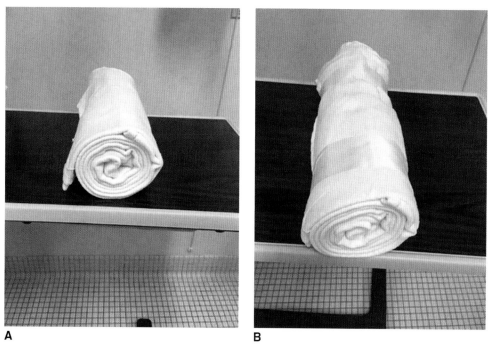

A   **B**

Figure 1-55 ▌ **A, B:** Blanket is rolled tightly and secured with 3-inch silk tape.

- For the bolster that will be removed, a "pull-tab" is made with tape (Fig. 1-56).

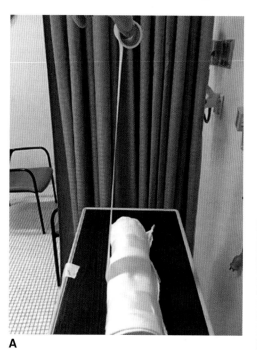 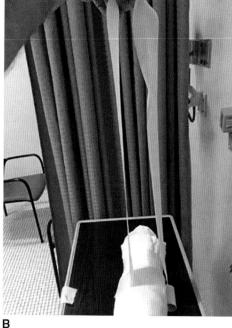

A   **B**

Figure 1-56 ▌ **A–E (left to right):** Tape is placed around the central portion of a bolster and a 24- to 36-inch tail is made. The tail is fashioned by creating a second limb by rolling the tape backward on the first limb and return it to the bolster. The two "tails" are compressed together and secured. The pull-tab is now ready.

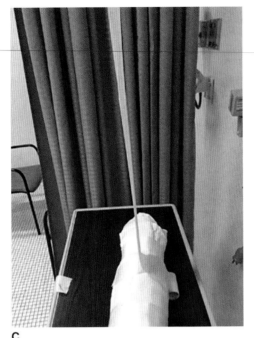

C

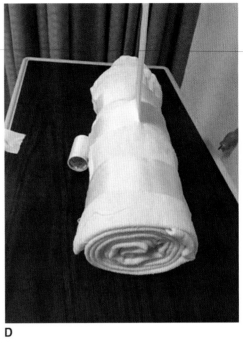

D

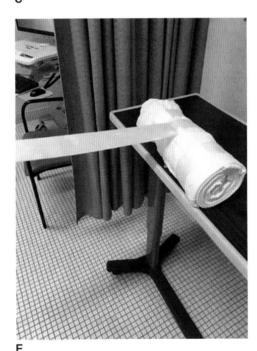

E

Figure 1-56 I (*Continued*)

- The bolster for the left hemipelvis is positioned first and checked for size. In general, a correctly sized bolster should result in the limb resting with the patella pointing directly anteriorly. Surgeon preference may dictate more or less rotation (Fig. 1-57).

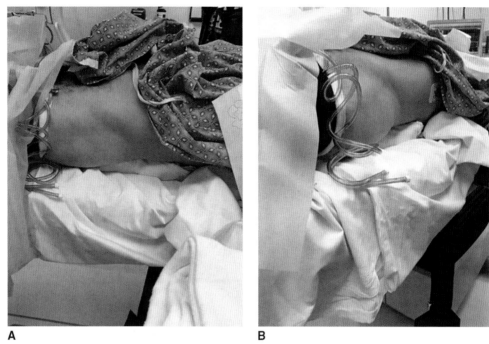

A   **B**

Figure 1-57 | **A, B:** Two views of left hip bolster. Note that the bolster is placed under the hemipelvis and directly under the patient and not under the OR table's sheet.

- Once the bolster under the left hemipelvis is checked and secured, attention is taken to the right bolster and hemipelvis. The patient's right hemipelvis is rolled to the left, and the "larger" bolster is placed under the ischium and hemitorso (Fig. 1-58).

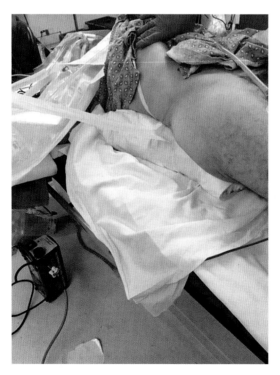

Figure 1-58 | The larger bolster is placed under the right hemipelvis. Note that the pull-tab is directed laterally, allowing easy removal during the surgery.

- The left lower extremity position is reevaluated and then prescrubbed followed by prepping and draping (Fig. 1-59A and B).
- Following ORIF of the medial plateau, a moistened sponge is placed in the medial incision, which is loosely approximated with 3.0 nylon suture or closed definitively.
- Using its pull-tab, the bolster under the right hemipelvis is removed without disturbing the sterile drapes.
- The position of the C-arm, surgeon, and scrub are switched.
- Exposure of the lateral plateau ensues.

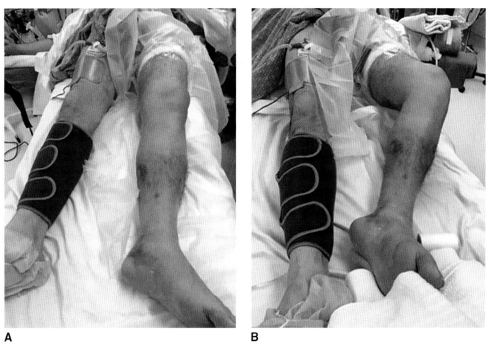

A   **B**

Figure 1-59 I **A,B:** Both bumps are placed, and access to the medial plateau is assessed.

Tibial Nail

- Radiolucent cantilever-type table.
- Bump under the flank (rolled towels, wedge, IV bag).
- C-arm from the opposite side.
- Radiolucent triangle to facilitate knee flexion and fracture reduction.
- Patient positioning for nailing in the semiextended position is the same as that for standard nailing although a radiolucent triangle is not required.

Calcaneus Fractures

- Lateral decubitus position.
- Radiolucent cantilever-type table.
- Patient as far distal on the table as possible.
- C-arm from posterior side of patient.
- Up arm in "airplane" sling positioned with foam padding underneath the arm to protect ulnar nerve and bony prominences.

- Foam padding underneath down arm.
- Bean bag with "axillary" roll or thoracic wedge with down arm relief cutout.
  - Alternatively, use rolled blankets wedged against the abdomen and spine to maintain lateral position (Figs. 1-60 and 1-61).

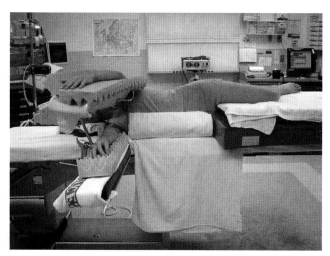

Figure 1-60 | Lateral position for lower extremity procedures.

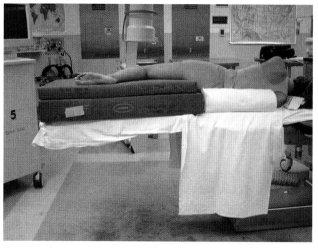

Figure 1-61 | Lateral position for lower extremity procedures, posterior view.

- Three foam pads around the legs
  - First pad between the table and patient to protect the greater trochanter, peroneal nerve at the fibular neck, and lateral malleolus.
  - Second pad surrounds the opposite lower limb, which is placed in "down-leg cutout" with calf compression device applied (Fig. 1-62).
  - Top pad is foam platform over the cutout and "down leg" and serves as an operating table (Fig. 1-63).

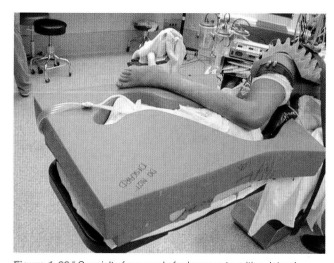

Figure 1-62 | Specialty foam pads for lower extremities, lateral position.

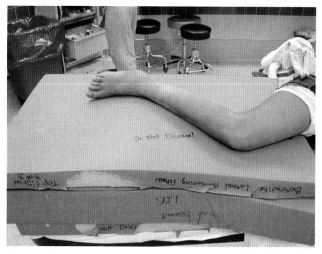

Figure 1-63 | Specialty foam pillows for lateral positioning for lower extremity procedures. Flat top pillow for working operative platform.

- Blankets on top of foam pads and taped to minimize slipping (Figs. 1-64 and 1-65).

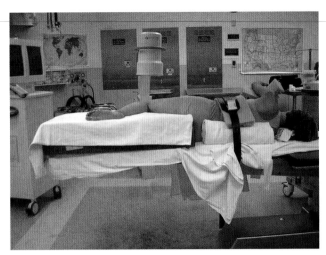

Figure 1-64 I Lateral position, posterior view with blanket on foam pillows prior to securing with tape.

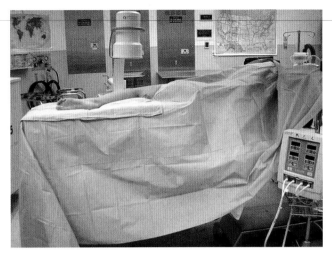

Figure 1-65 I Final lateral positioning after draping.

Calcaneus: Percutaneous Reduction and Fixation

- Same patient positioning as ORIF calcaneus.
- C-arm from the foot.
  - For axial heel view, C-arm almost aligned with long axis of the table, but swivels just enough toward patient's posterior to allow transmitter to clear table and come parallel to the floor.

Chapter 2
Intraoperative Assessment of Lower-Extremity Alignment

MITCHELL BERNSTEIN
HOBIE SUMMERS
CLAY A. SPITLER

Pathoanatomy

Malalignment of the lower extremity will lead to an alteration of gait and joint reaction forces and increase the potential for early and progressive posttraumatic arthritis.

Solution

Knowledge of the normal values of lower limb alignment (Figs. 2-1–2-4) and how to measure them will lead to restoration of anatomy and improved outcomes.

Technique

- Normal values and the reference ranges of lower extremity alignment have been well documented.[1]
- Anatomical alignment is one of the basic objectives in trauma reconstruction.
- Fractures about the knee (distal femur, proximal tibia) have the most influence on overall limb alignment.
- Knowledge of normal alignment values in the axial, sagittal, and coronal planes will allow the surgeon to master fracture reduction (Figs. 2-1–2-4).
- Intraoperative strategies should be used to evaluate alignment.
- Liberal use of intraoperative plain films (long cassettes) can be used to assess limb alignment in the coronal and sagittal planes.

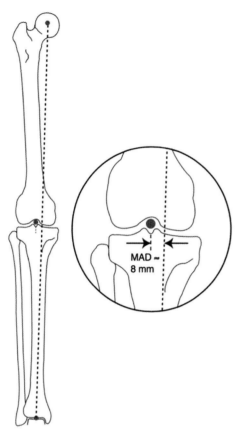

Figure 2-1 I Limb alignment (varus or valgus) is evaluated with a line drawn from the center of the femoral head to the center of the ankle. Normally, this line should pass medial to the knee's center by an average of 8 mm. MAD, mechanical axis deviation; medial MAD, varus limb alignment; lateral MAD, valgus limb alignment.[1]

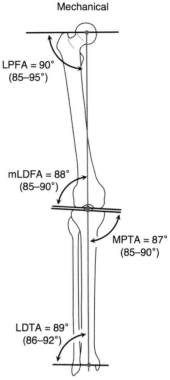

Figure 2-2 I Mechanical joint orientation angles. These are drawn from mechanical axis lines, which are derived from joint center points. By convention, the angles below are drawn on the lateral or medial side of the limb. Note, in the tibia, the mechanical and anatomic axes are collinear; thus, there is no prefix of mechanical (m) or anatomic (a) axes for the tibia. LPFA, lateral proximal femoral angle, which is always measured from the mechanical axis line; mLDFA, mechanical, lateral distal femoral angle; MPTA, medial proximal tibial angle; LDTA, lateral distal tibial angle.[1]

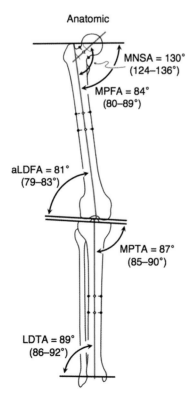

Figure 2-3 I Anatomic joint orientation angles. These are drawn from anatomic axis lines, which are derived from middiaphyseal lines. Note again in the tibia, the mechanical and anatomic axes are collinear; thus, there is no prefix of mechanical or anatomic axis for the tibia. MNSA, medial neck shaft angle, which is always measured from the anatomic axis line; MPFA, medial proximal femoral angle, which is always measured from the anatomic axis line; aLDFA, anatomic, lateral distal femoral angle; MPTA, medial proximal tibial angle; LDTA, lateral distal tibial angle.[1]

Sagittal

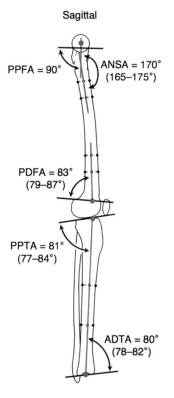

PPFA = 90°

ANSA = 170°
(165–175°)

PDFA = 83°
(79–87°)

PPTA = 81°
(77–84°)

ADTA = 80°
(78–82°)

Figure 2-4 I Sagittal limb alignment. These are drawn from anatomic axis lines, which are derived from middiaphyseal lines. ANSA, anterior neck shaft angle; PPFA, posterior proximal femoral angle; PDFA, posterior distal femoral angle; PPTA, posterior proximal tibial angle; ADTA, anterior distal tibial angle.[1]

Intraoperative Strategies to Assess Alignment: Length

- Use of radiographic ruler, templating off contralateral (normal) limb (Figs. 2-5–2-7)

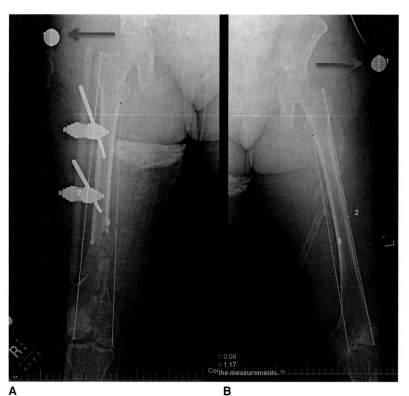

A   B

Figure 2-5 I A 46-year-old female sustained an open type IIIA distal femur fracture with 11 cm of metaphyseal bone loss after a motor vehicle crash. After the initial irrigation, debridement, and spanning external fixation, we obtained whole femur calibrated radiographs for templating. Note the calibration markers (*red arrows*) on the injured **(A)** and contralateral **(B)** normal limb. We arbitrarily chose the following radiographic landmarks to compare femur lengths: greater trochanter, lesser trochanter, lateral condyle, and medial condyle. Measurements indicated the injured limb was 12 mm shorter than the normal femur.

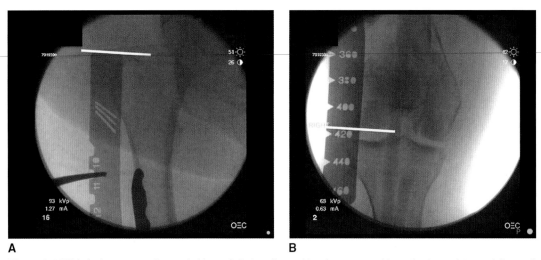

Figure 2-6 I This is the same patient as in Figure 2-5. A radiographic ruler was used from the femur intramedullary nail set. Preoperative assessment indicated that it would be necessary to lengthen the femur by 12 mm. **A,B:** Measuring from the greater trochanter to the lateral femoral condyle.

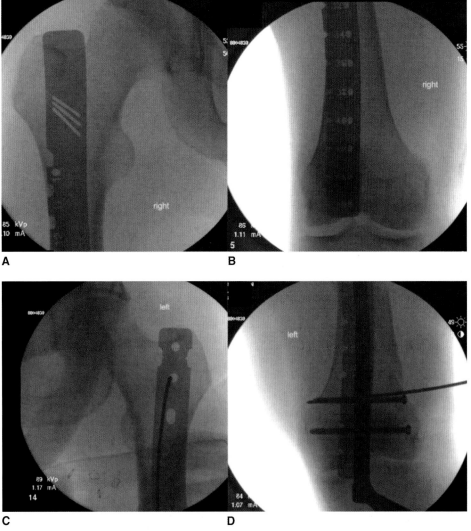

Figure 2-7 I Alternatively, prior to draping, a nonsterile radiographic ruler can be used to measure the length of the uninjured limb **(A,B)**. This measurement can then be used intraoperatively to confirm length of the injured extremity prior to fixation **(C,D)**.

Intraoperative Strategies to Assess Alignment: Rotation

- In certain clinical scenarios (segmental fractures of long bones, extensive comminution, bilateral injuries, or posttraumatic reconstruction), intraoperative assessment of rotation is not possible or practical (Fig. 2-8). CT cuts through the femoral necks, condyles, and ankle joints can accurately assess rotation.

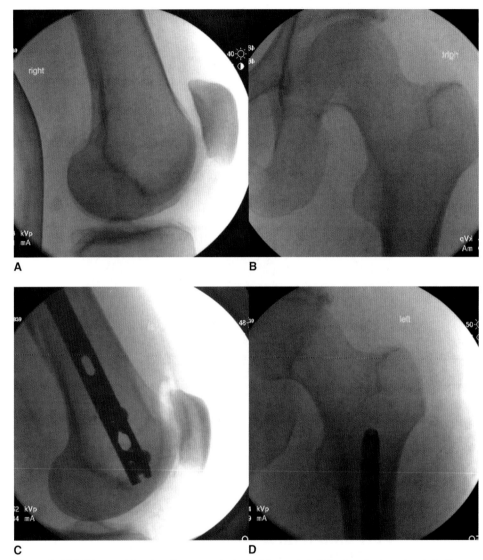

Figure 2-8 | A 54-year-old male with a comminuted left femoral shaft fracture that was treated with a retrograde intramedullary nail. At the beginning of the case, prior to draping, a perfect lateral of the contralateral distal femur is obtained **(A)**. The image intensifier is then rotated 90° and an AP image of the hip is obtained without moving the extremity **(B)**. Ensure this image is saved for use later in the case. Note that the image in **(B)** has been flipped horizontally 180° for ease of comparison to the injured extremity. After locking the nail in the distal segment, a perfect lateral is obtained of the distal femur **(C)**. The image intensifier is again rotated 90° to obtain an AP image of the hip, without moving the limb **(D)**, and the shape of the lesser trochanter is compared to the uninjured side **(B)**. If the lesser trochanter appears less prominent, the distal segment is externally rotated relative to the proximal segment. In order to correct this, the distal segment should be internally rotated and/or the proximal segment externally rotated. The radiographic assessment is then repeated until the shapes of the lesser trochanters appear similar.

- Interpretation of the CT rotational profile should be done by the treating surgeon, and one should not rely on the radiologist's interpretation alone.
- This interpretation is frequently done by two different surgeons to ensure the calculation of rotation is accurate (Fig. 2-9).

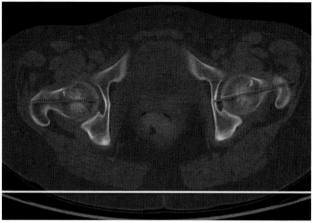

A

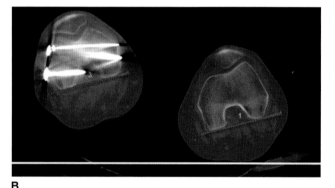

B

Figure 2-9 I This is the same patient as in Figure 2-5. Prior to second-stage bone grafting, a CT rotational profile was performed. **A:** The femoral neck line is drawn by connecting two points, generating a best-fit line through the center of the femoral head and neck (*red line*). The line of reference (*yellow line*) is drawn parallel in the same manner in both the proximal and distal images; this is frequently performed by making this line parallel to the bottom of the image. The right femoral neck measures 1.69° of external rotation relative to the reference line (*yellow line*). The left femoral neck measures 11.65° of internal rotation relative to the reference line (*yellow line*). **B:** At the level of the distal femur, the *red line* is drawn tangential to the posterior femoral condyles. Again, the reference line (*yellow line*) is drawn parallel to the bottom of the image. The right femoral condyle measures 15.92° of external rotation relative to the reference line (*yellow line*). The left femoral condyle measures 15.11° of internal rotation relative to the reference line (*yellow line*).

Right Side (Fig. 2-9)

A practical way to determine the deformity is to make the femoral neck line 0° relative to the reference line. On the right, one would need to rotate internally 1.69°. This would "remove" 1.69° of external rotation of the distal fragment. Therefore, the arithmetic would equate to 15.92° − 1.69° = **14.23° of external rotation**.

Left Side (Fig. 2-9)

Make the femoral neck line 0° relative to the reference line. On the left, one would need to rotate externally 11.65°. This would "remove" 11.65° of internal rotation of the distal fragment. Therefore, the arithmetic would equate to 15.11° − 11.65° = **3.46° of internal rotation**.

- Note in the above example, the terms anteversion and retroversion are not used; however,
  - Retroversion is an external rotation deformity of the distal femur.
  - Anteversion is an internal rotation deformity of the distal femur.

If one wanted to use the terms anteversion and retroversion, one could say that the right femoral neck is **retroverted 14.23°** and the left femoral neck is **anteverted 3.46°**.

In order to match the version of her right side to her normal left side, one would need to internally rotate the right distal femoral segment **17.69°** (14.23° + 3.46°). Intraoperatively, as a human, one cannot rotate 17.69°. Practically, this is performed by rotating >15° but <20° using a sterile goniometer and 2.5-mm or larger Steinman pins. Larger pins are stiffer and will be deflected less than smaller K-wires by the overlying soft tissues (e.g., IT band).

- Intraoperative execution correcting rotational differences (Fig. 2-10)

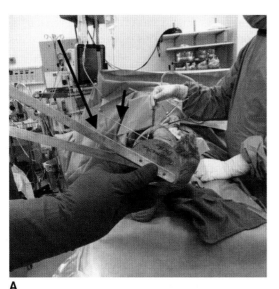 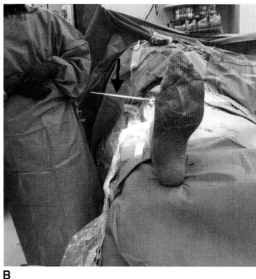

A   **B**

Figure 2-10 ▌Intraoperative execution. **A:** 2.5-mm Steinman pins (*black arrows*) are placed in the proximal and distal fragments. The distal Steinman pin is placed in >15° but <20° relative external rotation to the proximal pin. Since one is internally rotating the distal segment, they will become collinear upon correction. **B:** The distal segment is rotated internally so that the Steinman pins become collinear (*black arrow*).

Calculation (Fig. 2-11)

Make the femoral neck line 0° relative to the reference line. One would need to internally rotate 30.87°. This would "add" 30.87° of internal rotation of the distal fragment. Therefore, the arithmetic would equate to 30.87° + 28.24° = **59.11° of internal rotation**. Another way, the femoral neck anteversion on the right hip is **59.11°**

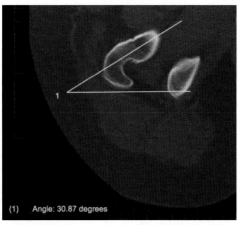

Figure 2-11 ▌This is another example of a patient with femoral malrotation. CT scan through the right femoral neck **(A)** and condyle **(B)**. **A:** The right femoral neck measures 30.87° of external rotation to the reference line (*green horizontal line*). **B:** The right femoral condyle measures 28.24° of internal rotation relative to the reference line (*green horizontal line*).

(1)   Angle: 30.87 degrees

A

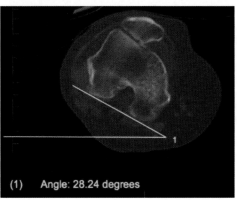

(1)   Angle: 28.24 degrees

B

- Normal anteversion is 10°
  - This equates to 10° of internal rotation of the femoral condyles relative to the femoral neck.
- This patient's deformity, assuming a "normal" value of 10° of anteversion, is **49.11°** (59.11° − 10°).
- This patient has excessive femoral anteversion. This equates to increased distal femoral internal rotation.
- In order to correct the deformity, one would need to **externally rotate** the distal segment **49.11°**.

Tibial Torsion

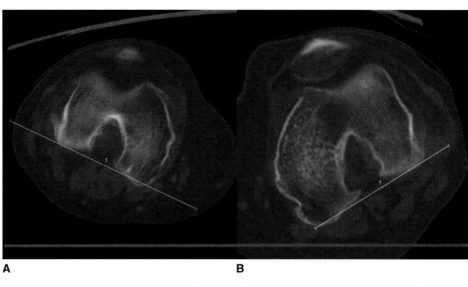

A   B

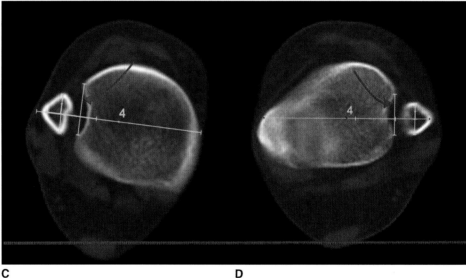

C   D

Figure 2-12 I Tibial malrotation. CT rotational profile through bilateral femoral condyles **(A,B)** and ankles **(C,D).** The calculation of the proximal tibial segment is performed using the femoral condyles as described in Figures 2-9 and 2-11. Since we are using the femoral condyles as a surrogate for the proximal tibia, it assumes no intra-articular pathology (e.g., rotational instability of the knee). **C,D:** At the level of the ankle, one needs to generate a best-fit line through the ankle syndesmosis. A method to perform this reproducibly is to first generate a perpendicular line to a line drawn from the anterior and posterior margin of the incisura (*red arrow*). Line 4 in image **C** and **D** is collinear with the perpendicular line to incisura and midway between the anterior and posterior diameter of the fibula. **A:** The right femoral condyle measures 26° of internal rotation relative to the reference line (*red line*). **B:** The left femoral condyle measures 31° of internal rotation relative to the reference line (*red line*). **C:** The right ankle measures 7.18° of internal rotation relative to the reference line (*red line*). **D:** The left ankle measured 0.31° of external rotation relative to the reference line (*red line*).

Right Side (Fig. 2-12)

Make the femoral condyle line 0° relative to the reference line. One would need to rotate externally 26°. This would "remove" 26° of internal rotation of the distal fragment. Therefore, the arithmetic would equate to 7.18° − 26° = −18.82° internal, or 18.82° of external tibial torsion. Note normal tibial torsion is 10 to 15° external.

Left Side (Fig. 2-12)

Make the femoral condyle line 0° relative to the reference line. One would need to rotate externally 31°. This would "add" 31° of external rotation of the distal fragment. Therefore, the arithmetic would equate to 0.31° + 31° = 31.31° of external tibial torsion.

Intraoperative Strategies to Assess Alignment: Mechanical Limb Alignment (Fig. 2-13)

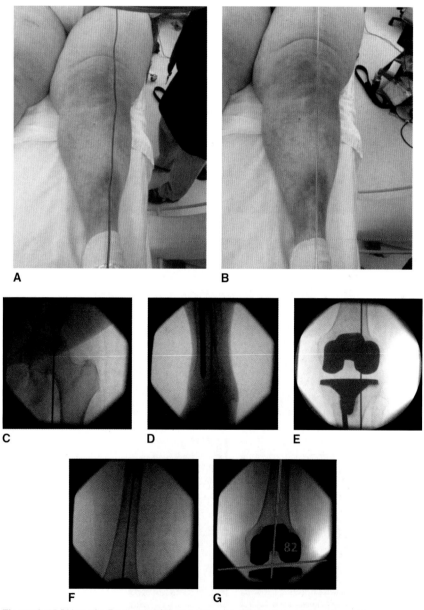

Figure 2-13 | Use of a Bovie cord **(A)** or a long wire **(B)** can be used to assess the mechanical axis of the limb. Fluoroscopy is used to locate the center of the femoral head **(C)** and the center of the ankle **(D)**. In this patient, the mechanical axis line passed lateral to the center of the knee **(E)**—valgus limb alignment. Upon analysis of the distal femur, the aLDFA is 82° (normal 79 to 83°); therefore, the deformity must be in the proximal tibia **(F,G)**.

Intraoperative Strategies to Assess Alignment: Femur— Coronal Plane (Figs. 2-14–2-23)

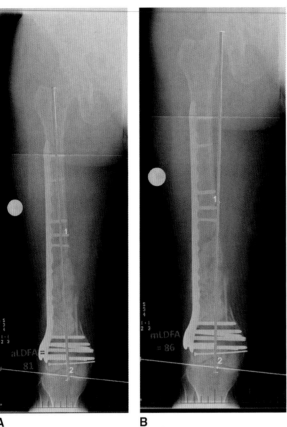

A   **B**

Figure 2-14 | Intraoperative use of long scoliosis cassettes, or stitched images, can aid in drawing the anatomic **(A)** and mechanical **(B)** angulations to assess coronal alignment.

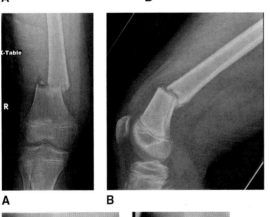

A   **B**

Figure 2-15 | An 11-year-old skeletally immature male sustained a displaced closed distal femoral shaft fracture **(A,B)**. A periarticular 3.5-mm medial distal tibial locking plate was chosen for fixation. **C:** After the initial reduction was achieved using conventional (nonlocking) screws, the aLDFA measured 76°, which is 5° of valgus. This was identified intraoperatively with the use of AP X-rays. **D:** The lateral X-ray did not reveal any malreduction, PDFA = 82°.

aLDFA = 76°   PDFA = 82°

C   **D**

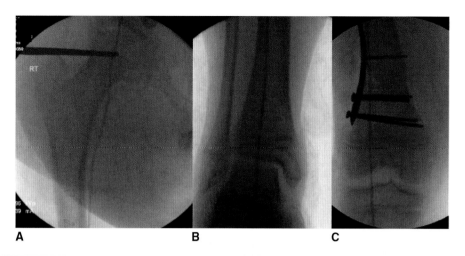

A   B   C

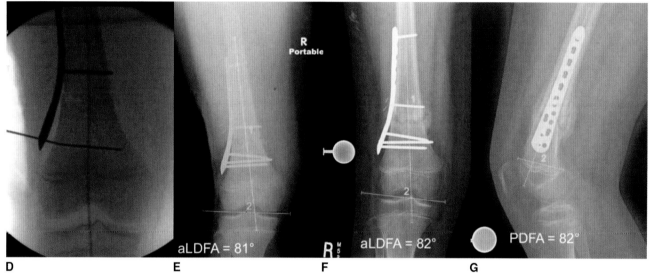

D   E   F   G

Figure 2-16 I This is the same patient as in Figure 2-15. In order to recreate the mechanical axis of the limb and assess our alignment, a Bovie cord was used from the center of the femoral head **(A)** to the center of the ankle **(B)**. Note confirmation of valgus malalignment **(C)** as this line passed lateral to the center of the knee. Removal of the screws in the distal segment and reassessment of the mechanical axis of the limb demonstrated neutral alignment **(D)**. The Bovie cord now passed through the center of the knee, mechanical axis deviation (MAD) = 0 mm. Locking screws in the distal fragment were used to maintain the reduction. Intraoperative **(E)** and postoperative X-rays **(F,G)** demonstrated anatomic coronal and sagittal alignment.

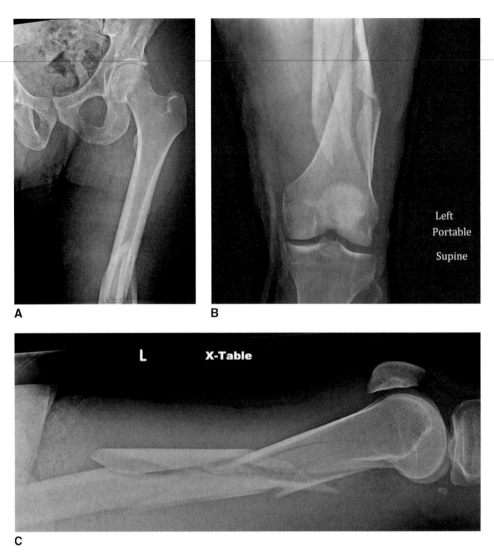

Figure 2-17 ▎ A 53-year-old male who sustained a comminuted distal femoral shaft fracture after a 1,000-lb cabinet fell onto his left thigh **(A–C)**.

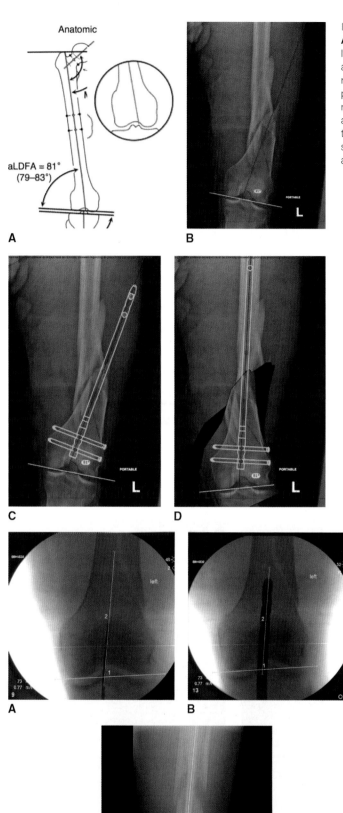

A

aLDFA = 81°
(79–83°)

Anatomic

B

C

D

Figure 2-18 ▌ Preoperative planning using the anatomic axis. **A:** The anatomic axis of the femur is defined as a middiaphyseal line. Note this line extends distally in-line with the medial tibial spine and not through the center of the knee. Preoperative planning for a retrograde femoral nail **(B,C)**. In this case, the isthmus of the femur proximal to the fracture site was intact allowing the nail to guide reduction in the proximal segment **(D)**. As long as the entry point and trajectory are in-line with the anatomic axis of the femur, then the final alignment should be anatomic. Therefore, the entry point should be in-line with the medial tibial spine and in 9° of valgus (i.e., aLDFA = 81°) from a line tangential to the joint.

A

B

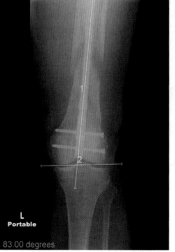

C

Figure 2-19 ▌ Intraoperative execution. The critical and most important step is ensuring a starting point collinear with the medial tibial spine **(A,B)** and a trajectory that is 9° in valgus. An 8.5-mm DHS (Synthes, Paoli, PA) rigid reamer was used to open the femoral canal to maintain anatomic trajectory **(B)**. A goniometer can be used on the C-arm screen to confirm the correct trajectory. The angle in **(A)** and **(B)** measured 82°. Final aLDFA = 83°. Note in **(C)** the femoral nail is collinear with the medial tibial spine (as a surrogate of middiaphyseal line extension).

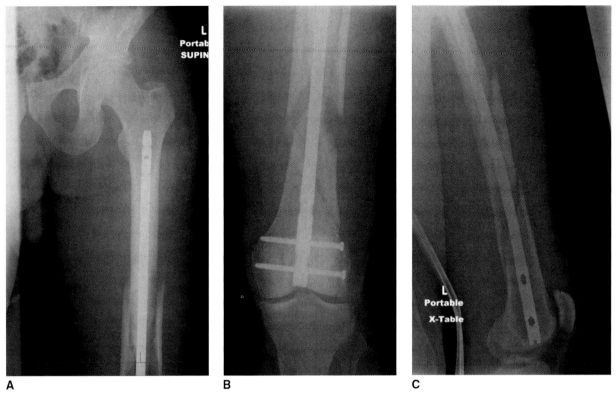

Figure 2-20 | Immediate postoperative X-rays demonstrating anatomic alignment in the coronal and sagittal plane **(A–C)**. aLDFA = 83°. PDFA = 82°. Length assessment was performed with a radiographic ruler. The rotation was assessed using preoperative fluoroscopic views of the lesser trochanter from the normal side.

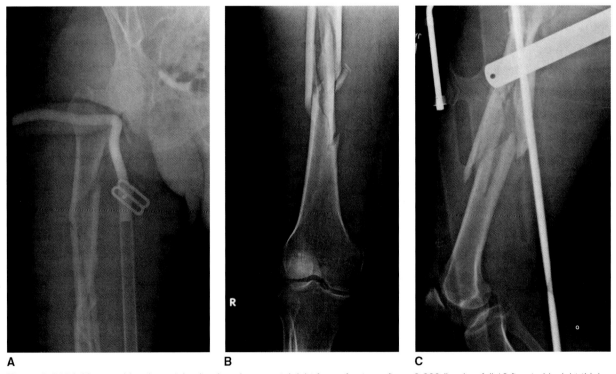

Figure 2-21 | A 23-year-old male sustained a closed segmental right femur fracture after a 2,000-lb rebar fell 10 ft onto his right thigh at work **(A–C)**.

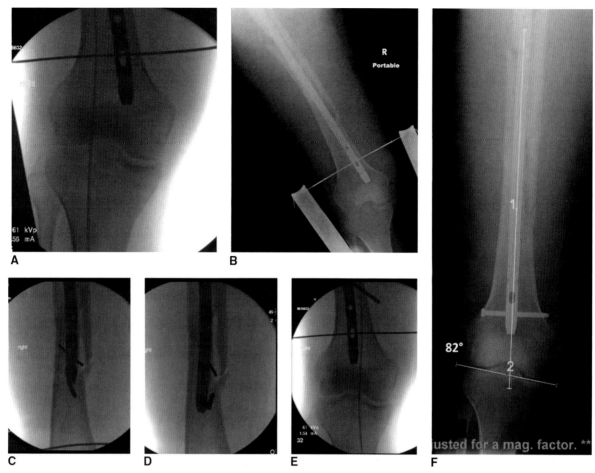

Figure 2-22 | Anterograde, piriformis fossa entry nailing was chosen. The distal target of the nail was nonanatomic. **A:** Bovie cord technique to determine mechanical alignment revealed valgus deformity, as the cord passed lateral to the center of the knee. **B:** Intraoperative X-ray prior to distal interlocking screws confirmed the malreduction in valgus. **C,D:** Blocking wires were used to adjust the alignment and to centralize the nail in the distal segment. **E:** Repeat Bovie cord testing demonstrated improved distal nail targeting and correct mechanical alignment of the limb. **F:** Repeat intraoperative X-rays confirmed normal alignment aLDFA 82°.

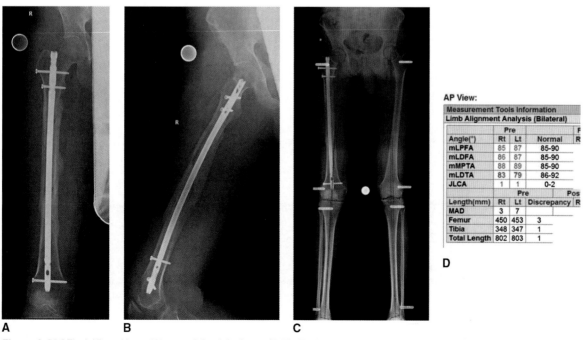

AP View:

Measurement Tools Information				
Limb Alignment Analysis (Bilateral)				
	Pre			F
Angle(°)	Rt	Lt	Normal	R
mLPFA	85	87	85-90	
mLDFA	86	87	85-90	
mMPTA	88	89	85-90	
mLDTA	83	79	86-92	
JLCA	1	1	0-2	

	Pre			Pos
Length(mm)	Rt	Lt	Discrepancy	R
MAD	3	7		
Femur	450	453	3	
Tibia	348	347	1	
Total Length	802	803	1	

Figure 2-23 | Final AP and lateral X-rays of the right femur **(A,B)**. Final standing hip-to-ankle X-ray **(C)**, and associated AP view limb alignment analysis **(D)**.

Clamshell Osteotomy
Clay Spitler

Pathophysiology

Preexisting lower extremity deformity in the setting of acute fracture can make fracture reduction and intramedullary fixation challenging. This typically requires the use of either a ringed external fixator or plate fixation.

Solution

Clamshell osteotomy of the malunion site can allow for the use of a medullary nail and improvement of the overall mechanical alignment of the deformed segment. Plate fixation without corrective osteotomy may result in bony union, but the preexisting deformity is not corrected and the lower extremity mechanical axis remains out of alignment. Ringed external fixators can be used to correct the overall mechanical axis alignment through the fracture, but shortening must be corrected through distraction osteogenesis. Clamshell osteotomy of the deformed segment, followed by intramedullary nail placement using the unaffected proximal and distal segment, can allow for effective fracture treatment with an intramedullary implant as well as angular and rotational deformity correction (Fig. 2-24).

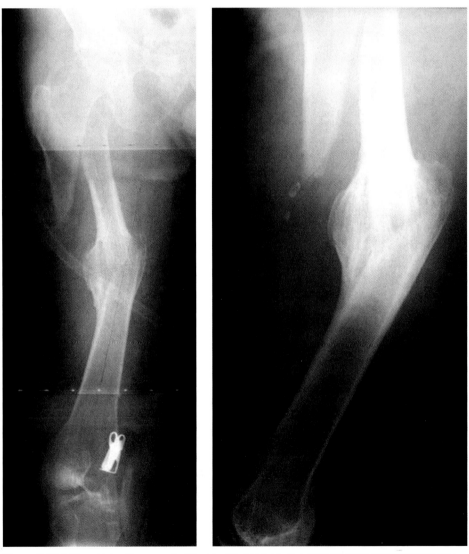

Figure 2-24 | AP and lateral images of a 62-year-old man's acute subtrochanteric femur fracture. The patient had a history of a femoral shaft fracture treated previously in traction.

Technique

- The clamshell osteotomy is performed via extraperiosteal dissection to the deformed segment and the transection of the normal diaphysis adjacent to the deformity in both the proximal and distal segments (Fig. 2-25).

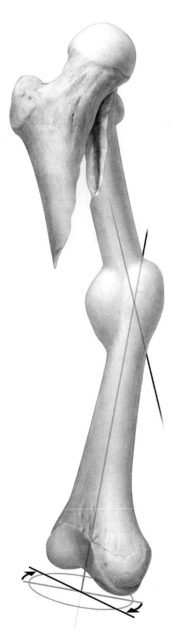

Figure 2-25 ▌ To successfully perform the clamshell osteotomy, the underformed proximal and distal segments must be identified for the location of the transverse portion of the osteotomy in the proximal and distal segments.

- The malunited segment is then osteotomized along its long axis on one side and laminar spreaders are used to open the osteotomy site with the far cortex cracking as a hinge, leaving intact periosteum on the far cortex (Fig. 2-26).

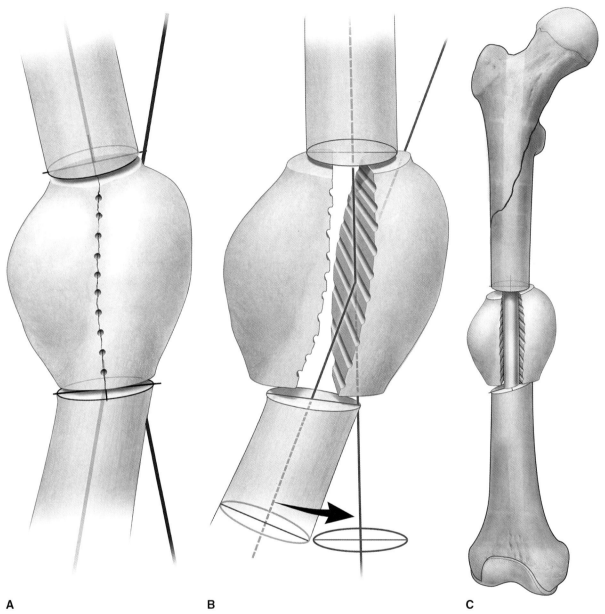

A   **B**   **C**

Figure 2-26 I Schematic representation of the clamshell osteotomy.

- A starting point in-line with the anatomic intramedullary axis is obtained with an entrance angle in-line with the medullary canal, and a ball tip guide wire is introduced into the center-center position of the distal segment.
  - The proximal and distal segments are reamed, but no reaming through the osteotomized segment is performed.
- Reaming is done with the muscle overlying the clamshell segment to trap the reamings. At the termination of nail insertion, the reamings are placed along the gaps of the osteotomy segments to encourage union.
- The contralateral extremity is used as a template for length and rotation, and interlocking screws are placed in the proximal and distal segments with the osteotomized fragments allowed to rest around the nail.
- The procedure has been used successfully in diaphyseal malunions of the femur and tibia without associated fractures (Figs. 2-27 and 2-28) (Russell et al., JBJS Am 2009).

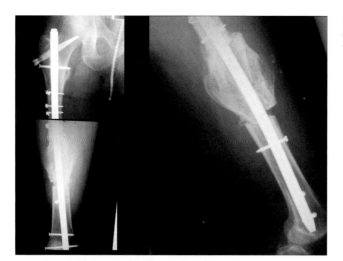

Figure 2-27 I AP and lateral of the 62-year-old man s/p clamshell osteotomy and IMN of the right subtrochanteric femur fracture.

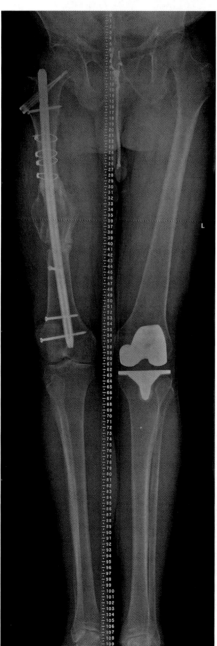

Figure 2-28 I Scanogram after healing demonstrates restoration of lower extremity mechanical axis with minimal shortening of the affected extremity.

Intraoperative Strategies to Assess Alignment: Tibia—Coronal Plane (Fig. 2-29)

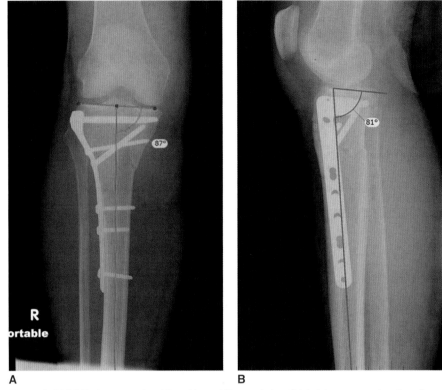

Figure 2-29 | **A,B:** Intraoperative AP and lateral X-rays during tibial plateau reconstruction allow for accurate measurement of coronal and sagittal alignment. The medial proximal tibial angle, MPTA 87°; and the proximal posterior tibial angle, PPTA 81°.

Intraoperative Strategies to Assess Alignment: Tibia—Sagittal Plane (Fig. 2-30)

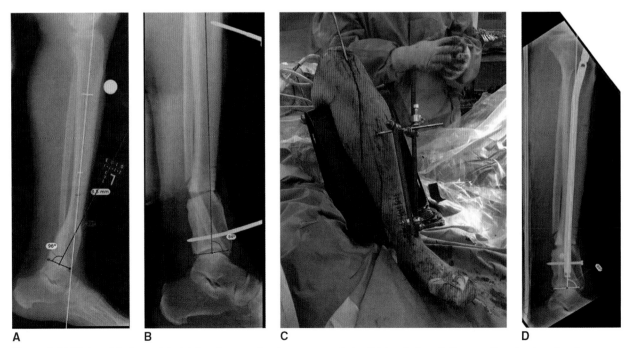

Figure 2-30 | External fixator-assisted deformity correction for an apex anterior tibial malunion. **A:** Preoperative planning aimed for a correction to an ADTA of 84°. **B:** Intraoperative plain film prior to nail insertion assessing the ADTA. **C:** Intraoperative clinical photograph demonstrating an anteriorly based external fixator assisting in deformity correction. **D:** Immediate postoperative X-ray after intramedullary nail insertion. ADTA = 84°, which was slightly undercorrected.

Intraoperative Strategies to Assess Alignment: Distal Femur and Proximal Tibia Combined (Figs. 2-31–2-33)

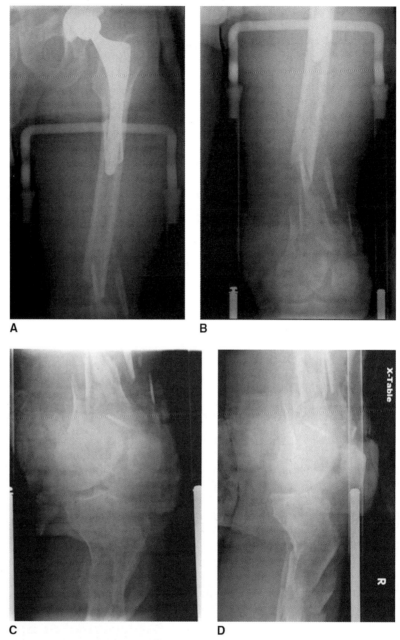

Figure 2-31 | A 55-year-old male was in a high-speed motorcycle collision and sustained an open left AO 33-C3 distal femur fracture with metaphyseal bone loss, left open intra-articular bicondylar tibial plateau fracture, and a right closed bicondylar tibial plateau fracture. He had a left total hip arthroplasty that was well functioning **(A–D)**.

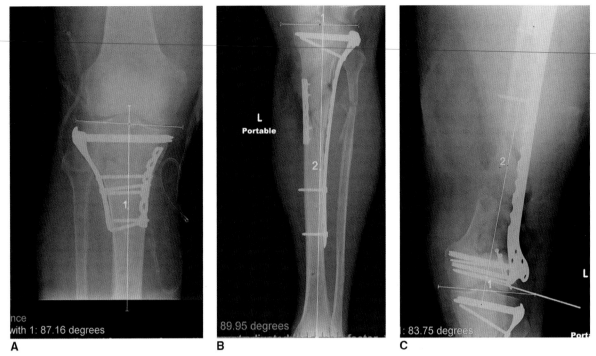

Figure 2-32 ▍The use of intraoperative X-rays confirmed coronal alignment on the right and left knee. **A:** MPTA = 87.16°.
B: MPTA = 89.95°. **C:** aLDFA = 83.75°.

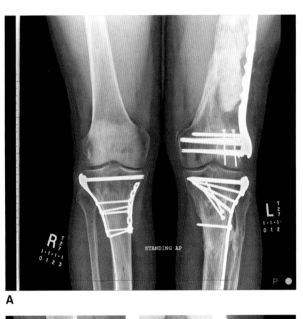

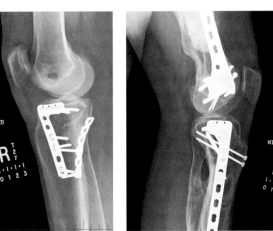

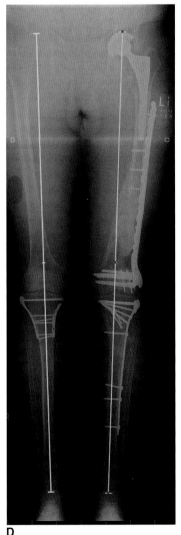

Figure 2-33 ▍Final standing X-ray of the knee **(A–C)**. MPTA, right = 89°; MPTA, left = 89°; PPTA, right = 84°; PPTA, left = 80°. **D:** Standing hip-to-ankle X-ray confirming neutral mechanical alignment of both limbs, MAD = 0. Note mechanical axis lines passing through the center of the knees and equal limb lengths.

Intraoperative Strategies to Assess Distal Tibia/Ankle Alignment: Coronal and Sagittal Planes (Figs. 2-34 and 2-35)

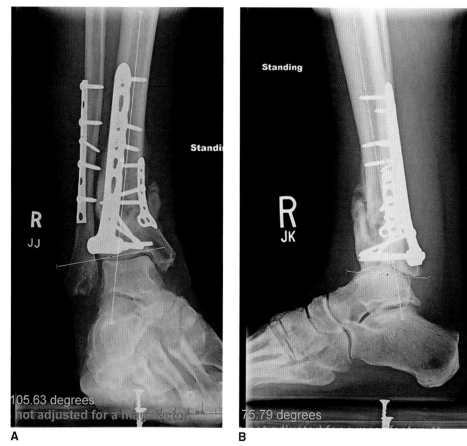

A   **B**

Figure 2-34 | A 64-year-old male presented with a distal tibial varus malunion. **A,B:** Preoperative distal tibial X-rays demonstrated varus and recurvatum deformity (LDTA of 106°, ADTA of 76°).

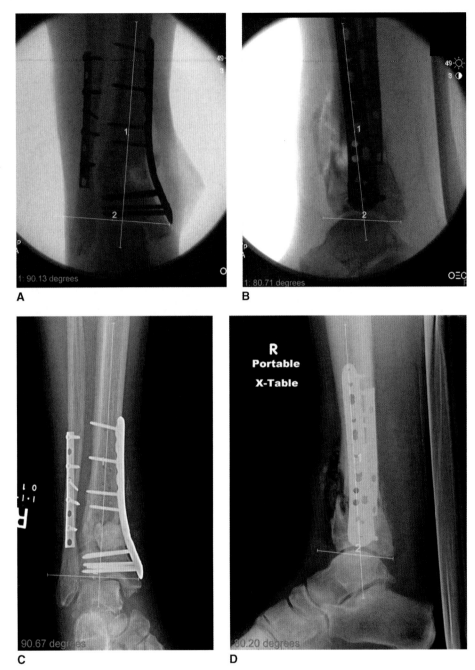

Figure 2-35 | Intraoperative correction of 17° varus deformity (106° − 89°) with a goal of a normal LDTA of 89°. **A,B:** Intraoperative fluoroscopy was used to calculate correction. **C,D:** Immediate postoperative X-rays with final LDTA = 90° and ADTA = 80°.

Reference

1. Paley D. *Principles of Deformity Correction*. New York, NY: Springer-Verlag Berlin Heidelberg; 2002.

Chapter 3
Management of Open Fractures, Compartment Syndrome, Bone Defects, and Infection

DAVID BROKAW

ERIC D. FARRELL

REZA FIROOZABADI

MICHAEL F. GITHENS

STEPHEN A. KOTTMEIER

RANDALL DREW MADISON

JOHN A. SCOLARO

CLAY A. SPITLER

MATTHEW P. SULLIVAN

Irrigation and Débridement of Open Fractures

Sterile Instruments/Equipment

- Cystoscopy tubing or pulsatile lavage system
- ≥6 L of sterile saline
- Multiple small and large retractors, typically "L" shaped, such as Sofield, Langenbeck, or Army-Navy
- Large curettes (straight and curved)
- Small curettes (straight and curved)
- Dental picks
- Shoulder hooks, bone hooks
- Rongeurs (pituitary, etc.)
- Occasionally or available: motorized burr
- Polymethylmethacrylate cement
- Heavy braded suture for beads
- Calcium sulfate beads
- Vancomycin, tobramycin, gentamicin powder

Management of Traumatic Wounds

- Elongate transverse lacerations that do not cross the tibial border in a Z-shaped fashion to maximize skin viability.
  - T-shaped or cruciform wounds may be contraindicated in compromised tissues.
    - Tendency to break down at the corners, and with ≥2 corners, can leave a sizeable defect that may not close or granulate sufficiently

- Try to avoid incorporating transverse or oblique wounds that cross the anteromedial tibial border in an extensile longitudinal approach, as these will gap when fracture is brought back out to length. Instead consider creating a separate longitudinal approach (either anterolateral or posteromedial to the tibial border) to use for débridement and fracture reduction.
- Open femoral shaft fractures mandatorily require delivery of the fracture ends out of the skin for examination and excisional débridement.
  - Even when skin wound is small, the distal end of the proximal femoral fragment may be grossly contaminated.
- For a Type I or II open wound over the medial tibial border, it may be reasonable to consider leaving this wound alone and instead using a separate anterolateral or posteromedial surgical approach for excisional débridement and irrigation of the open fracture.
  - It is best not to reconcile these "pretibial" open wounds into an extensile exposure over the medial aspect of the tibia; instead, only debride/excise the dermis, epidermis, and subcutaneous tissue (from outside in).
  - Debride the open fracture and deeper tissues via a separate surgical approach—from the inside out (Fig. 3-1).

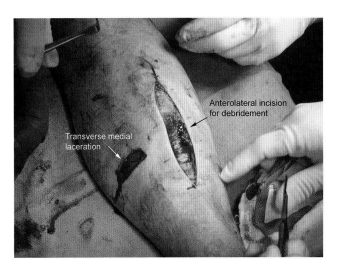

Figure 3-1 I In this patient with an anteromedial transverse traumatic laceration associated with an open tibial fracture, an anterolateral counterincision was used for the fracture débridement. This avoided extension of the medial traumatic wound, which has a more tenuous soft tissue envelope.

- Rationale: if edema precludes primary closure, anterolateral wound over the anterior compartment musculature will be amenable to skin graft, whereas a wound on the medial face may require rotational or free soft tissue flap for coverage.
- Do not use this technique if it is already clear that a free flap will be necessary.
  - Consider a discussion with a plastic surgeon to avoid compromising options for soft tissue repair.
- Expose the proximal and distal bone ends for débridement.
  - Be mindful that the zone of injury may extend in any direction further than the fracture and skin wounds themselves.
  - Evaluate all sheared tissue planes for the presence of dirt and other foreign debris.
  - Aggressively debride all foreign material and contamination.
  - Excise necrotic skin, avascular or loose subcutaneous tissue and fascia, noncontractile muscle, and cortical bone fragments lacking soft tissue attachments.
  - As skin may be an important resource in patients who are not flap candidates, consider being somewhat conservative in the débridement of skin, removing only what is ischemic/nonviable.
  - Marginally viable skin may serve at least temporarily as a biologic dressing if sufficiently cleaned.
  - Remove, but do not discard, large, devitalized bone fragments that may be used to facilitate an anatomical reduction.
  - Irrigate all wounds and bone ends after débridement with multiple liters of sterile saline to decontaminate.
- Sizeable soft tissue and/or osseous defects can be managed with creation of a bead pouch or application of a wound VAC (KCI Inc., San Antonio, TX) over a bone defect containing antibiotic beads.
- The risk of compartmental syndrome must be considered prior to, during, and following the stabilization of tibial shaft fractures (Fig. 3-2).

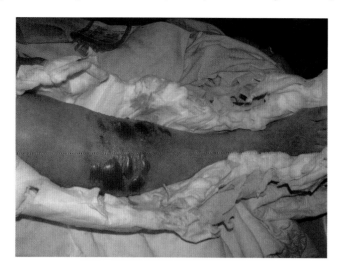

Figure 3-2 I In this patient with a high-energy proximal tibial fracture and a significant soft tissue injury, suspicion for acute compartment syndrome should be high.

TIP
Custom Extremity Irrigation Basin
David Brokaw

Pathoanatomy

Large volumes of fluid containing possible blood-borne pathogens are produced during irrigation and débridement surgeries for upper and lower extremity open fractures. Safe collection, containment, and disposal of these liquids is mandatory for maintaining sterile technique as well as protecting OR personnel from potential harmful exposures.

Solution

A custom, reusable, autoclavable, stainless steel débridement pan, also known as the "Lasagna Pan," was designed to maintain sterility and collect effluent. It safely holds the limb in a position amenable to irrigation and débridement surgeries while collecting, containing, and disposing of large volumes of blood-borne pathogen–contaminated fluids. It allows the use of intraoperative fluoroscopy, and it is easily disassembled for cleaning and sterilization.

Technique

● The débridement pan was constructed by a professional welding fabricator using medical-grade stainless steel sheet stock and ½ inch screen wire mesh (Figs. 3-3 and 3-4).

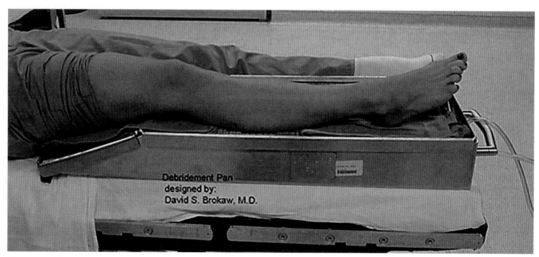

Debridement Pan
designed by:
David S. Brokaw, M.D.

Figure 3-3 I Clinical image demonstrating the debridement pan and limb positioning.

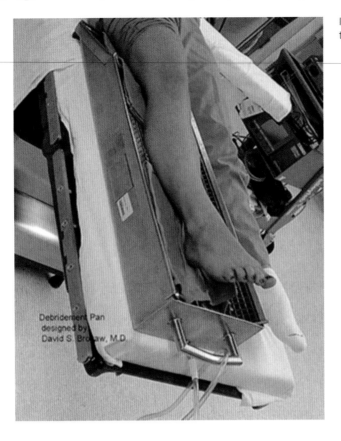

Figure 3-4 I Clinical image demonstrating the debridement pan and limb positioning.

- The dimensions were developed by measuring the limbs of multiple patients, surgical staff, and colleagues. It was proportionally sized to disassemble for cleaning and to fit inside a standard-size OR autoclave. The corners were rounded to allow sterile wrapping in blue wrap without causing perforations.
  - The dimensions are 32 inches/82 cm length, 10 inches/25 cm width, 4 inches/10 cm depth at the distal end tapering to 1½ inches/1.25 cm depth at the proximal end.
  - This proximal tapering allows the limb to rest in an ideal supine position under the popliteal fossa without pressure points. The collection pan is tapered from proximal to distal with a 1-inch fall to allow passive drainage of liquids (Figs. 3-5–3-8).

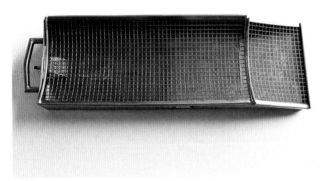

Figure 3-5 I Fully assembled debridement pan with mesh in place.

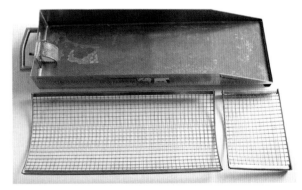

Figure 3-6 I Debridement pan with mesh removed.

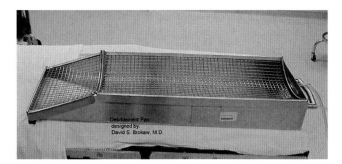

Figure 3-7 | Clinical image demonstrating position of the pan on the surgical table.

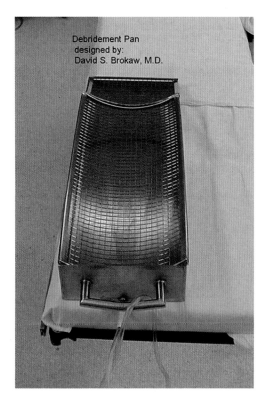

Figure 3-8 | Clinical image demonstrating position of the pan on the surgical table.

- A removable mesh strainer is attached at the distal end to prevent clogging of the suction tubing with debris and clotted blood (Fig. 3-9).

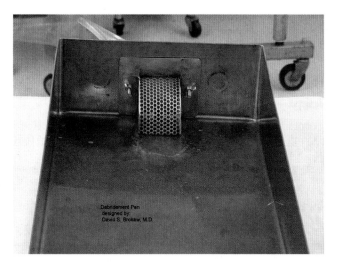

Figure 3-9 | The removable mesh strainer is attached at the distal end to prevent clogging of the suction tubing.

- Standard, sterile, and suction tubing is attached to an external drain nipple to allow egress of contaminant irrigate to a wall-mounted suction canister or the larger free-standing fluid collection units commonly used in arthroscopy.

- The 1 ½-inch mesh, stainless steel screen is fabricated into two pieces for cleaning and gently curved from medial to lateral to allow nesting support of the soft tissues of the upper and lower extremities (Fig. 3-10).
  - The pan will hold approximately 12 L of fluid, allowing OR personnel time to transfer suction tubes to empty suction containers as they fill during surgical procedures.
  - A large handle is attached at the distal end to allow positioning during setup and surgery as well as to allow scrub personnel to easily pass the contaminated pan off the sterile field after the débridement portion has been completed.
  - Sterile surgical towels can be used to support portions of the upper extremity while using this débridement pan to prevent pressure points.
  - Intraoperative fluoroscopy will penetrate the pan well enough to visualize all but the most covert fracture lines. This is a useful attribute to check intraoperative fracture alignment during applications of external fixators.

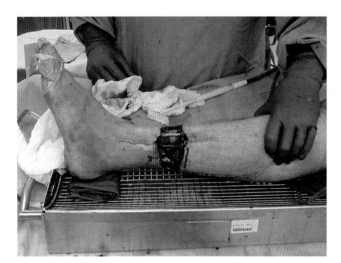

Figure 3-10 ▌ Debridement pan in use for treatment of an open tibia fracture.

- The original design has withstood thousands of autoclave cycles without damage. Its dimensions have accommodated every size extremity encountered over many years. Clinically, the sterile OR field has been kept cleaner and safer for the patient and OR personnel. The original cost was approximately $1,500.00 including materials and fabrication costs. Based on the thousands of times of use, the cost per use metric is very small.

TIP

Irrigation Technique: Keeping the Surgical Field Clean
Eric D. Farrell

Pathophysiology

Irrigation of clean or contaminated orthopaedic wounds is a common practice; however, collection of the used fluid can be difficult and messy. Traditionally, a kidney or round basin has been used but often leads to spillage.

Solution

A technique using blue towels and Ioban to divert all of the fluid into a basin or bag of choice.

Technique

Equipment
- Blue towels are rolled lengthwise to make the sides of the "gutter."
- Ioban is cut into strips approximately 16 cm in length. Larger pieces may be needed for the floor (Fig. 3-11).

- A collection bag (drain bag) is used for patients in the lateral decubitus position and for shoulder and hip surgery (Fig. 3-12).
- A large basin is used for distal extremity procedures (Fig. 3-13).

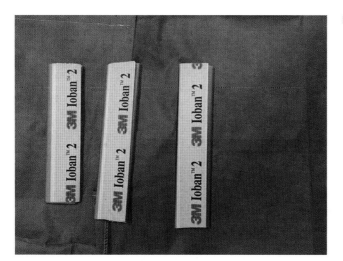

Figure 3-11 | Ioban cut into strips.

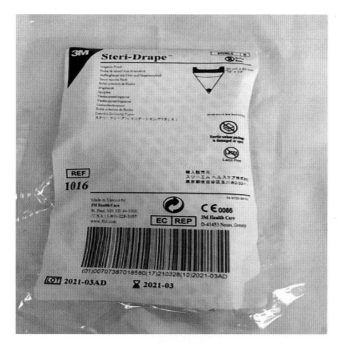

Figure 3-12 | Triangular-shaped drainage bag.

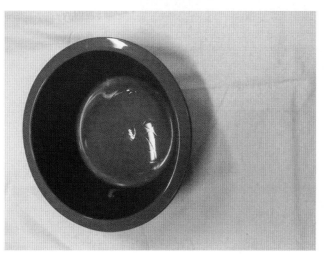

Figure 3-13 | Large basin.

Shoulder/Elbow Procedures

- An open distal one-third diaphyseal humerus fracture serves as an example (Fig. 3-14).

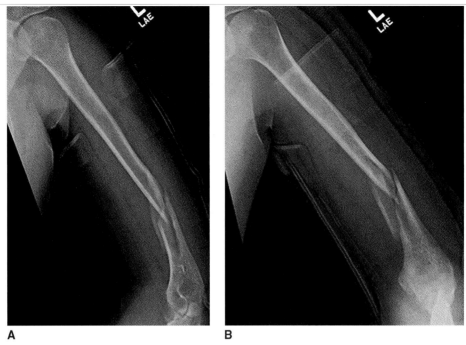

A   **B**

Figure 3-14 I A,B: Preoperative images of patient with a left distal one-third humerus fracture treated through a paratricipital posterior approach. The patient was positioned in the lateral decubitus position.

- A triangular drainage bag is placed prior to making incision ensuring good adhesive seal. The bag is positioned to allow the patient's hand to rest in neutral position without wrist flexion/extension (Fig. 3-15).

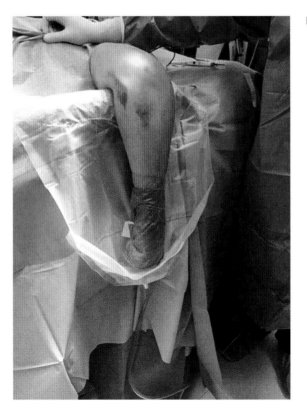

Figure 3-15 I Drain bag extending below wound.

- The forearm is then covered with a towel secured with towel clips during the case to prevent contamination of the hand (Fig. 3-16).
- When ready for irrigation, rolled blue towels are placed parallel to the extremity with the ends placed into the drainage bag. Ioban is then used to seal the towels to the field and drainage bag (Fig. 3-17).

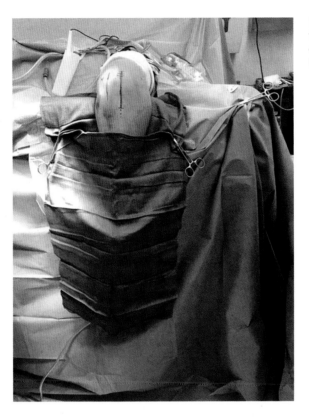

Figure 3-16 | Arm covered with blue towel during the case to prevent contamination. One towel clip can be removed to create a "door" to access the hand.

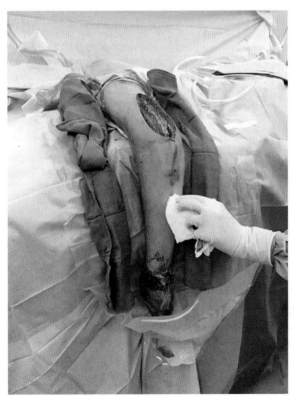

Figure 3-17 | New drapes have been applied and surgical gloves changed with the placement of a new drainage bag. Blue towels rolled parallel to extremity and extra towel placed superiorly to fill depression.

- A strip of Ioban is placed over each of the rolled towels extending into the drainage bag. A third wide strip of Ioban is placed under the extremity making the "floor" of the gutter. Note: blue towel(s) can be placed proximally and used to fill any voids or pockets to facilitate gravity flow of fluid into the bag (Fig. 3-18).
- Irrigation of the wound can now commence with all of the fluid draining into the drain bag, which is connected to suction (Figs. 3-19 and 3-20). Following débridement and irrigation, the fracture is treated definitively with fixation (Fig. 3-20).

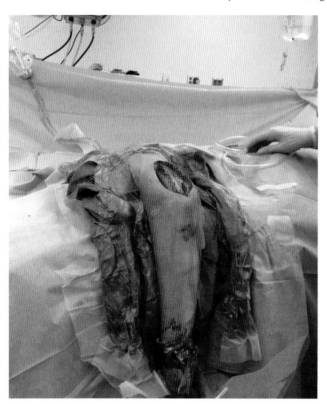

Figure 3-18 ▌ Blue towels lined with Ioban with care taken to not flatten the rolls and maintain the sides of gutter. The Ioban is sealed to skin and blue towels above the incision and extends into the drainage bag.

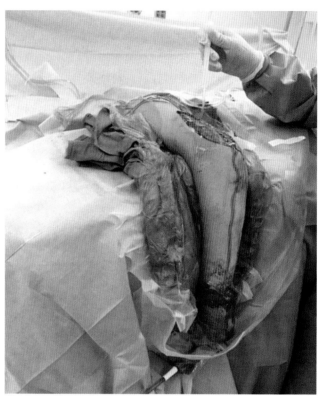

Figure 3-19 ▌ Cysto tube gravity irrigation in progress with fluid draining into bag. Ioban "floor" is noted in this photo.

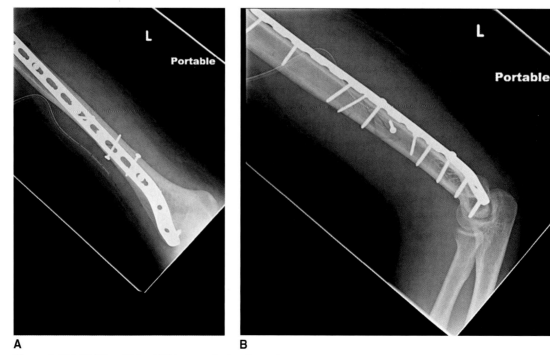

A   **B**

Figure 3-20 ▌ AP **(A)** and lateral **(B)** intra-op final radiographs.

Lower Extremity Technique

For wounds involving the knee or lower extremity, a basin can be placed directly underneath the wound and towels draped proximally and distally. Ioban is then used to seal the towels to the skin directing fluids into the collection basin. Suction is placed directly into the basin (Fig. 3-21A and B).

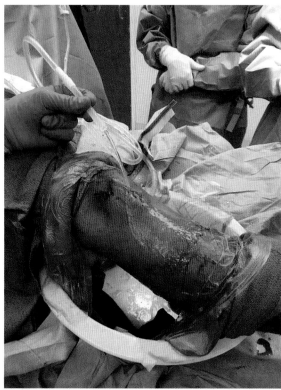

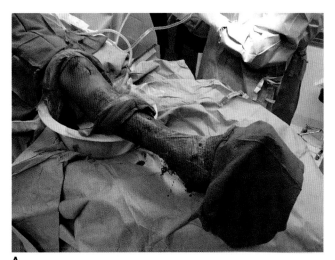

A

B

Figure 3-21 I A,B: Lower extremity placed over basin with towels wrapped around extremity and placed into the basin. Towels then sealed with Ioban.

Wound Management

TIP

Allgöwer (Modified Donati) Sequentially Tensioned Skin Closure

Matthew P. Sullivan
Reza Firoozabadi

Pathophysiology

Skin closure of traumatized tissues can be extremely challenging, particularly when soft tissue swelling is present prior to, or has occurred over the course of, surgery.

Solution

Certain surgical and traumatic wounds require advanced closure techniques in order to meticulously protect and close edematous tissues. These situations often include the following:

- Volar Henry approach to the forearm
- Anteromedial and anterolateral approaches to the distal tibia
- Posterolateral approach to the fibula
- Dual approaches to the talus
- Extensile lateral approach to the calcaneus
- Open fracture wounds

Surgical Goals

- Meticulous soft tissue handling so as to limit iatrogenic injury to the delicate tissues around traumatic open wounds and high-risk approaches
- Tension-free closure, which allows for wound healing and avoids the need for skin grafting or composite vascularized tissue transfer

Technique

Required instrumentation/materials:

- 3-0 or 4-0 nylon suture (Fig. 3-22A).
- 4 × ¼ inch uncut adhesive strips (Fig. 3-22B).
- Mosquito hemostats × 10 to 25 (Fig. 3-22C).

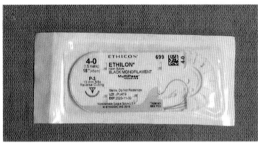

A

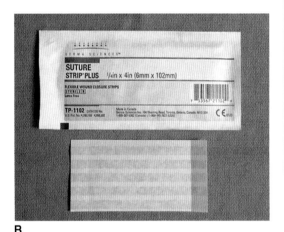

B

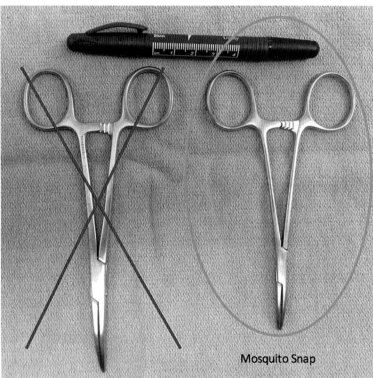

C

Figure 3-22 I Suture **(A)**, adhesive strips **(B)**, and the mosquito snaps **(C)** required for sequentially tensioned skin closure.

Illustrative Case

- A 24-year-old male involved in a high-energy motorcycle crash. Operative orthopaedic injuries include bilateral open both bone forearm fractures.
- Right type 3a open both bone forearm fracture (Fig. 3-23). Open wound over the subcutaneous border of the ulna. Significant soft tissue stripping about the radius and ulna.

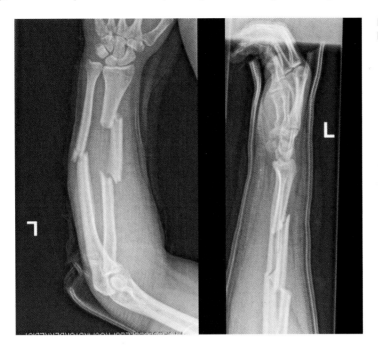

Figure 3-23 I Type 3a open both bone forearm fracture.

- Ulna fracture treated first using surgical extension incorporating the open wound. This surgical wound was subsequently closed prior to treating the radius fracture.
- Radius treated next through a formal volar Henry approach.
- Unable to close this incision at the time of internal fixation due to significant swelling. As such, the volar surgical wound was covered with a negative pressure wound dressing set to 125 mm Hg (Fig. 3-24).
- The patient returned to the operating room for irrigation and débridement followed by delayed primary wound closure 2 days later.

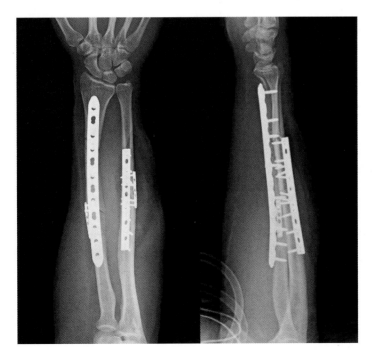

Figure 3-24 I Definitive fixation performed on day of admission. Unable to close volar Henry wound due to significant soft tissue swelling in the volar compartment.

Allgöwer-Donati Technique

- Multifaceted suturing method
  - Stitch technique
  - Tensioning technique
- Stitch technique
  - Half vertical mattress stitch.
  - Half-buried vertical dermal stitch.
  - The suture material enters and exits the epidermis on one side of the wound.
  - The knot is the most ischemic element of the stitch.
  - Must identify if there is a flap or undermined aspect of the wound. If there is any microvascular compromise to the skin, the knot should be placed on this least compromised side of the wound (Fig. 3-25).

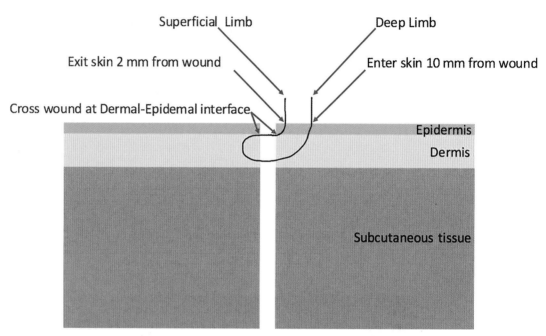

Figure 3-25 Schematic demonstrating the technique for placing the Allgöwer stitch. Notice that the suture enters the skin 10 mm from the wound and forms the deep limb. It then makes an abrupt turn in the dermis on the far side of the wound and exits as the superficial limb at the dermal-epidermal interface. It then reenters the near side of the wound at the dermal-epidermal interface and immediately exits the skin on the near side. Notice that the knot does not lie across the wound.

- Tensioning technique
  - The first stitch should be placed in the center of the wound. Each subsequent stitch should bisect the wound. Ultimately sutures should be spaced 5 to 10 mm apart (Fig. 3-26). This ensures the wound is evenly re-approximated.
  - Once each suture is placed, the tails of the suture are snapped with a small mosquito snap. Several sutures are placed prior to tensioning and tying (Fig. 3-26).

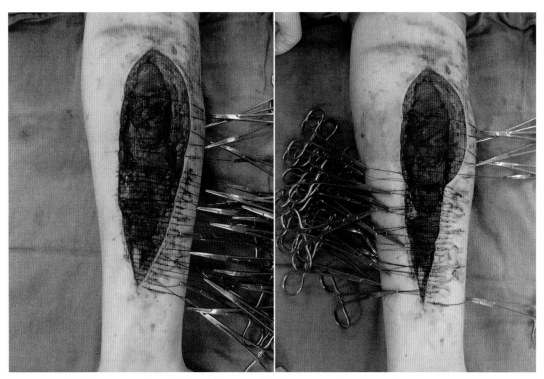

Figure 3-26 | The first suture placed bisects the wound (*). Sutures are placed and tails are snapped. Mosquito snaps are then brought to the other side of the wound to begin tensioning the soft tissues closed. Notice that initially sutures are placed over half of the incision only.

- The assistant holds 3 to 5 mosquito snaps, pulling the suture tails up and away from the side of the wound that the knots will be tied down to. This distributes the force required to close a tight wound over several stitches, allowing the surgeon to tie each knot across a relatively tension-free incision (Fig. 3-27).

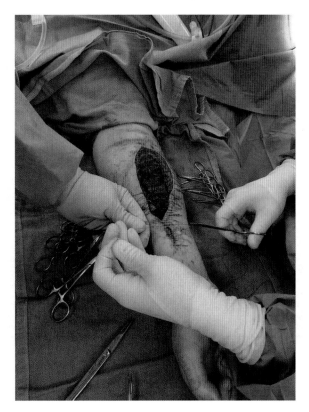

Figure 3-27 | Once sutures to half of the wound have been placed, the assistant holds 3 to 5 sutures pulling them up and away from the side of the wound the knots will be placed on. This allows wound edges to be approximated "in front of" the suture being tied by the surgeon. Notice that by pulling the subsequent five sutures the assistant is creating a "tension-free" environment for the surgeon to tie down each knot in.

- Sutures for only half of the wound should be placed at a time (Fig. 3-28). This prevents the surgeon from wasting time placing sutures along the entire wound only to realize when he/she begins tying that the wound will not eventually be closable.

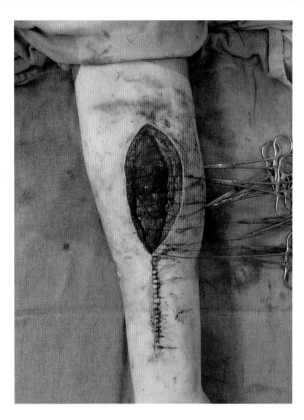

Figure 3-28 ‖ Half of the wound is closed at a time. Notice that the wound edge is well approximated and there is no ischemic eversion of the edges, which occurs with both horizontal and vertical mattress techniques.

- "Mosquito snap management" will greatly facilitate efficient wound closure. This can be done with the aid of long surgical forceps (DeBakey Tissue Forceps) (Fig. 3-29).

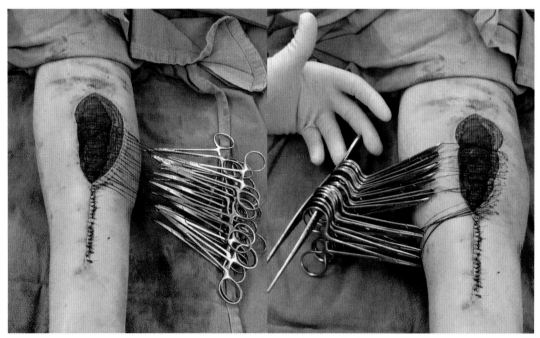

Figure 3-29 ‖ Sutures are placed in the proximal aspect of the wound and organized with DeBakey forceps.

● The remainder of the wound is closed by splitting each section in half and placing sutures along 50% of the incision and then tensioning and tying. Again, this prevents the surgeon from getting into a situation in which significant time has been dedicated to placing sutures across a stretch of the wound that is not ready for primary closure (Fig. 3-30).

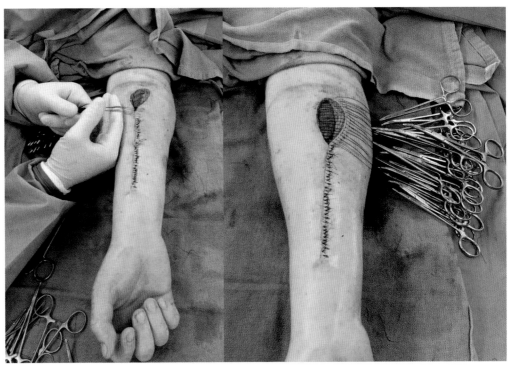

Figure 3-30 ▌ The technique is used for sequentially tensioning and closing the remainder of the wound.

● When done properly, the wound edges are perfectly apposed and not everted, as is typical of both horizontal and vertical mattress techniques (Fig. 3-31). This provides the most biologically friendly environment for ultimate healing.

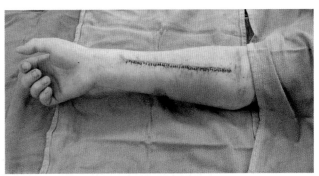

B

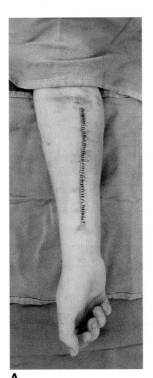

A

Figure 3-31 ▌ Final wound closure **(A and B)** demonstrating apposed wound edges, without skin eversion or evidence of necrosis.

- Prior to leaving the operating room, the surgeon should ensure that compartments are all compressible and there is no evidence of vascular compromise in the limb distal to the injury (Fig. 3-32).

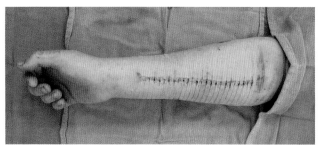

A

Figure 3-32 | Full-length Steri-Strips are placed along the length of the wound **(A)**. These should be kept long so as to distribute the tension away from the closed wound if there is swelling postoperatively. Also, notice that the surgeon is able to easily compress the forearm and the hand is pink and well perfused **(B)**.

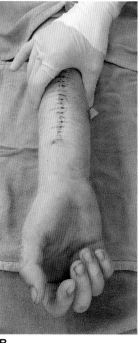

B

- Long (4 inch), uncut ¼-inch adhesive strips play an essential role in wound repair strength during healing, particularly when postoperative wound swelling may occur. By maintaining their length (4 inches), the tension forces that are created by soft tissue swelling are distributed over the length of the strips, thus preventing the wound edges from gapping.
- The entire wound should finally be covered with Betadine-moistened Adaptic gauze followed by dry sterile gauze.
- Sutures will be ready for removal between 2 and 4 weeks after surgery. At three months, the wound is well healed (Fig. 3-33).

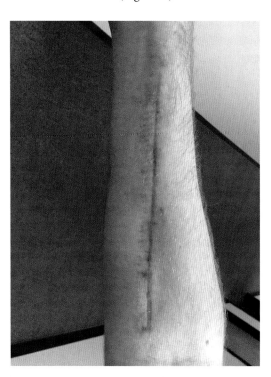

Figure 3-33 | Clinical follow-up at 3 months demonstrates a well-healed incision.

Compartment Syndrome: Single-Incision Fasciotomy

- Supine position.
- Long, straight, longitudinal incision along the posterolateral aspect of the leg in line with the fibula, from 4 to 7 cm distal to the proximal aspect of the fibular head to approximately 5 cm proximal to the distal tip of the fibula (Fig. 3-34).

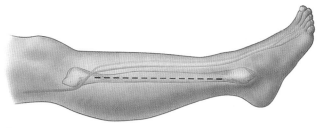

A

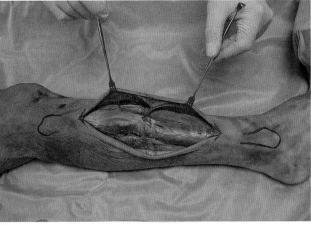

B

Figure 3-34 I **A:** Schematic representation of the right leg and the incision location relative to the fibula. **B:** Cadaveric dissection of the right leg demonstrating elevation of full-thickness anterior and posterior skin flaps. The anterior, lateral, and superficial posterior compartments can be identified at this point in the dissection. Note the presence of fascial perforating vessels. (From Maheshwari R, Taitsman LA, Barei DP. Single-incision fasciotomy for compartmental syndrome of the leg in patients with diaphyseal tibial fractures. *J Orthop Trauma.* 2008;22:723–730, with permission.)

- Full-thickness anterior and posterior skin flaps are elevated.
  - Elevation of these flaps is facilitated with the use of a sponge to separate the skin and subcutaneous layer from the underlying fascia.
  - Perforating arterial vessels are encountered, often located adjacent to the intermuscular septa, and are preserved.
  - During distal elevation of the anterior skin flap, the fascial perforation of the superficial peroneal nerve from the lateral compartment is identified and the nerve is protected.
  - Skin flap elevation is continued until the anterior, lateral, and superficial posterior compartments are identified definitively.
    - Identification of these compartments is aided by the direct palpation of the anterior and lateral intermuscular septa.
  - A long longitudinally oriented incision is then made in the fascia overlying the superficial posterior compartment followed by the lateral compartment, and finally the anterior compartment. Proceeding in this order will limit the amount of blood obscuring posterior (lower) operative sites.

- Transfascial entrance into each of the superficial posterior, lateral, and anterior compartments is verified by direct inspection of their muscular contents during ankle dorsiflexion, hind foot inversion, and ankle and metatarsophalangeal plantar flexion, respectively (Fig. 3-35).

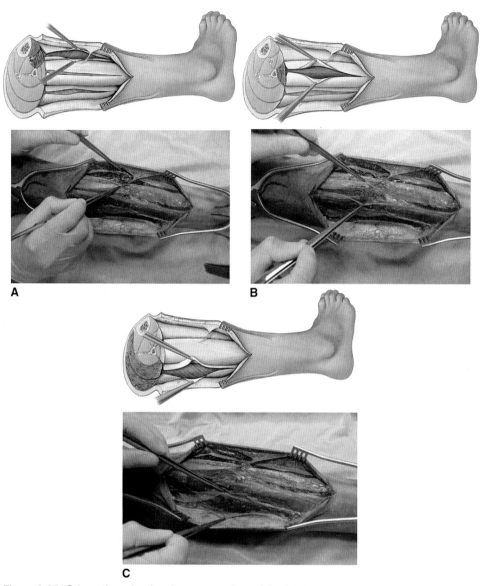

Figure 3-35 | Schematic and cadaveric representations of the right leg demonstrating fasciotomy of the anterior compartment **(A)**, lateral compartment **(B)**, and superficial posterior compartment **(C)**. (In this example, self-retaining retractors are used for illustrative purposes only and are typically not required during the actual procedure.) (From Maheshwari R, Taitsman LA, Barei DP. Single-incision fasciotomy for compartmental syndrome of the leg in patients with diaphyseal tibial fractures. *J Orthop Trauma.* 2008;22:723–730, with permission.)

- The posterior portion of the incised lateral compartment fascia is grasped with an Allis clamp, and the lateral intermuscular septum is placed under tension by sustained gentle traction toward the surgeon.
- The posterior aspect of the peroneal musculature is then bluntly elevated from the anterior aspect of the lateral intermuscular septum until the insertion of the lateral intermuscular septum into the posterolateral aspect of the fibula is fully identified along the length of the surgical incision.
- The deep posterior compartment of the leg is entered by incising the posterolateral fibular insertion of the lateral intermuscular septum sharply or with electrocautery.
  - Fascia is incised immediately adjacent to the posterolateral fibula.

● The posterolateral fibular insertion of the lateral intermuscular septum is incised along the entire length of the fibula until the distal limit of the surgical wound is encountered, exposing the deep posterior compartment.

  ▪ This dissection is facilitated by maintaining hemostasis, by lateral tension on the lateral intermuscular septum and with anterior retraction of the peroneal musculature (lateral compartment).

  ▪ Adequate entrance into the deep posterior compartment is verified by identification of the FHL musculature noted with dorsiflexion and plantar flexion of the metatarsophalangeal and interphalangeal joints of the hallux (Figs. 3-36 and 3-37).

● Fasciotomy incisions require sterile management after internal fixation.

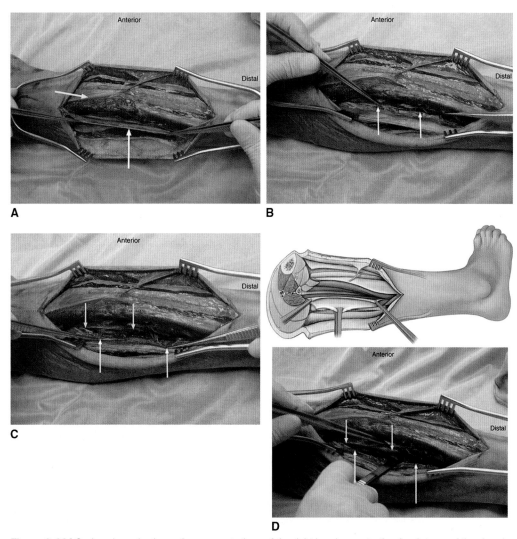

Figure 3-36 I Cadaveric and schematic representations of the right leg demonstrating fasciotomy of the deep posterior compartment. **A:** The lateral compartment fascia has been incised. The posterior aspect of the incised fascia has been grasped with two forceps (*white arrow*) and has been retracted toward the surgeon. The *yellow arrow* demonstrates the lateral compartment musculature (peroneal) that has been elevated from the deep surface of the lateral compartment fascia and the anterior aspect of the lateral intermuscular septum. **B:** The insertion of the lateral intermuscular septum on the posterolateral aspect of the fibula is indicated by the *white arrows*. **C:** The insertion of the lateral intermuscular septum (*white arrows*) has been incised and retracted posteriorly from the posterolateral aspect of the fibula (*yellow arrows*). The deep posterior compartment has now been opened. **D:** An instrument has been placed beneath the posterolateral aspect of the fibula (*yellow arrows*) into the deep posterior compartment. The incised insertion of the lateral intermuscular septum is marked by the *white arrows*. (In this example, self-retaining retractors are used for illustrative purposes only and are typically not required during the actual procedure.) (From Maheshwari R, Taitsman LA, Barei DP. Single-incision fasciotomy for compartmental syndrome of the leg in patients with diaphyseal tibial fractures. *J Orthop Trauma.* 2008;22:723–730, with permission.)

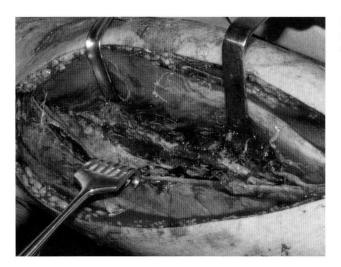

Figure 3-37 I Clinical example of complete release of all four leg compartments through a single lateral incision.

Management of Segmental Bone Defects

- Many options exist to manage bone defects. The method selected depends on location of defect and timing of treatment.
- Metaphyseal defects are typically treated with antibiotic-impregnated PMMA beads at the time of débridement and external fixation and transitioned to a formal cement spacer for initiation of the Masquelet technique at the time of definitive fixation.
  - If definitive fixation is planned at the time of initial débridement, a cement spacer or beads may be used to manage the defect.
- Often, diaphyseal defects may be treated at the time of initial débridement with a cement spacer and definitive fixation with IM nailing.
  - If the defects are heavily contaminated and serial débridements are planned, a bead pouch may be used for ease of removal.
- Very large segmental bone defects or heavily contaminated open fractures may be treated with tensioned fine wire circular external fixation and bone transport as an alternative to staged bone grafting.

Extracorporeal Fabrication of a PMMA Spacer to Treat Intercalary Long Bone Deficits with Induced Membrane and Intramedullary Fixation Techniques (A Minor Masquelet Modification)

Stephen A. Kottmeier
Randall Drew Madison

Pathoanatomy

- Traumatic skeletal defects pose a considerable therapeutic challenge. Soft tissue and osseous deficits must be remedied simultaneously, often with unpredictable outcomes and without established treatment algorithms. Several methods of osseous regeneration exist, most of which require advanced skill sets and resources. The induced membrane technique of Masquelet is elegant in its simplicity. It offers predictable and successful outcomes while obviating the need for microvascular techniques or distraction osteogenesis.
- However, introduction and extraction of a cement spacer surrounding an intramedullary device has proven difficult. Attempting in vivo spacer fabrication around an implanted IM nail can result in undesirable spacer shape or dimension and subjects the surrounding soft tissues to the exothermic reaction of cement polymerization. During subsequent extraction of the spacer, avoiding damage to the newly formed membrane can be challenging and time consuming.

Solution

- A cylindrical cement spacer matching the intercalary defect's shape and dimensions can be fabricated extracorporeally (on the back table).
  - The spacer can be bivalved prior to cement hardening.
  - The two halves can then be easily implanted and cerclaged after cement polymerization is complete.
- Facile and atraumatic extraction of the spacer, followed by bone grafting, can then be performed at a later date.
- The inclusion of intramedullary fixation with this technique may resolve conflicts associated with external fixation and perhaps even plating efforts.
- Advantages of extracorporeal spacer fabrication:
  - Exothermic process and threat to regional soft tissues during cement polymerization are circumvented.
  - A spacer of uniform design encourages the evolution of a membrane of predictably desirable dimensions.
  - The posterior dimension of the spacer is controlled, and the resultant void is accordingly more capacious.
  - Atraumatic spacer extraction is afforded with diminished hazard to the newly formed membrane.

Technique

- The described technique is most frequently used to address segmental defects in the femur and tibia, but may be used in other long bones. Case examples discussed here pertain to the tibia.
- Wide, aggressive, serial débridement of devitalized soft and osseous tissues is performed. Initial assessment (left) may fail to discern devitalized bone, which is more readily appreciated after subsequent débridement (right) (Fig. 3-38A).
  - Caveat: Cases complicated by infection are often the results of inadequate resection of necrotic bone and ischemic soft tissues. Adequate resection of necrotic bone commonly results in a resultant intercalary defect (Fig. 3-38B).

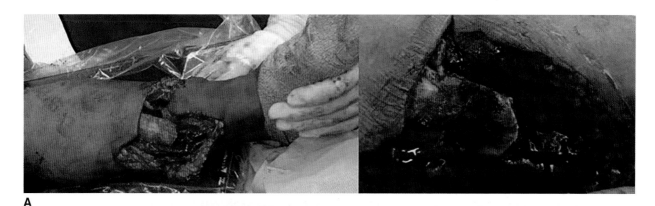

A

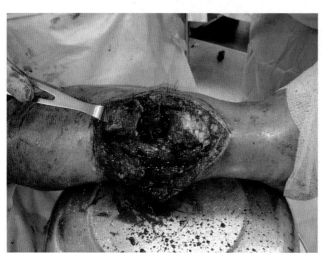

B

Figure 3-38 I **A:** A type III open tibial shaft fracture at presentation and a few days later. Note the ischemic diaphyseal bone. **B:** The same patient after excisional débridement and resection of necrotic bone.

- This initial step is commonly performed with contemporaneous application of a spanning external fixator and inclusion of standard open fracture antimicrobial prophylaxis
- After wide segmental osseous resection (excisional débridement) with provisional and external fixator application, intramedullary fixation is performed in conjunction with soft tissue coverage (Fig. 3-39).
  - For type IIIB open fractures, soft tissue coverage typically consists of regional or free soft tissue transfer.

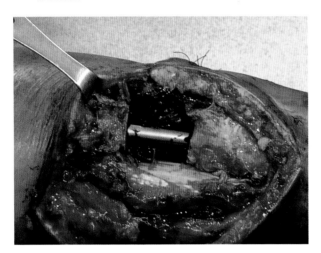

Figure 3-39 I Intramedullary nail is visible in osseous defect. Note the vascularized bone ends and soft tissues.

- An extracorporeal PMMA spacer is then fabricated at the back table.
  - While in a doughy state, mold cement to desired size and shape around the intended nail (prior to insertion), or use another tool with a similar size and shape.
    - Some IM nailing systems' drill guide sleeves may be appropriate.
  - Prior to hardening, opposing sides of the cement spacer are longitudinally sectioned with a scalpel (Fig. 3-40A and B).

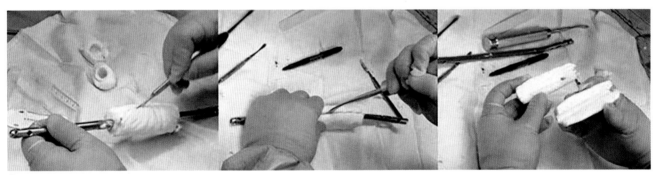

A

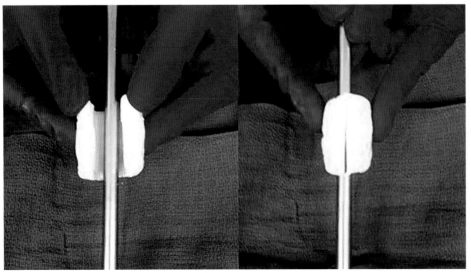

B

Figure 3-40 I A: Prior to hardening, the cement spacer is split longitudinally into two halves. B: The open and closed "clamshell" cement spacer modeled on an IM nail.

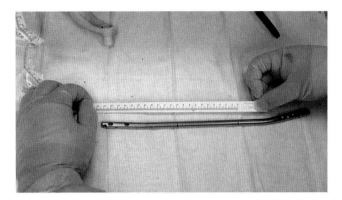

Figure 3-41 I Measure the bone defect and then create a spacer of slightly shorter length around the nail or a device of similar circumference.

- Caveat: Make the spacer slightly shorter than the defect to ensure it will fit (Fig. 3-41).
- Individual spacer halves are introduced into the skeletal defect separately to surround the nail and lashed with a circumferential PDS suture (Fig. 3-42).

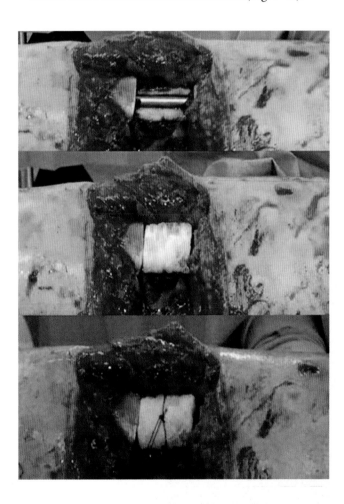

Figure 3-42 I Bone defect is first filled with one half and then the second half of the clamshell spacer. The two halves are stabilized with a circumferential monofilament.

- A separate batch of antibiotic cement is then mixed to form cement caps.
  - When in the doughy state, they are applied at each end of the defect so as to overlap the cement spacer and the accessible ends of the fracture.
  - Bathe the caps in cool saline to reduce the exothermic heat created by polymerization.
  - The caps are made to overlap the fracture margins thereby ensuring formation of a contiguous membrane (red arrows) (Fig. 3-43).

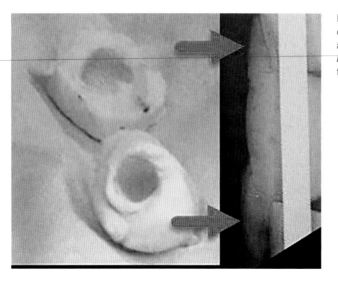

Figure 3-43 I Antibiotic spacer caps are created and applied to overlap the spacer and the accessible fracture cortical surfaces. *Red arrows* demonstrate the placement of the cement caps on x-ray.

- Antibiotics are usually added to the cement spacer.
  - A combination of tobramycin and vancomycin is common.
  - Each antibiotic's heat stability/lability should be considered.
  - Antibiotic type should be tailored to known infection and pathogen.
  - Caveat: The volume of antibiotics used may affect the cement's mechanical properties, though this is generally unimportant.
  - Caveat: Use of bacteriostatic versus bactericidal antibiotics may suppress rather than eradicate undiagnosed infection.
- At the desired time interval, spacer extraction is then performed (typically within 1 to 2 months).
  - Atraumatic extraction (Fig. 3-44) allows preservation of an intact membrane (Fig. 3-45).
- Atraumatic spacer extraction is facilitated by creating a sectioned spacer with two hemicylindrical halves at the time of implantation. This precludes the use of chisels or other aggressive methods of removal that may disrupt the induced membrane. Yellow arrows denote induced membrane, which is contiguous with the fracture margins.

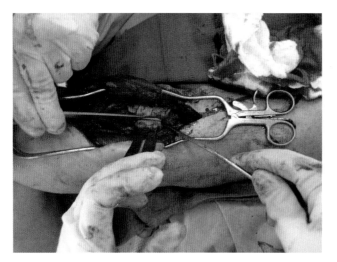

Figure 3-44 I The open approach for removal of a tibial diaphyseal spacer.

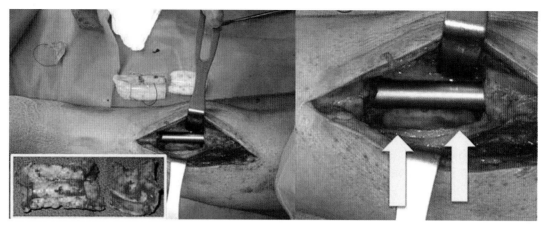

Figure 3-45 I The spacer is atraumatically removed by exploiting the hemisectioned spacer. *Yellow arrows* denote induced membrane, which is contiguous with the fracture margins.

- The robust intact membranous chamber is then filled with the selected graft or bone void filler combination (Fig. 3-46).
  - Caveat: Avoid overstuffing the membrane as this may lead to undesirable diminished porosity of the graft, which may impede osseous regeneration.
  - Weight bearing is initiated when the radiographic opacity of the evolving bone approaches 50% of that of intact neighboring bone.

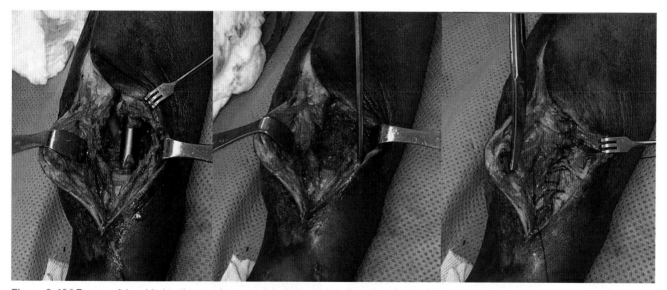

Figure 3-46 I Bone graft is added to the membranous chamber, which is then closed with suture.

Case Example #2

- As a result of a motorcycle crash, a patient sustained a high-energy open tibial fracture with bone loss. Excisional débridement of devitalized bone resulted in a larger intercalary osseous deficit (Fig. 3-47A).
- After removal of the external fixator and locked intramedullary nailing, a cement spacer of specific dimensions is fabricated around either a tibial nail (prior to insertion) or interlocking screw guide sleeves.
  - It is divided in half prior to hardening (Fig. 3-47B).
  - The spacer is then inserted to bridge the segmental defect (Fig. 3-47C).
- The spacer is extracted atraumatically 4 to 6 weeks subsequent to insertion (Fig. 3-47D).
  - Graft material and/or bone void filler is introduced within the formed membrane (Fig. 3-47E).
  - The induced membrane technique regenerated bone 6 months postoperatively with satisfactory clinical outcome (Fig. 3-47F).

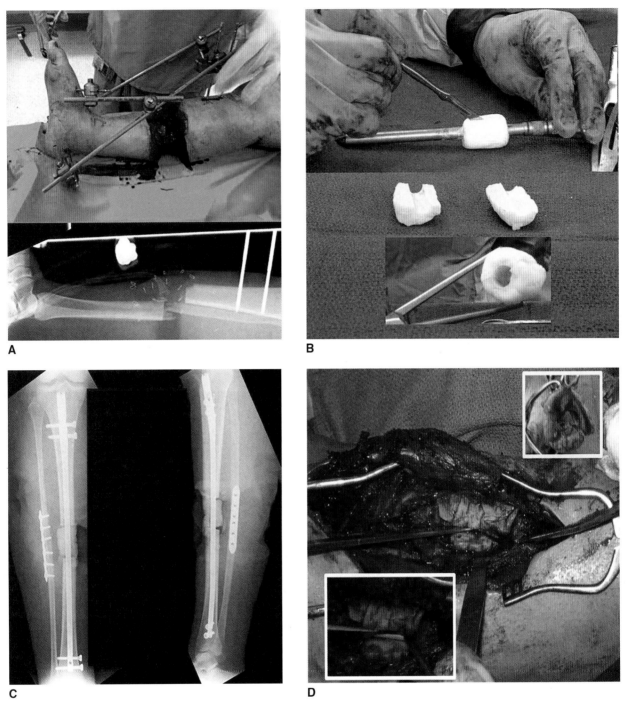

A

B

C

D

Figure 3-47 | **A:** Type IIIB open tibial shaft fracture stabilized with an external fixator. Note the segmental tissue and bone loss after excisional débridement. **B:** The bone defect size is measured, and a spacer of similar size (reduced by a few millimeters in its cranial-caudal length) is created around a drill guide sleeve. **C:** Postoperative radiographs after restoration of limb length, IM nail stabilization, and insertion of the spacer. Note both the soft tissue and osseous defects. **D:** The induced membrane has been incised longitudinally exposing the bone ends and cement spacer. The two halves of the spacer are removed atraumatically preserving the induced membrane.

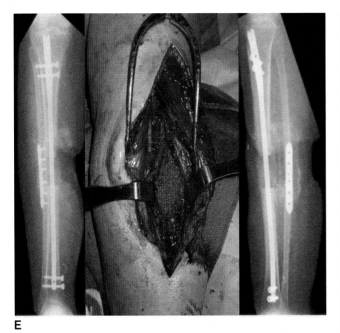
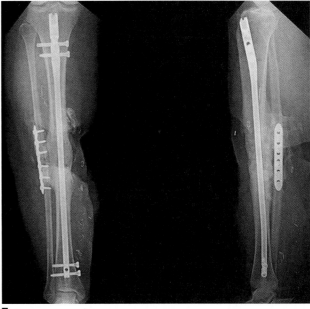

E   F

Figure 3-47 I (*Continued*) **E:** In this patient, autogenous cancellous bone graft was placed within the cavity of the induced membrane after atraumatic spacer removal. **F:** These radiographs demonstrate bridging bone regenerated 6 months after grafting.

Infection Management

- Infection may occur at any time point after an operation.
- If an infection occurs before osseous union, infection management with maintenance of implants versus conversion to external fixation is usually necessary.
  - Skeletal instability will significantly decrease the ability to clear infection.
  - Maintaining skeletal stability prevents progressive deformity that can be catastrophic.
- Additionally, if a septic nonunion develops, treatment of the infection and nonunion in concert will require some form of implant or external fixator.
- Naturally, fighting infection in the presence of implants is difficult due to bacterial biofilm production.
- Several strategies exist to mitigate this problem.

TIP | Creation of Antibiotic-Impregnated Cement-Coated Plates and Nails

John A. Scolaro
Clay Spitler

Pathophysiology

Periarticular and long bone infections are treated with parenteral antibiotics. Local antibiotics are adjunctive though less effective in the presence of metallic implants.

Solution

Metallic implants may be modified by covering much of their surfaces with antibiotic impregnated bone cement, thereby enhancing antibiotic delivery and providing stable fracture fixation. This often creates an environment conducive to fracture healing.

Technique for Making an Antibiotic-Impregnated Cement-Coated Plate

Gather the sterile instruments and equipment needed for fixation (Fig. 3-48).

- Plate and instruments for desired anatomic area.
- Multiple drill bits.
- Freer elevator.
- Dental pick.

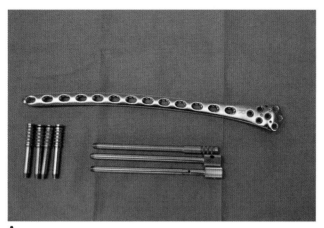

A

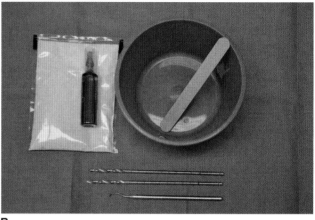

B

Figure 3-48 I Required equipment for fashioning an antibiotic-impregnated PMMA coated plate. **A:** Desired implants and associated instrumentation. **B:** Cement kit, extra drill bits and dental pick.

- Standard tongue depressor.
- Polymethylmethacrylate cement powder and monomer.
- Desired antibiotic powder to be implanted.
- Place locking towers in the desired screw holes to be used in the plate (Fig. 3-49).

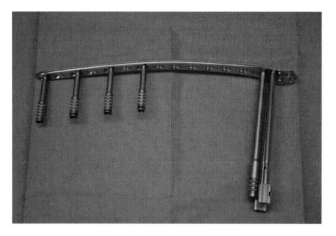

Figure 3-49 I Locking towers are placed before cement application.

- Fill all holes if the desired screw configuration cannot be determined before implant application.
- A second implant tray or small/large fragment locking set may be needed to acquire the desired number of locking towers.
- If the percutaneous insertion guide will be used, mark the footprint of the attachment handle on the plate so cement is not applied to this area.
- Mix the desired antibiotic powder to the PMMA cement powder, add liquid monomer, and mix cement.

- Apply antibiotic-impregnated cement to the plate using the tongue depressor in a uniform manner (Fig. 3-50).

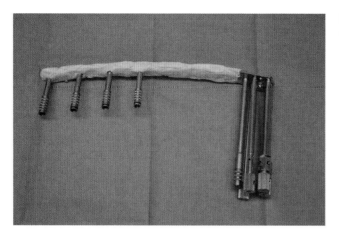

Figure 3-50 I Cement is used to circumferentially coat the plate.

- The undersurface of the plate is covered with cement at the surgeon's discretion; if cement is not applied in a circumferential manner around the plate, the potential for cement dissociation with the plate is greater.
- Place cement around the locking towers, but make sure there is no buildup of excessive cement around the tower.
- A Freer elevator can be used to contour the cement around each locking tower and remove cement from the screw holes on the undersurface of the plate.
- Prior to final cement setting, the locking tower should be removed from the plate and the Freer elevator used to gently remove any excess cement from around each screw hole. The dental pick can be used for fine manipulation of cement away from the locking threads of the plate (Fig. 3-51).

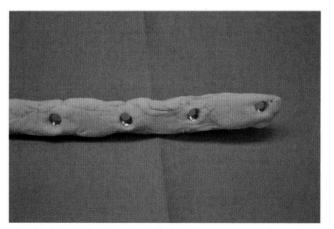

Figure 3-51 I Locking towers are removed, and the locking threads are cleaned.

- After the cement has set completely, a drill bit should be passed through each desired plate hole to ensure that a drill and screw can be placed into the plate hole.
- The dental pick can again be used to clear any cement away from threads within the plate.

- The percutaneous insertion guide can then be applied if needed prior to plate application (Fig. 3-52).

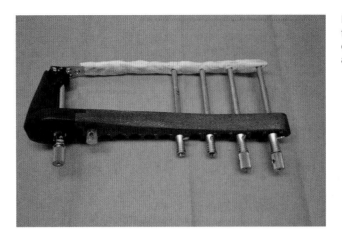

Figure 3-52 I If using a targeting arm, the footprint for the arm is placed to avoid cement application precluding targeting arm application.

- The fracture is then reduced and provisionally held.
- Although a locking or nonlocking screw can theoretically be used through each maintained screw hole, locking screws are most commonly used as the implant functions primarily as an internal external fixator (Fig. 3-53).

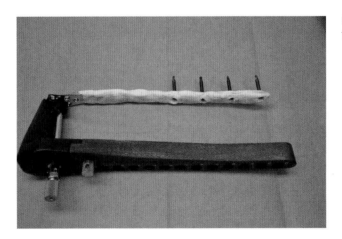

Figure 3-53 I Locking screws are placed through the targeting arm for stable fixation.

Pearls
- The locking towers should be removed from the plate prior to cement setting but not too early as the cement is difficult to handle early and can be stringy.
- Consider keeping cement off plate areas that are typically prominent (distal humerus, distal femur, distal tibia, etc.)
- Use of an antibiotic-impregnated cement–coated locking plate is most beneficial when an intramedullary implant cannot be used (Figs. 3-54 and 3-55) or when short bone segments must be controlled (Figs. 3-56 and 3-57).

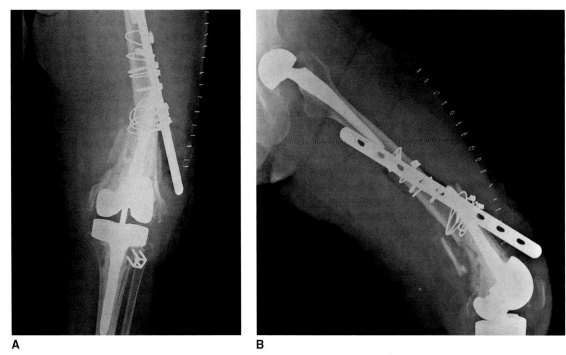

Figure 3-54 I AP **(A)** and lateral **(B)** radiographs demonstrate a chronically infected nonunion of an interprosthetic femur fracture.

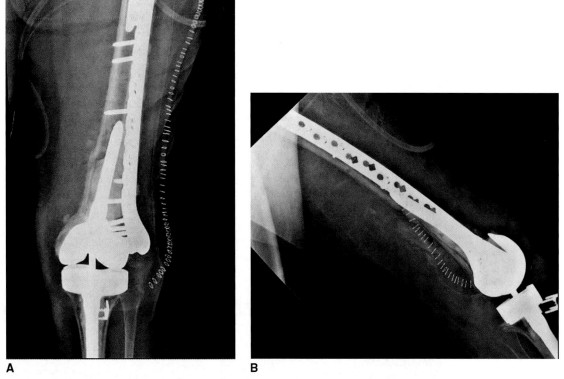

Figure 3-55 I Postoperative AP **(A)** and lateral **(B)** radiographs after implant removal and nonunion repair with an antibiotic-coated lateral locking plate.

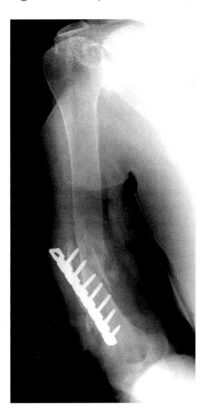

Figure 3-56 ▌ AP radiograph of an infected distal 1/3 diaphyseal humerus nonunion.

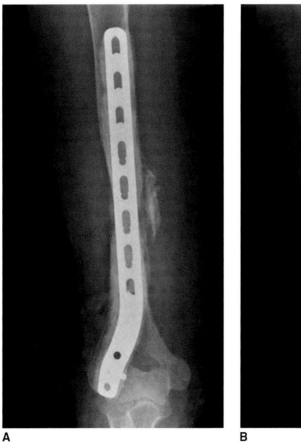

A

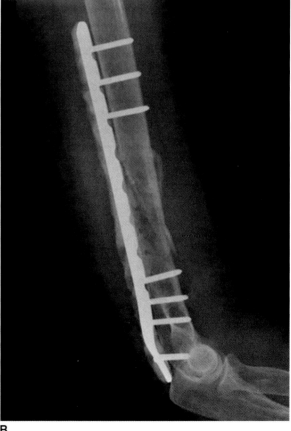

B

Figure 3-57 ▌ Postoperative AP **(A)** and lateral **(B)** radiographs demonstrating implant removal and nonunion repair with an antibiotic-coated locking plate.

- Plates can be used temporarily as a staged management technique while appropriate infection control interventions are under way, or they may be definitive if osseous healing occurs and the plate remains asymptomatic.

Technique for Antibiotic-Impregnated Cement-Coated Intramedullary Nail

Sterile Instruments/Equipment
- Desired core implant (Fig. 3-58)
  - Standard intramedullary nail
  - Threaded ring fixator connecting rod with or without threaded eyelet and corresponding nut
  - Rush rod/smooth guidewire
- Desired outer nail mold (Fig. 3-59)
  - 40-French chest tube
  - Perfusion tubing (various diameters)

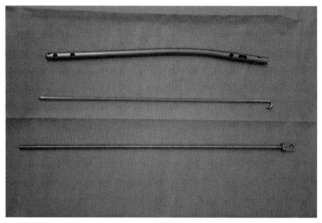

Figure 3-58 | Various types of intramodullary implants may be coated with antibiotic cement. From left to right, locking IM nail, Rush rod, Ilizarov threaded rod with female hinge.

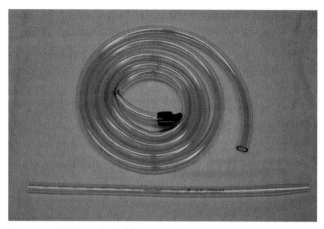

Figure 3-59 | Pertusion tubing of varying diameters can be used as an alternative conduit for cement application.

- Mineral oil (Fig. 3-60)
- Polymethylmethacrylate cement powder and monomer
- Desired antibiotic powder to be implanted
- Cement mixing apparatus

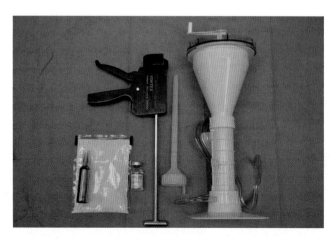

Figure 3-60 | Cementing kit including a cement gun for creating a cement-coated nail.

- Cement injection gun
- No. 10 or larger scalpel blade × 2
- Freer elevator
- If standard locked intramedullary nail used
  - Multiple drill bits
  - Guidewire for intramedullary nail

Technique

- Determine the desired core implant to be used.
  - If the fracture is unstable or not healed, a small-diameter intramedullary nail should be used as it permits interlocking (8 to 10 mm).
  - If the long bone is stable, a smooth wire or threaded rod can be used instead of an IM nail.
- Determine the desired final diameter of the intramedullary nail (Fig. 3-61).
  - The inner diameter of a 40-French chest tube is typically just over 10 mm.
  - The inner diameter of standard perfusion tubing is variable and measured to determine the final outer diameter of the created cement nail.

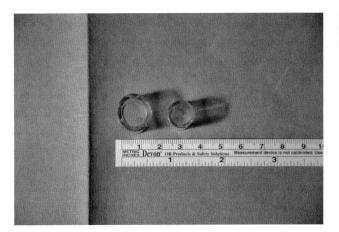

Figure 3-61 I Different diameter chest tubes and perfusion tubing are available and selected based upon desired nail diameter.

- If a wire or rod is used, measure the approximate intramedullary length of the bone and cut the core implant to the appropriate length.
- Cut the selected tubing to a length slightly greater than the length of the core implant.
- Coat the inside of the tubing with mineral oil, ensuring that oil coats the entire circumference of the tube (Fig. 3-62).
- Place the nail or rod within the tube (Fig. 3-63).

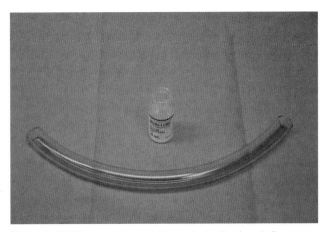

Figure 3-62 I The cement conduit is coated with mineral oil.

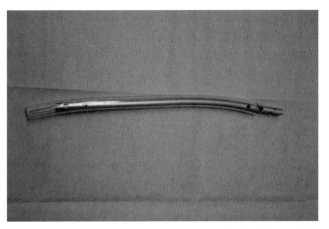

Figure 3-63 I The rod is placed within the tube, leaving the proximal end free to keep threads for the insertion jig cement free.

- Mix the desired antibiotic powder and a reduced amount of PMMA cement powder, add liquid monomer, and mix cement within the cement mixing apparatus.
- Once the cement has been mixed and is uniform in consistency, deposit the cement into the cement injection gun immediately.
- Place the end of the tube over the nozzle of the injection gun and inject cement into the plastic tube (Fig. 3-64).
- Once the cement has been placed within the tube, manually manipulate the tube around the core implant so that there is uniform distribution of cement over its surface (Fig. 3-65).

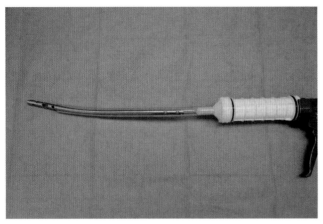

Figure 3-64 | After cement mixing, the cement gun is loaded into the tubing.

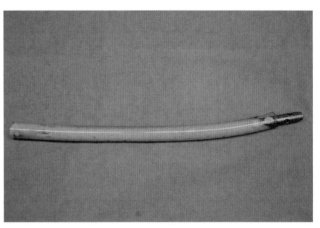

Figure 3-65 | Cement is injected until the tube is filled.

- If the cannulation of a standard locked nail needs to be maintained, insert, remove. and reinsert the ball tip guidewire repetitively while the cement sets so as to create a path for the guidewire (Fig. 3-66).
- After the cement has set completely and returned to room temperature, use a no. 10 blade and make a decisive cut along the length of the plastic nail mold (Fig. 3-67).

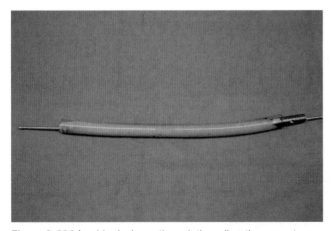

Figure 3-66 | A guidewire is run through the nail as the cement hardens.

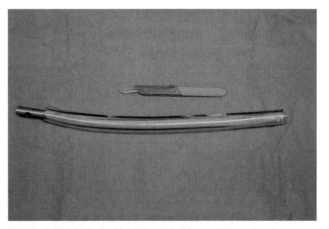

Figure 3-67 | A 10- or 20-blade scalpel is used to section the tubing.

- Use a Freer elevator to carefully remove the plastic mold.
- A sharp drill bit can be used to restore the interlocking holes if a standard locked nail is used (Fig. 3-68).

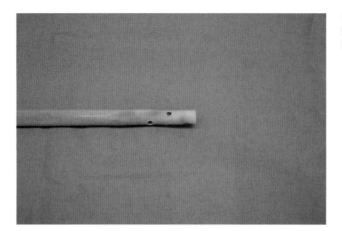

Figure 3-68 | If interlocking bolts are intended, a drill is used to reconstitute the holes.

Pearls

- Cement should be injected into the tubing as soon as possible after mixing so that the liquid cement can flow easily along the whole length of the nail within the tubing.
- The threaded rod, Rush nail, or smooth guidewire can be contoured to conform to the Herzog bend or radius of curvature of the removed intramedullary implant (Fig. 3-69).

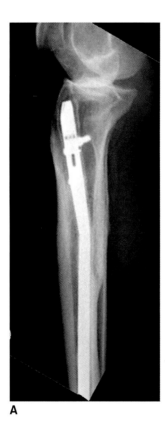
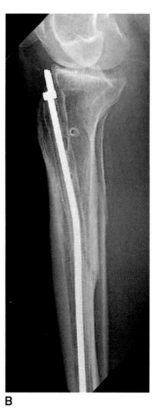

Figure 3-69 | Lateral radiograph view **(A)** of a standard tibial nail coated in cement and a lateral view **(B)** of a smaller diameter threaded rod coated in cement.

A

B

- A nut can be placed at the bottom of the threaded rod to provide a cap to the bottom of the created implant.
- An eyelet (e.g., female Ilizarov hinge) can be placed at the top of the threaded rod to either (a) facilitate easy insertion and removal or (b) function as an opportunity for an interlocking screw/bolt.
- The cement must be allowed to set completely before the mold is cut, or the cement will stick to the mold or dissociate from the core implant.
- At the surgeon's discretion, a portion of the nail can be left uncovered or removed (by chipping away the brittle cement once it has set) especially when it is desired to use multiple interlocking screws (Fig. 3-70).

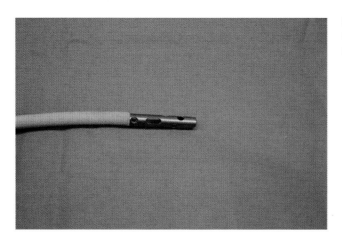

Figure 3-70 I The distal aspect of this nail has been left cement free in anticipation of using multiple interlocking bolts.

Section 2
Shoulder/Arm

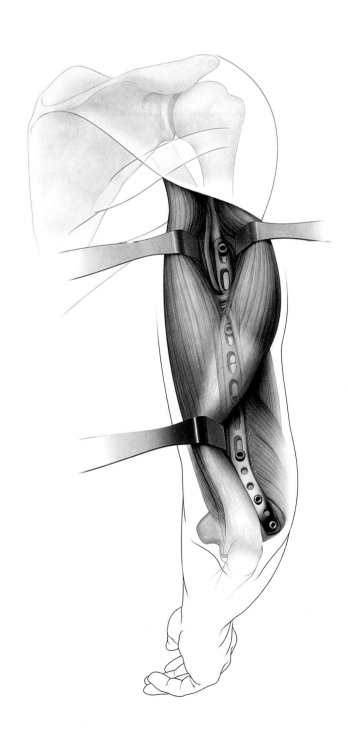

Chapter 4
Scapula and Glenoid Fractures

PETER A. COLE
ANTHONY J. DUGARTE
ZACHARY V. ROBERTS

Sterile Instruments/Equipment

- Sterile drapes, including impervious stockinette and 4-inch elastic bandage wrap for forearm and hand
- 1/4% bupivacaine, with epinephrine for posterior incision (minimizes skin bleeding)
- Large and small pointed bone reduction clamps ("Weber clamps")
- Implants:
  - 2.7- and 3.5-mm reconstruction plates and screws
  - 1/4 and 1/3 tubular plates
  - 2.0- and 2.4-mm plates and screws
  - Extra long screws (2.0, 2.4, 2.7, and 3.5 mm)
- K-wires and wire driver/drill
- Femoral distractor(s) if reducing displaced fractures, especially if >20 days after injury

Positioning

- Lateral: modified Judet approach
  - Lateral positioning is preferred to prone.
  - The lateral position allows for better palpation of the coracoid for screw placement, percutaneous "joystick" placement in the coracoid as needed, and facilitates reduction maneuvers.
  - Place the patient on the cantilevered end of a radiolucent operating table (reversed), which facilitates intraoperative imaging.
  - Chest roll for axillary protection, using a beanbag and appropriate padding.
  - A padded Plexiglas board supports the uninjured, dependent arm; the operative arm is prepped free and supported on a padded (pillow) sterile Mayo stand.
    - This enables intraoperative limb manipulation and positioning to aid in reduction and imaging.
    - Pad Mayo stand and tray with a taped pillow; cover with a sterile Mayo stand cover.
  - Alternatively, the operated upper extremity may be supported by an adjustable radiolucent arm board under the drapes (Figs. 4-1 and 4-2).
  - Fluoroscopy should be positioned perpendicular to the patient and table, entering from the patient's anterior/front side, opposite from the surgeon.
    - This allows a rollover image for a scapular Y view and a rollback to image a Grashey AP view.

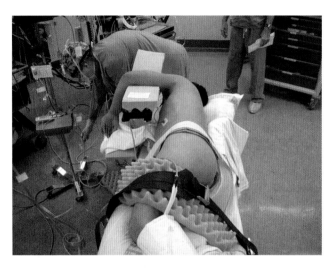

Figure 4-1 ‖ The lateral decubitus position for modified Judet surgical approach.

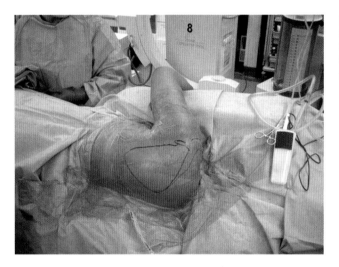

Figure 4-2 ‖ Prepped and draped. The arm is prepped into the field so it can be manipulated sterilely. There should be a clear path for the C-arm to come in from the opposite side.

Surgical Approach

- Modified Judet.[1]
- The incision is curvilinear and parallels the scapular spine and the medial scapular border (Fig. 4-3).
- Prior to incision, injection of Bupivacaine 0.5% with epinephrine can help minimize cutaneous bleeding.

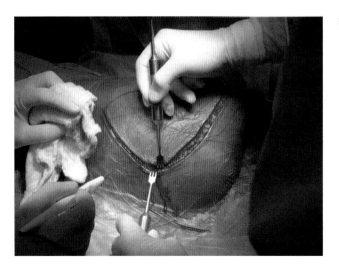

Figure 4-3 ‖ Curvilinear incision.

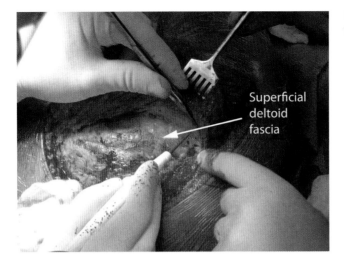

Figure 4-4 | A full-thickness flap is elevated from the deltoid fascia.

- Develop a full-thickness skin and subcutaneous flap, taking care to leave the fascia intact over the posterior scapular muscles and latissimus dorsi (Fig. 4-4).
- Identify the lower border of the deltoid, and incise the fascia sharply (Fig. 4-5A and B).
- Separate the inferior border of the posterior deltoid from the infraspinatus from medial to lateral.
  - Keep the deep fascia with the deltoid as reflected (Fig. 4-6).

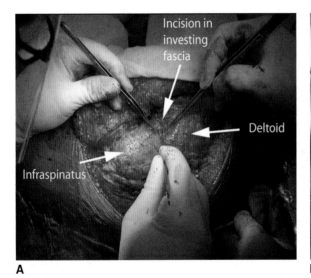

A

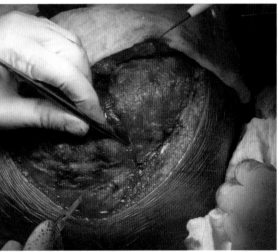

B

Figure 4-5 | **A,B:** The investing fascia is incised along the inferior border of the posterior deltoid.

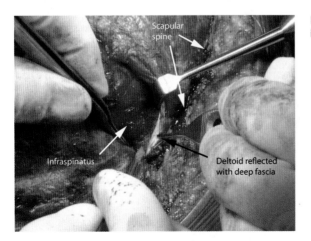

Figure 4-6 | The deltoid is reflected from the infraspinatus with the deep fascia.

- Sharply release the deltoid origin from the scapular spine.
  - A tag stitch in the superomedial corner aids in retraction and identifies this area for later repair (Fig. 4-7).
- Retract the posterior deltoid superolaterally (Fig. 4-8).
- Developing the interval between teres minor and infraspinatus will allow exposure of the lateral border of the scapula and inferior glenoid neck (Figs. 4-9A,B and 4-10).

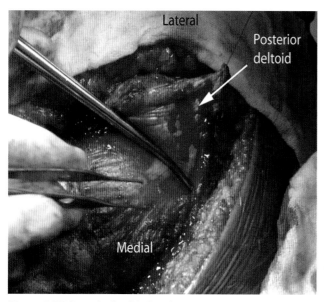

Figure 4-7 I Once the fascial plane is developed, the posterior deltoid is incised from the scapular spine.

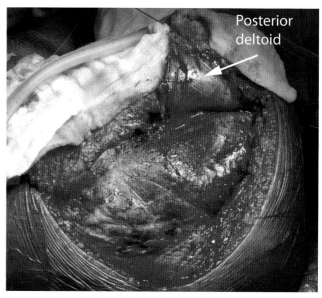

Figure 4-8 I The deltoid is mobilized and reflected from medial to lateral to the lateral border of the scapula.

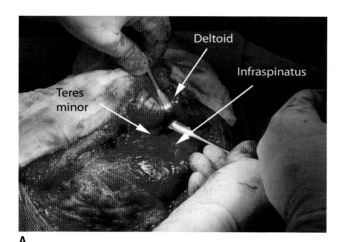

A

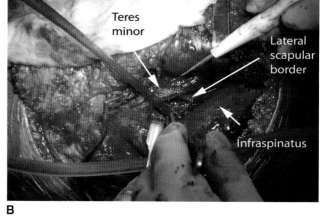

B

Figure 4-9 I **A,B:** Deltoid reflection allows complete exposure of the infraspinatus teres minor interval for lateral scapular access.

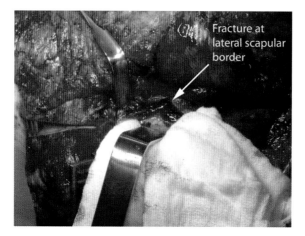

Figure 4-10 I The fracture site is further exposed and cleaned of hematoma and periosteum.

- If visualization of the articular component of the fracture is required, a longitudinal posterior capsulotomy can be performed in the interval between infraspinatus and teres minor.
- To access the superomedial extent of the fracture line, elevate the origin of the infraspinatus to create a limited medial window as needed.
- If the fracture presents >2 weeks postinjury, a formal Judet approach, with reflection of the infraspinatus on its neurovascular pedicle, is usually necessary to clean and reduce the fracture.

Minimodified Judet

Peter A. Cole
Anthony J. Dugarte

Pathoanatomy

A transverse scapular body fracture, with exit sites at the scapular neck and vertebral border, is the most commonly encountered scapular fracture pattern. Fractures involving the scapular neck, which exit/enter through the scapular spine, are less common but allow for a significant reduction in the size of a Judet incision.

The classic extensile Judet approach uses an incision following the spine of the scapula from the acromion to the vertebral angle and caudal along the vertebral border. Elevation of the rotator cuff and deltoid in one muscular periosteocutaneous flap is then performed protecting its suprascapular neurovascular pedicle.

The modified Judet Approach is a variation, which uses the same skin incision, but raises a subcutaneous flap off the muscular fascia. Intermuscular intervals are then used to access the lateral border, as well as the spine and medial border for reduction and fixation.

Solution

A new variation of the classic posterior approach is the "minimodified Judet," which can reduce the incision size by as much as one-third, limit soft tissue trauma, and decrease the difficulty of the procedure. It can be used for specific fracture patterns, which do not exit medially, but remain lateral by extending from the lateral border proximally through the spine of the scapula.

Technique

Optimal Indications

- Extra-articular fractures
- Intra-articular fractures associated with the glenoid neck, in which fracture pattern extends through lateral border and proximally through the spine of the scapula, lateral to the superior angle/vertebral border (Figs. 4-11 and 4-12)

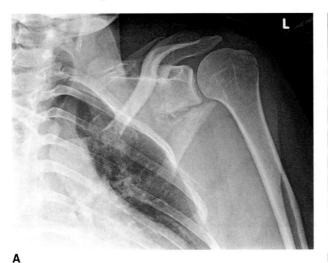
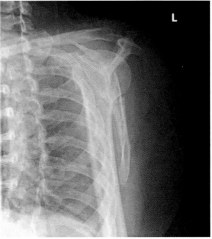

A   B

Figure 4-11 ▌ Anterior-posterior (AP) **(A)** and Scapula Y **(B)** X-ray views demonstrating a comminuted fracture of the scapula that extends through the base of the glenoid neck without articular extension. Additionally, there are multiple left-sided rib fractures.

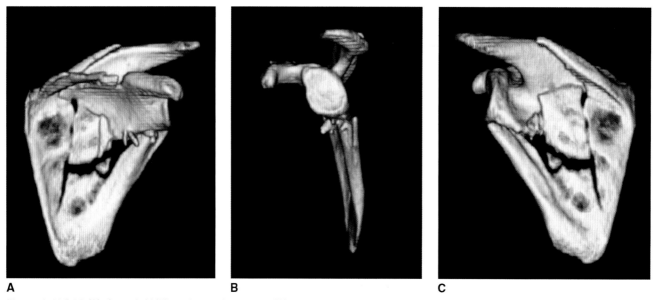

A   B   C

Figure 4-12 ❚ AP **(A)**, Scapula Y **(B)**, and posterior-anterior **(C)** three-dimensional computerized tomography scans of the injury shown in Figure 4-11.

Approach

- Similar to standard Judet approach, except it doesn't extend as far medially as the vertebral border.
- Standard "boomerang" incision (Fig. 4-13A) can be reduced by 1/2 or 1/3 (Fig. 4-13B) while still allowing appropriate exposure to the acromion, lateral portion of the scapula spine, scapula neck, and posterior glenoid as needed.

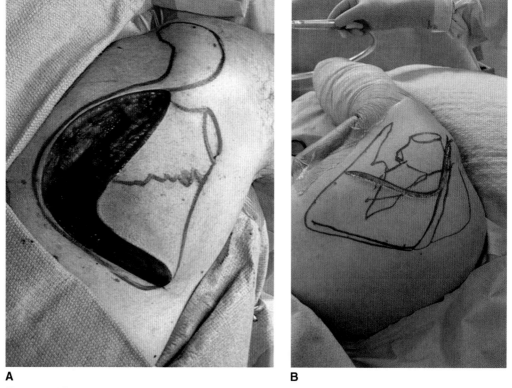

A   B

Figure 4-13 ❚ **A:** The classic Judet incision is a curved, "boomerang" incision that extends from the lateral lip of the acromion, continues along the spine, and finishes along the medial border. **B:** The minimodified Judet incision reduces the incision by nearly 50%. Note the classic Judet incision drawn along the medial border of the scapula.

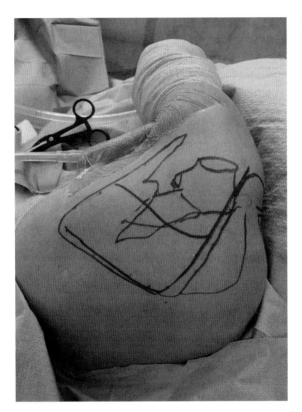

Figure 4-14 I Patient in left lateral decubitus position, with landmarks demarcated by the surgeon, highlighting the glenoid, acromion, spine, inferior and superior angles, as well as the medialized lateral border.

Patient Positioning
- Lateral decubitus position, "sloppy forward" (Fig. 4-14)
- Prep and drape the entire forequarter

Surgical Approach
- Establish landmarks (Fig. 4-14).
- Palpate acromion, from its most lateral border, and follow along the spine.
- Incision is then directed caudally, allowing for a subcutaneous flap that can be raised over the deltoid and rotator cuff musculature.
- Dissection taken through the subcutaneous tissue to fascia overlying deltoid (Fig. 4-15).

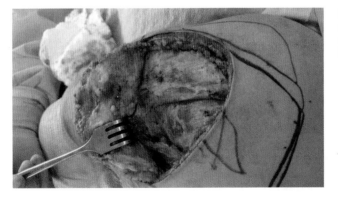

Figure 4-15 I Subcutaneous flap is elevated over the deltoid fascia and corresponding muscle, exposing the underlying fascia over the infraspinatus and teres minor muscles.

- The inferior posterior surface of deltoid is established. An incision is then made in this fascia allowing for superior or cephalad retraction of deltoid (Fig. 4-16).
  - Exposes underlying fascia over infraspinatus and teres minor muscles
- Fascia overlying the infraspinatus and teres minor is incised in line with the fibers of the musculature, and the interval between teres minor and infraspinatus is developed (Fig. 4-16).
  - This allows access to posterior glenoid and glenoid neck.
- This approach allows for fixation of the acromion, spine of scapula, scapula neck, and posterior glenoid.

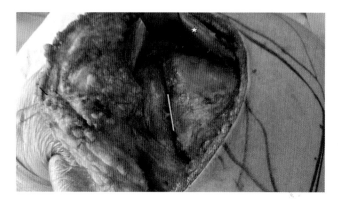

Figure 4-16 ▌ With deltoid (*white star*) retracted cephalad, the interval (*green line*) between infraspinatus and teres minor muscles is revealed.

Reduction
- Reduction of glenoid neck proceeds first to reestablish the lateral border.
- Reduction of scapular spine subsequently to reestablish curve of the spine.
- Reduction aids:
  - A shoulder hook can be used to manipulate lateral border of caudal segment.
  - A Schanz pin in glenoid neck can be used to manipulate cranial fragment, which is attached to and contains the glenoid.
  - A pointed bone reduction tenaculum can then be used on lateral border.

Implants (Fig. 4-17)
Typical implants include:
- 2.7-mm reconstruction and compression plates for the scapular spine and lateral border, respectively.
- Minifragment fixation with 2-mm screws may be useful for butterfly fragments or other comminution.
- A 3.5 lag screw from the lateral spine of the acromion (or base of the acromion spine) with a vector into the glenoid neck is powerful.

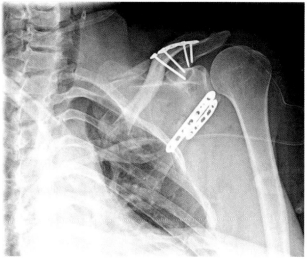
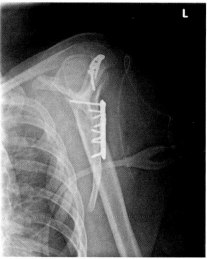

A   **B**

Figure 4-17 ▌ AP **(A)** and scapular Y **(B)** X-ray views demonstrating a 4-hole 2.7-mm dynamic compression, combination plate on the tension surface of the acromion, a 3.5-mm cortical lag screw with washer across the fracture site, a 7-hole, 2.7-mm dynamic compression plate, and a 5-hole 2.0-mm plate on the lateral border adjacent to the 2.7-mm combination plate.

Wound Closure
- Lateral border
  - The fascia is repaired with running 0 braided, absorbable suture.
- Acromion spinal border
  - Fascia repaired with 0 braided, absorbable suture.
- Subcutaneous tissue approximated with 2-0 absorbable suture.
- Skin closed with running 3-0 absorbable subcuticular stitch.

TIP

A Minimally Invasive Operative Approach for Scapula Body and Neck Fractures

Peter A. Cole
Anthony J. Dugarte

Pathoanatomy

The majority of scapular fractures warrant a posterior operative approach for fixation. Classically, Judet described a large, angled incision that parallels the scapular spine and vertebral border followed by elevation of a muscular flap off the infraspinatus fossa.

Solution

An enhanced understanding of scapula body and neck fracture patterns has allowed for variations to the classic approach that employ smaller incisions to accomplish reduction and fixation from posterior approaches.

Technique

Optimal conditions for this approach

- Simple fracture patterns with a single exit at both the lateral and vertebral borders (Ada and Miller IIC/ Revised AO/OTA Classification A3) (Fig. 4-18)
- Date of surgery <1 week from date of injury

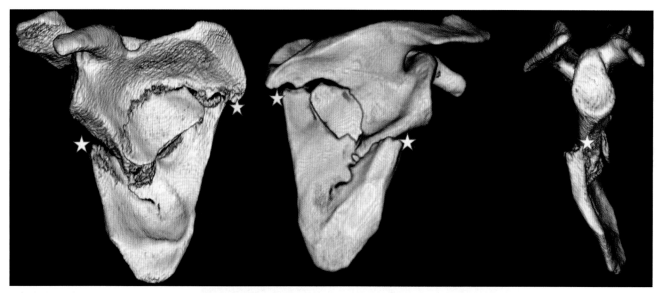

Figure 4-18 Three-dimensional computed tomography of a Revised AO/OTA Classification A3 right scapula fracture, with its medial border exit point (*yellow star*) and lateral border exit point (*white star*) demarcated.

Patient Positioning and Prep

- Lateral decubitus, with body leaning slightly anteriorly ("sloppy forward") (Fig. 4-19)
- Prep and drape the entire forequarter
  - Place at 90 degree over an upper extremity bolster

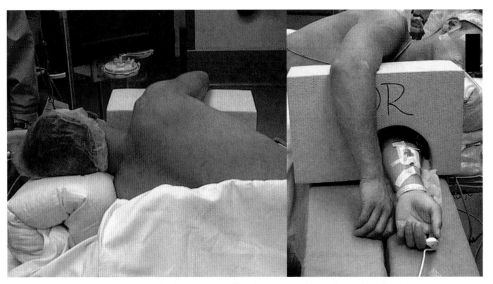

Figure 4-19 ▌ Patient is positioned "sloppy forward" to be prepped and draped for fixation.

Approach
- After careful study of 3D computerized tomography (CT) and palpation of bony landmarks, the incisions are marked.
- Two 6 cm straight incisions
  - First incision: at glenoid neck or lateral border:
    - Dissect down to deltoid fascia and divide fascia in line with muscle fibers on the inferior border of the posterior head of the deltoid.
    - Reveal fascia overlying infraspinatus and teres minor by retracting deltoid fibers superiorly.
    - Divide this fascia in line with its muscle fibers and bluntly dissect down to lateral scapula border between the infraspinatus and teres minor, which is often noted by a stripe of fat.
    - Use mindful retraction of infraspinatus to avoid injury to the suprascapular nerve, either from traction or from tip of retractor.
    - Cauterize circumflex scapular artery at the lateral scapular border as necessary.
  - Second incision: at vertebral border or spine:
    - At medial angle, take dissection down to the fascia and periosteum.
    - Elevate infraspinatus fascial origin from borders to visualize fracture.
- The lateral and medial windows provide visualization of both fracture exit sites and allow for reduction and fixation (Fig. 4-20).

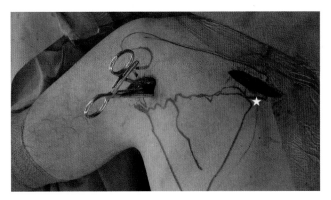

Figure 4-20 ▌ Intraoperative image demonstrating the surgeon's rendering of the Revised AO/OTA Classification A3 this patient sustained. Both the glenoid neck (*blue star*) and vertebral border (*yellow star*) incisions are seen. Each allowed for identification of muscle planes, and visualization, but two assistants are often needed for such exposures.

Reduction Tips
- A Schanz pin with T-handle chuck in the glenoid neck, along with a shoulder hook in a hole drilled at the lateral border of the caudad segment, can be used to achieve reduction.
  - Mobilize the cephalad fragment laterally and the caudad segment medially.
- Pointed bone reduction forceps can be used through pilot holes at the vertebral border, on either side of the fracture.

Implants

- Lateral border.
  - 2.7-mm dynamic compression plate
- Medial border.
  - 2.7-mm reconstruction plate
- Locking plate(s) recommended since small windows are used for fixation.
- Lateral border plate fixation is typically performed first since no contouring is necessary. Additional plates can be used to augment fixation (Fig. 4-21).

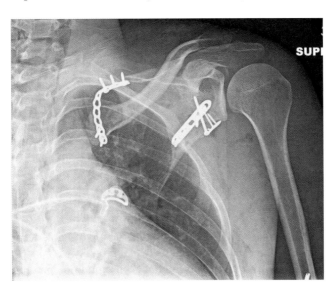

Figure 4-21 I Postoperative anterior-posterior (AP) X-ray image demonstrating a 3-hole, modified, 2-mm locking plate with locking screws for provisional reduction to allow clamp removal, a 2.7 locking dynamic compression plate along the lateral border with two locking screws on each side of the fracture, and an 8-hole, 2.7-mm recon plate, contoured to the vertebral border, and fixed using locking screws at the superior angle at the base of the scapular spine and vertebral border.

Wound Closure

- Lateral border.
  - Muscular fascia repaired with running 0 braided, absorbable suture
- Medial border.
  - Fascia repaired with #1 braided, absorbable suture
- Subcutaneous tissue approximated with 2-0 braided, absorbable suture.
- Skin closed with a running 3-0 absorbable subcuticular stitch (Fig. 4-22).
- Drains may not be necessary.

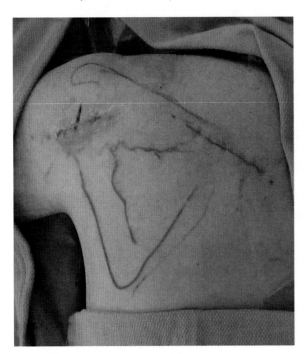

Figure 4-22 I Medial and lateral border wound closure upon completion of the case.

Fracture Assessment

- Most operative scapula fractures involve a transverse fracture line caudal to the scapular spine with the caudal segment displaced laterally (Fig. 4-23).

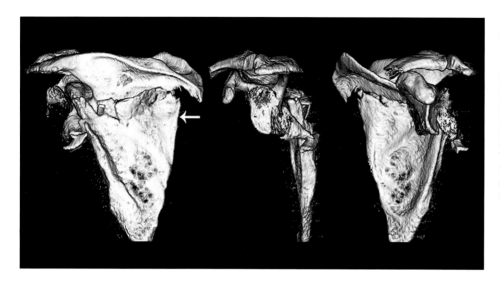

Figure 4-23 ▮ 3D CT reconstructions of a scapular body and neck fracture with a displaced glenoid component. Note that the caudal segment of the scapula is lateralized, owing to the pull of the infraspinatus, teres major and minor, and latissimus dorsi. In most cases, this displacement should be reduced initially to allow space for the articular reconstruction. The medial extent of the transverse fracture line at the medial scapular cortex often offers an excellent reduction assessment (*white arrow*).

- Frequently, the lateral scapular border must be reconstructed to enable accurate reduction of the glenoid neck component.
  - This region should be scrutinized for the amount of comminution present, which can range from none to severe (Fig. 4-24).

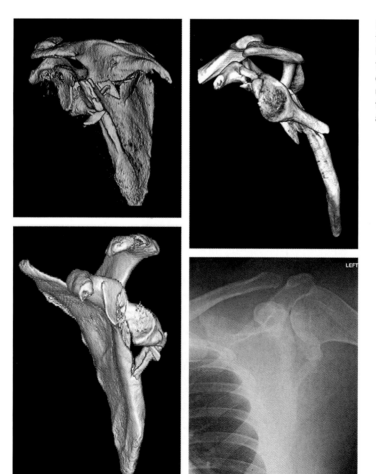

Figure 4-24 ▮ Comminution along the lateral margin of the scapula and inferior neck of the glenoid affects the ability to accurately reduce the extra-articular fracture lines and ultimately may determine the need for an arthrotomy to assess the articular reduction.

- Occasionally, the caudal scapular segment is divided into medial and lateral halves by a vertical fracture in the sagittal plane.
- These fractures will disrupt the relationship between the medial and lateral borders of the caudal scapular segment and should be recognized, since reduction of the medial scapular border alone will not affect an accurate reduction of the lateral margin of the caudal scapular segment.

Reduction and Fixation

- Clean the fracture of hematoma, granulation tissue, and infolded periosteum.
  - Because of its broad muscle origins and insertions, the scapula has a rich vascular supply.
  - Scapular fractures tend to heal quickly, and there can be considerable interfragmentary callus that will prevent reduction if left within or surrounding the fracture.
- Work from medial to lateral.
  - When a displaced transverse body component is present, accurate reduction of the vertebral border and scapular body component medially can improve the quality of reduction and restore the appropriate defect along the lateral border and at the glenoid neck for articular segment reductions (Fig. 4-25).

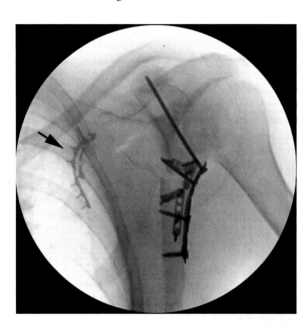

Figure 4-25 I The initial reduction and provisional plate fixation at the medial infraspinatus fossa (*arrow*) maintain the position of the caudal scapular body and allow the lateral margin and glenoid neck to be reconstructed accurately.

Scapular Fracture Reduction Strategies

Peter A. Cole
Anthony J. Dugarte

Pathoanatomy

Deforming forces on individual scapula fragments after fracture and the displacement of these fracture fragments often require technically demanding solutions to achieve fracture reduction.

Solution

Several tricks and aids have been developed, which simplify and facilitate scapular fracture reduction. Strategically located Schanz pins, shoulder hooks, lamina spreaders, or a minidistractor may be beneficial.

Techniques

- Deforming forces on the lateral border cause significant displacement; this is the largest challenge during reduction (Fig. 4-26).

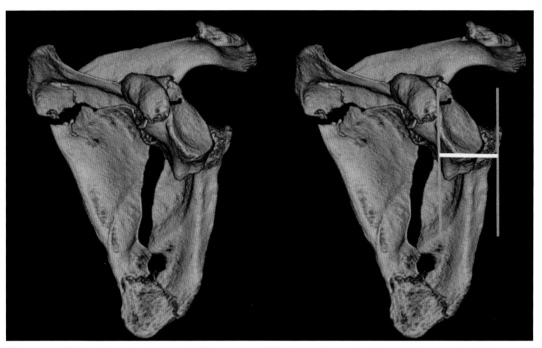

Figure 4-26 | Three-dimensional computed tomography (CT) of the left scapula demonstrating an extensively comminuted fracture, with fracture lines extending into the superior rim of the glenoid, base of the coracoid process, and medially across the body of the scapula. Note the lateral border offset (medialization, *yellow*).

- Achieving reduction may be further hindered by the need to work around muscular flaps.
- Prior to attempting fracture manipulation, ensure that adequate visualization is attained and soft tissue is removed from fracture edges to clearly delineate fracture lines (Fig. 4-27).

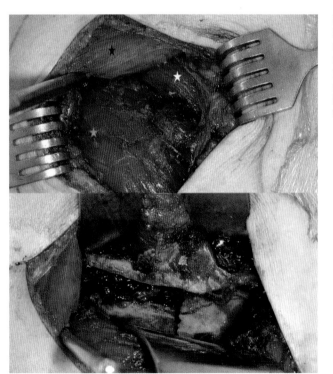

Figure 4-27 | **Above:** Intraoperative image demonstrating superior retraction of the deltoid (*black star*), to expose the intermuscular interval between the infraspinatus (*blue star*), and the teres minor (*yellow star*). **Below:** Development of the interval between the aforementioned rotator cuff musculature reveals the fracture lines.

- Soft tissue often includes callus, which forms rapidly in these fractures, as well as adhesions and periosteum.
  - Osteogenic proteins found in callus can be advantageous for fracture healing if saved and used for grafting.
- It is vital to understand the most common deformities before manipulating fracture fragments.
  - Typically, the proximal fragment is medialized and flexed relative to the body of the scapula.
  - Five techniques may be used separately, or in concert, to accomplish reduction at the lateral border, restore angulation, and normalize glenopolar angle.

1. **Schanz Pin**
   - Can be used in the glenoid neck to joystick proximal fragment.
     - Helps achieve alignment with the distal lateral border segment by allowing for derotation and translation at the neck
   - 4.0- or 5.0-mm Schanz pin with a T-handled chuck is helpful (Fig. 4-28).

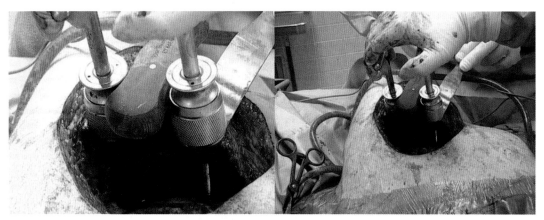

Figure 4-28 I Schanz pins with a T-handle chucks.

2. **Shoulder Hook**
   - To achieve alignment, drill a pilot hole in distal fragment at the lateral border and insert hook and joystick to proximal fragment (Fig. 4-29).

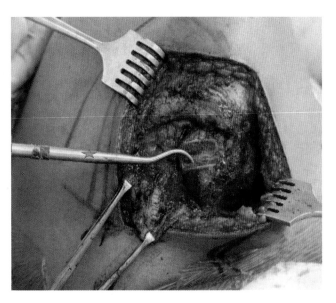

Figure 4-29 I Shoulder hook.

3. **Pointed Bone Tenaculum**
   - Anchor tines in drill holes placed across the primary fracture line, in a serial fashion, at lateral border (Fig. 4-30).

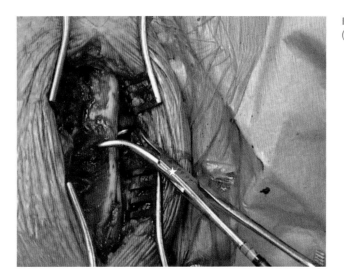

Figure 4-30 I Pointed bone tenaculum (*white star*).

4. **Lamina Spreader and pelvic reduction clamp**
   - Insert between proximal and distal fragments (Fig. 4-31).

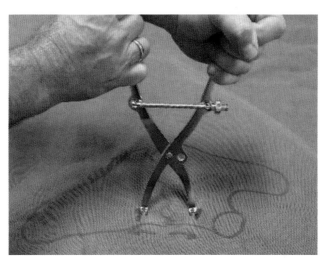

Figure 4-31 I Pelvic reduction clamp or lamina spreader.

   - Mobilize fragments to achieve reduction.
   - Soft tissue callus forms after a few days and progresses to harder, well-developed callus after 2 weeks.
     - In this case, callus must be overcome via mobilization with lamina spreader or mobilizing clamp.
     - A 3.5-mm cortical screw inserted in the glenoid is helpful to serve as a post to push against with lamina spreader.

5. **Small Ex-Fix and 4.0-mm Schanz Pins**
   - Helpful to maintain reduction and/or length when use of pointed bone tenaculum is not possible due to orientation of fracture line or extensive comminution (Fig. 4-32).
   - Can also be useful if acceptable reduction is not attained with previous four techniques.

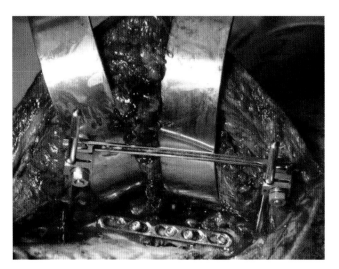

Figure 4-32 I Small Ex-Fix and 4.0 mm Schanz pins.

- If acceptable reduction is achieved, stabilization of the lateral border is obtained with a 4- or 5-hole 2.4-mm locking reconstruction plate.
   - Provisional fixation should be placed medial enough to allow for 2.7-mm compression plate to be definitively placed along lateral border.
- Medial border can be reduced in a similar manner.
   - A contoured 12-hole 2.4-mm locking reconstruction plate is clamped to the scapula with pediatric Kocher clamps for provisional and definitive stabilization.
      - Place one tine of clamp deep to scapula and the opposite tine to clamp the plate to the dorsal surface of the scapula.
      - Clamps are also used to contour the plate: the nose of each clamp is inserted into specific holes to achieve desired twist and bend to allow for fixation into scapular spine.
   - 8- to 10-mm screws placed along the medial border typically only provide unicortical feel during drilling so it is important to consider potential risk for iatrogenic injury at thoracic cavity.
- Less common variants can include a scapular inferior angle fracture.
   - Small fragment 3.5-mm locking T-plate can be used to maximize the number of screws in the distal fragment.

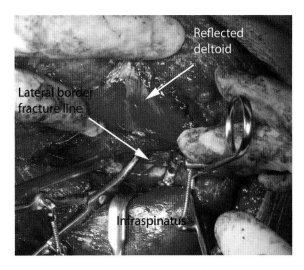

Figure 4-33 ‖ A typical clamp application is to place one tine on the lateral scapular border and the other clamp tine in a unicortical drill hole in the dorsal scapula. Minifragment plates provide adequate provisional stabilization and allow clamp removal.

- Use minifragment plates (e.g., 2.0 mm, 1/4 tubular) or small fragment (e.g., 1/3 tubular) to provide provisional fixation (see Figs. 4-25 and 4-33).
- While a 3.5- or 2.7-mm plate along the lateral border of the scapula provides the strength of the construct, reduction clamps frequently utilize this surface as well, becoming an obstruction to the correct positioning of this implant.
- A strategy to allow use of the lateral border for both clamp application and implant placement employs the use of minifragment (2.0-mm) plates.
  - The smaller plates typically provide sufficient fixation to allow removal of the reduction clamps, for subsequent placement of larger, 1/3 tubular or similar plates.
  - The smaller plates can be left in place to supplement the construct.
- Use the coracoid for docking longer implants to improve stability.
  - Use the scapular Y view to assist with placing the coracoid screw.
  - Palpation of the coracoid is useful to triangulate the appropriate screw trajectory (Fig. 4-34).

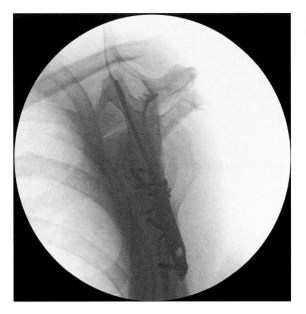

Figure 4-34 ‖ The scapular Y view is used to help direct the placement of the coracoid screw.

- A posterior sublabral glenohumeral arthrotomy can be used to visualize the articular reduction and ensure extra-articular position of implants.
- To enhance articular visualization in patterns with significant articular displacement or comminution, a distractor may be applied across the glenohumeral joint (Fig. 4-35).

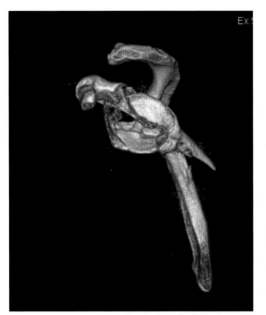
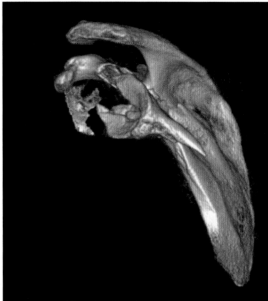

Figure 4-35 I 3D CT reconstructions demonstrating a glenoid fracture with intercalary articular comminution.

- Place a 4.0-mm Schanz into the base of the acromion process and a 5.0-mm Schanz pin into the proximal humerus percutaneously, confirming position under fluoroscopy (Fig. 4-36).

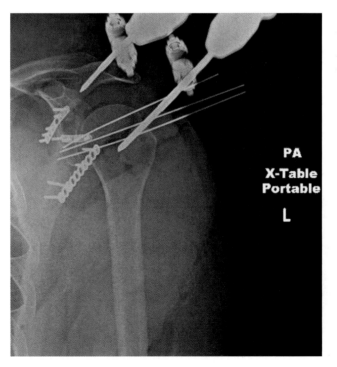

Figure 4-36 I Intraoperative radiograph demonstrating placement of the distractor pins. A 4.0-mm pin is placed in the base of the acromion and a 5.0-mm pin is placed in the proximal humerus.

- Use a single external fixator bar with the open compressor device or a small universal distractor to distract across the joint (Fig. 4-37).
  - The Grashey AP is also useful to confirm extra-articular screw location and articular reduction (Fig. 4-38).

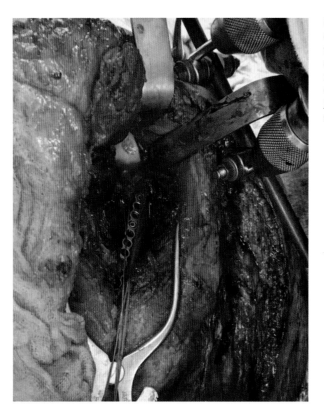

Figure 4-37 I An intraoperative photograph demonstrating the utility of distraction across the glenohumeral joint. A modified Judet approach with a posterior capsulotomy was used to expose the fractures. Application of controlled distraction across the glenohumeral joint allows enhanced visualization of the glenoid surface.

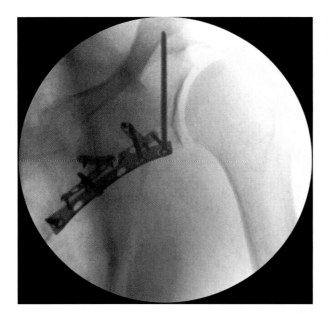

Figure 4-38 I The Grashey AP view confirms the extra-articular location of the coracoid screw.

Closure and Postoperative Management

- Anatomically repair the fascial deltoid origin to the scapula using drill holes in the scapular spine to prevent detachment.
- Use interrupted, nonabsorbable, or slowly resorbable sutures in the fascia.
- Close skin in layers over a closed suction drain.
- Rehabilitation should consist of Codman's exercises and passive range of motion only for 6 weeks to protect the deltoid repair.

Anterior Glenoid Fractures

- Typically occur during anterior glenohumeral joint dislocations and can be seen in isolation or concurrently with proximal humerus fractures (Fig. 4-39).
  - They may include the coracoid process.
- The fragment can be of variable size, and the most common indication for surgical fixation is instability of the glenohumeral joint.

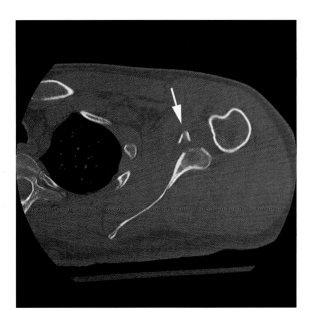

Figure 4-39 | Anterior glenoid fracture (*arrow*).

Position

- Supine or beach chair

Surgical Approach, Reduction, and Fixation

- Deltopectoral.
- Visualization usually requires that the subscapularis be tenotomized.
  - The location of the subscapularis tenotomy should be 1 cm from its insertion on the lesser tuberosity to facilitate repair.
  - Stay sutures are placed to prevent medial retraction and to assist with retraction and reattachment.
- The glenohumeral capsule may be intact anteriorly or may be avulsed from either the humerus or the glenoid labrum.
- If intact, an arthrotomy will be required to visualize the articular surface and should be performed laterally to avoid damage to the labrum.

- Occasionally, the fragment will be of sufficient size so that a reduction can be obtained from cortical interdigitation at the anterior glenoid neck.
  - Fluoroscopic reduction assessment is usually difficult because of the relatively small size of the anterior inferior fragment, and if articular impaction is present, it may go unrecognized if an arthrotomy is not performed.
- Fixation can often be accomplished using 2.7-, 2.4-, or 2.0-mm cortical lag screws, with or without buttress plates, depending on the fragment's size (Fig. 4-40).

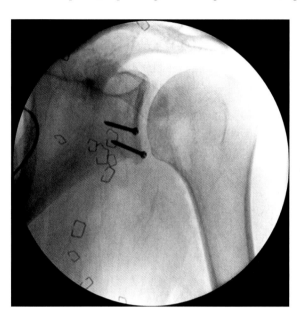

Figure 4-40 I Fixation accomplished using 2.4-mm cortical lag screws.

- Anterior glenoid fracture pathology cannot be addressed through a deltoid-splitting approach. Thus, combined injuries to the proximal humerus and anterior glenoid should both be repaired using a deltopectoral approach.

Reference

1. Nork SE, Barei DP, Gardner MJ, et al. Surgical exposure and fixation of displaced type IV, V, and VI glenoid fractures. *J Orthop Trauma.* 2008;22(7):487–493.

Chapter 5
Clavicle Fractures

JULIUS BISHOP
MICHAEL L. BRENNAN
MICHAEL F. GITHENS
ERIC G. PUTTLER

Sterile Instruments/Equipment

- Draping to include impervious stockinette and 4-inch elastic bandage wrap for the forearm and hand
- Selection of bone clamps for reduction:
  - Large and small pointed bone reduction clamps ("Weber clamps")
  - Plate-holding clamp (Verbrugge, self-centered)
  - Small serrated bone-holding clamp (small "lobster claw")
- Threaded K-wires or 2.5-mm Schanz pins (e.g., from small external fixator) for manipulation and intramedullary fixation
- Small distractor (especially for delayed treatment, nonunions or malunions)
- Implants
  - Open reduction and internal fixation:
    - Anatomically contoured plates
    - 3.5-mm compression or reconstruction plates
    - 2.7-mm compression or reconstruction (nonheat annealed)
    - 2.0-mm and 2.4-mm straight plates for provisional fixation
    - 2.0-mm and 2.4-mm screws for independent lag screw fixation
  - Intramedullary fixation:
    - Stainless steel or titanium small diameter flexible intramedullary nails typically 2.5 to 3.5 mm.
    - Intramedullary screw fixation: long 4.5-, 5.0-, 5.5-, or 6.5-mm cannulated screws (use largest size possible to gain endosteal purchase).
  - Consider partially threaded screws for compression or using cortical screws placed using a lag screw technique.
- K-wires and wire driver/drill.

Positioning

- Captain's chair (beach chair position) or supine, with patient on radiolucent table (e.g., a reversed position on radiolucent cantilever table).
  - A reversed cantilever table is used for clavicle fractures amenable to nail fixation.
  - A beach chair or reversed cantilever table is used for clavicle fractures amenable to either plating or intramedullary screw fixation.
    - A flat radiolucent table, typically supported at the head and foot, is not used for clavicle fractures due to difficulties obtaining "inlet" and "outlet" radiographs of the clavicle because of the table's end-based support structure.
- Entire ipsilateral extremity prepped and draped circumferentially to allow freedom of movement and facilitate reduction.

Surgical Approaches

Anteroinferior approach

- The incision is centered over the fracture site and extended in line with the inferior border of the clavicle.
- Care is taken to preserve the three to five branches of the supraclavicular nerve that run obliquely or perpendicular to the clavicle.[1]
- Laterally, the deltoid origin is taken sharply off the anterior border of the clavicle.
  - It should be repaired at closure.

Anterosuperior approach

- Skin incision similar to anteroinferior.
- Deep dissection elevates platysma from clavicle.

Intramedullary fixation approach

- Small incision 1.5 cm distal to ipsilateral sternoclavicular joint for medial to lateral flexible nail stabilization
- Small incision posterior to the acromion, collinear with the lateral clavicular shaft, for lateral to medial intramedullary screw placement

Reduction and Implant Techniques

- The reduction strategy depends on the fracture location and pattern.
- For simple patterns (long oblique or simple butterfly), obtain an anatomic reduction and interfragmentary compression with small Weber clamps and independent 2.0- or 2.4-mm lag screws. A 3.5-mm neutralization plate is then applied in either the superior or anterior inferior position.
- For comminuted fractures, restore length and alignment of the clavicle while planning for a bridging construct (Fig. 5-1).

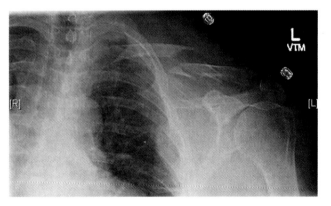

Figure 5-1 I AP radiograph demonstrating a comminuted clavicle fracture.

- This can be achieved by manipulating the proximal and distal segments with serrated clamps and provisionally stabilizing with a long 2.0- or 2.4-mm plate on the osseous surface that is not planned for the definitive implant.

- The clamps can then be removed, and bridge plate of choice is applied to the free surface (Fig. 5-2).

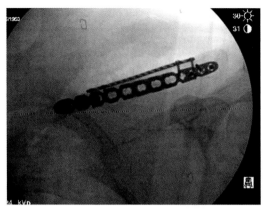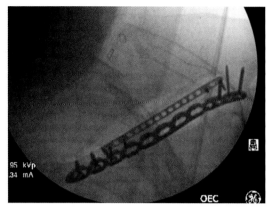

Figure 5-2 ▌ Intraoperative fluoroscopic images demonstrate bridge plating of a comminuted clavicle fracture. Length, alignment and rotation are reestablished and then provisionally held with a long 2.0-mm plate followed by summative fixation with a 3.5-mm anatomically contoured plate applied to the anterior clavicle.

- The provisional plate can be left in for additional stability or removed, again depending on fracture pattern (Fig. 5-3).
  - When deploying dual plating for comminuted or segmental patterns, one of the plates should be a 3.5-mm plate for sufficient construct strength.

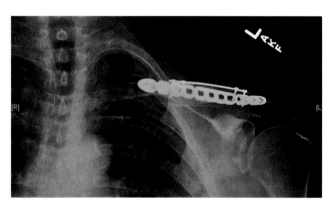

Figure 5-3 ▌ The provisional plate used for intraoperative reduction aid was left in place to augment fixation for this clavicle with a long segment of comminution.

- Use an anatomically contoured plate or contour a 2.7- or 3.5-mm compression plate or a non–heat annealed (i.e., stiff) 2.7- or 3.5-mm reconstruction plate so that it lies on the superolateral or anteroinferior surface.
  - Plate selection depends on the patient size, anticipated patient compliance, fracture morphology, and acuity.
    - Avoid smaller (2.7-mm) or flexible (reconstruction) plates for larger patients and for delayed fracture treatments.
    - Combined 90-90 plating with a 2.7- and 2.4-mm plate can be employed for a sufficiently strong construct in simple patterns and perhaps decrease the risk of implant related symptoms (Fig. 5-4).
    - This strategy should not be used in comminuted patterns or in large patients.

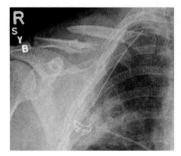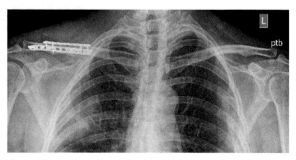

Figure 5-4 ▌ Injury and postoperative radiographs demonstrate a simple clavicle fracture treated with 90-90 plating with a superior 2.4-mm plate and an anterior inferior 2.7-mm plate.

- In general, anteroinferior plates are less prominent and may be better tolerated by patients (Fig. 5-5), especially those who carry loads on their shoulder and those wearing backpacks.

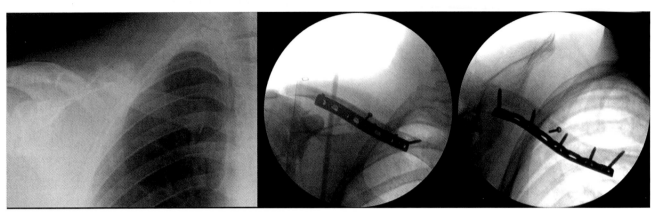

Figure 5-5 ‖ Use of a 3.5-mm compression plate for anteroinferior clavicle plating.

- They have the added advantage of much longer screws in the distal segment where fixation is often most tenuous, by virtue of the cross-sectional osteology.
- Distal screws in the AP direction are typically 22 to 28 mm long as compared to 10 to 14 mm long when superior plating is performed (Fig. 5-6).

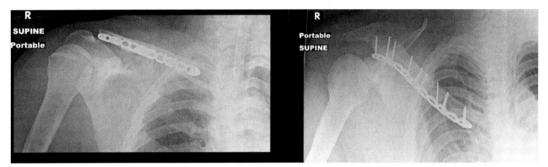

Figure 5-6 ‖ Postoperative radiographs demonstrate screw trajectory for an anterior inferior plate. The osteology of the distal clavicle allows significantly longer screws in the distal segment as compared to superior plating.

- Superior plate placement may provide some mechanical advantage, being on the tension surface, especially for some nonunions, and precludes the need to take down the deltoid laterally (Fig. 5-7).

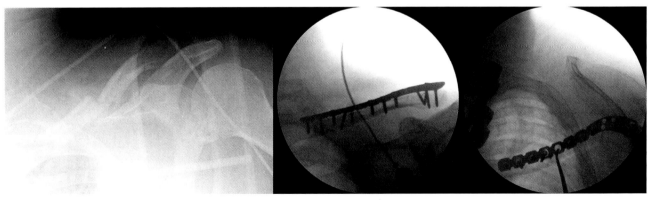

Figure 5-7 ‖ Segmental clavicle fracture treated with an anatomically contoured superior plate.

- Tips
  - Avoid annealed reconstruction plates that are flexible and deform easily.
  - If using a reconstruction plate, be aware that these plates are designed to be less stiff than their paired compression plates.
  - They are also weaker and may deform or break, especially in segmentally comminuted fractures, if several holes are left empty when used in a bridging application.
  - When using a 2.7- or 3.5-mm plate to bridge the comminution, it is best to choose a stiff plate, either compressed or anatomically contoured.
  - Consider contouring the plate to fit a skeletal model's clavicle before the procedure to save intraoperative time.
- On occasion, a plate can be torsionally contoured for placement on the superior surface laterally and the anteroinferior surface medially.
  - This allows safe bicortical screws medially and minimizes the deltoid reflection laterally (Fig. 5-8).

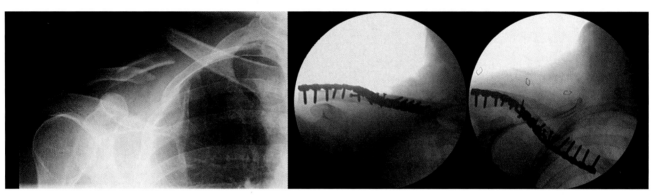

Figure 5-8 ▎ One clavicle plating option involves multiplanar contouring to allow the medial plate to sit anteroinferiorly and the lateral plate superiorly, avoiding interference with the anterior deltoid origin.

- For lateral clavicle fractures with poor bone quality or difficult fixation due to peripheral comminution, consider several options.
  - Anatomically contoured distal clavicle plates with a cluster of screws distally (locking screws may be beneficial in osteoporosis).
  - Intramedullary screws or several threaded Steinmann pins to partially fill the canal.
    - The intramedullary device(s) can be inserted lateral to medial prior to reduction and plate fixation.
    - The screw or pins act as a stable post, such that the plate screws interdigitate with the IM wires, as well as the cortex to gain improved fixation (Fig. 5-9).

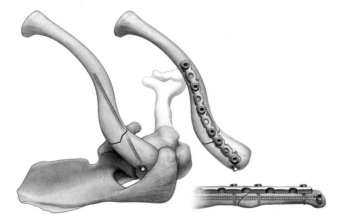

Figure 5-9 ▎ To augment fixation of lateral clavicle fractures, an intramedullary screw can be placed for interdigitation of subsequent plate screws.

- Extend the fixation (plate or IM screw) across the AC joint and include the acromion.
  - In general, hardware that spans the AC joint will need to be removed after healing.
- A hook-type plate may be positioned under the acromion (Fig. 5-10).

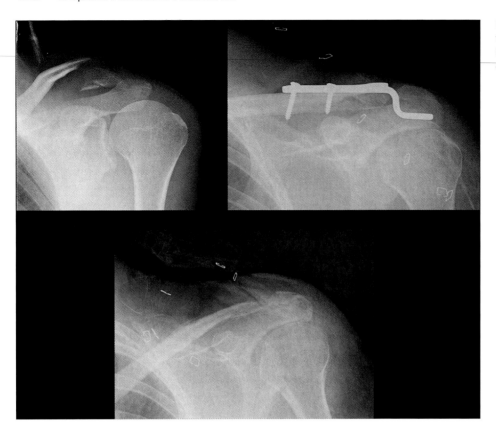

Figure 5-10 I Hook plate used for distal clavicle fracture. After healing and plate removal, anatomic alignment is maintained.

TIP

Temporary Coracoclavicular Suture/Cable Fixation in the Management of Unstable Lateral Clavicle Fractures

Eric Puttler

Pathoanatomy

Displaced lateral clavicle fractures with disruption of the coracoclavicular ligaments (AO/OTA Type 15.3C1 and 15.3C2) can be unstable injuries with little bone available laterally for fixation. Previous solutions employing fixation to the acromion (e.g., the hook plate, pinning or plating across the acromioclavicular joint) introduce the opportunity for potential complications due to implant migration, loss of fixation, or erosion of the acromion due to motion at the acromioclavicular joint. These complications can be minimized through early removal of implants but at the risk of loss of reduction.

Solution

Repair the fracture with a precontoured superiorly placed locking implant, and engage the scapula for fixation via the coracoid process instead of the acromion by using an orthopedic cable (or large nonabsorbable suture) as temporary coracoclavicular fixation. Circumferential placement of the cable, as opposed to a suture button construct through the coracoid, minimizes the risk of coracoid fracture and allows for plate placement optimized for fracture fixation as opposed to accessing to the base of the coracoid through the plate. The cable/suture is removed 8 to 12 weeks postoperatively to minimize the risk of implant complications due to motion between the clavicle and scapula, while the plate remains in place (augmented by early fracture consolidation) to maintain control of the fracture until solid union.

Technique

- Position the patient supine on a radiolucent operating room table. The arms may be tucked at the patient's side or alternatively the ipsilateral arm may be prepped and draped into the surgical field "free."

- A reversed cantilever table is ideal, but a radiolucent table supported at the head and foot can be used. When using the latter, position the patient as far down (caudad) on the table as possible to allow for adequate imaging.
- The C-arm is positioned orthogonally on the opposite side of the table to obtain an AP and at least 30-degree cephalad and caudal tilt views ("inlet" and "outlet" views).
  - Alternatively, the C-arm may be positioned ipsilateral to the surgical field.
- The patient is draped using a pediatric laparotomy sheet centered over the fracture, with the fenestration expanded as needed and secured with an impervious adhesive drape.
- The fracture is exposed via an anterosuperior approach while protecting the supraclavicular nerves. The exposure is extended as far medially as required based on the fracture pattern and laterally to the acromioclavicular joint to allow for complete access to the lateral segment. The acromioclavicular joint is left intact.
- Prior to reducing the fracture, a cable/suture is passed under the coracoid anterior to the clavicle.
  - The cable/suture passer is passed from medial to lateral to avoid injury to the nerves of the brachial plexus.
    - The cable/suture passer is applied directly to the medial aspect of the coracoid under direct visualization and then passed immediately adjacent to the undersurface of the coracoid using palpation and C-arm control.
    - An appropriately sized cable passer minimizes the amount of soft tissue capture lateral to the coracoid.
  - The cable is then passed from end hole in the passer laterally and retrieved from the shaft hole medially through the passing device, which is then removed.
- The posteromedial end of the cable is then shuttled under and posterior to the medial segment using careful blunt dissection.
  - The cable passes anterior and superior to the rotator cuff.
- Fracture reduction and fixation is then performed as dictated by the fracture pattern using a superior clavicular plate and standard AO/ASIF techniques (Fig. 5-11).

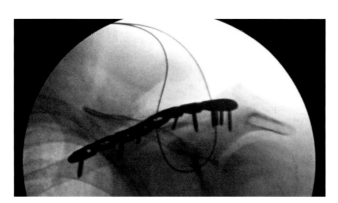

Figure 5-11 | The cable is passed initially, and then open reduction and internal fixation proceeds as indicated based on the fracture pattern. After the fracture is reduced access to the base of the coracoid is restricted.

- For markedly unstable fractures, the plate can be carefully applied to the medial segment, and the cable provisionally tensioned to assist in maintaining the reduction, while lateral fixation is performed.
  - Soft tissue attachments and blood supply to comminuted lateral fracture fragments are carefully preserved to facilitate early fracture healing.
- After the plate and screw fixation is complete, the cable is adjusted to position the cable crimp anterosuperiorly to facilitate later removal with minimal dissection.
- The cable is then tensioned using anatomic and radiographic landmarks as opposed to a desired cable tension.
  - The coracoclavicular interval should be approximately 11 to 13 mm or similar to the uninjured contralateral side.
  - The acromioclavicular joint should appear reduced, and not over reduced.
    - Supine positioning facilitates imaging of the contralateral side for comparison.
  - The cable should appear tensioned as opposed to slack on image intensification.
  - The cable should feel tensioned when manipulated adjacent to the clavicle.

- The cable is secured with the crimper and cut.
- Routine closure is performed.
- Postoperative protocol.
  - The patient is discharged on the day of surgery, unless precluded by concomitant injuries or medical condition.
  - A sling is worn for 4 weeks and is removed only to perform daily elbow, forearm, wrist, and finger range of motion exercises.
    - Gentle Codman's exercises may be performed if isolated to the glenohumeral articulation.
    - Aggressive pendulum exercises should be avoided so as to minimize shearing friction between the cable and coracoid.
  - Radiographs are taken at the first postoperative visit 7 to 14 days after surgery to evaluate the reduction of the fracture and acromioclavicular joint, as well as cable tension and its relationship to the base of the coracoid (Figs. 5-12 and 5-13).

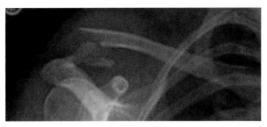 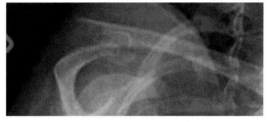

Figure 5-12 ▮ Displaced lateral clavicle fracture with diminutive, comminuted, lateral segment.

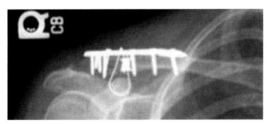 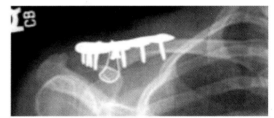

Figure 5-13 ▮ One week postop.

- The sling is discontinued at 4 weeks postop, and light waist level activities of daily living are allowed.
- Repeat radiographs are obtained 6 weeks postoperatively, and if the fracture is provisionally united both radiographically and clinically, cable removal is scheduled on an outpatient basis for 8 to 12 weeks after the index procedure (Fig. 5-14).
  - Cables can be left in for longer; however, patient compliance is needed to minimize the risk of coracoid fracture

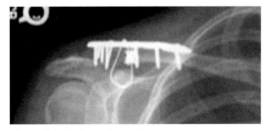 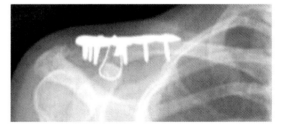

Figure 5-14 ▮ Six weeks postop.

- At the time of cable removal, the previous incision is reopened and the cable crimp is exposed with a limited exposure. The cable is cut and removed
  - Image intensification is use to confirm no immediate loss of reduction.
  - Sutures are removed at 10 to 14 days postop and repeat radiographs are taken to confirm no loss of reduction (Fig. 5-15).
- After the cable is removed, motion is progressed to full, with progressive activities based on continued clinical and radiographic union. Physical therapy is typically not required (Fig. 5-16).

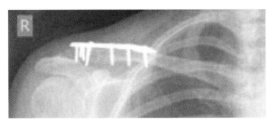
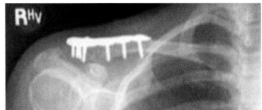

Figure 5-15 ▌ Eight weeks postop.

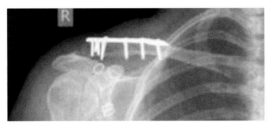
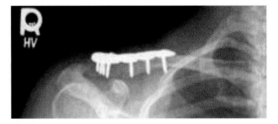

Figure 5-16 ▌ One year postop.

- Lateral to medial intramedullary screw (Fig. 5-17).
  - A small incision with clamp reduction may be necessary if unable to be reduced closed.
  - 4.5, 5.0, 5.5 to 6.5-mm cannulated screws.
    - Use larger diameter screws for patients with larger IM canals and osteoporosis.
    - In young patients with narrow IM canals, consider a 4.5- or 5.0-mm cortical screw placed using lag technique for fracture compression.

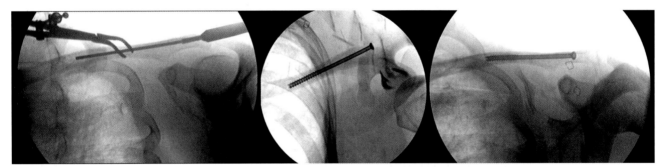

Figure 5-17 ▌ Example of a medullary screw for internal fixation of a clavicular fracture.

- If an open reduction is performed, consider using an "inside-out" (retrograde) technique by inserting the guide pin via the fracture into the medullary canal of the lateral fracture and out of the posterolateral cortex until soft tissues are tented.
- Fracture is then reduced and the guide pin is advanced across the fracture "antegrade" into the medial fragment.
- Cannulated drill bit and screws are inserted over the guide pin from lateral to medial while maintaining the fracture reduction and compression (Fig. 5-18).

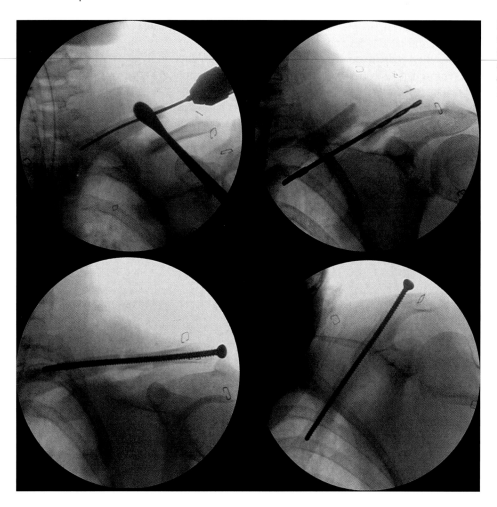

Figure 5-18 ∥ The medullary canal of the medial fragment is first cannulated through a small incision at the fracture site. Antegrade drilling of distal segment then helps localize lateral entry point.

- ▪ A modified point-to-point Weber clamp inserted via unicortical drill holes is helpful to maintain fracture reduction and compression during intramedullary screw fixation.
- Flexible titanium nails (Fig. 5-19)
  - For nail insertion, the surgeon stands on the contralateral side and the assistant is ipsilateral to the fractured clavicle.
    - ▪ These roles may be alternated during different phases of the procedure.
  - Typically, a 2.5-, 3.0-, or 3.5-mm diameter flexible nail may be used.
  - Select the largest titanium nail accepted by the medullary canal, or stack several smaller flexible nails to fill the intramedullary canal for rotational and bending stability.
  - Drill the anteroinferior medial cortex obliquely with a 2.5-, 2.8-, 3.2-, or 3.5-mm bit, depending on the diameter of the nail selected (Fig. 5-19, top left image).
  - Use of a cannulated drill bit may be helpful in confirming the K-wire's position prior to creation of the entry site with the cannulated drill bit
  - If necessary, contour the nail prior to insertion then advance to the fracture.
  - Reduce the fracture by manipulating the arm and confirming reduction on fluoroscopy with "inlet" and "outlet" views.
    - ▪ If reduction is difficult to obtain using a closed technique, consider placing threaded K-wires or small Steinmann pins (2.5 to 4.0 mm) into the distal and proximal segments as joysticks for manipulation of one or both fragments.
  - If unable to obtain closed reduction, then proceed to an open reduction.
  - Impact nail into distal segment near acromion.
    - ▪ Take care not to penetrate the lateral cortex.
  - Confirm the position of the nail on orthogonal views.

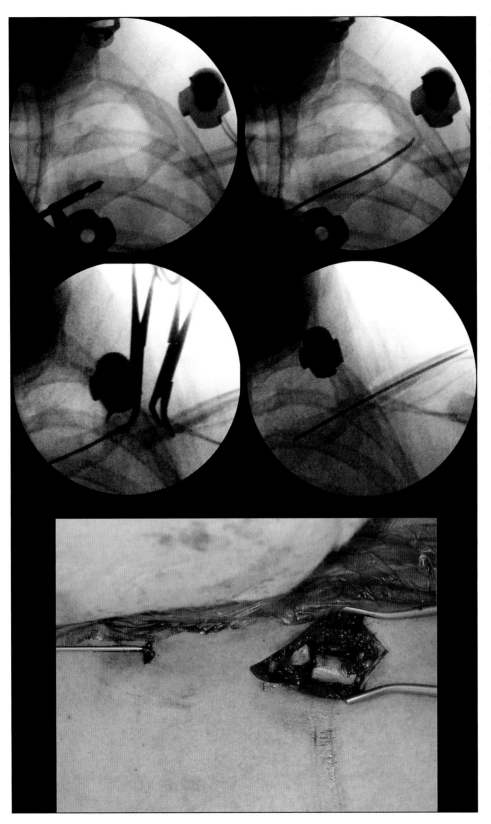

Figure 5-19 ∎ Medullary nailing of a left midshaft clavicle fracture. Through a small medial incision, the medial cortex is drilled and the nail is inserted to the fracture site. If closed or percutaneous reductions are unsuccessful, a miniopen approach is made for clamp placement and medullary canal realignment, followed by nail passage. The nail is cut short medially.

Reference

1. Collinge C, Devinney S, Herscovici D, et al. Anterior-inferior plating of middle-third fractures and nonunions of the clavicle. *J Orthop Trauma*. 2006;20:680–686.

Chapter 6
Proximal Humerus Fractures

MICHAEL J. GARDNER
JONAH HÉBERT-DAVIES
M. BRADFORD HENLEY
ANNA N. MILLER

Sterile Instruments/Equipment

- Impervious stockinette and 4-inch elastic bandage wrap for arm, forearm, and hand
- Large and small pointed bone reduction clamps ("Weber clamps")
- Threaded K-wires, and 2.5/4.0-mm Schanz pins for fragment manipulation
- Implants
  - Anatomically contoured periarticular plates, consider locking plates for osteoporotic fractures
  - Minifragment screws and plates for provisional/definitive fixation of metaphyseal cortical or tuberosity fragments
  - Number 2 or number 5 nonabsorbable suture for rotator cuff/tuberosity fixation augmentation, generally required
  - Fibular strut allograft (fresh frozen) for deficient medial column, if required
  - Morcellized cancellous allograft bone, autograft, or osteobiologic substitute for metaphyseal bone defects (e.g., valgus impacted four-part fractures)
- K-wires and wire driver/drill

Surgical Approaches and Positioning

- Positioning for percutaneous pinning/plating or for ORIF using deltopectoral or deltoid-splitting approach.
  - Supine with the patient reversed on cantilever radiolucent table (i.e., head and upper extremities at the cantilevered end of table).
  - Consider small bump under the ipsilateral shoulder.
  - Move the patient so that the head is at the proximal and lateral corner of the table, ipsilateral to operated extremity.
  - Place the arm on radiolucent Plexiglas sheet (70 cm × 40 cm × 1 cm).
    - Plexiglas is placed on the table and under the table pad and is supported by the patient's torso.
    - Approximately 1 ft of Plexiglas, protrudes beyond the table's edge.
    - Blankets or foam padding are taped to Plexiglas to match its height to that of the table's padding.
  - Rotate table 90 degrees so that the operative arm faces the main operating space.
  - C-arm should be placed at the head of the OR table to allow for axillary view with arm abducted 70 to 90 degrees (assess sagittal plane fracture alignment and plate position on humeral head and shaft) (Fig. 6-1).

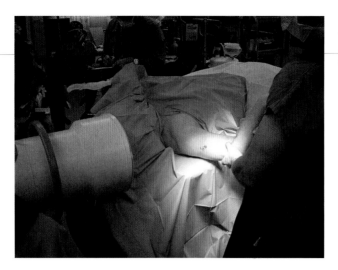

Figure 6-1 I With the patient moved to the edge of the table and the arm on a radiolucent extension, a reliable axillary view can be obtained intraoperatively.

- Positioning for intramedullary nailing of proximal fractures and for repair/ORIF of greater tuberosity fractures.
  - Positioning for nailing
    - Use Jackson table, which is narrow in width and allows C-arm to come in from the opposite side.
    - Scapular Y lateral view of proximal humerus is used instead of axillary lateral view, since arm cannot be abducted as implants (guide wire(s)/nail/targeting jig) interfere with acromion.
    - Patient is positioned in center of the OR table or slightly to the side of the injured extremity so that contralateral arm can be adducted to the patient's side and rests on table top.
    - No arm board is attached to the side of the table for uninjured upper extremity.
      - This affords maximal C-arm excursion across OR table for AP/Grashey imaging views.
    - Patient is supine with bump under the ipsilateral scapula.
      - Either a foam wedge or folded blankets placed under both the shoulder and the hip can be used.
      - Alternatively, place the rolls/wedge under the contralateral side.
        - This rolls the patient's body toward the side of injury allowing an AP C-arm image without the same degree of "roll back."
        - This accommodates the normal retroversion of the humeral head and anteversion of glenoid, thereby obviating external rotation of the arm for an orthogonal view of proximal humerus and glenoid.
        - The scapular Y view is also improved in this position as long as the C-arm can roll forward, over-the-top far enough.
    - Place the radiolucent Plexiglas sheet between the table and the cushion, under the patient's torso and ipsilateral arm, protruding in long dimension approximately 4 to 6 inch to support arm in adduction if the patient is large or obese.
      - This may not always be necessary in thin patients, as both upper extremities can be placed on the table adducted, next to the patient's torso.
    - C-arm rotates between 45 degrees roll back and 45 degrees roll over views to obtain orthogonal AP and scapular Y views, respectively.
    - These views are important in confirming that the entry portal is collinear with intramedullary canal.

- If needed, a modified axillary view can be obtained by tilting the C-arm maximally such that the cathode (receiver end) of the image intensifier is near the patient's head.
  - This position looks like the C-arm position for a pelvic inlet view.
  - The arm can be extended at the shoulder to facilitate an axillary lateral of the proximal humerus.
  - Use C-arm to guide the location of skin incision in anterior-posterior and medial-lateral planes relative to ideal entry portal in proximal humerus.

Reduction and Implant Techniques

- For proximal humeral fracture dislocations, reduction of the humeral head fragment is facilitated by manual manipulation, multiple K-wire joysticks, or one or more 2.5-mm terminally threaded Schanz pins (Fig. 6-2).

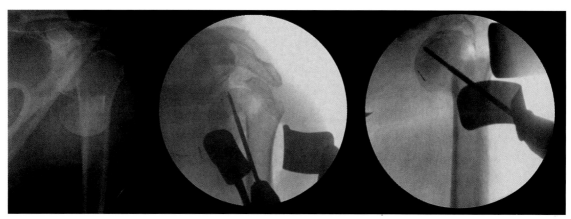

Figure 6-2 | For proximal humeral fracture dislocations, the humeral head fragment can be manipulated using a small threaded Schanz pin.

- This is best accomplished by placing a Schanz pin through the fracture into the head fragment and using this to manipulate the fragment directly while simultaneously facilitating a reduction with manually applied external pressure.
- Once the head fragment is reduced in the glenoid, reduction of the metaphysis to the head can proceed.
  - The metaphyseal fracture deformity is most often apex anterior at the surgical neck and in varus angulation (except in three- and four-part valgus impacted patterns).
  - The shaft is commonly adducted and shortened.
    - Fracture reduction is achieved by traction and forward flexion (elevating the arm) while simultaneously applying posterior and lateral pressure to the proximal end of the humeral shaft.
    - The laterally directed force vector applied to the proximal shaft will neutralize the deforming adducting force of the pectoralis major (Fig. 6-3).

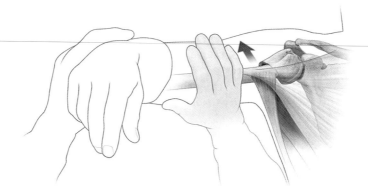

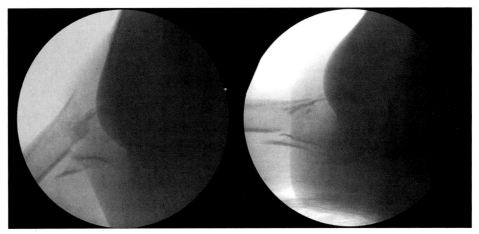

Figure 6-3 ‖ A common sagittal plane deformity includes apex anterior displacement. Thus, typical reduction maneuvers involve a laterally and posteriorly directed force on the proximal portion of the humeral shaft fragment to overcome muscle displacements **(top)**. This reduction is visualized on the axillary fluoroscopic view **(bottom row)**.

- Place several nonabsorbable sutures through the enthesis of the supraspinatus, infraspinatus, and teres minor tendons to mobilize and stabilize greater tuberosity or its composite fracture fragments.
  - Mobilize the greater tuberosity and provisionally reduce the tuberosity using the sutures for traction (Fig. 6-4).

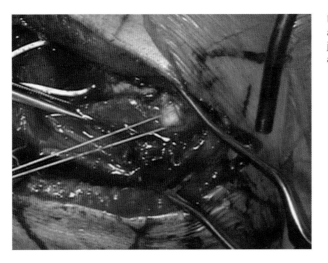

Figure 6-4 ‖ Several locking sutures are placed through the bone-tendon junction of the rotator cuff to mobilize and control the greater tuberosity.

- Place K-wires from the anterior humeral shaft, posteriorly into the humeral head fragment to provisionally stabilize the fracture, followed by a plate and screws (Fig. 6-5).

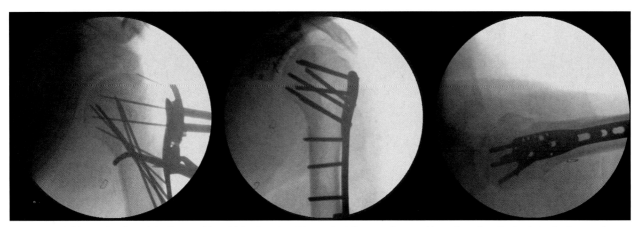

Figure 6-5 After reduction of the humeral head into the glenoid, manipulation can be used to reduce the diaphysis to the humeral head.

- For nondislocations, use K-wires to manipulate and reduce the humeral head fragment laterally and in valgus.
- Use a nonlocking screw to draw the humeral shaft to the plate if required to indirectly reduce the greater tuberosity and humeral head (Fig. 6-6).

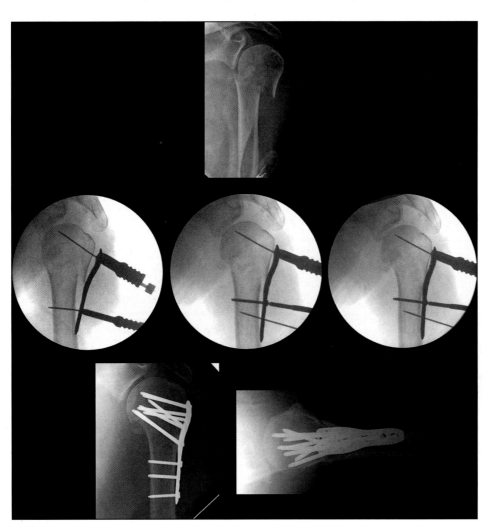

Figure 6-6 One strategy is to overreduce the proximal fragment in valgus, with direct manipulation of the greater tuberosity using rotator cuff traction sutures. With the plate provisionally applied in the appropriate position, a nonlocking screw is then inserted into the proximal shaft to complete the reduction while elevating the head fragment. Fixation is concentrated in the inferomedial humeral head region.

● Provisional K-wires should be placed anteriorly to avoid conflict with subsequent lateral plate placement (Fig. 6-7).

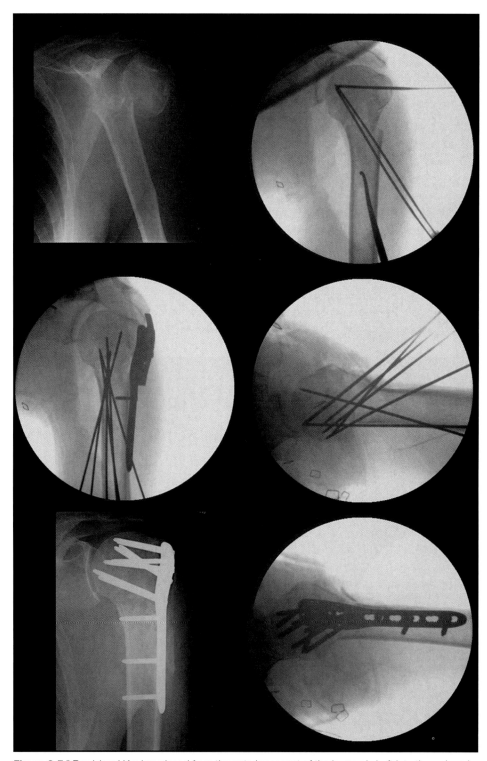

Figure 6-7 | Provisional K-wires placed from the anterior aspect of the humeral shaft into the reduced humeral head greatly facilitate plate placement without K-wire removal.

- It is important to place screws into the inferomedial humeral head to optimize fixation stability.
  - The locking plate should be positioned such that the screws may be placed in this region.
  - If this is not possible due to plate design or other factors, a nonocking screw should be placed inferomedially (Fig. 6-8).

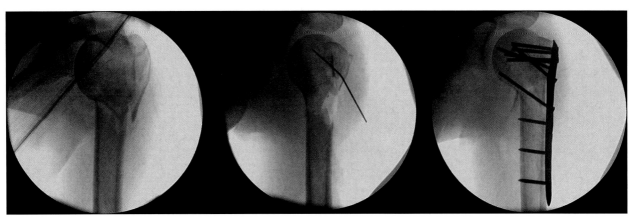

Figure 6-8 ▍ In this case, the plate was placed slightly too proximally for optimal locking screw placement into the inferomedial humeral head along the calcar. A nonlocking screw was used instead.

- In four-part valgus impacted patterns, one strategy is to place clamp tines on the greater and lesser tuberosities to provisionally reduce to each other (Fig. 6-9).
  - Next, use an elevator or spiked pusher to disimpact and elevate the humeral head fragment while simultaneously reducing both tuberosities so that they begin to support the elevated head fragment.
  - Graft the underlying defect with allograft or bone graft substitute, if required.
  - Complete the tuberosity clamp reduction to support the humeral head.
  - Place additional K-wires and remove the clamp.
  - Lesser tuberosity screws or a separate plate may be placed independent of the lateral humeral plate, if lesser tuberosity fragment is large.
  - Support the tuberosity reduction with suture fixation.

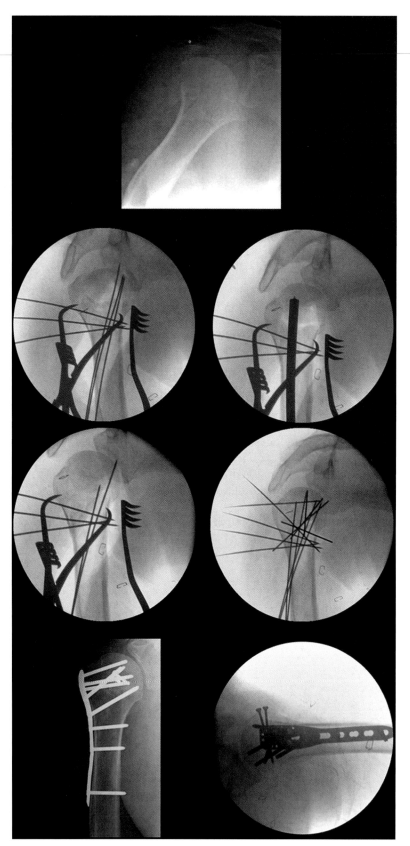

Figure 6-9 Four-part valgus impacted patterns can be reduced by first using a large Weber clamp on the tuberosities, with subsequent elevation of the humeral head fragment. Lesser tuberosity screws can be used in addition to sutures passed through rotator cuff bone-tendon junction if the fragment is large and unstable.

- If the greater tuberosity is a large fragment, it may be reduced and stabilized provisionally with 2.4- or 2.7-mm screws, placed posteriorly to the plate.
  - It is crucial to support the fixation with sutures through the rotator cuff enthesis which are then tied to the plate or through bone tunnels (Figs. 6-10 and 6-11).

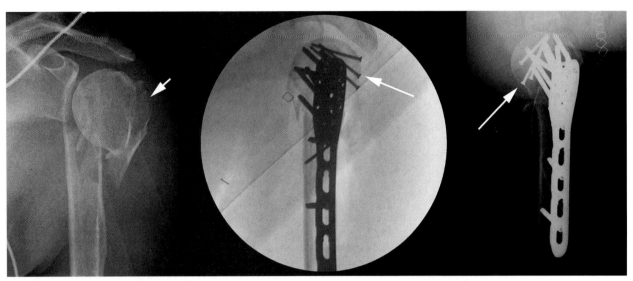

Figure 6-10 ▮ Using screws in addition to sutures for fixation of large greater tuberosity fractures (*arrows*) can supplement fixation.

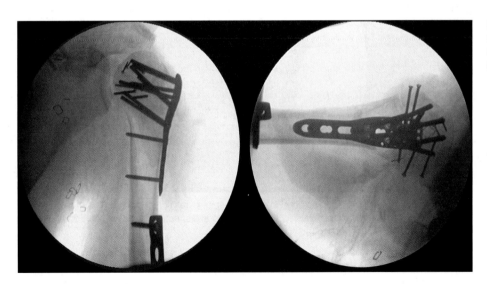

Figure 6-11 ▮ Another example of small screws used to stabilize a multifragmentary humeral neck and head fracture.

- In some instances, the fracture may be too short and it is difficult to manually restore appropriate length (Fig. 6-12).
    - A femoral distractor placed from the coracoid (4.0-mm Schanz pin) to the humeral shaft (4.0-mm Schanz pin) can greatly facilitate length restoration.

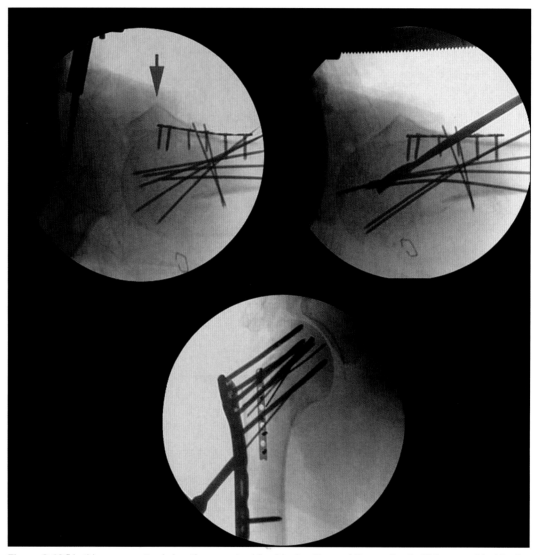

Figure 6-12 I In this case, anatomic length was not achievable despite paralytic anesthesia. This was evident by the inability to reduce the lesser tuberosity (*upper left, red arrow*). A femoral distractor placed from the coracoid to the humeral shaft greatly facilitated anatomic length reduction (*upper right*).

TIP

Utility of a Distractor in the Reduction and Fixation of Proximal Humeral Fracture

M. Bradford Henley
Anna Miller

Pathophysiology

Displaced and comminuted proximal humeral fractures are commonly treated using an open approach. Obtaining fracture reduction can be challenging, especially in younger, muscular individuals with shortening, bayonet apposition and/or impaction (Fig. 6-13). The humeral shaft may be completely separated at the surgical neck from the remaining humeral head and metaphyseal fragments. The multiple muscular attachments to the humerus can pull the diaphysis or metaphyseal fragments proximally, medially, and anteriorly, resulting in further fracture displacement; this also interferes with visualization and reduction.

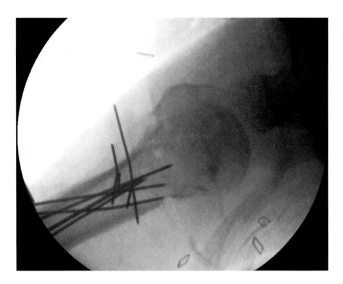

Figure 6-13 | Unsatisfactory reduction: This postreduction axillary lateral of a comminuted proximal humerus fracture was made after provisional K-wire fixation of the metaphysis. Note that the humeral head appears to be reduced to the metaphysis; however, the lesser tuberosity fragment and a portion of the humeral head's articular surface remains unreduced. There is also persistent impaction.

Solution

A distractor can be an effective tool in the restoration of humeral length and fracture reduction.

Technique

This technique uses a universal distractor with placement of two 4.0-mm, terminally threaded Schanz pins.

- One pin is placed in the base of the coracoid process.
  - When the humeral head is a single fragment, the proximal pin may be placed into the humeral head, from anterior to posterior at the level of the lesser tuberosity.
- The second pin is placed in the anterior portion of the humeral shaft.
- In the placement of the humeral diaphyseal pin, it is important to avoid interference with planned placement of final fixation.
  - This pin is usually placed in the sagittal plane, just lateral to the biceps and in the proximal humeral diaphysis.
  - The coracoid (or proximal humeral) pin is placed in the same anterior to posterior plane, with the arm abducted between 60 and 90 degrees.
  - Both pin trajectories are first predrilled with 2.5 mm drill bits, and fluoroscopic imaging is used to confirm these trajectories, as well as depth of insertion. Figure 6-14 shows an intraoperative anteroposterior radiographic view with the universal distractor in place after restoration of length and a provisional reduction.

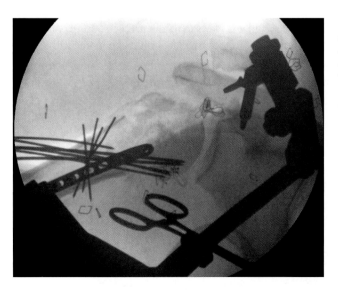

Figure 6-14 | Grashey's AP view after application of an anterior distractor. Additional distraction creates sufficient space for reduction of the lesser tuberosity fracture fragment, which has been stabilized provisionally with a unicortical anterior 2.7-mm plate.

- If a laterally placed proximal humeral plate is used for definitive fixation, it should be of sufficient length to extend beyond the distal 4.0 mm distractor pin site to protect this potential stress riser.
- The universal distractor should be placed so that it does not interfere with intraoperative fluoroscopic imaging. Figure 6-15 shows an intraoperative axillary view with the distractor in place prior to proximal humeral locking plate fixation.

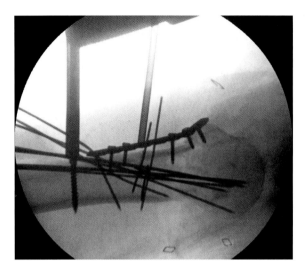

Figure 6-15 ▌ Axillary lateral radiograph, after distraction and provisional fixation. After applying the definitive lateral proximal humeral locking plate, the 2.7-mm unicortical screws were replaced with bicortical 2.7-mm screws in the humeral shaft segment, and locking 2.7-mm screws were placed in the humeral head.

Deltoid-splitting approach:

- A deltoid-splitting approach can be very useful for certain fracture types.
- Simple two-, three-, and four-part fractures are easily managed through this approach.
- Care should be taken to palpate and protect the axillary nerve, usually found 3.5 cm distal to the greater tuberosity.
- Once the nerve is identified, a second distal incision can be made to insert screws into the humeral shaft.

Specific points for Greater tuberosity fractures:

- Split-type fractures are treated with ORIF and reinforced with rotator cuff sutures.
- Standard proximal humerus plates may be used; however, often smaller fragment-specific (2.7 mm T-plates or mesh plates) implants offer better "capture."
- Avulsion-type fractures are treated as "boney" rotator cuff repairs with suture anchors or bone tunnels.

Proximal Humeral Nailing

- Use guide wire on AP and scapular Y views to obtain precise starting point medial to the insertion of the rotator cuff, at the lateral edge of the articular surface and in line with the humeral shaft (Fig. 6-16).

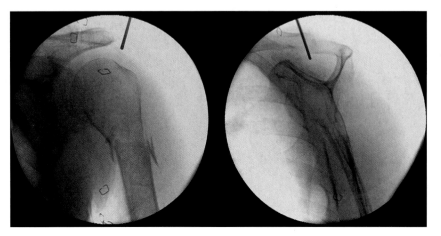

Figure 6-16 ▌ When placing a humeral nail, the starting point is assessed using AP and scapular Y orthogonal fluoroscopic views.

- Make skin incision based on the radiographic starting point.
- Split deltoid and retract.
- Identify the starting point again radiographically with guide pin and confirm by subdeltoid palpation using anatomical landmarks.
- Incise the rotator cuff longitudinally, in line with its tendinous fibers and tag each side with heavy nonabsorbable sutures (e.g., no. 2 Ti-Cron) for retraction and cuff protection.
- Open canal with an awl or a cannulated drill bit (Fig. 6-17).

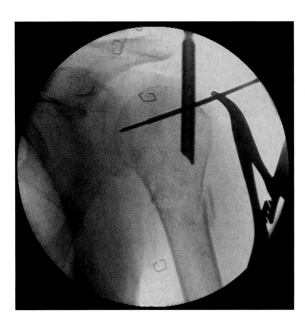

Figure 6-17 ‖ The starting point is opened with an awl.

- Reduce fracture using two Schanz pins as joysticks or with manipulation of the arm and bump placement.
  - Schanz pins should be placed anterior and posterior to nail insertion site (as "goal posts" on either side of the entry portal) (Fig. 6-18).
- Ream and place nail (Fig. 6-19).

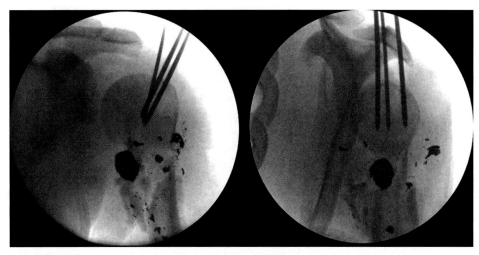

Figure 6-18 ‖ Two Schanz pins are placed in the humeral head on either side of the anticipated starting point. These are used for reduction and also assist in soft tissue retraction. The starting guide wire is inserted between the two Schanz pins.

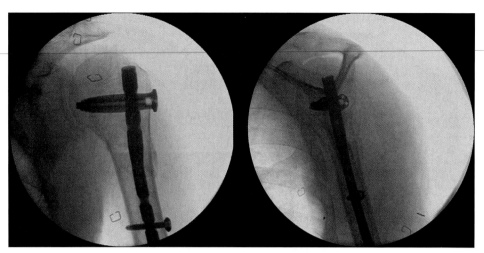

Figure 6-19 I The nail path is then reamed with the fracture reduced, and the nail is placed.

Shoulder Arthroplasty for Proximal Humerus Fractures

- Some fractures, either because of the type (head split, four part with comminution) or because of patient factors (osteoporosis, advanced age), are better served by proximal humeral replacement (Fig. 6-20).
- Treatment options include hemiarthroplasty (HA) and more recently reverse shoulder arthroplasty (RSA) (Fig. 6-20).
- RSA is generally reserved for older, lower demand patients, whereas HA is used for younger patients with nonreconstructable fractures.
- An important aspect of both procedures is to securely fix the tuberosities.
- A combination of vertical (through the implant and humeral bone tunnels) and horizontal (from the greater to the lesser tuberosity) fixation allows for optimal stability.

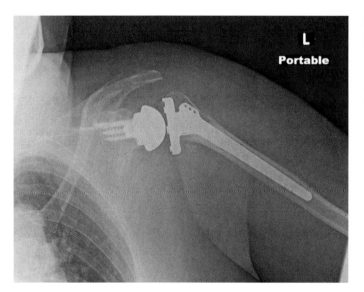

Figure 6-20 I Postoperative radiograph demonstrating treatment of a four-part proximal humerus fracture with reverse total shoulder arthroplasty. Note the accurate reduction of the greater tuberosity fragment to the proximal humerus.

Chapter 7
Humeral Shaft Fractures

MARK R. ADAMS
ANDREW R. EVANS
MICHAEL S. SIRKIN
EDWARD R. WESTRICK

Sterile Instruments/Equipment

- Impervious stockinette and 4-inch elastic bandage wrap for forearm and hand
- 1/4% Marcaine with epinephrine for arm incision, if desired
- Sterile tourniquet for distal diaphyseal fractures, if desired
- Vessel loop for identification and gentle retraction of radial nerve
- Articulated tensioner for transverse and short oblique fractures
- Variety of bone reduction clamps, including large and small pointed bone reduction clamps ("Weber clamps")
- Extra Mayo stand cover or adhesive plastic bag to collect irrigation fluids
- Implants
  - 4.5-mm broad or narrow compression plates, depending on the humeral size
  - Anatomically contoured humeral plates
  - 3.5-mm compression plates for smaller stature individuals
  - Small (3.5-mm) and minifragment (2.0/2.4/2.7-mm) screws for lagging butterfly fragments
- K-wires and wire driver/drill

Surgical Approaches

Modified posterior approach to the humeral shaft

- Prone position
  - Patient is positioned at the cantilever end of a radiolucent table.
  - Use a Wilson frame or blanket rolls to prevent abdominal compression.
  - Alternatively, place two smooth double-blanket rolls or gelatin rolls longitudinally on each side of the torso, separated enough to accommodate the patient's abdomen and breasts.
    - Rolls should extend from the level of inferior axillary fold to anterior superior ilium.
    - Consider placing a transverse roll across the pelvis in patients with large abdomen, to decrease abdominal pressure and optimize respiration.
  - The affected upper extremity should be positioned with the shoulder abducted approximately 90 degrees and draped over a radiolucent arm board with the forearm hanging freely.
    - To prevent edema of the dependent forearm, place the operative forearm and hand in a stockinette and overwrap with an elastic bandage.
  - The unaffected upper extremity should be positioned with the shoulder either adducted at the side of the patient's body or abducted <90 degrees and comfortably externally rotated (<70 degrees) to protect the brachial plexus and ulnar nerve.

- ▪ Build up the padding height of the arm board so that the arm rests at the level of the torso.
  - ▪ The elbow, forearm, and hand should be well padded on an arm board with attention given to protection of the ulnar nerve.
  - Place padding under the knees and a pillow under the distal legs to prevent pressure on the toes.
- Lateral decubitus position
  - Drape the affected arm over a radiolucent arm board anchored to the head of the table above the patient's head and oriented longitudinally to the table's axis.
  - Bean bag with gel pad or similar lateral positioning device; high chest roll to protect axilla.
  - Plexiglas table extension.
    - ▪ Inserted so that it protrudes 6 inches from the edge of the bed, under cushion to support down arm.
    - ▪ Position and protect the arm with blankets and foam.
  - Position down arm with elbow flexed to 90 degrees, with forearm and hand in "natural" position, and with shoulder forward flexed just enough so that down elbow does not interfere with affected humeral imaging (Fig. 7-1).

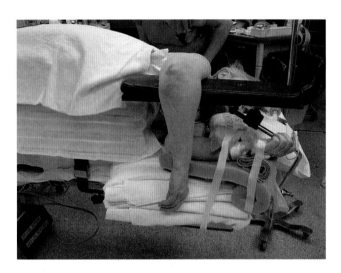

Figure 7-1 I Lateral positioning for plate fixation of a humeral shaft fracture.

- For both lateral and prone positioning, rotate the OR table (usually 90 degrees) such that the affected extremity is maximally accessible by surgeons and fluoroscopy.
  - Fluoroscopy comes in from head of patient; AP and lateral imaging are accomplished by 90 degrees rotation of the C-arm without rotation of extremity.

Technique

- Make a longitudinal incision in the midline of the dorsal aspect of the arm.
  - Subcutaneous injection of 1:10,000 epinephrine, prior to the incision will help control bleeding of this vascular layer.
  - Curve incision slightly radially for distal extension beyond the olecranon process.
  - Access the distal diaphyseal and supracondylar regions of the humerus through the lateral paratricipital posterior approach.[1]
    - ▪ Dissect full-thickness skin/subcutaneous flap directly to the deep posterior compartment (triceps) fascia and then laterally to the intermuscular septum.
    - ▪ Identify the radial nerve as it penetrates the lateral intermuscular septum, approximately 10 cm proximal to the lateral epicondyle.
    - ▪ Follow the radial nerve course proximally and obliquely.
    - ▪ Distal to the nerve, release the lateral triceps border and anconeus from intermuscular septum and lateral epicondyle, if distal exposure is required.
    - ▪ Identify the course of the radial nerve, and decompress if displaced or dislocated with respect to the fractured humerus.

- Access proximal shaft and metadiaphyseal region posteriorly by splitting the long and lateral heads of the triceps proximally (Fig. 7-2).
    - Radial nerve is deep and distal to their confluence, generally near the medial border of the humeral shaft at this level.
    - Take care to avoid injury to the axillary nerve and posterior humeral circumflex vessels if a limited dorsal deltoid release is necessary.

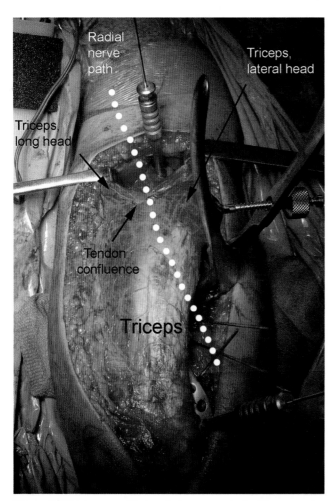
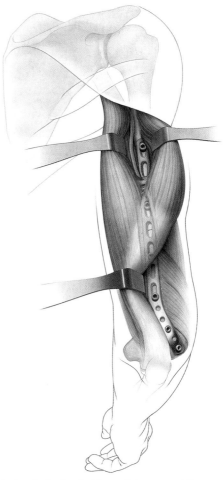

Figure 7-2 | Using a modified posterior approach, the triceps can be reflected up to the level of the radial nerve and the fracture. To avoid additional dissection to the proximal extent of the plate, the interval between the long and lateral triceps heads can be developed proximally. At this proximal tendon confluence, the radial nerve is usually adjacent to the medial edge of the plate and humerus.

- Alternatively, continue reflecting triceps from lateral to medial proximally for full extension of modified posterior (Gerwin) approach.

Anterolateral approach to the humeral shaft

- Supine position.
    - Place small one-blanket bump beneath the patient's affected shoulder, posterior thoracic wall, and pelvis.
    - Position the endotracheal tube to the side opposite the fractured extremity, and position the patient's head facing anteriorly or away from the affected extremity.
        - Secure the head to the table with foam and tape.
    - Radiolucent Plexiglas extension with long dimension protruding 4 to 6 inches beyond the bed cushion; place blankets on Plexiglas to equal bed cushion height, and position patient such that affected extremity is supported by Plexiglas extension.
    - The affected extremity may be positioned "naturally" over the torso.
    - Rotate OR bed such that the patient's affected extremity is maximally accessible by surgeons and fluoroscopy.

- Place fluoroscope on the opposite side of the radiolucent table; AP and lateral imaging are accomplished by rotating the C-arm through a 90-degree arc (Fig. 7-3).

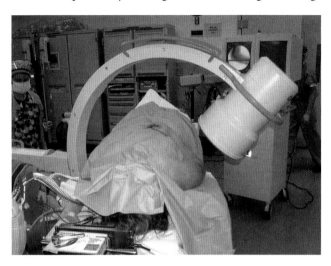

Figure 7-3 | With the patient's scapula elevated on the blanket or towel bumps, a lateral fluoroscopic view of the humerus can be obtained by rolling the C-arm "over the top."

- An excellent approach for operative fixation of middle and proximal one-third fractures of the humeral shaft.
- Allows for extensile exposure of the humeral shaft.

Lateral approach to the humeral shaft[2]

- A small open lateral approach may be used for insertion of Schanz pins for humeral external fixation or for limited exposure during intramedullary nailing to avoid injury to the radial or axillary nerves.
- The radial nerve is easily identified throughout the length of a lateral approach.
- Patient positioned supine.
  - Plexiglas extension may be used as described above (or a Mayo stand may be used as a broader, adjustable radiolucent working surface [Note: Mayo stands are metal and not radiolucent]).
- Incise the skin longitudinally along the line connecting the center of deltoid insertion and the lateral epicondyle (Fig. 7-4).

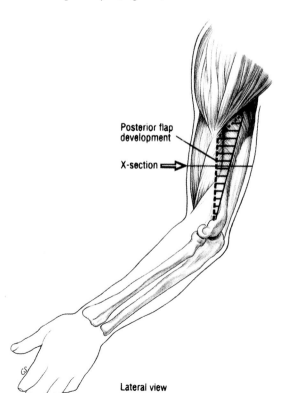

Posterior flap development

X-section

Lateral view

Figure 7-4 | A skin incision is made in line with the center of the deltoid insertion and the lateral epicondyle. The posterior flap is developed to expose the underlying fascia and intermuscular septum. (Adapted from Mills WJ, Hanel DP, Smith DG. Lateral approach to the humeral shaft: an alternative approach for fracture treatment. *J Orthop Trauma.* 1996;10(2):81–86, with permission.)

- Create a small posterior skin flap, and incise the fascia of posterior compartment, approximately 1 cm posterior to intermuscular septum (Fig. 7-5).

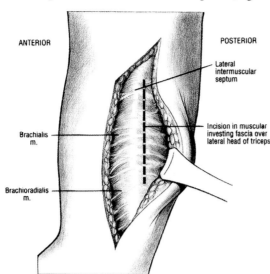

Figure 7-5 | Incise the fascia ≈1 cm posterior to the intermuscular septum, ensuring that the dissection proceeds in the posterior compartment of the arm. (Adapted from Mills WJ, Hanel DP, Smith DG. Lateral approach to the humeral shaft: an alternative approach for fracture treatment. *J Orthop Trauma.* 1996;10(2):81 86, with permission.)

- Dissect the lateral head of triceps off of the septum down to the level at which radial nerve pierces lateral intermuscular septum (Fig. 7-6).

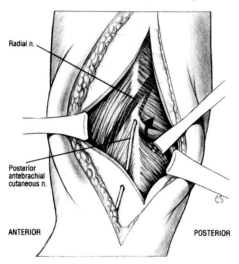

Figure 7-6 | Sharply elevate the lateral head of the triceps from the intermuscular septum, dissecting down to the humerus. The radial nerve will be found within investing fat in the proximal extent of the incision. The posterior antebrachial cutaneous nerve may be found in the distal subcutaneous dissection or as it pierces fascia; follow it proximally to its origin from the radial nerve proper. (Adapted from Mills WJ, Hanel DP, Smith DG. Lateral approach to the humeral shaft: an alternative approach for fracture treatment. *J Orthop Trauma.* 1996;10(2):81–86, with permission.)

- Identify and protect the posterior cutaneous branch of the radial nerve and motor branches of the radial nerve innervating the lateral head of the triceps.
- Retract radial nerve and associated branches carefully to expose the distal two-thirds of the humerus as needed for reduction of fractures or the placement of Schanz pins for external fixation (Fig. 7-7).

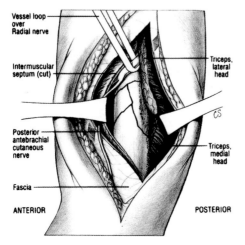

Figure 7-7 | Complete elevation of the triceps from intermuscular septum, retraction of the brachialis and brachioradialis anteriorly, and isolation of the radial nerve with a vessel loop; the humerus fracture is exposed. Division of the intermuscular septum allows visualization of the radial nerve distally. (Adapted from Mills WJ, Hanel DP, Smith DG. Lateral approach to the humeral shaft: an alternative approach for fracture treatment. *J Orthop Trauma.* 1996;10(2):81–86, with permission.)

- The anterior, lateral, and/or posterior surfaces of the humerus may be exposed as potential sites for plate application.
- The exposure is extensile, both proximally (anteriorly) and distally, although access is limited to the proximal third of the humeral shaft by the deltoid insertion.

Anterolateral approach to the shoulder (antegrade humeral nailing)

- For full technique, see Chapter 6

Implant/Reduction Techniques

Humeral Shaft Plating

- Dissect to humerus, clean fracture edges of hematoma, and infolded periosteum; avoid devitalization of comminuted or intercalary fracture fragments.
- Use small or large Weber or serrated reduction clamps to obtain an anatomical reduction.
- Recommend lag screw fixation with countersunk 2.0, 2.4, or 2.7-mm cortical lag screws between fragments that can be anatomically reduced, depending on the fragment size.
- Use large plates for fixation of diaphyseal fractures, when possible.
  - 4.5-mm narrow plates fit most humeri, but 4.5-mm broad plate is best in large male patients.
  - Posterior plates must be positioned under the radial nerve after sufficient nerve mobilization.
  - The radial nerve typically drapes directly over the plate (Fig. 7-8).

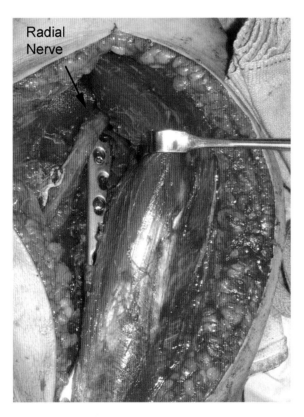

Radial Nerve

Figure 7-8 ▮ For posterior plating of the humerus, the plate must be carefully placed deep into the radial nerve.

- At the conclusion of the procedure, it is helpful to dictate the position of the radial nerve relative to the plate by noting over which plate hole it lies.
  - This facilitates identification, if future surgery is required.

- Consider using a lateral column distal humeral metaphyseal plate for distal one-fourth to one-third diaphyseal or metadiaphyseal fractures in which distal fixation options using conventional large fragment plates are limited (Fig. 7-9).

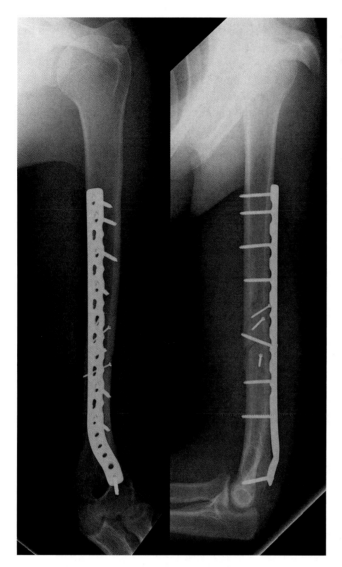

Figure 7-9 I Extra-articular distal humeral diaphyseal fractures are often treated effectively with specialty plates that extend to the lateral condyle.

- For transverse fracture patterns, interfragmentary compression is achieved by eccentrically drilling the compression holes of the plate on one side of the fracture. When using this technique, preloading the plate with a gentle concave bend in the sagittal plane is critical to achieve symmetric fracture compression. If the plate is not prebent, the near cortex will be overcompressed and the far cortex will gap, creating an extension deformity.
- In addition, plate contouring may require a torsional bend in the plate to fit the humeral contour anatomically.
- Bridge plating of the humeral shaft may be preferable for extensively comminuted fracture patterns, as long as the radial nerve is identified and protected.

Modified Triceps Split for a Submuscular Humerus Bridge Plate

Mark R. Adams
Michael S. Sirkin

Pathoanatomy

- Segmentally comminuted distal humeral fractures (Fig. 7-10) may be treated by fragment specific, open reduction and internal fixation, or they may be bridge plated to achieve union.
- Fragment-specific ORIF may result in delayed union or nonunion due to devascularization.

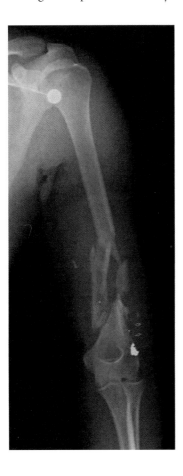
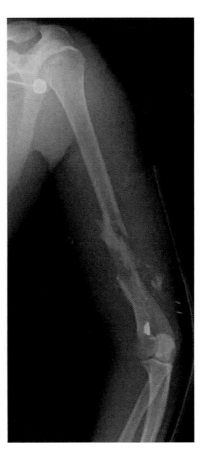

Figure 7-10 | AP and lateral radiographs demonstrate a comminuted distal one-third humeral shaft fracture.

Solution

- Bridge plating of a comminuted long bone fracture relies upon maintaining the biology of the fracture site in order to achieve union.
- Ideally, the soft tissue attachments on the comminuted intercalary fracture fragments are left undisturbed.

Technique

- A posterior plate for a humeral shaft fracture is typically applied through either a triceps splitting or a triceps reflecting approach. An open procedure, as opposed to a percutaneous plating, is necessary to place a posterior plate on the humerus as the radial nerve needs to be visualized and protected.
- With extensive comminution, a "fully" open approach with either method may lead to devitalization of some of the fracture fragments as the muscle is elevated to apply the plate.
- A modified triceps splitting approach involves locating the nerve proximally, prior to the confluence of the more superficial (long and lateral) heads of the triceps. It is usually found just medial and adjacent to the shaft between the long and lateral heads and adjacent to the medial head and humeral shaft. As it courses distally, it crosses the radial shaft under the triceps three conjoined muscle bellies (Fig. 7-11).

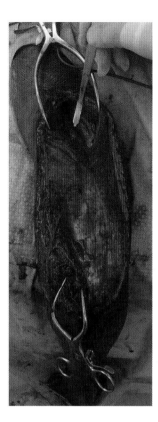

Figure 7-11 Intraoperative photograph demonstrating a split in the triceps proximal to the aponeurosis and a reflection of the distal lateral triceps. The small Hohmann retractor is pointing toward the radial nerve.

- The proximal portion of the plate is affixed to the humerus through this interval, prior to the confluence of the three tricep's heads. The aponeurosis is not incised as the two long and lateral heads may be parted bluntly. The fracture site is not directly exposed (Fig. 7-12).

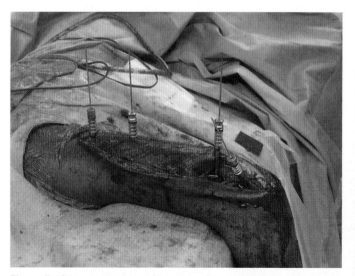

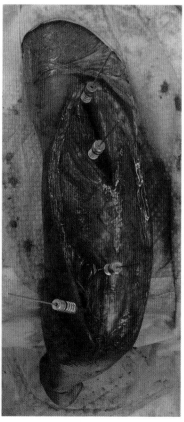

Figure 7-12 Intraoperative photographs of wires maintaining the plate on the humerus through locked drill sleeves proximally and distally.

- The fracture fragments maintain their muscular attachments. At the distal humerus, the triceps is elevated off of the posterior aspect of the lateral epicondyle, in a lateral to medial direction. This facilitates plate placement.
- The plate is introduced from distal (under the elevated anconeus and triceps) and advanced proximally. It is passed deep to the radial nerve and is visualized proximally between the heads of the triceps.
- The plate is used as a reduction tool, as the length, alignment, and rotation of the humerus are set by the plate (Figs. 7-13 and 7-14).

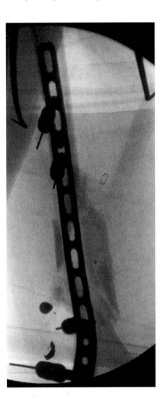
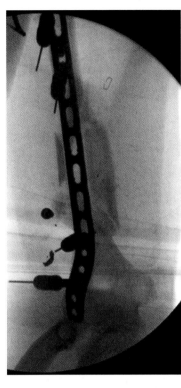

Figure 7-13 I Fluoroscopic images of the plate centered on the proximal and distal humeral segments, confirming restoration of length and alignment.

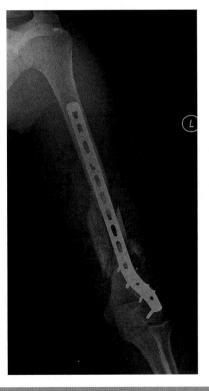
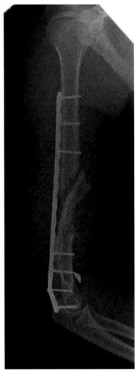

Figure 7-14 I Postoperative AP and lateral radiographs of the humerus demonstrating posterior plate fixation.

- Open and ballistic distal diaphyseal injuries with segmental comminution or bone loss may be at risk for implant failure when a single plate is used.
  - When an extended healing time or planned staged bone grafting is anticipated, consider 90-90 dual plating.

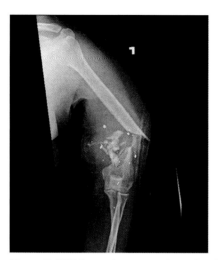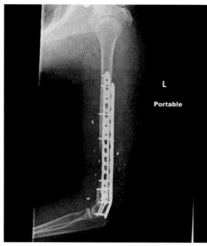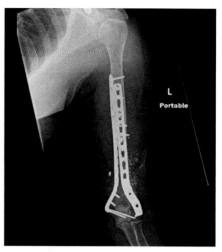

Figure 7-15 I Injury and postoperative radiographs demonstrating dual column plating for a distal humeral shaft fracture with segmental bone loss.

- A long posterior lateral column metaphyseal plate combined with a long medial column plate provides multiplanar fixation in the short distal segment (Fig. 7-15).
- Posterolateral and medial plating allows easy direct lateral access of the bone void for staged bone grafting.
- Shortening of the humerus may be advantageous in accelerating time to union and is well tolerated up to 2 cm. This should be considered preoperatively and discussed with the patient.

Antegrade Humeral Nailing

- For full technique, see Chapter 6.
- Prior to humeral nailing, consider the radial nerve function and the potential for shoulder discomfort.
- Transverse or short oblique fractures which can be anatomically reduced prior to reaming may be nailed using closed technique.
  - Otherwise, consider making a small lateral incision posterior to the intermuscular septum for radial nerve identification and protection during a nailing procedure.
- Antegrade technique (Fig. 7-16).

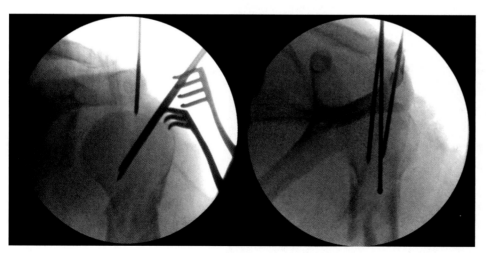

Figure 7-16 I The intramedullary nail starting point is determined based on the AP and scapular Y views. This should be medial to the sulcus of the greater tuberosity on the AP view (*left*) and collinear with the diaphysis on the lateral view (*right*).

- Skin incision should begin at the anterolateral corner of the acromion, extending at least 1 to 2 cm distally.
- Incise the deltoid fascia, at the junction of the anterior and middle thirds of the muscle.
- Insert guide wire fluoroscopically to identify the nail insertion point.
- Incise rotator cuff at the point of entry, splitting the supraspinatus tendon in line with its fibers.
  - The edges of the tendon should be retracted with sutures, which can later be used for repair.
  - The starting point should be just posterolateral to the biceps tendon.
  - Usually one can palpate the bicipital groove.

TIP — Obtaining a Difficult Starting Site
Edward R. Westrick

Pathoanatomy

A properly placed starting point is critical for avoiding malalignment, maintaining reduction, and concentric nail placement. The patient's body habitus, soft tissue contractures, additional musculoskeletal injuries, and previous soft tissue trauma (i.e., previous surgical field, radiation, soft tissue coverage, etc.) increase difficulty in obtaining the proper nail entry site.

Solution

The surgeon can obtain an ideal nail entry portal using a retrograde technique. This is obtained using a distal surgical approach, to avoid displacement of fracture fragments and excessive soft tissue disruption. This allows the surgeon to obtain the ideal starting point in an otherwise challenging extremity, due to a multitude of potential factors (Figs. 7-17 and 7-18).

Technique

- See the legends of Figs. 7-17 and 7-18 for specific details.

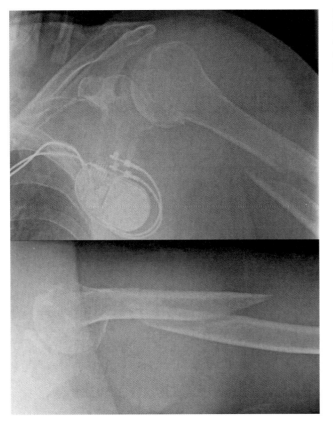

Figure 7-17 I An ipsilateral proximal humerus fracture (surgical neck) and humeral shaft fracture, in a morbidly obese patient with previous shoulder melanoma resection, breast surgery, and pacemaker placement.

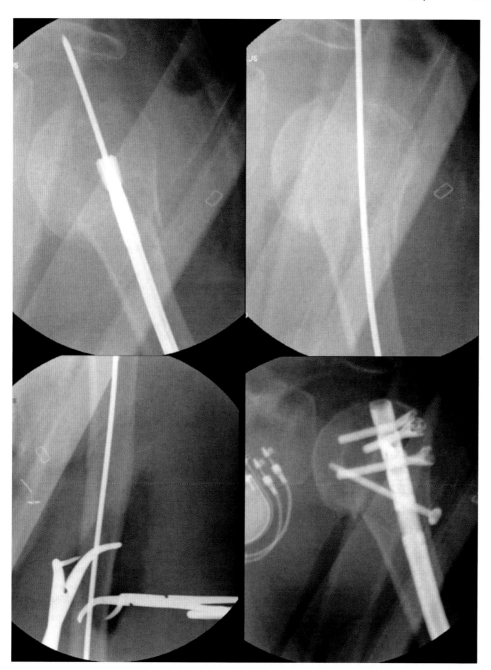

Figure 7-18 I A retrograde approach was used to identify the nail entry point. The humeral shaft fracture was accessed with an open approach, and the starting guide wire passed in retrograde fashion to obtain the ideal nail entry site. The opening reamer was passed retrograde as well. The ball tip guide wire was then passed retrograde, and a small skin incision was made to control the wire and pass reamers. Both fractures were reduced, and the ball tip guide wire advanced in the usual fashion. The previously passed ball tip guide wire is then advanced antegrade, across the proximal humerus and humeral shaft fractures. The reduction is maintained, and the remainder of the case proceeds in the usual fashion.

- Overream guide wire with cannulated drill bit.
- For segmentally comminuted humeral shaft fractures, measure length, alignment, and rotation based on the contralateral humerus if not fractured as a guide to fracture reduction.
  - Length—radiolucent ruler to measure from top of humeral head to trochlea.
  - Alignment—normal humeral diaphyseal alignment has minimal varus/valgus or flexion/extension angulation.
  - Rotation—may assess through comparison of greater and lesser tuberosity morphology with the contralateral side.
- For fractures with proximal extension, two 2.5-mm Steinmann pins can be useful to control the proximal segment.
  - These are placed anterior and posterior to the anticipated nail start point.
  - Guide wire and nail are placed between pins like "goal posts."
  - Pins also retract rotator cuff (Fig. 7-19).

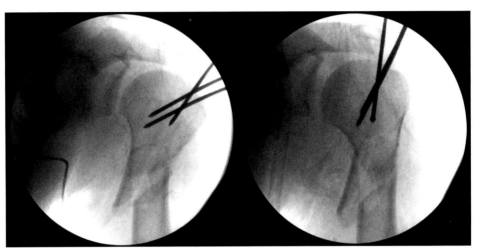

Figure 7-19 I For more proximal fractures, 2.5-mm Steinmann pins are very useful for manipulation of the proximal fragment. These are positioned such that the guide wire, reamers, and nail are placed between the pins.

- Avoid eccentric reaming of the canal by reaming the humerus with the fracture reduced.
- When considering nail length, remember that the humeral canal narrows and tapers just proximal to the olecranon fossa.
  - Using a nail that is too long will result in distraction and/or iatrogenic extension of the fracture.
  - Avoid retracting the nail and positioning it prominently the subchondral bone of the humeral head.
- In open fractures, or if a fracture is opened to identify/protect the radial nerve, consider placing a modified small Weber clamp in two 2.0-mm drill holes to maintain reduction of transverse or oblique fractures during reaming[3] (Fig. 7-20).

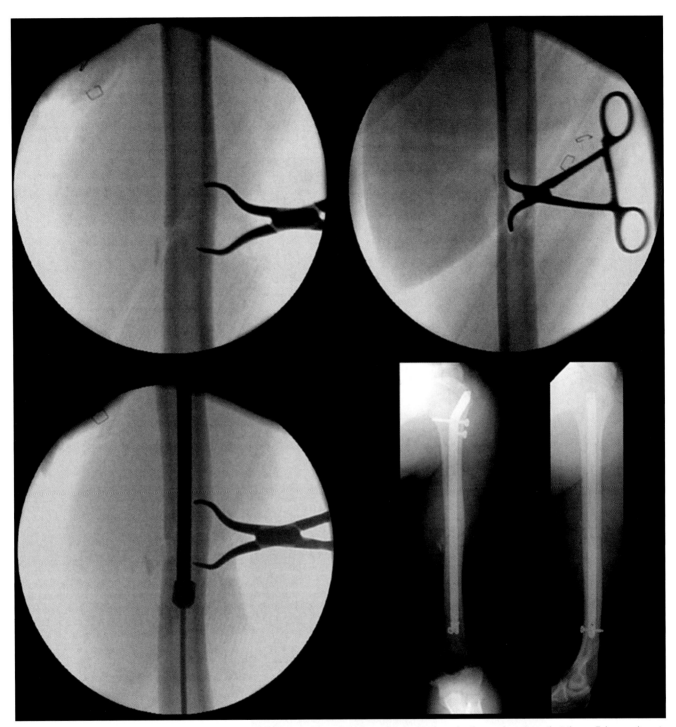

Figure 7-20 I Direct identification of the fracture site with clamp placement allows for anatomic reduction and ensures that the radial nerve is not at risk with reaming.

- When locking proximally, create safe paths for drilling and interlocking using a blunt muscle splitting technique to avoid injury to the axillary nerve.
  - Alternatively, extend the proximal incision, used for nail entry, to the anterolateral deltoid until the nerve is identified by palpation or visualization.
- When locking distally, anterior to posterior, use a sleeve system or ample exposure with retraction; consider an oscillating drill to protect surrounding soft tissue structures.
  - When placing distal interlocking screws from lateral to medial, make an incision to allow sufficient visualization of the humerus to avoid injury to the lateral antebrachial cutaneous or radial nerves.
- Distally, the lateral humeral border has a narrow border and drill bits tend to slip off of this ridge.

External Fixation of the Humeral Shaft

- An option for provisional or definitive treatment of humeral shaft fractures, particularly in mangled upper extremity injuries (Fig. 7-21).
- Perform a limited lateral approach to the distal humeral shaft for pin placement to avoid injury to cutaneous or deep nerves (e.g., radial nerve).
- Avoid injury to the axillary nerve through blunt dissection and use of sleeve systems for proximal pin placement.

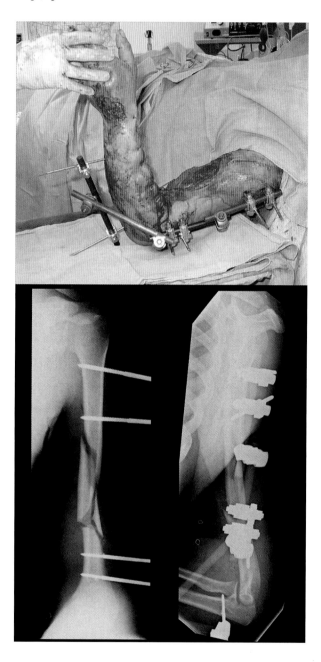

Figure 7-21 I Typical external fixation pin positions in the humerus. Proximally, the axillary nerve must be avoided around the surgical neck. Distally, the radial nerve must be protected.

References

1. Schildhauer TA, Nork SE, Mills WJ, et al. Extensor mechanism-sparing paratricipital posterior approach to the distal humerus. *J Orthop Trauma.* 2003;17(5):374–378.
2. Mills WJ, Hanel DP, Smith DG. Lateral approach to the humeral shaft: an alternative approach for fracture treatment. *J Orthop Trauma.* 1996;10(2):81–86.
3. Schoots IG, Simons MP, Nork SE, et al. Antegrade locked nailing of open humeral shaft fractures. *Orthopedics.* 2007;30(1):49–54.

Section 3
Elbow/
Forearm

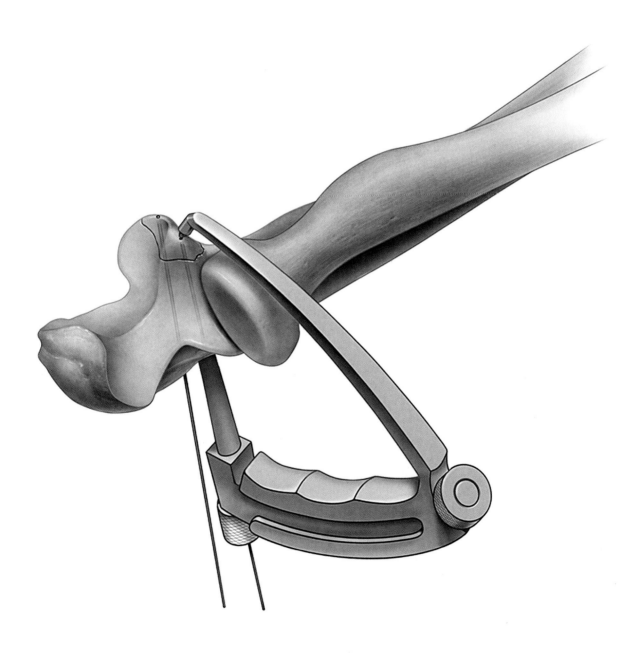

Chapter 8
Distal Humerus Fractures

MICHAEL J. GARDNER
JONAH HÉBERT-DAVIES
M. BRADFORD HENLEY
MATTHEW A. MORMINO
JUSTIN C. SIEBLER

Sterile Instruments/Equipment

- Extra Mayo stand cover or adhesive bag as fluid collection drape
- Impervious stockinette and 4-inch elastic bandage wrap for forearm and hand
- Bipolar cautery for ulnar neurolysis dissection, if required
- 1/4% Marcaine with epinephrine for posterior arm skin and subcutaneous tissues prior to incision
- Tourniquet if desired
- Large and small pointed bone reduction clamps ("Weber clamps")
- If planning proximal ulnar osteotomy: micro oscillating saw, small osteotomes (e.g., Hooke osteotomes)
- Implants:
  - Anatomically contoured periarticular plates for application to the medial and lateral humeral columns, 2.7/3.5 reconstruction plates, 3.5 compression plates
  - Consider cannulated 3.5- or 4.0-mm screw(s) for stabilizing the intercondylar split.
  - Consider small and minifragment screws and minifragment plates (2.0/2.4 mm) if comminuted medial and/or lateral columns.
- K-wires and wire driver/drill

Patient Positioning

- Position the patient either prone or lateral.
  - Radiolucent table extension; cantilever type.
  - Patient is placed backwards so that the patient's head is toward the radiolucent and "foot end" of the table.
  - U-drape to exclude the axilla and thorax.
  - If prone, support fractured arm by radiolucent (e.g., Plexiglas) board placed orthogonally to table so that board is supported by patient's torso and weight; Plexiglas board is placed under table's "mattress pad."
    - Most arm tables are too long and do not permit sufficient elbow flexion when patient is prone.
    - Center Plexiglas on patient's shoulder so that arm is abducted at a right angle to torso; this aids in obtaining lateral images.
  - If positioned laterally, an elevated arm board that can be adjusted for height is needed.
  - In either position, the contralateral arm is supported by an arm board designed for prone positioning, so excessive abduction and external rotation are avoided.

- OR table is rotated 90 degrees with respect to usual position in room, to provide unimpeded access to shoulder, arm, and elbow.
- C-arm is positioned above patient's head, parallel to long axis of patient's body and perpendicular to the injured extremity which is abducted 90 degrees. This permits AP and lateral imaging without moving the extremity (Figs. 8-1 and 8-2).

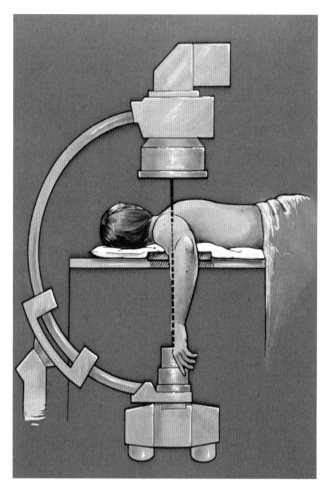

Figure 8-1 | Prone positioning with arm supported by radiolucent Plexiglas board allows for unimpeded AP and lateral images from shoulder to elbow. The contralateral upper extremity may be positioned at the patient's side or abducted comfortably. Also, it is not near the operative field being imaged with X-ray.

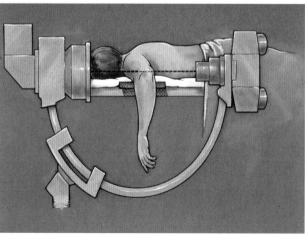

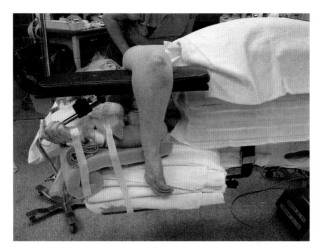

Figure 8-2 I In the lateral position, the contralateral upper extremity may impede some AP images. This can be avoided by carefully positioning the contralateral extremity and by canting the C-arm anode toward the patient's torso. After draping, the forearm and hand of the injured extremity are placed in an impervious stockinette and over wrapped with an elastic bandage to reduce dependent edema. The extremity is contained in a second Mayo stand cover which is used to collect irrigation fluid and to keep the operative field tidy. A fenestration is made in the dependent end of the Mayo stand cover; it is weighted with a clamp and placed in a kick bucket as a fluid collection reservoir.

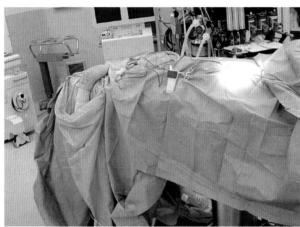

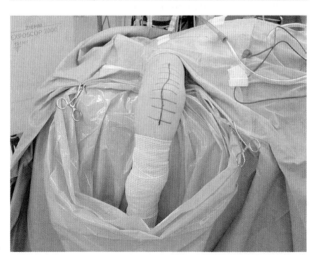

Surgical Approaches

- Place hand and forearm in impervious stockinette, over wrap with ACE.
  - Take extra Mayo stand cover and create fenestration at the closed end.
  - Attach weighted clamp (e.g., Ochsner/Kocher) at this fenestration (to keep it open and dependent).
  - Place this dependent portion of the Mayo stand cover, with clamp, into a kick bucket to collect irrigation fluids.
  - Place extremity in normal opening of Mayo stand cover (Fig. 8-2).
  - Alternatively, use commercially available, triangular, irrigation fluid collecting drape.
- Posterior midline incision skirting the radial side of the olecranon (Fig. 8-3).

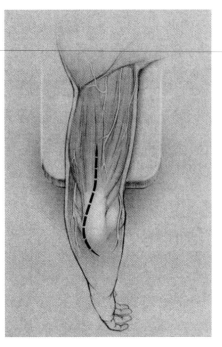

Figure 8-3 I Posterior midline skin incision between the lateral and medial brachial cutaneous nerves, curving laterally around the olecranon. (Adapted from Schildhauer TA, Nork SE, Mills WJ, et al. Extensor mechanism-sparing paratricipital posterior approach to the distal humerus. *J Orthop Trauma*. 2003;17(5):374–378, with permission.)

- Develop medial and lateral soft tissue flaps.
  - Open in the midline and retract skin and subcutaneous tissues in flap.
  - Over the elbow and forearm, include the olecranon bursa in the radial flap, but exclude the anconeus fascia.
    - Medially, the flap is superficial to the fascia/tendinous insertion of the flexor-pronator muscle mass.
- Identify and protect the ulnar nerve and superior and inferior ulnar collateral arteries.
  - Consider using a vessel loop or small Penrose drain around the nerve (Fig. 8-4).

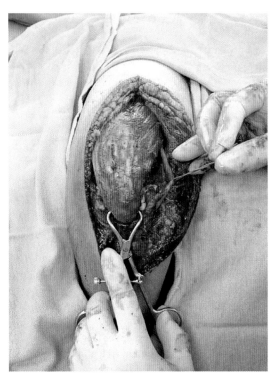

Figure 8-4 I The ulnar nerve is protected with a vessel loop.

- If an olecranon osteotomy is not needed (type A and type C1 fracture patterns):
  - Elevate the triceps and anconeus off of the lateral and medial intermuscular septae to the posterior aspect of the humerus (Figs. 8-5 and 8-6).

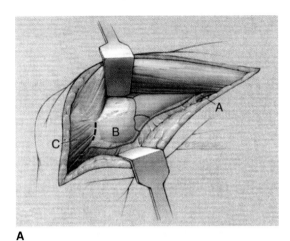 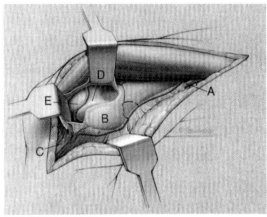

A   **B**

Figure 8-5 | Lateral dissection along the lateral triceps border to the intermuscular septum with an elevation of the triceps muscle off the lateral humerus. In the proximal wound, the radial nerve can be identified **(Left)**. The deep dissection can be distally extended anterior to the anconeus muscle (*dotted line*). Lateral view presenting the arthrotomy. The anconeus muscle is elevated in conjunction with the triceps muscle **(Right)**. *A,* radial nerve; *B,* lateral epicondyle; *C,* reflected anconeus muscle, and capsule; *D,* trochlea; *E,* olecranon tip. (Adapted from Schildhauer TA, Nork SE, Mills WJ, et al. Extensor mechanism-sparing paratricipital posterior approach to the distal humerus. *J Orthop Trauma.* 2003;17(5):374–378, with permission.)

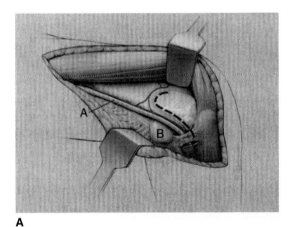 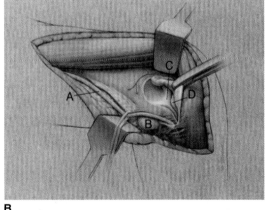

A   **B**

Figure 8-6 | Medial dissection along the medial triceps border to the medial intermuscular septum. The ulnar nerve is released from the cubital tunnel and dissected distally to its first motor branch **(Left)**. Medial deep dissection and arthrotomy. The arthrotomy is performed posterior to the humeroulnar ligaments **(Right)**. *A,* ulnar nerve; *B,* medial epicondyle; *C,* trochlea; *D,* olecranon tip. (Adapted from Schildhauer TA, Nork SE, Mills WJ, et al. Extensor mechanism-sparing paratricipital posterior approach to the distal humerus. *J Orthop Trauma.* 2003;17(5):374–378, with permission.)

- Locate and protect the radial nerve and profunda brachii (deep brachial) artery and its branches (radial and medial collateral arteries).
- In the distal arm and elbow, elevate the anconeus off of the posterior aspect of the lateral epicondyle.
  - May dissect through the proximal portion of the anconeus, but avoid straying too radially or joint visualization becomes difficult.
- Perform lateral and medial elbow joint arthrotomies until the olecranon fossa, olecranon, posterior-inferior portion of the capitellum, and posterior trochlea are all visualized.
- A bone clamp placed on the proximal ulnar allows elbow joint distraction for the medial and lateral capsulotomy and improved joint visualization.

TIP

Distal Humeral Fracture Fixation with an Extensor Mechanism-On Approach

Matthew A. Mormino
Justin C. Siebler

Pathoanatomy

Supracondylar-intercondylar distal humerus fractures are difficult to access due to position of the extensor mechanism and olecranon. As such, an olecranon osteotomy is often used to access the articular surface, although this brings with it its own set of potential pitfalls.

Solution

Using the extensor mechanism-on technique, it is possible to perform ORIF without an olecranon osteotomy.

Preoperative Planning/Case Selection

A. Planning

- An AP radiograph with gentle manual traction applied is often helpful in defining each fracture fragment. Look specifically for:
  - Intra-articular comminution
  - Fracture lines separating the trochlea and capitellum
  - Comminution of either or both the lateral and medial columns
  - On the lateral image look for evidence of coronal shear fractures (Fig. 8-7)

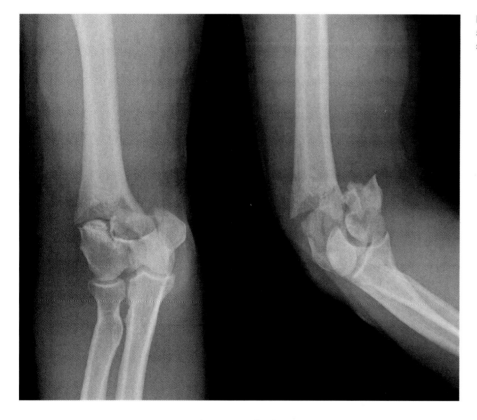

Figure 8-7 ▌ AP and lateral images of a 55-year-old male after a fall at construction site.

- Computed tomography (CT) scan with axial, coronal, and sagittal views with or without three-dimensional reconstructions may better define fracture complexity and configuration.
  - Look for fracture lines involving the capitellum or trochlea, as these fractures will make reduction and fixation more difficult.

B. Case Selection

- Appropriate approach for AO/OTA type A and simple type C fractures.
- With greater experience, it can be extended to include more complex type C fractures.
- An olecranon osteotomy can be added to increase visualization if needed during the procedure.

Surgical Approach

- A posterior skin incision is made, slightly lateral to the midline and extending distal and lateral to the olecranon tip (Fig. 8-8).
- Full-thickness flaps are elevated medially and laterally (Fig. 8-9).

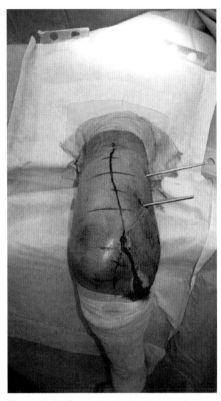

Figure 8-8 ‖ Posterior skin incision made slightly lateral to midline, incorporating open wound. Note previously placed external fixation pins.

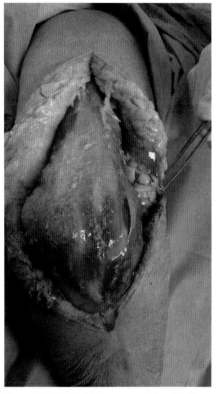

Figure 8-9 ‖ Full-thickness posterior skin flaps are made exposing the triceps and anconeus muscles.

- Medial dissection is usually accomplished first.
  - The ulnar nerve is identified along the medial intermuscular septum and dissected along its course from the arcade of Struthers to the first motor branch in the flexor carpi ulnaris muscle belly.
  - The ulnar nerve is left in situ. Circumferential dissection is only needed to pass plates/screws under it.
  - Allow the nerve to rest in this retro-epitrochlear position at the time of closure.
  - Rarely, will a subcutaneous anterior transposition be needed unless implant proximity will cause postoperative irritation.
  - Elevate the medial borders of the triceps muscle from its intermuscular septum and use extra-periosteal dissection to expose the back of the humerus (Fig. 8-10).
- The lateral dissection is carried out next.
  - Incise the triceps fascia posterior to the intramuscular septa and continue the distal dissection anterior to the anconeus muscle and elevate it with the triceps muscle.
  - Elevate the lateral border of the triceps and anconeus muscles from the posterior aspect of the humerus in an extraperiosteal fashion and connect the medial and lateral windows under the triceps (Fig. 8-11).

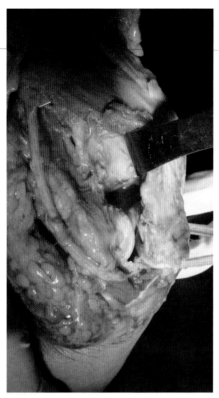

Figure 8-10 | Medial dissection is performed, identifying the ulnar nerve, resecting the olecranon fat pad, and distracting the distal triceps and olecranon with a lap sponge. In this example, the ulnar nerve was mobilized from its groove.

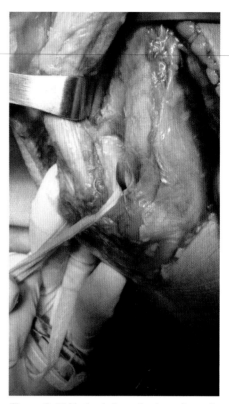

Figure 8-11 | Lateral dissection is performed, resecting the olecranon fat pad and distracting the olecranon with a lap sponge to improve intra-articular visualization.

- Excise the olecranon fossa posterior fat pad and posterior aspect of the capsule. This is helpful to visualize the articular surface.
- Perform medial and lateral elbow arthrotomies posterior to the collateral ligament complexes. This will allow visualization of roughly 60% of the overall articular cartilage surface of the distal humerus.
  - The posterior band of the ulnar collateral ligament may be released to allow better trochlea visualization without compromising elbow stability.

Fracture Reduction and Fixation

- Visualization and reduction of the joint are facilitated by placing a sponge or small Penrose drain into the ulnohumeral joint allowing distraction of the joint by pulling distally on the olecranon via the sigmoid notch. Alternatively, a small Weber clamp can be used to grasp and distract the proximal ulna.
- By increasing elbow flexion, the most distal portions of the trochlea and capitellum may be viewed.
- The intact sigmoid notch serves as a template for articular reduction under direct visualization posteriorly and indirectly with fluoroscopy.
- Reduce and temporarily fix the fracture fragments with clamps, Kirschner wires, and/or small plates to strategically achieve the desired stable provisional fixation that should not interfere with final plate and screw placement (Fig. 8-12).
  - Often reduce one column first (usually the one with the simplest fracture configuration), and then reduce the rest of the joint to that column.
  - Kirschner wires, used as joysticks in each condyle, can be helpful to reduce condylar segments that are rotated by the weight of the forearm via the collateral ligaments and the attached epicondylar muscle origins.

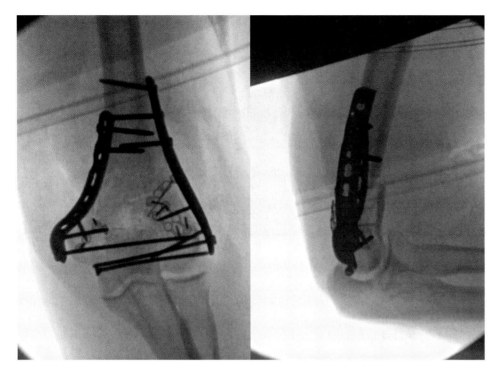

Figure 8-12 I Intraoperative AP and lateral image during ORIF of intra-articular distal humerus fracture with extensor mechanism-sparing approach.

- Place parallel or orthogonal plates based on the fracture pattern and/or your preference.
  - One or two long transcondylar "spool" screws can be placed through or outside the plate as lag screws or stabilization screws if there is intercondylar comminution.
  - Apply a proximal screw in compression mode and place and tighten the remainder of the diaphyseal screws in each plate.
  - Bridge plating should be used in cases of comminution at the metadiaphyseal region.
- Look for intra-articular implants with direct visualization and with fluoroscopy. Then assess fixation stability and smooth motion arcs prior to closure.

Wound Closure and Postoperative Management

- Repair the triceps fascia laterally with an absorbable suture followed by skin closure.
  - Subcutaneous anterior ulnar nerve transposition is performed rarely and only if plate contact is excessive (Fig. 8-13).

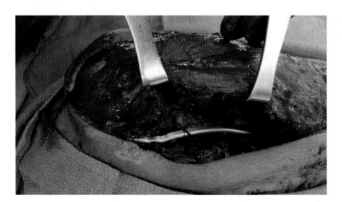

Figure 8-13 I Direct lateral plate shown in situ on the lateral column.

- The medial fascia is not closed to allow the ulnar nerve to "find" its position (Fig. 8-14).

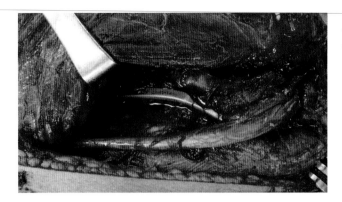

Figure 8-14 ▌ Medial plate shown in situ with the ulnar nerve left to find its position, adjacent to the medial epicondyle.

- A drain is not typically required.
- The elbow is placed in a bulky dressing with the elbow in extension.
- Remove the dressing on postoperative day two and begin active and active-assisted elbow range of motion and grip-strengthening therapy.
- Fractures are typically healed and range of motion has plateaued at 3 months postoperatively (Fig. 8-15).

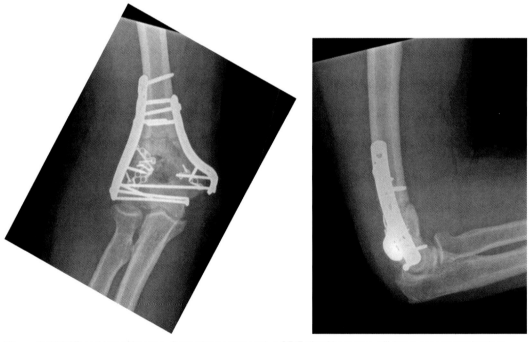

Figure 8-15 ▌ AP and lateral images, 3 months postoperative ORIF distal humerus utilizing extensor mechanism sparing on approach.

Olecranon Osteotomy Localization and Technique
Jonah Herbert-Davies

Pathoanatomy

Many distal humerus fractures are amenable to fixation through a standard triceps sparing, paratricipital approach. Some complex AO/OTA 13.C-type fractures, however, will require an olecranon osteotomy to allow proper articular visualization and repair. Creating a new "fracture" may be associated with complications including nonunion, malunion, and prominent hardware. These problems may make some surgeons hesitant to use an osteotomy and thereby may make surgery needlessly more complicated.

Solution

It is important to minimize potential complications. This begins with choosing the right location for the apex of a chevron osteotomy.

Technique

The following technique allows the surgeon to reliably choose the ideal location for the osteotomy. To decrease the potential impact of a slight mal reduction, the apex of the chevron should be centered on the olecranon bare area.

- Use a posterior skin incision; find and protect the ulnar nerve.
- Expose the distal humerus using a paratricepital approach.
- When the distal humeral fracture is judged to be inadequately visualized using this approach, the osteotomy is prepared. The proximal dorsal ulna is exposed. While planning the level of the osteotomy, a 2.5-mm drill is lined up with the bare area on a lateral fluoroscopy image (Fig. 8-16).

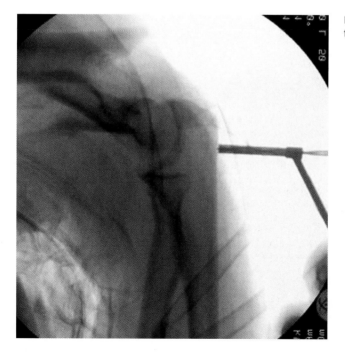

Figure 8-16 Lateral fluoroscopy showing the optimal position of the osteotomy apex.

- The drill is then advanced to the subchondral bone—without breaching the deep cortex (Fig. 8-17).

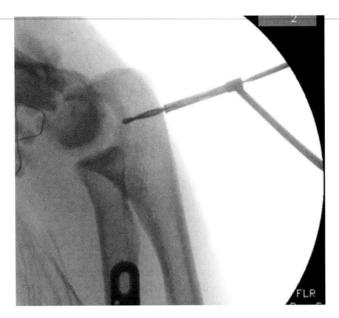

Figure 8-17 | Drilling to subchondral bone without perforating.

- A microsagittal saw is used to create the chevron osteotomy with a distally pointing apex, with both oblique limbs converging on the drill hole. The saw should be advanced only to the subchondral bone.
- Prior to completing the osteotomy, an olecranon plate is then fitted over the bone to its ideal position. The proximal screw and distal screws are drilled and inserted (Fig. 8-18).

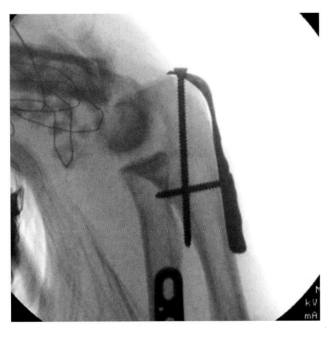

Figure 8-18 | Plating of the olecranon prior to completing osteotomy.

- The plate and screws are then removed and the osteotomy is completed with two fine osteotomes or chisels inserted in each limb of the chevron.
  - Allow for a controlled fracture of the articular (volar) subchondral bone and articular cartilage (break in tension).
    - This makes reduction easier and enhances its stability as it permits fracture interdigitation.
    - It also aids in the identification of complete healing postoperatively.

- Reflect olecranon, posterior fat pad, and triceps proximally.
  - Suturing the reflected olecranon and triceps to proximal skin or soft tissues aids in its retraction.
  - Wrapping or covering with a moist saline sponge will prevent desiccation (Fig. 8-19).

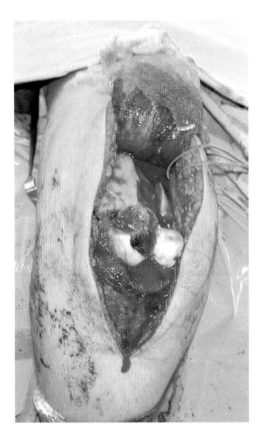

Figure 8-19 | The olecranon osteotomy fragment is retracted with a moist laparotomy sponge.

- After fixation of the distal humerus, the osteotomy is reduced and the plate is reinstalled using the previously created screw paths. One or more extra screws can be added for stability (Fig. 8-20).

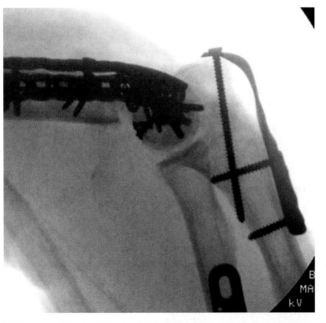

Figure 8-20 | Plating of the olecranon after fixation of humerus.

- If an olecranon osteotomy is needed, the paratricipital approach can be converted to an olecranon osteotomy.

Reduction and Implant Techniques

- For fractures with a simple intercondylar split, the joint reduction is usually performed first.
  - A large Weber clamp is useful to obtain interfragmentary compression when placed from lateral epicondyle to medial epicondyle or just below the medial epicondyle at the medial aspect of the trochlea's epicenter (Fig. 8-21).

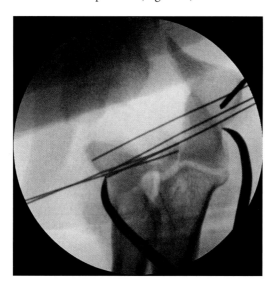

Figure 8-21 | Several examples showing clamp placement between the capitellum, the trochlea and the medial epicondyle.

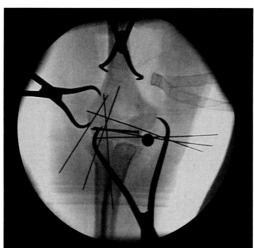

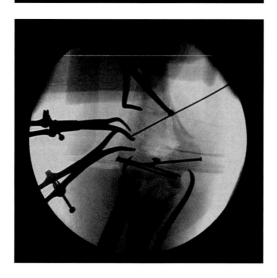

- Two transcondylar K-wires or a screw and K-wire are used for provisional stability, followed by definitive bicolumnar plate and screw fixation (Fig. 8-22).

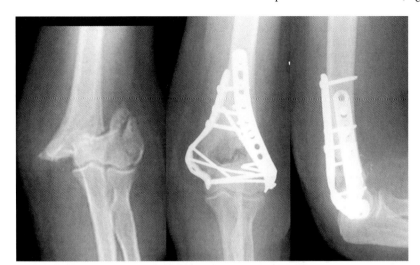

Figure 8-22 | Several case examples demonstrating definitive bicolumnar plate fixation of distal humerus fractures.

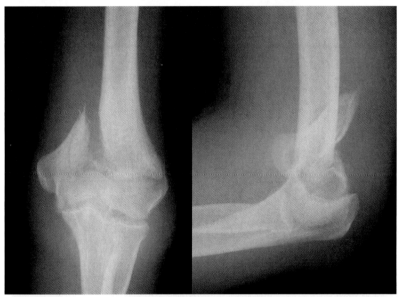

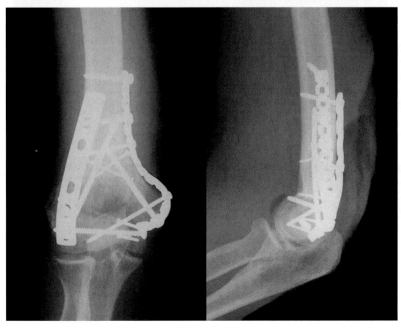

- For fractures with intercondylar comminution or bone loss, if associated with relatively simple epicondylar fracture patterns, the reduction of the medial and/or lateral epicondyles will aid in the reduction of the intercondylar components (in terms of length, width, and rotation).
    - Modified small Weber clamps may aid in the reduction when placed dorsally, medially, or laterally in unicortical 2.0- or 2.5-mm drill holes.
    - Provisional 0.062-inch K-wires can be inserted up the medial and lateral columns, from the distal aspects of the epicondyles, into the shaft.
        - These will usually provide sufficient stability to allow for definitive fixation without encumbering the plates.
    - Small osteochondral screws can be countersunk for articular fixation but must be placed strategically to avoid transverse screws (Fig. 8-23).

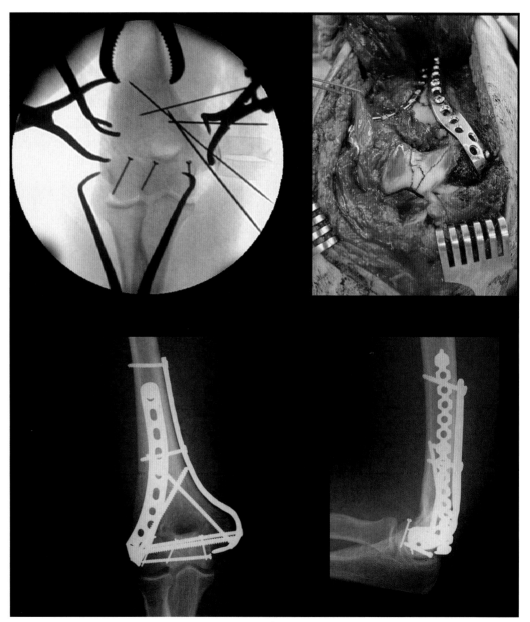

Figure 8-23 I Small osteochondral fragments stabilized with minifragment screws as the initial step.

- If comminution or bone loss of the medial or lateral epicondyles, consider supplementing the provisional axial 0.062-inch K-wire fixation with 2.0-mm plate(s) and screws prior to definitive plate and screw fixation (Fig. 8-24).

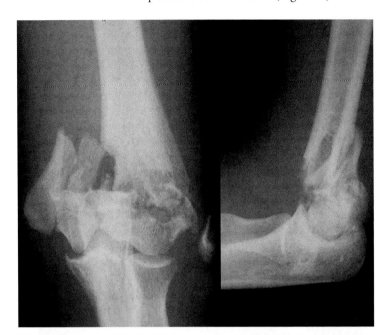
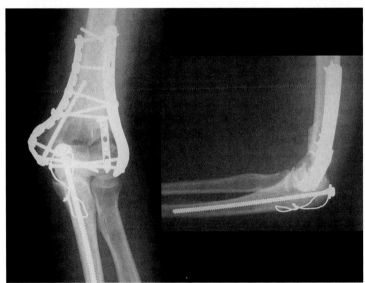
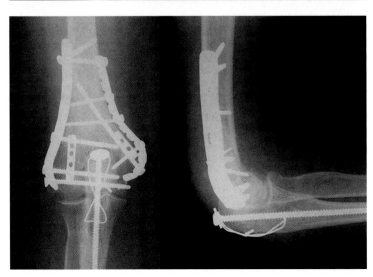

Figure 8-24 | Two case examples with multifragmentary articular surfaces stabilized with provisional minifragment plates. The plates were left in place following a definitive plate fixation.

- For fractures with supracondylar comminution, it is imperative that one of the definitive plates is at least a 3.5-mm compression plate or of equivalent thickness.
- Repair olecranon osteotomy with plate or modified tension band wire technique (Fig. 8-25).
- Repair triceps fascia, anconeus fascia, subcutaneous tissues, and the skin.

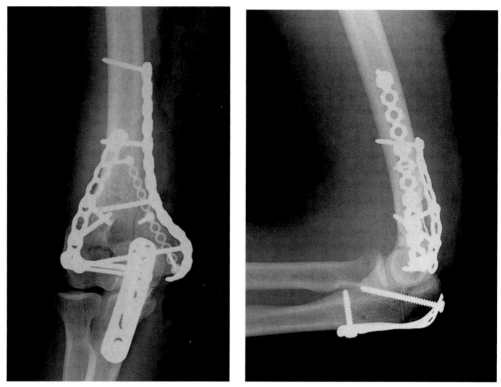

Figure 8-25 | Repair of olecranon osteotomy with periarticular plate.

Chapter 9
Proximal Radius and Ulna Fractures

DAPHNE M. BEINGESSNER
ANDREW R. EVANS
MICHAEL F. GITHENS
M. BRADFORD HENLEY
ANNA N. MILLER

Sterile Instruments/Equipment

Proximal Ulna Fractures

- Dental picks
- Freer elevators
- Small Hohmann retractors (narrow and wide)
- Small point-to-point clamps
- Kirschner wires
- Implants:
  - 3.5/2.7-mm head screws
  - 2.0- and 2.4-mm plate and screw sets
  - Proximal ulnar periarticular plating sets
  - 18-Gauge stainless steel cerclage wire or cable
  - 5.0-, 5.5-, 6.0-, or 6.5-mm cancellous intramedullary screw

Radial Head and Neck Fractures

- Dental picks
- Small point-to-point clamps
- Kirschner wires
- Implants:
  - 2.0- and 2.4-mm screw sets
  - Minifragment plate/screw set with T- and L-shaped plates
  - Radial head arthroplasty system of choice

Terrible Triad Injuries of the Elbow

- Dental picks
- Small point-to-point clamps
- Kirschner wires
- In-line ACL drill guide
- Implants:
  - 2.0- and 2.4-mm screw sets
  - Minifragment plate/screw set with T- and L-shaped plates
  - Nonabsorbable suture material (Ti-Cron or FiberWire)

- Radial head arthroplasty system of choice
- Suture anchors

Surgical Approaches

- *Dorsal extensile approach to the proximal ulna.*
  - For Monteggia fracture/dislocations, comminuted proximal ulna fractures, and olecranon fractures
  - Lateral or prone position
    - Drape affected arm over radiolucent arm board with the shoulder in a forward flexed (~90 degrees) and partially abducted (~90 degrees) position.
    - Verify that adequate C-arm imaging is possible prior to draping (Fig. 9-1).
      - The prone position provides improved C-arm access and imaging over the lateral position as there are fewer anatomical and positioning impediments (e.g., the opposite extremity, metal arm board support).
      - Alternatively, olecranon fractures can be treated with the patient in the supine position.

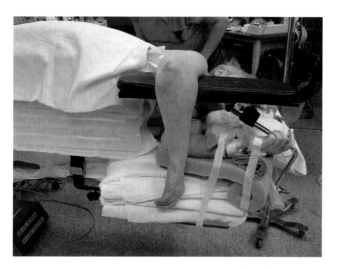

Figure 9-1 I Lateral positioning for a proximal ulna fracture.

TIP

Supine Positioning for Olecranon Fracture Fixation

M. Bradford Henley
Anna Miller

Pathoanatomy

Though the proximal ulna is typically approached with patients in a prone or lateral position, this may be imprudent in polytraumatized patients with concomitant neck, head, chest, lung, and or abdominal injuries.

Solution

A dorsal surgical approach with fixation may be performed easily with the patient in the supine position.

Technique

- When supine, the patient's head is positioned at the cranial corner of a radiolucent cantilever type OR table, ipsilateral to the injured extremity. The chest is moved laterally so that the shoulder on the affected side is just off the edge of the table.
- One (or two) arm board(s) usually used for prone positioning are attached at the head of the table, cranial to the patient's head, and extended distally parallel with the patient's body (Fig. 9-2).

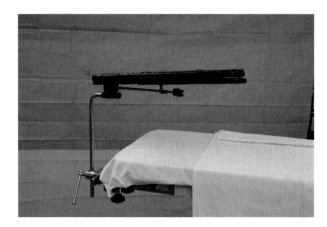

Figure 9-2 ‖ Set up for supine fixation of the proximal forearm and ulna. Note that the elevated armboard is attached to the head of the cantilever type OR table. Nothing is attached to the ipsilateral side of the table thereby allowing unencumbered C-arm access.

- The arm board(s) can be adjusted in height and medially or laterally so that the arm is balanced above the patient's thorax (Fig. 9-3).

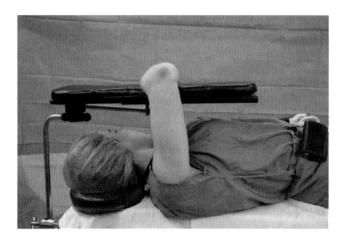

Figure 9-3 ‖ The arm board can be translated medially or laterally to balance the upper extremity. This reduces the need for an assistant to hold the arm in a stable position.

- For patients with large or long forearms, two arm boards may be placed side-by-side (Fig. 9-4).

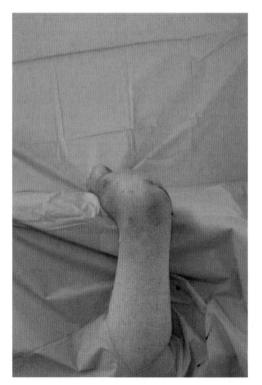

Figure 9-4 ‖ A clinical photograph of arm balanced on arm board after prepping and draping.

- Prepping and draping are done with the drapes placed over the arm board(s) and under the arm and forearm. This permits a circumferential prep resulting and a large sterile field. The arm is forward flexed 90 degrees at the shoulder and rests in a balanced position on the arm board(s).
- A dorsal exposure is performed and lateral images can be obtained by bringing the C-arm's anode under the drapes (Figs. 9-5 and 9-6).

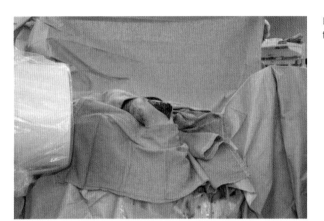

Figure 9-5 I Clinical photograph of positioning for lateral imaging.

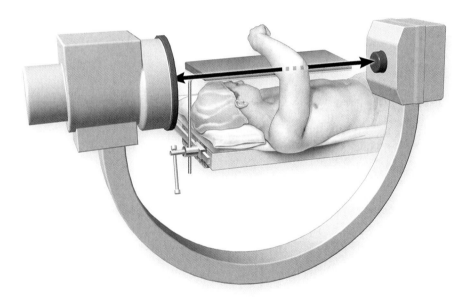

Figure 9-6 I Intraoperative lateral imaging.

- Internal fixation is also facilitated, as the forearm is supported by the arm board for posterior to anterior, medial to lateral, or lateral to medial drilling and screw placement in the proximal ulna.
- AP imaging is easily accomplished by manually abducting the arm with simultaneous extension of the elbow away from the table and arm board while bringing the C-arm to a vertical position.

- Skin incision located directly over subcutaneous border of the ulna, deviating radial to the olecranon process and returning to the dorsal midline.
  - Avoids dissection of the olecranon bursa
  - Places incision away from contact with desks and tables when extremity is resting on these surfaces
- Create full-thickness skin flaps radially and ulnarly to visualize the proximal ulnar shaft and olecranon process.
- If visualization of the medial aspect of greater sigmoid notch (semilunar fossa) is required, the ulnar nerve should be identified in the cubital tunnel and protected.
  - Ensure that the path of the ulnar nerve is known, either by palpation or direct visualization.[1]
- Avoid dissection of soft tissue attachments to fracture fragments.

- *Posterolateral (Kocher) approach to the elbow joint.*
  - For terrible triad injuries and radial head fractures and posterolateral elbow dislocations
  - Supine position:
    - Radiolucent hand or arm table.
    - Shift patient to the edge of the table so that elbow rests away from the junction of the hand table and OR table.
    - Prep and drape the entire involved upper extremity.
    - Be sure that the patient has adequate shoulder abduction and external rotation if access to the medial joint is required.
  - Two possible skin incisions to access the deep Kocher interval:
    - Obliquely across the radial head and radiocapitellar joint.
    - Posterior midline incision used with distal skin incision located directly over the subcutaneous border of the ulna.
      - Deviate radially around the tip of the olecranon.
      - Return incision to central dorsal location just proximal to lateral epicondyle.
      - Elevate a full-thickness flap laterally (radially), sufficiently to locate the fascial septum separating the extensor carpi ulnaris and anconeus, and incise the fascia sharply just ulnar to the septum.
  - Gently elevate anconeus off of the fascial septum, which often leads directly into the elbow joint if the capsule has been traumatically compromised due to the dislocation.
  - In terrible triad injuries, the lateral humeral epicondyle will often be "bald" due to avulsion of the lateral ligament complex.
    - The superficial fascial layer may be intact, and thus, the injury may appear to have an intact lateral ligament complex.
    - Raising full-thickness flaps will ensure that the full extent of the deep soft tissue injury is appreciated.
  - Identify the annular ligament, lateral ulnar collateral ligament, and the origin of the mobile extensor mass.

Reduction and Implant Techniques

Radial Head Fractures

- Locate all fractured fragments of the radial head (reassemble to confirm restoration of full head circumferentially).
  - Check olecranon, radial, and capitellar fossae for any unaccounted fragments or other fracture debris.
  - Take care while retracting distally over the radial neck and keep the forearm pronated.
    - This relaxes the posterior interosseous nerve (PIN) and rotates it into a safer position.
    - Do not place Hohmann retractors blindly around the radial neck or retract excessively, especially anteromedially.
  - The radial head is reconstructed in situ whenever possible (Fig. 9-7).

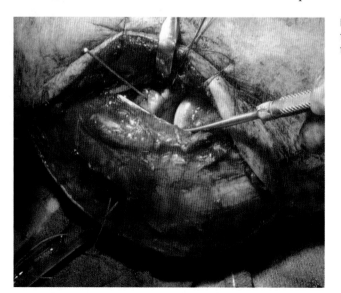

Figure 9-7 | In situ reduction and K-wire fixation of a comminuted radial head fracture.

■ The reduction is achieved with "joystick" wires and dental picks. Careful positioning of the "joystick" wire will allow them to be advanced for fragment fixation (Fig. 9-7).

■ Definitive fixation is typically achieved with countersunk 1.5- or 2.0-mm lag or position screws.

● If radial head is multifragmentary and fragments are displaced, remove displaced fragments and place on the back table in a saline moistened gauze or saline solution.

● On the back table, attempt to reduce the radial head fragments such that they may either be stabilized to the intact portion of the radial head/neck or sized appropriately for radial head arthroplasty.

■ Reassembling the radial head also confirms that all fracture fragments have been identified (Fig. 9-8).

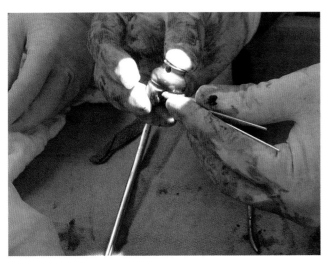 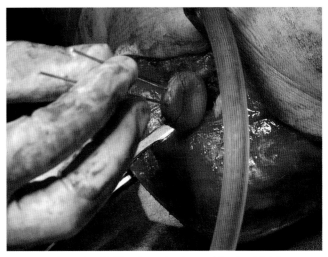

Figure 9-8 ▌The radial head is reassembled either in preparation for arthroplasty replacement **(left)** or for reduction and fixation **(right)**.

■ If the radial head fractures can be reduced for repair, a plate is used for fixation of the radial head to the neck segment. The plate must be placed in the safe zone to avoid implant impingement with the PRUJ (Fig. 9-9).

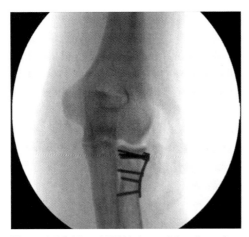 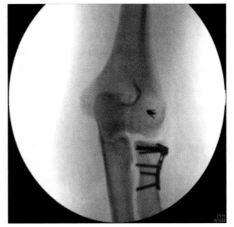

Figure 9-9 ▌AP and PRUJ views of the elbow demonstrating plate fixation of a comminuted radial head fracture. The PRUJ view demonstrates screws are not in the PRUJ.

● If the radial head fracture(s) cannot be reduced for repair, plans are made for arthroplasty. Determination of the height of the radial head implant should be made based upon AP and lateral fluoroscopic views of the elbow confirming that the articular surfaces of the coronoid (at the level of the trochlear groove) and radial head are at the same level.

■ On the AP view, the medial half of the ulnotrochlear joint should be concentric to avoid "overstuffing."

■ The joint space across the ulnohumeral articulation should be symmetric, accounting for the thickness of the articular cartilage on the coronoid portion of the greater sigmoid notch (Fig. 9-10).

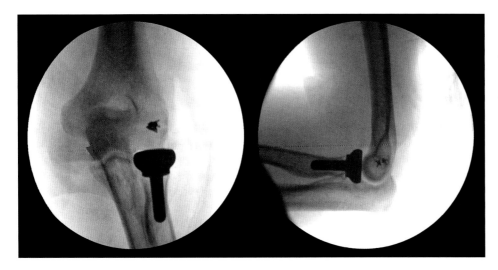

Figure 9-10 | Radial head arthroplasty. To ensure that the radiocapitellar joint is not "overstuffed," the medial ulnotrochlear joint should be symmetric (*left*, *arrowheads*).

- When the patient is supine, positioning of the arm for posterolateral access to the radial head causes an obligatory varus moment across the elbow.
  - This can improve access, but care must be taken to neutralize this stress when assessing the radial head height relative to the capitellum.
- The indication for radial head fixation versus arthroplasty is based upon intraoperative assessment of comminution, the ability to achieve an anatomic reduction with stable fixation of fracture fragments, and overall stability of radial head within the elbow joint.
  - In the setting of gross elbow instability associated with radial head fracture, secure fixation of the radial head is mandatory to maintain elbow stability during rehabilitation.
    - If it cannot be achieved, then radial head arthroplasty should be performed.

Radial Neck Fractures

- Reduction and fixation strategy depends on the fracture pattern.
  - Simple fractures without neck comminution may be treated with screw fixation alone.
  - 2–3 Bicortical countersunk 2.0- or 2.4-mm screws are place in an antegrade fashion from the rim of the radial head into the distal segment. These screws may be placed as lag or strut screws (Fig. 9-11).

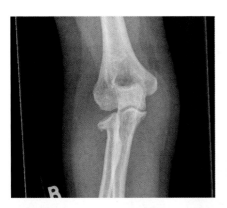
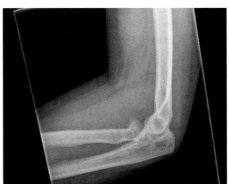
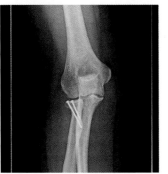
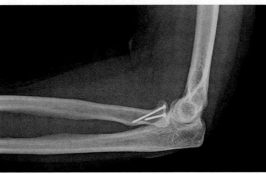

Figure 9-11 | Injury and postoperative AP and lateral radiographies demonstrating screw only fixation for a displaced radial neck fracture.

- Screw-only fixation avoids the potential problem of implant impingement in the PRUJ.
- When neck comminution is present, a bridging plate is placed in the safe zone. Anatomically contoured plates or a 2.0-mm T- or L-plate work well.

Olecranon Fractures and Transolecranon Fracture/Dislocations

- Fixation of the olecranon process
  - Modified tension band wiring
    - Only for noncomminuted simple transverse or short oblique fracture patterns proximal to the center of the greater sigmoid notch.
    - Either paired intraosseous K-wires or an intramedullary lag screw and washer may be used in combination with the tension band wire or cable.
    - Currently, plates are generally preferred over either tension band wire technique as plating provides secure fracture fixation with early ROM and a reduced chance of fixation failure.
  - Olecranon and proximal ulnar plating (Fig. 9-12)
    - Unicortical drill holes in on either side of the ulnar crest allow for anchorage of medial and lateral pointed reduction clamps for concentric reduction force.
    - K-wires to provisionally stabilize plate to bone
      - The reduced fracture is then stabilized provisionally with two or more 0.062-inch K-wires placed across the fracture in an oblique fashion. Ideally, these enter the medial and lateral proximal corners of the olecranon in an area that will not impede plate placement.
    - Alternatively, a centrally placed point-to-point reduction clamp may be used to achieve an interfragmentary reduction
      - After provisional stabilization with two crossed K-wires, the centrally placed bone reduction clamp may be removed and the chosen plate is then applied to the proximal ulna relying on the two crossed 0.062-inch K-wires to maintain fracture reduction.
    - A small longitudinal split in triceps insertion allows plate to lie flush with bone to avoid hardware prominence and tendon necrosis
    - Unicortical screw is placed through proximal portion of the plate, usually at the bend of plate as it curves around the olecranon. If this is placed at 45 degrees to the long and vertical (proximal olecranon) axes of the plate, it will nestle the plate to the olecranon tip.
      - Ideally, this screw will exert an equal force in the anterior and distal directions, orthogonal to the surface at the tip of the olecranon, thereby positioning the plate in intimate contact with the proximal ulna.
    - The second screw should be placed in the metadiaphysis, just distal to the fracture.
      - This screw is effective in neutralizing any anterior displacement of the proximal radius and ulna as is seen in Monteggia and transolecranon fracture dislocation patterns.
      - The plate's dorsal position will assist in neutralizing the deforming forces of the brachialis and biceps.

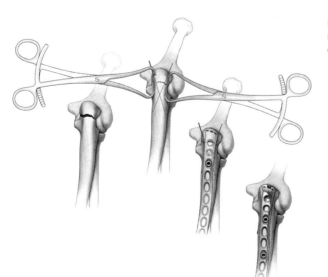

Figure 9-12 | Typical reduction and fixation sequence for facilitating plate fixation of olecranon fractures.

- Save all articular and cortical bone fragments, even when displaced in surrounding soft tissues or loose in fracture hematoma, so that they may be used to as aids in achieving an anatomical reduction.
    - Place an appropriately sized K-wire into small articular or cortical fragments for joystick manipulation to assist with reduction.
- Use minifragment plates on the lateral or medial surface of the proximal ulna for provisional metaphyseal fixation (Fig. 9-13).

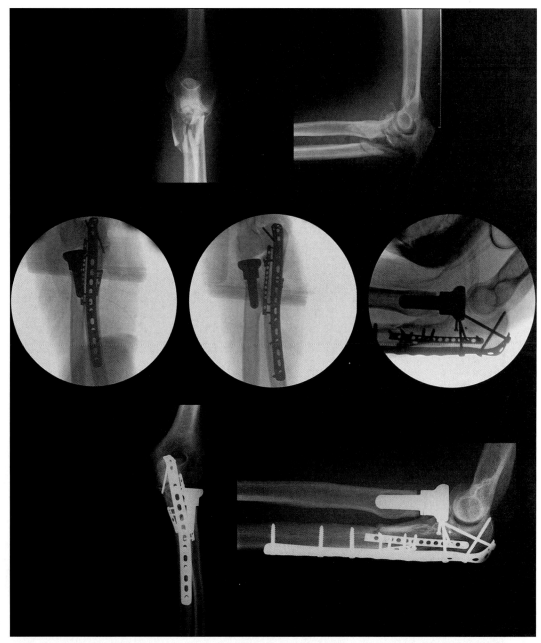

Figure 9-13 I Minifragment plates are frequently used in the reconstruction of the metadiaphyseal component of complex proximal ulnar fractures.

- Restore the articular congruity of the greater sigmoid notch prior to reduction and compression of fracture lines in the dorsal ulnar cortex.
    - Visualization of the articular reduction is accomplished through mobilization of the elbow capsule radially and/or ulnarly off of the proximal ulna as needed.
    - Do not detach the collateral ligaments.
    - Use the humeral trochlea as a "template" for articular reduction of the greater sigmoid notch/olecranon.

■ Bone graft osseous defects, using structural autograft, allograft, or an osteobiologic substitute, and then reduce the main olecranon fragment to the reconstructed articular segment.

■ Place a screw from the posterior olecranon anteriorly toward the coronoid.
  ○ This screw can be subchondral to support the articular surface, if previously impacted.
  ○ This screw should end on the anteromedial ulna to avoid the proximal radioulnar joint (Fig. 9-14)

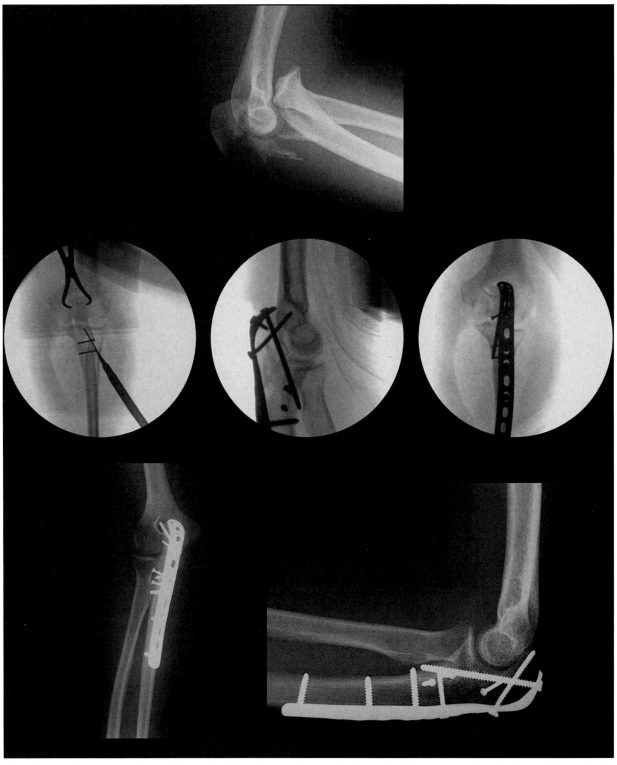

Figure 9-14 ▏ Transolecranon fracture/dislocation. The articular surface of the sigmoid notch was reconstructed initially and supported with a subchondral screw into the coronoid. A bicortical screw was also placed into the tip of the olecranon.

○ Alternatively, a long intramedullary screw can be inserted from this site or through one of the other proximal plate holes.

■ Place a bicortical screw into the proximal tip of the olecranon fragment to ensure rotational control and secure fixation, particularly when that fragment is small.

● By restoring the sigmoid notch in transolecranon fracture/dislocations, elbow stability is restored.

■ Ligament injuries are rare with this fracture pattern.

■ The proximal radioulnar joint remains reduced.

● In few ballistic injuries or open fractures with substantial bone loss, the olecranon cannot be repaired (Fig. 9-15).

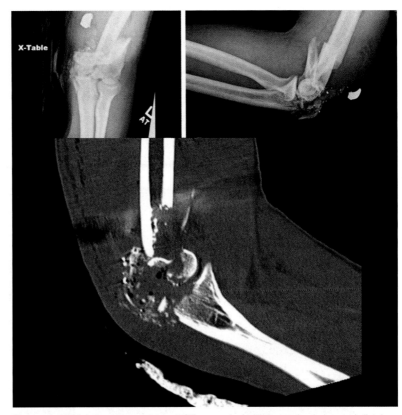

Figure 9-15 | Injury radiographs and CT scan of a ballistic proximal ulna and distal humerus fracture. The proximal ulna is not reconstructible given the comminution and bone loss.

● Restoring the extensor mechanism is critical for patient function

● In this case, an olecranon excision and triceps advancement can be performed.

▪ A last result salvage option

▪ Requires the triceps tendon to be good condition and in continuity with the triceps muscle.

▪ Additionally, the tendon must be of sufficient length to successfully advance to the proximal ulnar segment.

▪ The coronoid must be intact on the proximal ulnar segment to provide osseous stability, particularly to anterior humeral translation.

▪ All cortical, cancellous, and osteoarticular fragments are debrided.

▪ Two heavy (#5) braided sutures are placed in the triceps tendon using a running locking technique so that four limbs are available to secure to the proximal ulna.

- The sutures are passed through two long oblique osseous tunnels and tied over bone bridges (Fig. 9-16).
- The patient is splinted for a sufficient duration to allow associated soft tissue and wound healing. Early passive motion is initiated when soft tissue healing allows.

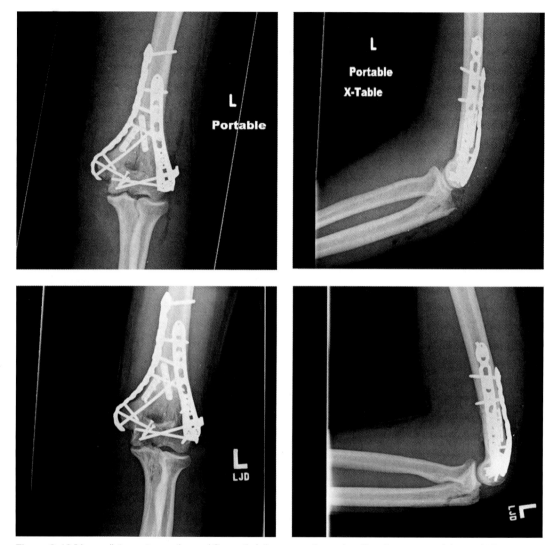

Figure 9-16 | Immediate postoperative and 3-month follow-up radiographs after olecranon excision and triceps advancement. The patient has a stable elbow with functional motion and no extensor lag.

Monteggia Fractures

- Provisionally reduce and stabilize the proximal ulna initially to allow for accurate sizing of radial head arthroplasty if necessary.
  - Anatomical restoration of ulnar length is also important in assuring stability and congruity of radioulnar and radiocapitellar articulations (Fig. 9-17).

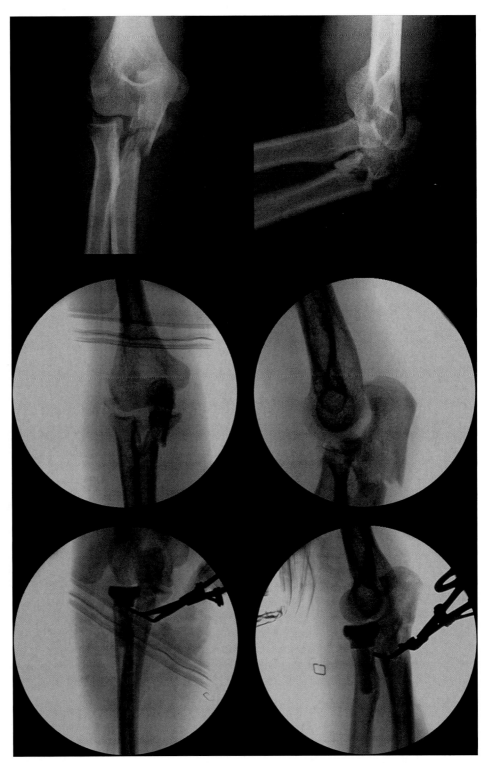

Figure 9-17 I Provisionally reducing the ulna is necessary prior to sizing the radial head arthroplasty to ensure proper height restoration.

- After radial neck cut has been made and trial components have been sized, disassemble the ulna and implant the definitive radial head prosthesis.
- Minifragment plates can be helpful to sequentially stabilize selected fracture lines and cortical fragments containing ligament insertions (Fig. 9-18).

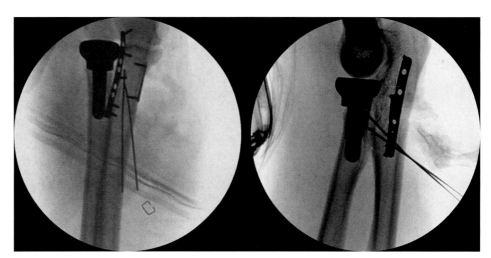

Figure 9-18 ‖ Following placement of the final radial head implant, the ulna is progressively reduced and stabilized.

- Finally, definitive ulnar fixation is applied (Fig. 9-19).

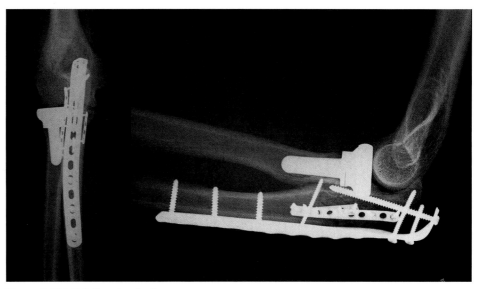

Figure 9-19 ‖ Definitive ulnar fixation.

- In most Monteggia fracture/dislocations, reduction and fixation of the proximal ulnar shaft fracture reduces the dislocated radial head indirectly.
  - Malreduction of the ulnar shaft can contribute to persistent subluxation or dislocation of the radial head after ulnar shaft reduction and must be addressed (Fig. 9-20).

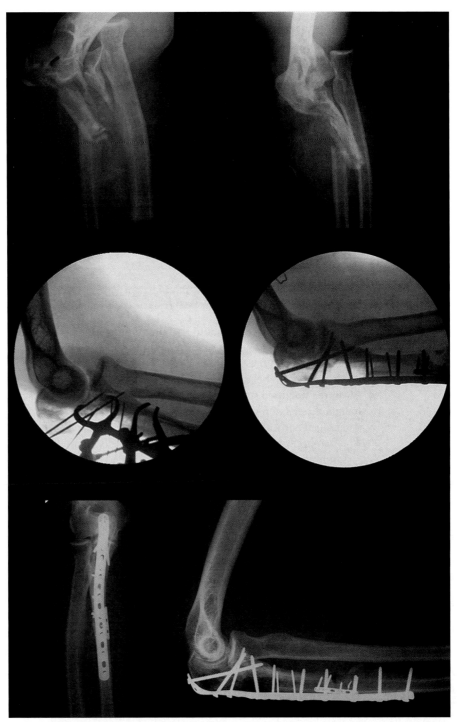

Figure 9-20 ▌ In this Monteggia fracture/dislocation, the initial ulnar reduction attempt led to subluxation of the radiocapitellar joint, indicating ulnar malreduction (*middle row, left*). Improving the ulnar reduction resulted in a concentric radiocapitellar reduction.

Terrible Triad Injuries

- A wrist examination and wrist radiographs should be performed routinely, to identify an Essex-Lopresti injury pattern.
- Treatment of the radial head fracture with fixation or arthroplasty should be deferred until after the coronoid fracture has been addressed.
  - However, if the radial head cannot be repaired, then perform the neck cut for the arthroplasty to improve visualization of the coronoid fracture reduction.
  - With partial articular radial head fractures that will undergo open reduction and internal fixation, address the coronoid injury anterior to the radial head/neck (e.g., through the displaced fracture).

- May subluxate the elbow dorsally to facilitate visualization of the coronoid fracture bed for preparation of drill holes for sutures or screws.
  - Fracture reduction is carried out with the elbow joint reduced (Fig. 9-21).

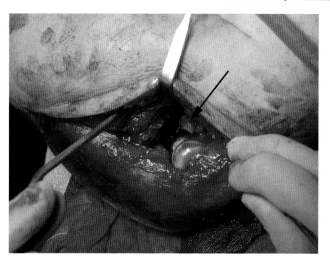

Figure 9-21 I With the elbow joint reduced, the coronoid fragment can be visualized though the resected radial head defect (*arrow*).

- Evaluate the size of the coronoid fracture fragment by direct visualization to determine whether it is sizeable enough to accept screw fixation (e.g., 2.0- or 2.4-mm lag screws × 2) or whether it will require wire or suture fixation.
  - A head lamp is helpful.
- Clean the fractured surface of the proximal ulna and reduce the coronoid fragment(s) to it and maintain reduction with Kirschner wires and/or clamps.
  - Confirm cortical and articular surface reduction reads.
  - When performing this reduction, reduce the elbow and flex it to reduce tension on the displaced coronoid (Fig. 9-22).

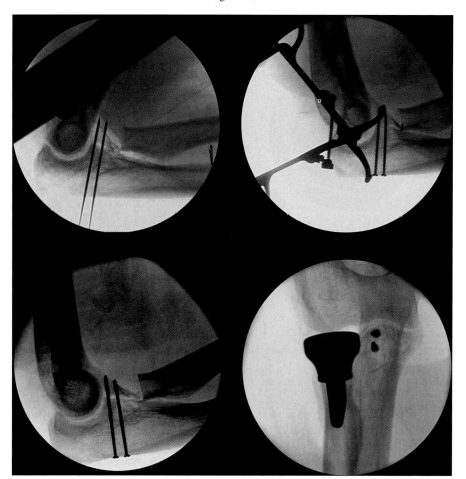

Figure 9-22 I Through the radial head defect, the coronoid can be clamped and provisionally stabilized with K-wires. Definitive screws are placed from the dorsal cortex of the ulna.

- Place drill holes through the dorsal ulna and into the coronoid fragment if possible for screw placement or for the passage of suture.
  - Drill hole placement for screw or suture fixation of the coronoid can be facilitated by the use of an in-line ACL drill guide to accurately position the gliding and pilot drill holes for lag screws or the two to three drill holes for suture(s) repair (Fig. 9-23).

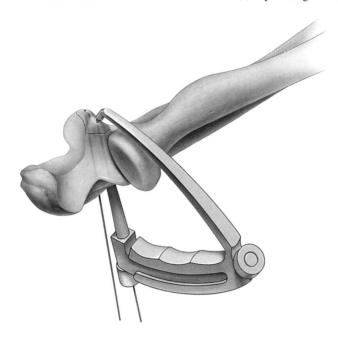

Figure 9-23 | An in-line ACL guide can be used to assist in coronoid reduction and for directing drill holes from the dorsal ulna for suture fixation.

- For suture fixation of the coronoid and/or anterior elbow capsule, use a durable, nonresorbable suture, such as Ti-Cron or FiberWire.
  - Drill two 2.0-mm holes with the in-line ACL drill guide (as above for screw fixation).
    - Suture should be passed through the ulna and the coronoid fragment.
      - Often helpful to also repair anterior capsule to extra-articular portion of coronoid.
      - If the bone fragment is too small or comminuted, then a suture placed into the anterior capsule and around the fragments will often suffice.
    - May use suture passer (e.g., Huson suture passer) to assist in passing suture from the coronoid through the proximal ulnar drill holes.
  - If using a nonmodular radial head replacement system or if operative fixation of radial head is facilitated through the visualization gained by elbow subluxation, perform those steps prior to definitive reduction of the elbow joint and securing of the coronoid sutures.
  - Secure fixation through the ulna into the coronoid fragment and/or anterior elbow capsule (Fig. 9-24).

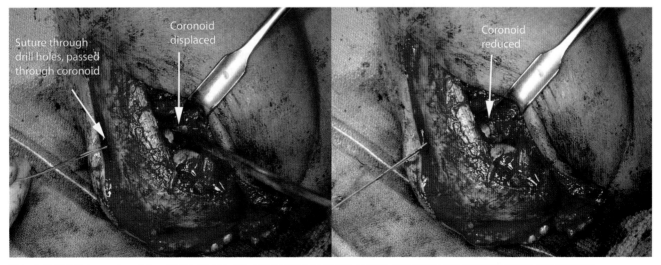

Suture through drill holes, passed through coronoid

Coronoid displaced

Coronoid reduced

Figure 9-24 | Sutures placed though the dorsal ulnar cortex can be used to capture and reduce the anterior capsule and coronoid.

- Tie sutures over cortical bridge between drill holes on the dorsal ulna with the elbow flexed.
  - Do not tie these sutures until radial head fixation or arthroplasty is complete, to avoid stressing the suture fixation or losing fracture reduction during implantation of radial head and reduction.
  - Several knots in heavy braided suture can cause discomfort when knot is subcutaneous.
  - To avoid this, make a small incision in the adjacent fascia, tuck the knots below the fascia, and oversew the fascia with absorbable suture.
- The repair of the lateral ligamentous complex is critical for elbow stability.
  - Identify the lateral ulnar collateral ligament (LUCL) remnant.
  - Gain sufficient visualization of extracartilagenous portion of lateral condyle and lateral epicondylar ridge to identify placement points for bone fixation through drill holes or with suture anchors within the lateral epicondyle.
  - Typically, one of these anchor points is placed at the center of rotation of the lateral epicondyle, and another proximally on the epicondylar ridge for fixation of the extensor/supinator/anconeus conjoined muscle-fascial origins.
    - For the repair of the avulsed soft tissues from the lateral epicondyle, spread the epicondylar fixation point(s) apart from the center of the condylar fixation point sufficiently.
      - If bone tunnels or suture anchors are used, this will avoid interference of fixation points for each suture or suture anchors.
  - Determine the appropriate location/tension for LUCL repair, and perform suture fixation of the LUCL to its lateral epicondylar origin.
    - Avoid a varus or valgus moment across the elbow joint when tying these sutures to achieve anatomic ligament repair.
    - Forearm midpronation also allows the sutures to be tied with the appropriate ligamentous tension.
- Clinically and fluoroscopically, evaluate elbow joint stability in the flexion/extension, varus/valgus, and pronation/supination axes.
  - Posterolateral rotatory instability must be assessed.
  - Ulnohumeral stability is assessed on the lateral view with the elbow taken through a full arc of motion in flexion and extension, in both supination and pronation to confirm stability.
  - If any subtle subluxation is present in one position, note this so as to determine the most appropriate static and/or dynamic splinting parameters (e.g., range of motion; extension block bracing).
  - The elbow should be stable through an arc of at least 20 to 130 degrees with the forearm in neutral rotation prior to leaving the operating room.
    - The most unstable position typically is full extension, with the forearm supinated with posterolateral dislocations.
  - Do not force the last 10 to 20 degrees of extension motion intraoperatively to avoid disruption of the coronoid repair, particularly if suture fixation was used.
    - Passive extension using gravity is the best test for terminal extension.
- Clinically and fluoroscopically evaluate the radial length at the wrist, as well as the distal radioulnar joint (DRUJ) stability.
  - Instability at the wrist or DRUJ may occur in the presence of an Essex-Lopresti injury to the forearm.
  - Repair this if necessary.
- If elbow remains unstable, proceed to the medial elbow through the same skin incision to evaluate the integrity of the flexor-pronator origins, the medial collateral ligament, all of which may be persistent sources of elbow instability.
  - Instability requiring medial ligament repair is uncommon, if the coronoid and medial aspect of the ulnohumeral articulation are unfractured or anatomically repaired and stable.
  - Valgus instability alone is not an indication for medial ligament repair.
  - If instability persists, verify the integrity and accuracy of the lateral repair.

Anteromedial Coronoid Facet Fractures

- The sublime tubercle of the anteromedial coronoid serves as the insertion for the medial collateral ligament (Fig. 9-25).
- Thus, anteromedial coronoid facet fractures render the elbow joint unstable and should be surgically repaired.

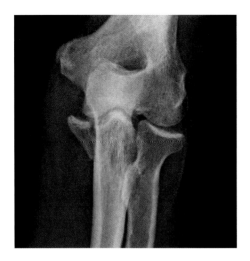
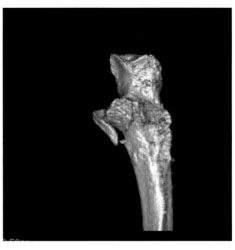

Figure 9-25 | AP radiograph and CT scan demonstrating a displaced two-part anteromedial coronoid facet fracture.

- Often require plating with a small four to six hole 2.0-mm plate, or an anatomically precontoured plate, with or without bone grafting of the articular impaction injury[2] (Fig. 9-26).

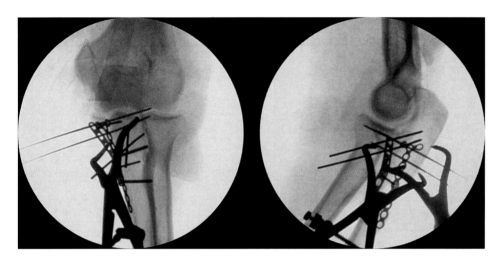

Figure 9-26 | Reduction and provisional fixation of a displaced anteromedial coronoid fragment.

- Posterior midline incision used and then medial approach is used to access the coronoid base, medial collateral ligament (MCL) insertion, medial elbow capsule, and anteromedial facet.
  - Supine position.
  - Ulnar nerve identified, dissected free, and protected.
  - Elevate or split flexor-pronator mass taking care to avoid injury to the MCL (Fig. 9-27).

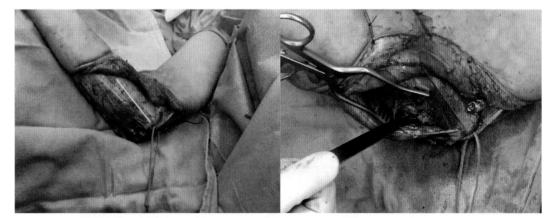

Figure 9-27 | After a long posterior incision is made and a subcutaneous flap is raised, the ulnar nerve is identified and protected. The *yellow* strip indicates the location of the fascial incision for the flexor-pronator mass split. The proximal medial ulna is carefully exposed.

- Suture anchors may be required for suture fixation of the MCL, which is most commonly avulsed from its ulnar attachment onto the base of the coronoid process.
- Alternatively, if the coronoid fragment is large enough, it is fixed with a 2.0-mm T-plate or straight plate (Fig. 9-28).

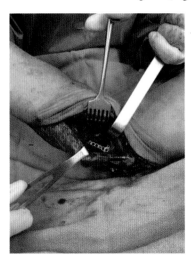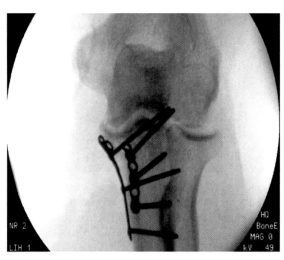

Figure 9-28 | Intraoperative photograph and fluoroscopic images demonstrating plate fixation of an anteromedial coronoid facet fracture.

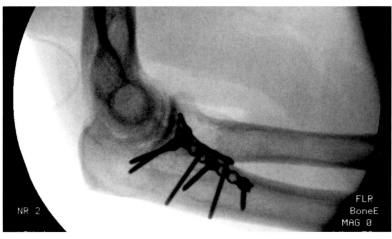

- Plate fixation may be augmented with suture fixation of the MCL.
- Additionally, the lateral ligaments may be injured concomitantly, so stability assessment and ligament repair should be performed if necessary.
  - Can elevate lateral full-thickness skin flap through same incision if lateral ligament repair is needed (see above for technical tips) (Fig. 9-29).

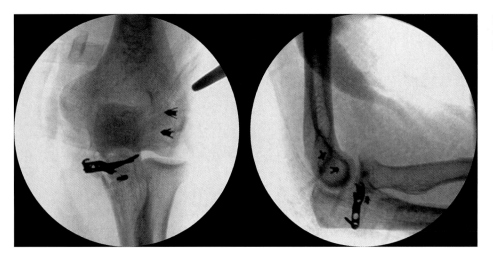

Figure 9-29 | Anteromedial coronoid fracture with concomitant lateral ligament repair.

References

1. Lindenhovius AL, Brouwer KM, Doornberg JN, et al. Long-term outcome of operatively treated fracture-dislocations of the olecranon. *J Orthop Trauma*. 2008;22(5):325–331.
2. Ring D, Doornberg JN. Fracture of the anteromedial facet of the coronoid process. Surgical technique. *J Bone Joint Surg Am*. 2007;89(suppl 2 Pt 2):267–283.

Chapter 10
Forearm Fractures

MARK R. ADAMS
CHRISTOPHER DOMES
MICHAEL F. GITHENS
MICHAEL S. SIRKIN
MATTHEW P. SULLIVAN
LISA A. TAITSMAN
RAYMOND D. WRIGHT JR

Sterile Instruments/Equipment

- 3.5-mm compression plates with 3.5-mm cortical screws
- Alternatively, a curved 3.5-mm compression plate (pediatric femur plate) for the radius
- 2.7-mm plates, especially for distal ulnar diaphyseal fractures
- 2.0- and 2.4-mm screws
- On-table plate-bending press or handheld bender and torqueing irons
- Small pointed bone reduction clamps
- Small serrated bone reduction clamps
- K-wires and wire driver/drill

Patient Positioning

- Supine position with a radiolucent arm table.
- May use proximal arm tourniquet, if desired.
- Surgeon is usually seated in the patient's axilla.

Surgical Approaches

- Ulna: direct approach to subcutaneous border of ulna. Use interval between ECU and FCU.
  - If the ECU or FCU has been traumatically disrupted, continue elevation of this muscle to avoid plating directly on the subcutaneous ulnar ridge.
  - Plate may be placed on the volar surface (under FCU), on the dorsal surface (under ECU), or directly on the subcutaneous border of ulna.
    - The ideal location should depend primarily on the fracture morphology.
- Radius: volar Henry's approach for exposure of the radius
  - Allows extensile exposure from proximal to distal radial shaft
    - Retract radial artery ulnarly
  - Alternatively, through sheath and bed of FCR tendon, then, retract radial artery radially.

Reduction and Fixation Techniques

- For both bone forearm fractures, usually approach and reduce the fracture with the simpler pattern first.
  - Restores length of the forearm anatomically.
  - This facilitates anatomic reduction with the other bone and subsequently facilitates reduction of the more complex fracture.

- Multiple independent 2.0- or 2.4-mm lag screws are useful for fractures with comminution (e.g., butterfly, segmental). After interfragmentary lag screw fixation, a neutralization plate is applied spanning the area of injury.
- Usually, plates are placed on the volar surface of the ulna (under FCU, in the flexor compartment) to avoid implant irritation as patients rest their forearms on their direct ulnar border.
  - However, if either the extensor carpi ulnaris or the flexor carpi ulnaris is stripped/disrupted more than the other, this muscle should be elevated preferentially.
  - The plate should be placed under the elevated muscle, preserving the soft tissue attachments and, hence, the blood supply of the intact muscle (Fig. 10-1).

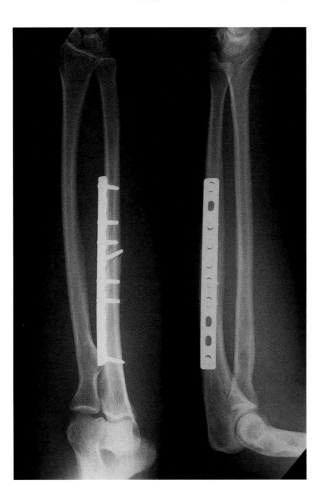

Figure 10-1 I Ulnar plate placed on the flexor surface.

- For distal one-fourth ulnar fractures, consider a 2.7- or 2.4-mm compression or locking plate, especially for individuals of small stature or with osteoporosis.
  - Hole spacing of the plate will allow more points of fixation in a short distal segment.
  - Additionally, a 2.7-mm plate may have a better coronal plane fit than a 3.5-mm plate (Fig. 10-2).

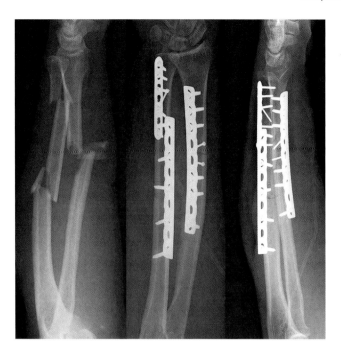

Figure 10-2 I A segmentally comminuted ulnar fracture stabilized with two plates. A smaller plate was used for distal ulnar shaft fracture as it permitted fixation with more screws and offered a lower-profile plate fit.

- Once length and stable fixation is obtained in one bone, the wound should be closed prior to performing the second approach to the other forearm bone.
  - In acute trauma, generally only the skin and subcutaneous tissues are closed over the plate, to avoid compartmental syndrome.
  - However, in subacute fractures, consideration may be given to closing the fascia of the FCU to the fascia of the ECU over the border of the ulna.
  - If an anatomic reduction cannot be verified (e.g., in a comminuted fracture), the first incision may be left open to allow adjustment after reduction and fixation of the other bone.
- For segmental radial shaft fractures, for example, with distal extension, consider applying two overlapping plates.
  - Reconstruct the anatomic radial bow.
  - Fully supinated AP view with contralateral comparison is helpful to confirm symmetry of radii.
  - Additionally, account for several degrees of apex dorsal bow in contouring plate(s) (Fig. 10-3).

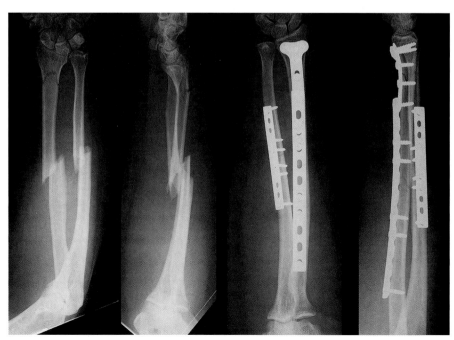

Figure 10-3 I Overlapping plates for a segmental radius fracture with distal extension. The distal plate is a thinner buttress plate, and shaft is stabilized with a thicker compression plate.

- A plate-bending press can be used to bend a 3.5-mm LC-DCP "on the flat" to contour the plate to match the radial bow and to allow a segmentally comminuted fracture to be stabilized with a long plate placed on its volar surface (e.g., 12 to 18 holes) (Fig. 10-4).

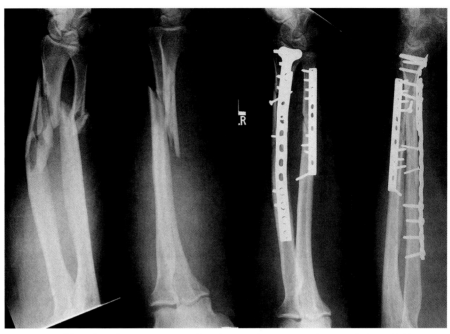

Figure 10-4 ▌ A 12-hole 3.5-mm compression plate can be contoured to match the radial bow. In this case, the 12-hole plate overlaps a short plate buttressing the distal radius. The contouring may also be achieved preoperatively using a skeletal model so that only a minimal amount of additional contouring is required intraoperatively.

- If segmental comminution is spanned using a bridge-plating technique, plate contouring may not be necessary.
  - When long straight plate is applied to the volar aspect of the radius in a bridge-plating mode, it should be translated slightly radially at each end, so that it is centered over the medullary canal of the radius in its central portion.
  - This will permit bicortical screws to be inserted in both fracture fragments, close to the fracture and at each end of the plate.
    - Because the radius is wider distally than proximally, the plate can be translated radially in its distal extent to a greater degree than it can be translated proximally.

- This technique allows for restoration of the anatomic radial bow (Fig. 10-5).

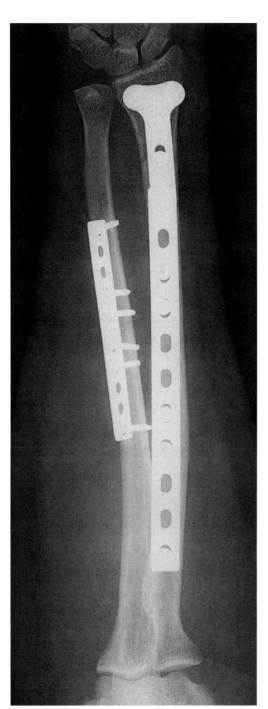

Figure 10-5 I If a straight plate is placed over a long curved segment of bone, and the radial bow is restored, the plate should be translated slightly radially at its proximal and distal ends, so that its central portion overlies the bone and not the interosseous membrane. This will permit the insertion of bicortical screws though nearly any hole in the plate.

■ Alternatively, use a long anatomically contoured metadiaphyseal plate for the radius with the concomitant restoration of radial bow (Fig. 10-6).

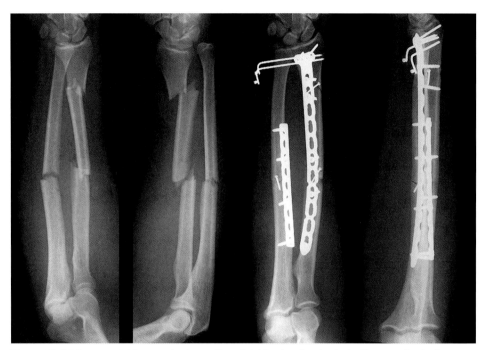

Figure 10-6 I A segmental forearm fracture with a distal fracture line treated with an anatomically contoured plate assists with the restoration of anatomical radial bow.

TIP

Operative Fixation of Radial Shaft Fractures with Curved 3.5-mm Compression Plate

Lisa Taitsman
Christopher Domes

Pathoanatomy

Restoration of radial bow in radial shaft fractures is important in restoring normal forearm rotation and biomechanics. Fracture fixation of the radius with the classically described 3.5-mm straight compression plate can be challenging due to its natural bow. This necessitates either eccentric plate placement on a portion of the radius or a malreduction (Fig. 10-7). This is more likely in fractures with extensive comminution or long fracture segments. Some surgeons are able to contour the standard compression plate, adding a bow in the plane of the plate, but this is difficult to achieve.

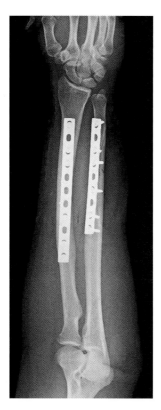
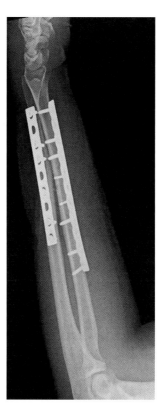

Figure 10-7 I Radial bow to plate mismatch that occurs when using the classically described 3.5-mm straight compression plate.

Solution

Precontoured, curved 3.5-mm compression plates are made by several manufacturers. Some are designed for fixation of pediatric femur fractures. These plates match the radius' native radial bow in adults and can be used for fixation of metaphyseal and diaphyseal fractures (Fig. 10-8).

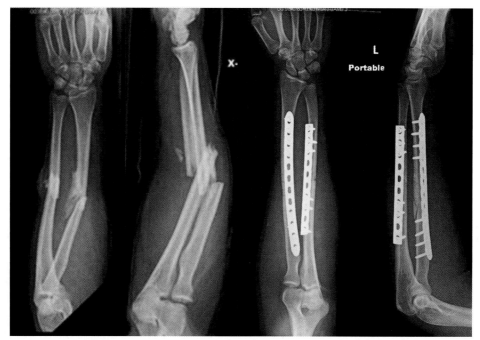

Figure 10-8 I A precontoured 3.5-mm curved plate better matches the native radial bow than does a 3.5-mm straight plate.

Technique

- The radial fracture is exposed via standard surgical approaches.
  - Typically, this is done through a volar Henry's approach.
- The fracture is reduced and provisionally stabilized with reduction clamp(s) and/or K-wire(s).
  - Alternatively, the fracture can be reduced to the plate during fixation.
- A curved 3.5-mm compression plate is chosen, placed provisionally on the volar surface of the radius, and secured at each end with unicortical K-wires.
  - Its position is verified with C-arm imaging.
  - A wide variety of plate length exists, which aids in plate selection.
- Once an acceptable reduction and position is achieved, the plate is affixed to the bone using the appropriate technique.
  - If the fracture pattern permits, compression of the fracture may be achieved using the plate.
  - Alternatively, the plate can also be used as a neutralization plate or bridge plate depending upon the extent of comminution and fracture pattern.
  - In comminuted fractures, the curve of the plate can be useful in facilitating a plate reduction.
- Radiographs of the contralateral intact side can be used for comparison to ensure restoration of native radial bow.
- If ulnar fixation is required, this is completed and forearm range of motion is checked and compared to the contralateral side.

- Sometimes, a mismatch between the contour of the plate and the surface of the bone will cause a malreduction when the screws are tightened (Fig. 10-9).

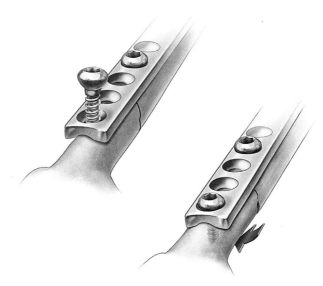

Figure 10-9 | Due to the relatively small ratio of the plate width to forearm bone shaft width, plate-derived malreductions can occur easily (*arrow*). Care should be taken to place the ends of the plate centrally on the bone and to place the plate on the flat portion of the radius to minimize this effect. If screw tightening causes fracture malreduction, this screw should be loosened and a different screw placed first in that fragment.

- This is usually a torsional problem and can be avoided by initially stabilizing the plate distally to the "flattest" volar portion of the radius.
  - If the flat undersurface of the plate is perfectly parallel to this flat osseous surface (after placing two or more screws through the distal portion of the plate), then screws placed perfectly orthogonally to the plate through the holes proximal to the fracture will not cause bone rotation as these screws are tightened.
  - Additionally, clamps placed on the plate near the fracture and their subsequent replacement by screws will minimize the torsional and translational malreductions.
- In oblique fracture patterns, it is preferential to place the first screw in the plate that creates an acute angle "plate-bone axilla."
- If the plate contour is acceptable and an anatomic or nearly anatomic provisional reduction has been achieved, place the far screws on both sides of the plate first, accommodating for the radial bow.

- The fracture pattern must be amenable to this technique (e.g., transverse or segmentally comminuted).
- This allows the plate to be centered precisely on the bone, so that all screws are bicortical, along the length of the plate.
- Screws can be placed in compression mode but not fully tightened.
- Clamps can then be placed near the fracture site to "fine-tune" the reduction (usually translational), followed by tightening of screws for fracture compression (Fig. 10-10).

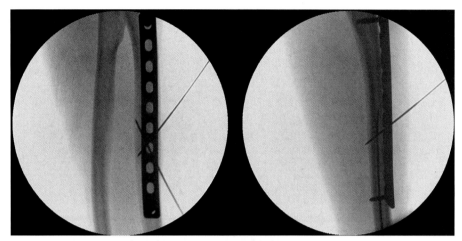

Figure 10-10 ▌ With a nearly anatomical reduction stabilized by crossed K-wires, screws are placed at each end of the plate. One is placed in a neutral mode, and the other in a compression mode. The screws are not fully tightened. The fracture reduction is then fine-tuned under the plate and the screws are tightened, providing interfragmentary compression, after achieving an anatomical reduction.

- Alternatively, place small bone reduction clamps so as to straddle each end of the plate such that the plate is contained between the two "arms" of the clamp.
  - This centers the plate on the bone directly.
  - The small serrated bone reduction clamps work best in this application.
- For long segmental fractures, particularly with distal extension, AO wrist fusion plates allow for a low-profile distal implant with appropriate screw hole clustering (Fig. 10-11).

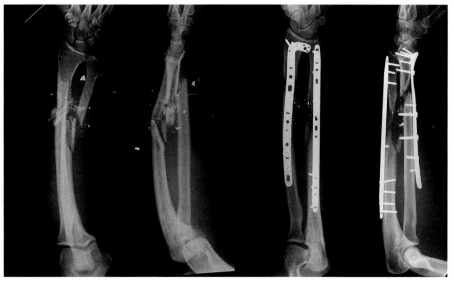

Figure 10-11 ▌ A wrist fusion plate for a segmental ulnar fracture with bone loss.

- In proximal radial shaft fractures, avoid placement of the plate too ulnarly on the bicipital tuberosity, since it may cause impingement of the biceps tendon insertion (Fig. 10-12).

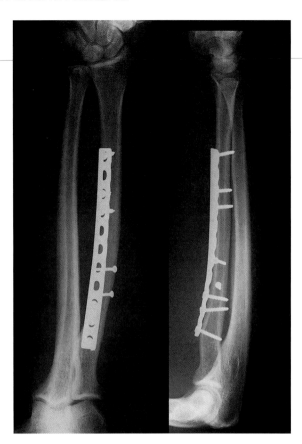

Figure 10-12 | Proximal radial plates should be placed so as to avoid the bicipital tuberosity. In this position, the plate is more likely to impinge on the proximal ulna in full pronation. This plate should have been translated more radially in its distal extent. Doing so would have allowed for screw placement in its central portion.

- Range of motion should be checked, particularly in pronation, prior to closing.
- For comminuted proximal ulnar shaft fractures, removing the proximal (olecranon) extension of a periarticular precontoured plate allows for a better plate fit over the diaphyseal portion of the plate.
  - This is particularly helpful in revisions, when a new plating surface over the dorsal ulnar spine is selected (Fig. 10-13).

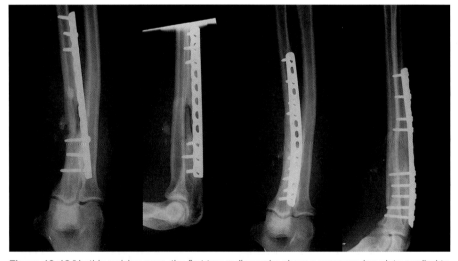

Figure 10-13 | In this revision case, the first two radiographs show a compression plate applied to the proximal ulna, under the ECU. This plate was removed because of inadequate fixation to the proximal fracture fragment. The plate was replaced with an anatomically contoured periarticular proximal ulnar plate applied to the dorsal, subcutaneous border of the ulna. The proximal olecranon portion of the plate was removed as sufficient fixation could be achieved without this portion. This may be beneficial as the olecranon portion of a dorsal plate is often subcutaneous and has the propensity to cause patients discomfort in this location.

- Alternatively, IM nailing can be an excellent solution for segmentally comminuted radius and/or ulna fractures.

Radius and Ulna Fractures: IM Nailing

Matthew Sullivan
Michael Githens

Pathophysiology

Fixation of proximal fractures of the forearm bones may not be easily amenable to plate fixation.

Solution

Certain fractures of the radius and/or ulna may lend themselves to intramedullary fixation. These clinical situations include

- Proximal comminution
- Segmental fractures
- Ballistic injury
- Osteopenic bone or osteolytic tumor (e.g., Brown's tumor)
- Low-demand patient
- Significant soft tissue injury in which a plate might best be avoided (Fig. 10-14)

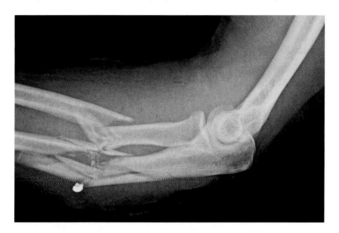

Figure 10-14 | Comminuted proximal radius and ulnar shaft fractures resulting from a low-velocity gunshot.

Surgical Goals
- Restoration of length, alignment, and rotation of each bone
- Restoration of radial bow
- Minimizing surgical soft tissue trauma

Forearm Nailing Pros
- Minimal iatrogenic soft tissue injury
- Indirect reduction with minimal biologic cost to fracture site

Forearm Nailing Cons
- Difficult to reestablish radial bow.
- Unlocked nails may not provide sufficient rotational stability.
- Depending on implant choice, rotation may be difficult to control.

Technique

Technique and Positioning for Nailing the Radius and/or Ulna
Supine on radiolucent hand table if one bone will be plated and one nailed:

- Initial control of the forearm may be difficult. If planning plate fixation of one bone and IM nailing of the other, plate first to provide restoration of forearm length and initial stability to limb for nailing.
- If nailing both bones, utilize an assistant for traction or consider nailing in the lateral position (see below).
- Finger traps can be hung off the end of the hand table (or from the ceiling) to provide longitudinal traction for retrograde nailing of the radius.

When only the radius is comminuted and plate fixation of the ulna can be achieved:

- Initiate treatment with open reduction and plate fixation of ulna in order to achieve length, alignment, and rotation.
- Then perform closed reduction and intramedullary fixation of the radius (Fig. 10-15).

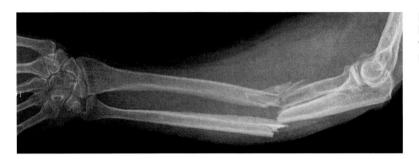

Figure 10-15 I Osteopenic both-bone forearm fracture with comminuted proximal radius fracture.

Surgical technique for proximal ulna fixation with minimal assistance:

- Positioning: supine with the arm prepped and draped on a radiolucent hand table.
- Sterile finger traps are applied to the digits, and the finger traps are then hung from the ceiling with sterile rope.
  - Flex the elbow approximately 90 degrees so the (upper) arm is still supported by the hand table. Once the forearm is positioned in this fashion, the surgeon has full access to the subcutaneous and medial and lateral borders of the forearm without requiring additional hands to hold the unstable forearm (Fig. 10-16).

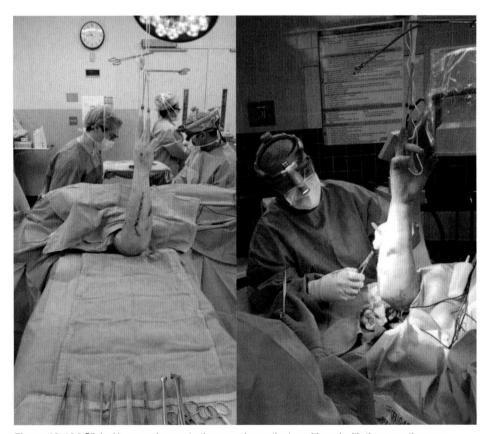

Figure 10-16 I Clinical images demonstrating a supine patient positioned with the operative arm over a hand table and fingers/forearm suspended from a ceiling hook with the aid of finger traps. No assistants are required to hold the arm, and the surgeon has full access to the ulnar aspect of the forearm. In addition to providing effortless positioning of the limb, the finger traps provide a moderate traction force, which assists in fracture reduction.

- Use of an anatomically contoured proximal ulna plate of which the olecranon extension is removed (cut off) is an excellent option for proximal ulna fractures that do not require fixation into the olecranon.
- These plates are anatomically precontoured to reproduce the varus bow of the proximal ulna, which can be challenging to contour in a stiff plate (Fig. 10-17).

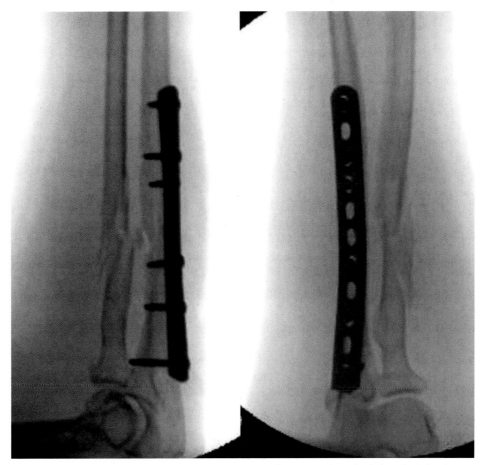

Figure 10-17 | Ulna fixation is achieved with an anatomically contoured proximal ulna plate showing that the proximal olecranon portion has been cut off. These plates are designed to fit the ulna's proximal varus bow.

Surgical technique for proximal radius fixation:

- The finger traps are released and the elbow is extended so that the forearm rests on the hand table. In-line traction applied via sterile finger traps if required with a weight suspended from the end of the table.
- For a radial styloid entry portal, a 3.5-mm drill is used to open the cortex with a longitudinal trajectory so as to minimize the risk of iatrogenic radial styloid fracture. The positions of the radial artery and dorsal cutaneous branch of the radial nerve should be noted (Fig. 10-18).

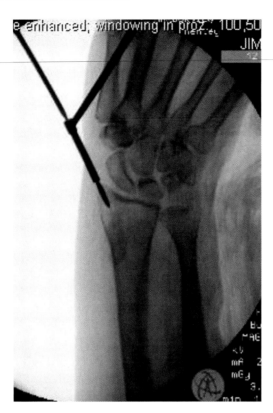

Figure 10-18 | The radial styloid is opened with a 3.5-mm drill bit. Notice that cortex is perforated just radial to the most distal aspect of the styloid and the trajectory aligned closely with the intramedullary canal of the radius. This mitigates the risk of iatrogenic radial styloid fracture when the intramedullary device is place.

- Preoperative templating will guide elastic nail size. Typically, a 2.5- to 4.0-mm nail will be appropriate.
- The nail should be contoured so as to reproduce the native radial bow.
- The nail should be passed under fluoroscopic guidance to avoid perforation or incarceration and ultimately should be advanced into the metaphyseal bone of the radial neck (Fig. 10-19).

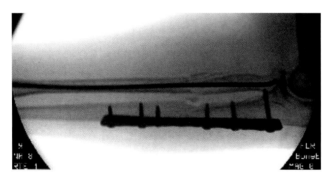

Figure 10-19 | The elastic nail is advanced into the metaphyseal bone of the radial neck/head.

- Upon completion of radius fixation, rotational alignment of the radius can be evaluated based on the relationship between the biceps tuberosity and the radial styloid. These two structures should lie within the same plane 180 degrees opposite from one another.
- Final plain x-rays (supinated AP and lateral) confirm anatomic rotational alignment of the radius as well as anatomic varus bow of the proximal ulna (Figs. 10-20 and 10-21).

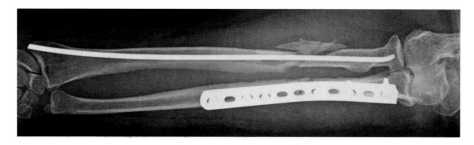

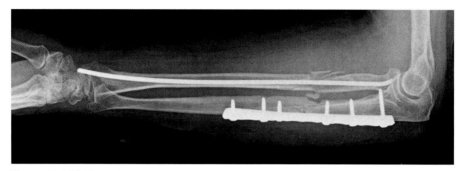

Figure 10-20 | AP and lateral images demonstrate restoration of radius' rotational alignment and proximal ulna bow.

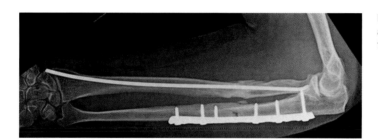

Figure 10-21 | Follow-up imaging at 3 months demonstrates excellent fracture healing.

Lateral positioning should be considered if both bones will be nailed as this will permit access to both bones and their entry portals should they be nailed simultaneously or sequentially:

- Lateral position with a traction device and sterile finger traps is an excellent option when nailing both bones.
- Provides easy access to both entry sites.
- Facilitates AP and lateral C-arm images solely by C-arm rotation without repositioning the forearm and without changing forearm rotation (and images can be obtained in pronation/neutral/supination as required).
- Traction via finger traps obtains and maintains an excellent reduction.
- Allows use of percutaneous or limited open techniques to fine-tune reduction if needed.
- Use of sterile finger traps can be advantageous if they may need to be removed to reposition arm intraoperatively (Figs. 10-22 and 10-23).

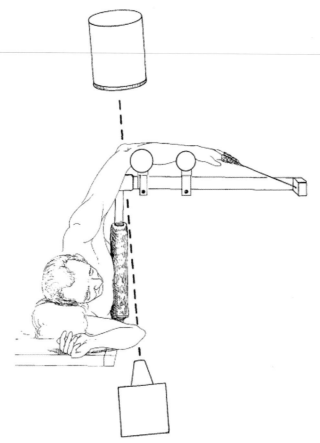

Figure 10-22 | Schematic of lateral positioning using OR table–mounted positioning frame, which permits antegrade nailing of the ulna and retrograde nailing of the radius. The forearm may be positioned in pronation, neutral, or supination as necessary as traction is maintained via finger traps.

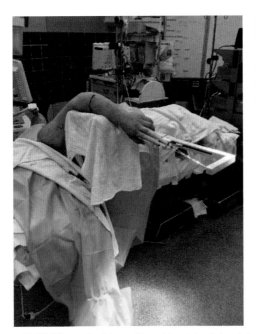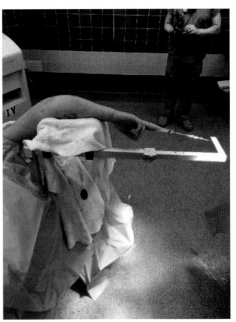

Figure 10-23 | The patient is positioned in a lateral decubitus position. Prior to draping, nonsterile finger traps and traction are applied to ensure adequate imaging and satisfactory provisional reduction.

- Prior to surgery, obtain supinated AP and lateral radiographs of the uninjured, contralateral forearm for intraoperative comparison.
- Depending on the implant being used, preoperative nail contouring may be advantageous. A sterile composite forearm model can be used as a template for contouring. The surgeon should also reference the contralateral forearm images when contouring the implants.

Reduction

- If planning plate fixation of one bone, perform this first as it will provide partial indirect reduction of the other bone.
- Closed reduction with traction is typically sufficient and ideal as the fracture site is not disrupted (Fig. 10-24).
- A hand reamer or the nail may be inserted into the near segment and used for manipulative reduction of the fracture to allow nail passage (Fig. 10-25).

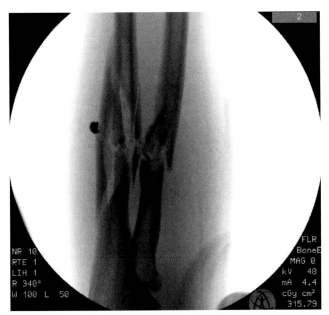

Figure 10-24 I Closed reduction with longitudinal traction in finger traps restores length and alignment.

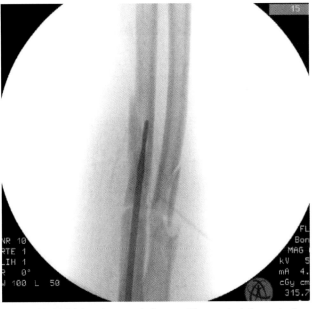

Figure 10-25 I A hand reamer being used for manipulative reduction to traverse the fracture using a "push-through" technique.

- If closed techniques do not provide an adequate reduction, percutaneous application of a shoulder hook or 2.5-mm Schanz pin as a pushing or pulling device allows manipulative reduction throughout the case.
- If these means remain insufficient, a limited open approach at the site of the fracture is performed. Fracture fragment stripping is kept to a minimum, and fracture hematoma is disturbed as little as possible.

Ulna entry portal for an antegrade nail:

- A 0.062-inch K-wire is used to localize the entry site, which is coaxial with the intramedullary canal on both the AP and lateral views. This is driven into the olecranon process approximately 1 cm (Fig. 10-26).

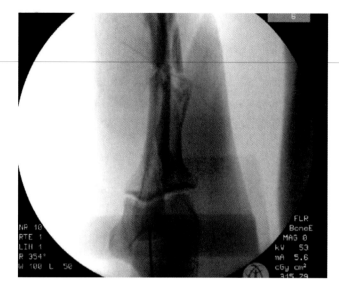

Figure 10-26 I Entry site is localized with a 0.062-inch K-wire.

- A 4.0-mm cannulated drill is used to create a coaxial entry portal. Once the wire is engulfed by the drill bit, its trajectory may be adjusted and advanced another 1 cm ensuring a coaxial entry portal on AP and lateral views (Fig. 10-27).

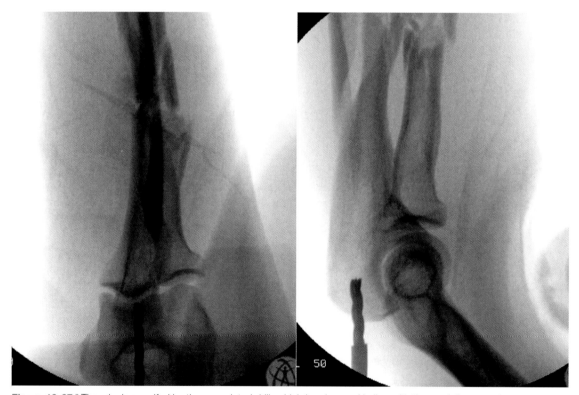

Figure 10-27 I The wire is engulfed by the cannulated drill, which is advanced in line with the medullary canal.

Radius entry portal for a flexible (e.g., titanium) retrograde nail:

- Depending on the implant chosen, one of two entry portals may be chosen.
  - Radial styloid entry site: Between first and second dorsal extensor compartments ("snuffbox")
    - Small open approach to the tip of the radial styloid to prevent iatrogenic radial artery injury
  - Second dorsal compartment entry site: In ulnar portion of second extensor compartment (retract ECRB and ECRL), and radial to Lister's tubercle and EPL (see below re precontoured rigid nail)

- A 0.062-inch K-wire is used to localize the entry site, which is on the most distal tip of the styloid on the AP and lateral view. This is driven in 1 cm.
- A 3.5- or 4.0-mm cannulated drill bit is passed over the wire and advanced another 1.5 cm ensuring correct trajectory on AP and lateral views.

Rigid Precontoured Nail
- Open approach to the second dorsal compartment. A 3-cm longitudinal incision is just radial to Lister's tubercle centered over the wrist joint. Retract ECRB/ECRL.
- A 0.062-inch K-wire is used to localize the entry site, which is just proximal to the dorsal rim of the distal radius on lateral view and in line with the canal on the AP view. This is driven in 1 cm.
- A 4.0-mm cannulated drill bit is used to drill over the wire and advanced another 1.5 cm ensuring correct trajectory on AP and lateral views.
- Nail diameter is determined preoperatively based on canal diameter.
- The nail is precontoured to reestablish the radial bow.
- Nail passage is performed under fluoroscopic guidance to avoid cortical perforation. If using a flexible titanium nail, it is seated into the metaphyseal bone and cut beneath the skin.
- Rotational alignment of the radius is best assessed based on the relationship between the biceps tuberosity and the radial styloid. They should be oriented 180 degrees from each other on a perfect AP view.

Interlocking If Available
- Ulna: lateral to medial proximal interlock, ulnar to radial distal interlock (small open approach to avoid injury to sensory dorsal cutaneous branch of ulnar nerve).
- Radius: no proximal interlock, radial to ulnar distal interlock.
- It is worth noting that the IM device depicted in Figures 10-28–10-30 (Smith & Nephew Foresight Nail System) is no longer commercially available in the United States.

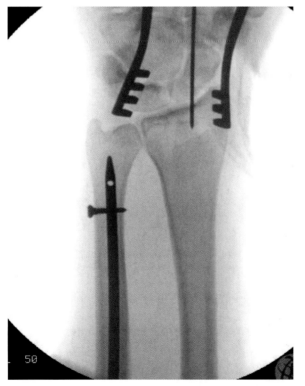

Figure 10-28 I For a second dorsal compartment entry site, the ECRB and ERCL are retracted and a localization K-wire is inserted in line with the medullary canal.

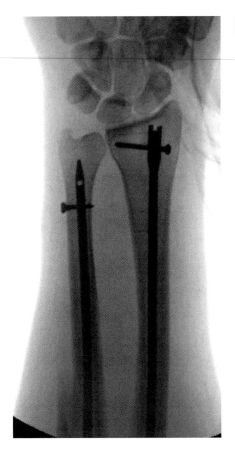
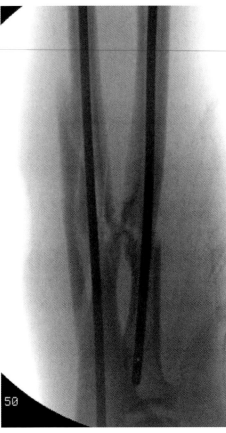

Figure 10-29 ▌ After radius fixation, rotational alignment is confirmed correct, with the profile of the biceps tuberosity 180 degrees from the radial styloid.

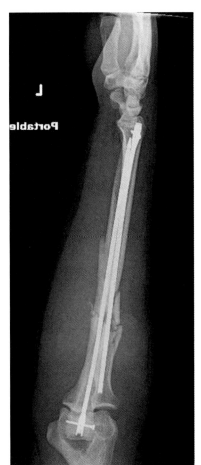
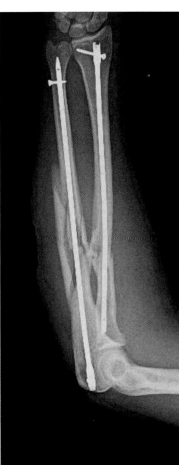

Figure 10-30 ▌ Final postoperative images after closed nailing of both the radius and ulna confirm restoration of length, alignment, and radial bow.

Flexible Nail for Comminuted Proximal Radial Shaft Fracture

Mark R. Adams
Michael S. Sirkin

Pathoanatomy

- The more proximal a radial shaft fracture is, the more difficult it is to perform an ORIF with a plate and screws (Fig. 10-31).

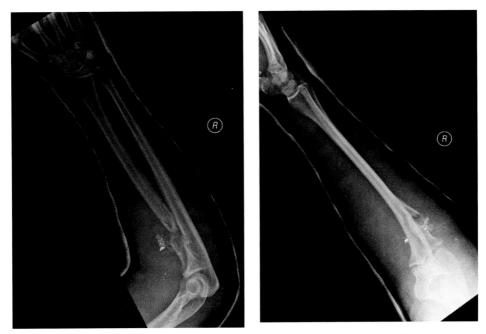

Figure 10-31 I AP and lateral views of forearm demonstrating a comminuted proximal fracture of the radius.

- The issues with proximal plates:
  - Difficult to contour plate avoiding the bicipital tuberosity
  - Plate impingement on proximal radioulnar joint limiting forearm rotation
  - Limited options for proximal fixation resulting in inadequate stability
  - May require Thompson approach and PIN mobilization with the potential for nerve injury

Solution

- Closed flexible nailing is an option that ideally avoids the above-mentioned issues.

Technique

- The preferred entry site is on the ulnar side of the second extensor compartment (contains the ECRL and ECRB) (Fig. 10-32).

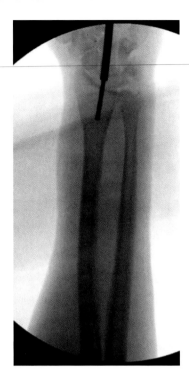

Figure 10-32 | Entry site for nail—3.5-mm cannulated drill placed over a guide wire at the dorsal distal radius, just radial to Lister's tubercle and in line with the radial shaft canal.

- This avoids the EPL and Lister's tubercle (ulnar to entry) thereby reducing the risk of late tendon irritation or rupture.
- The tendons of the ECRL and ECRB are much stouter than the EPL and their excursions are also less.
- A cannulated 3.5 drill bit may be used to facilitate entry.

When contoured correctly, the nail will provide improved alignment in the coronal and sagittal planes.

- A radial bow and distal bend or hook in the nail will improve rotational control of the proximal segment.
- Distal portion of nail left outside of cortex to maintain 3 points of fixation and facilitate later removal (Figs. 10-33–10-35).

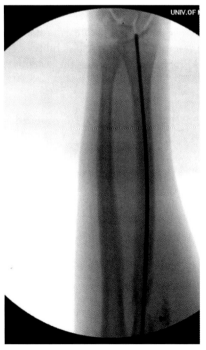
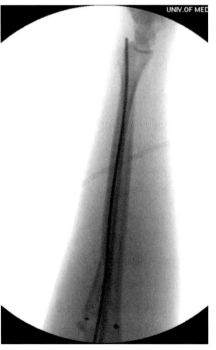

Figure 10-33 | Fluoroscopic images demonstrating the proximal radial shaft rotating with the distal shaft as a unit after insertion of the hooked end of the nail into proximal segment.

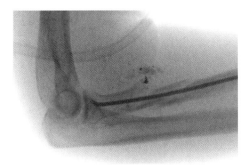
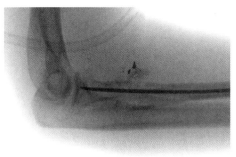

Figure 10-34 | AP and lateral views of forearm immediately post-op demonstrating improved radial shaft alignment and an intramedullary nail in the radius.

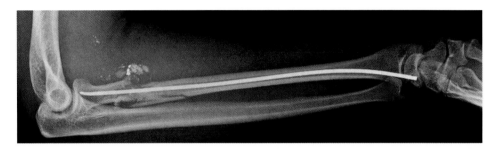
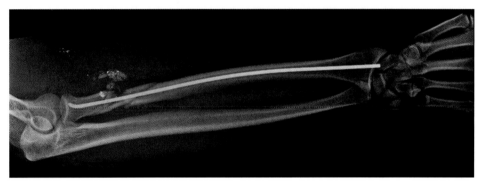

Figure 10-35 | AP and lateral views of forearm 3 months post-op demonstrating maintained alignment of the radius and callus formation about the fracture site. Forearm rotation at 3 months: supination 40 degrees, pronation 85 degrees.

Chapter 11
Distal Radius Fractures

DOUGLAS P. HANEL

E. J. HARVEY

STEPHEN A. KENNEDY

SARAH C. PETTRONE

Sterile Instruments/Equipment

- Finger traps
- Sterile rope for on-table traction
- Small pointed reduction clamps ("Weber" clamps)
- Implants
  - Precontoured volar locking distal radius plates and screws (most common, but does not work for all fractures)
  - Minifragment plates and screws (2.0 to 2.7 mm), locking or nonlocking
  - Wire-form or rim hook plate systems for fragment-specific fixation
  - Wrist spanning plate, such as 3.5-mm locking plates, or custom locking plate made specifically for spanning technique through the second compartment of the wrist
  - External fixator if necessary
- K-wires and wire driver/drill

Positioning

- Supine on a radiolucent hand table.
- Bring the patient to the lateral edge of the bed.
- Center the shoulder/elbow/hand on the hand table, with the shoulder abducted 90 degrees.
- Place a pneumatic tourniquet on the ipsilateral arm, if desired.
- A sterile traction device may be applied after draping (Fig. 11-1).
- Consider using a pulley system for the rope traction. This can be as simple as a metal kidney dish/emesis basin, a metal pulley attached to the hand table, or a commercially manufactured traction hand table. Generally limit weight to <10 lb to avoid overdistraction.

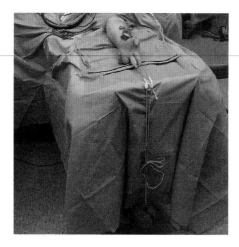
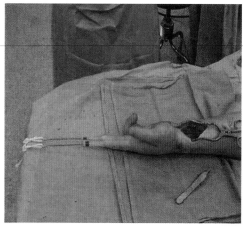

Figure 11-1 ▌ A sterile traction device for reduction assistance. Two "overhand" knots are tied at the ends of a 3-ft (100-cm) rope. One end is attached to finger traps, and 10 lb of weight is hung from the loop of the rope at the other end. A pulley can ensure consistent traction and improved maneuverability.

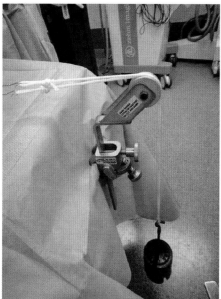

Reduction and Fixation Techniques

- Typical reduction maneuvers (described by Agee).
  - Longitudinal traction to restore length.
  - Palmar translation of the carpus relative to the forearm. This restores palmar tilt and demonstrates volar instability, when present.
  - Slight pronation of the hand relative to the forearm, combined with ulnar deviation. This corrects the supination deformity of a great majority of distal radius fractures.
- After reduction maneuvers, repeat fluoroscopic fracture assessment (AP, lateral, and oblique).
- Determine the fracture involvement of the three columns of the wrist (Rikli and Regazzoni).
  - Medial—ulnar head.
  - Intermediate—sigmoid notch, volar and dorsal ulnar lunate fossa, and lunate fossa die-punch.
  - Lateral—volar and dorsal scaphoid fossa and radial styloid.
  - Assess metaphyseal comminution.
- Determine the overall fracture stability.
  - Stable fractures are generally defined prior to reduction.
  - Factors, which may predict displacement after closed reduction, include:
    - Articular step off or gap >2 mm
    - Dorsal tilt >20 degrees prior to reduction
    - Metaphyseal comminution >1/3 of AP width (on lateral projection)
    - Involvement of the volar medial corner (critical corner)
    - Involvement of the distal ulna
    - Age >60 or any history of poor bone quality

- Treatment of stable fractures.
  - Cast or splint immobilization
    - If fracture reduction tenuous, then long arm with forearm in supination, otherwise short arm.
    - Wrist in neutral or slightly extended position.
    - Check X-rays weekly for a minimum of 3 weeks.
    - Compare the most recent X-ray with the immediate postreduction film.
      - Comparing X-rays from 1 week to the next can result in failing to recognize gradual loss of reduction. Follow-up X-rays must be compared to the initial reduction films.
    - If reduction becomes unacceptable, then proceed to rereduction and fixation.
- Three basic types of fixation for unstable fractures.
  - Closed manipulation with percutaneous fixation, with or without external fixation, or dorsal spanning plate fixation
  - Open reduction with volar locking plate, or less commonly dorsal buttress plate
  - Open reduction with fragment-specific implants, also referred to as "column specific" or "fragment specific"
- Closed techniques.
  - Percutaneous K-wire (interfocal through fracture fragments)
    - 1.5 mm or 0.062 inch
    - At least two pins, one in the radial column and the other in the dorsal aspect of the intermediate column (either through Lister's tubercle or between fourth and fifth dorsal compartments)
  - Percutaneous K-wire (intrafocal through fracture site)
    - The Kapandji technique of intrafocal pinning involves placement of biplanar K-wires.
      - Introduce a coronal plane K-wire into the fracture site in a radial to ulnar direction on the AP radiographic view.
      - A second sagittal plane K-wire is placed into the fracture site in a dorsal to volar direction.
      - Once in the fracture site, the wires are used as a lever to elevate the distal fragments, restoring the radial inclination, length, and volar tilt.
        - The wires are then driven into the opposite cortex of the radius.
        - Supplemental K-wires may be inserted to secure the fracture reduction and improve the fixation stiffness (Fig. 11-2). Intrafocal pins alone may not be adequate fixation due to comminution and diminished bone quality.

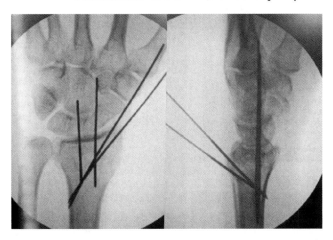

Figure 11-2 ▌ AP and lateral radiographs demonstrating the combined intrafocal and interfocal percutaneous pinning. Two pins were placed using the Kapandji technique to restore the volar tilt. Two additional percutaneous pins were placed in the radial styloid.

      - Supplemental fixation (external fixation or a dorsal spanning plate) is often required in older patients or in those with poor bone quality.
  - Wrist joint spanning external fixation.
    - Bridging external fixation may be used as a temporizing measure or as a definitive fixation for distal radius fractures.
    - Indicated for severe open fractures with soft tissue defects, as a temporizing measure in a polytrauma patient, unstable extra-articular fractures, and nondisplaced intra-articular fractures.
    - Spanning external fixation may be combined with internal fixation techniques to maintain length and added stability with internal fixation.
    - Contraindicated as isolated fixation of displaced intra-articular fractures, unless those fractures are irreparable and serve as a preamble to fusion.

- The reduction maneuver described by Agee is performed (described above).
- Pin placement:
  - Exposure to bone and soft protection is required.
  - Most fixator systems have a drill guide to ensure placement of parallel, bicortical pins spaced 3 to 5 cm apart.
  - Free hand systems also work well, although less convenient.
  - Forearm pins are placed in the bare area of the radius just proximal to the muscle bellies of the abductor pollicis longus (AbPL) and extensor pollicis brevis (EPB).
    - This is approximately 10 to 12 cm proximal to the radial styloid.
    - A 3- to 5-cm dorsal radial incision is made just proximal to the EPB and AbPL.
    - Using the interval between the extensor carpi radialis longus (ECRL) and the extensor carpi radialis brevis (ECRB), the superficial radial nerve is protected.
    - The interval between the ECRL and BR can also be used but has an increased risk of injury to the superficial branch of the radial nerve.
  - Hand (distal) pins are placed in the second metacarpal, parallel to the proximal pins.
    - The more proximal pin is placed through the metaphysis of the second metacarpal.
    - If this pin does not have adequate purchase, advance it through a third cortex into the third metacarpal.
    - The more distal pin is placed in the diaphysis of the second metacarpal.
- Fracture length and wrist alignment are restored with traction and fixator clamps, and bars are applied.
- After the fixator is applied, examine the midcarpal and radiocarpal joints to be sure that the extremity is not over distracted.
  - The fingers should fully flex and extend without excessive tightness.
- Residual dorsal angulation is difficult to correct, but can be managed by palmar translation of the hand relative to the forearm, prior to tightening the clamps and bars.
  - Increased traction often worsens the dorsal angulation.
  - Supplemental K-wires used as joysticks may be necessary to achieve reduction.
- Intra-articular depression.
  - Limited internal fixation may be necessary to reduce and maintain articular fragments (Fig. 11-3).

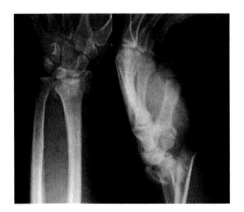
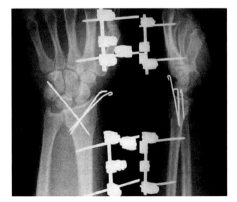
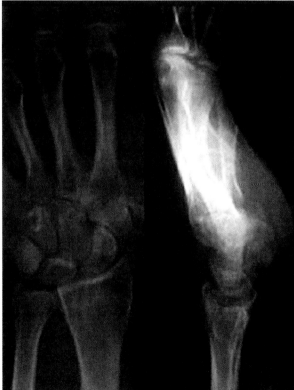

Figure 11-3 | Compression fracture involving all three columns, treated with closed reduction, percutaneous pin fixation, and external fixation. Final radiographs taken 2 years after injury demonstrated healing in accurate position.

- Nonspanning (joint sparing) external fixation.
  - Indicated for unstable extra-articular distal radius fractures.
  - Contraindicated when the distal fragments are too small for pin placement.
    - At least 1 cm of intact volar cortex is required for pin purchase.
  - A small external fixation set is recommended with 2.5-mm threaded tip pins.
  - A transverse incision is made over Lister's tubercle; tendons adjacent to the tubercle are retracted.
  - The dorsal cortex is predrilled and threaded tip pins introduced.
  - The pins are placed slightly convergent in the sagittal (dorsal to palmar) plane.
  - It is critical that the pins purchase the volar cortex.
  - Alternatively, one pin may be placed from dorsal to volar as described above, and a second pin may be placed in the subchondral bone, from radial to ulnar.
    - This pin cannot penetrate the medial cortex of the radius, the sigmoid notch.
  - The proximal pins are placed proximal to the muscle bellies of the EPB/AbPL, in line with and between the tendons of the radial wrist extensors.
  - The pins in the distal fragment are used to manipulate the fragment and reduce the fracture.
  - A standard frame is then applied (Fig. 11-4).

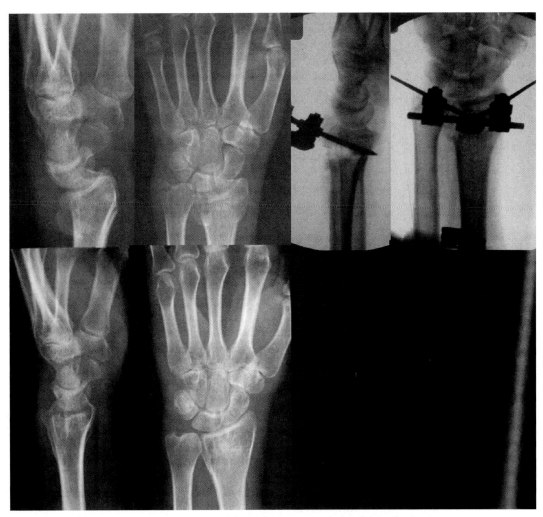

Figure 11-4 ▮ Example of a joint sparing external fixator for an extra-articular distal radius fracture.

- Open techniques.
  - Surgical approaches
    - Volar "FCR" approach (also called a "modified Henry" approach)
      - Most extensile for application of volar plates to all but volar medial corner, used for the great majority of radius fractures and volar plating techniques.

- Longitudinal incision centered over the flexor carpi radialis (FCR).
- Incision may be curved 45 degrees radially at the level of wrist crease.
- Incise the sheath of the FCR, retracting the FCR medially and the radial artery laterally.
- Avoid the palmar cutaneous branch of the median nerve by staying radial to the FCR.
- A longitudinal incision is made in the floor of the FCR sheath.
- Proximally, the flexor pollicis longus (FPL) is retracted ulnarly.
- Distally, the pronator quadratus (PQ) is elevated sharply off the radial border of the radius.
- The insertion of the brachioradialis (BR) is divided when needed to facilitate restoration of length and radial inclination at the radial styloid.

- Volar Henry approach
  - Most extensile for application of fragment-specific fixation to radial styloid volar, lateral or dorsal, most commonly used for combined wrist and radius shaft fractures.
  - Longitudinal incision centered between FCR and radial styloid; this is directly over the radial artery.
  - Incision may be curved 45 degrees radially at the level of wrist crease.
  - Dissect down to investing fascia and then mobilize all superficial structures as one flap.
    - The radial nerve is then protected.
  - Incise forearm fascia, and mobilize radial artery laterally at the wrist but medially in the proximal forearm.
  - FPL tendon is retracted ulnarly.
  - Distally, the PQ is elevated sharply off the radial border of the radius.
  - The insertion of the BR is divided.
  - Dorsal radial styloid can be approached by dividing all but the distal 1 cm off the first dorsal compartment.

- Volar ulnar approach
  - Best exposure for unstable volar medial distal radius fractures involving the intermediate column, which are rare injuries but vexing if missed.
  - Longitudinal incision just radial to the flexor carpi ulnaris (FCU) to the distal wrist crease.
  - If distal extension is required, direct the incision radially at a 60-degree angle until encountering the hypothenar crease, and then extend distally between the thenar and hypothenar eminences.
  - The contents of the carpal tunnel are retracted radially, and the ulnar neurovascular bundle is retracted ulnarly.
  - The PQ is elevated either from its ulnar insertion or from its radial insertion.
    - Leave the joint capsule attachments on the volar medial fracture fragment.

- Dorsal approach (fourth extensor compartment)
  - Although supplanted by the FCR approach, it still has application in the management of "die-punch" fractures that cannot be reduced from volar approach.
  - Longitudinal incision centered over the wrist, midway between the radial and ulnar styloids in line with the third metacarpal.
  - Blunt dissection down to the retinaculum of the extensor tendons and raise skin flaps that include all structures superficial to it.
    - Take care to elevate crossing branches of the superficial radial and dorsal ulnar nerves.
  - Incise the distal forearm fascia just distal to the muscle bellies of the EPB/AbPL and radial to the ECRL/ECRB tendons.
  - The radial most structure in the depths of this wound is the muscle belly of the extensor pollicis longus (EPL).
    - The EPL is followed distally, and the extensor retinaculum divided over the third compartment.
  - Mobilize the EPL and retract it radially.
    - The EPL is left out of its sheath during closure.
  - The interval between the residual second and fourth extensor compartments is developed.
  - The fourth compartment is retracted ulnarly and the second compartment radially.
  - Ulnar dissection stops when the fifth compartment is encountered.
    - Care is taken to leave soft tissues attached to the dorsal ulnar fragment.

- Dorsal approach (fifth extensor compartment)
  - ▪ Exposure used to reduce and fix isolated dorsal ulnar "die-punch" or avulsion fractures.
  - ▪ Incision in line with the fourth metacarpal at the level of the distal radioulnar joint.
    - Avoid damage to the dorsal cutaneous branch of the ulnar nerve.
  - ▪ Incise fifth compartment to mobilize the extensor digiti quinti (EDQ) ulnarly; leave soft tissues on the floor of compartment attached to bony structures.
  - ▪ Identify the ulnar dorsal border of distal radius, and follow distally into the fracture site.
  - ▪ Leave all soft tissue attachment to the dorsal ulnar fragment intact.
- Approach to ulnar head/styloid fractures
  - ▪ Indications: upon completion of radius reconstruction and in the setting of continued DRUJ instability.
  - ▪ This dissection is carried out with the elbow flexed 90 degrees and the forearm in maximum supination.
    - Doing so places the ulnar styloid collinear with the subcutaneous dorsal border of the ulna.
  - ▪ An incision is made along the dorsal ulnar subcutaneous border of the ulna, stopping at the ulnar styloid.
  - ▪ Elevate skin flaps from proximal to distal.
    - Avoid damage to the dorsal cutaneous branch of the ulnar nerve.
  - ▪ Identify fracture fragments but do not dissect soft tissue attachments.

Implants: Clinical Indications and Examples

Dorsal Spanning Plate

- Indicated for patients with high-energy injuries, who have fracture extension into the radius and ulnar diaphysis, and in patients with multiple extremity injuries who require load bearing for mobilization.
  - Acts as an "internal fixator" with the mechanical advantage of being immediately adjacent to the fracture with optimal pin (in this case screw) spread and is a closed system that is particularly helpful in eliminating the pin tract infections in critically ill trauma patients
  - May also be used as an adjunct to internal fixation or percutaneous fixation in highly comminuted fractures
- Uses a plate that spans the radiocarpal joint, from the intact radial diaphysis to an intact metacarpal.
  - If the plate is passed through the second retinacular compartment, it is fixed to the second metacarpal.
  - If the plate is passed through the fourth compartment, it is fixed to the third metacarpal.

- The choice of compartments is dictated by closed reduction maneuvers.
  - If the articular fracture reduces and can be held with simple wire fixation, use the second compartment.
  - If not, the articular fracture can be exposed through the fourth compartment, reduced, and secured with a plate and screws in this compartment.
- Reduction is performed as described previously (Agee's reduction maneuver).
  - The plate length and position are confirmed by fluoroscopy, by placing the plate on the dorsal skin of the distal forearm/wrist/hand.
  - The plate should be aligned such that at least three bicortical screws can be placed proximal to and three distal to the fracture.
  - More screws or increased screw spacing may be required in osteoporotic bone or in anticipation of diminished fixation strength.
- An incision is made at the base of the second or third metacarpal.
- A second incision is made just proximal to the EPB/AbPL.
- When the second compartment is used for passage of the plate, the interval for plate placement is between the ECRL and the ECRB.

- The plate is introduced in the proximal incision and advanced distally between the ECRL and ECRB.
- When the fourth compartment is used, the muscle belly of the EPL is retracted from the dorsal ulna aspect of the radius metadiaphysis, and the plate is passed deep into the muscle in the fourth compartment, to rest on the third metacarpal.
- The plate is secured with a 2.7-mm nonlocking screw in the distal and proximal most screw holes.
  - Although 2.4-mm screws can be used for plate fixation, we have found them to break with unacceptable frequency.
- The remaining holes may be filled with locking screws.
- At least three proximal and three distal screws are recommended in good quality bone.
- Plates are removed after fracture healing, at approximately 8 to 12 weeks (Fig. 11-5).

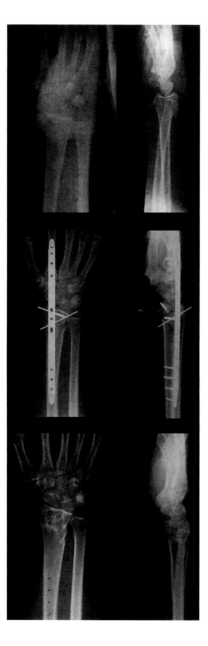

Figure 11-5 | Spanning plate used to secure fixation in a patient who sustained multiple injuries and required this limb to assist with weight bearing.

Volar Plate Fixation

- Indicated for most intra-articular distal radius fractures.
- Acts as volar buttress and with locking screws or preformed blades functions as a fixed angle device (Fig. 11-6).

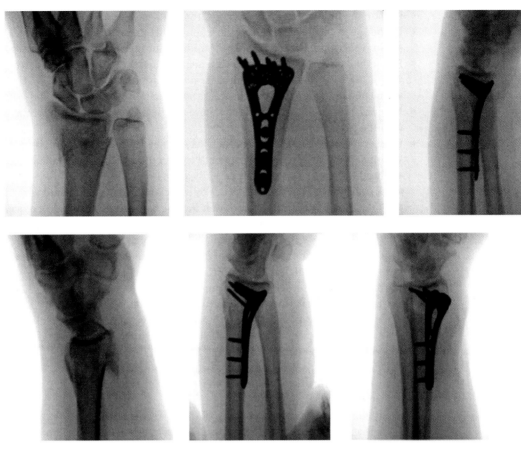

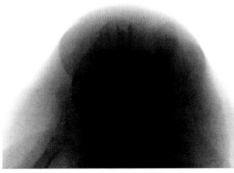

Figure 11-6 I Volar locking plate fixation of a distal radius fracture. Lifting the hand by approximately 10 to 15 degrees off the table allows for clear visualization of the lunate facet, to ensure adequate volar tilt and no intra-articular screw penetration. Oblique radiographs and the "dorsal horizon view" axial radiograph ensure no screw tip penetration on either side of the Lister's tubercle.

- Contraindicated in dorsal shear fractures or as sole fixation in complex dorsally displaced fractures.
  - Dorsal buttress plating is preferred in this fracture pattern.
- Sterile traction may be applied to aid in the initial reduction.
- Often, traction will be released later in the procedure to allow further manipulation and detension soft tissues for retraction.
- Placing the hand on rolled towel(s), with supinated forearm flat on the table, may help to restore volar tilt.
- The choice of incision is based on the location of the most complex and most comminuted fracture.
  - Comminuted intermediate column fractures are best exposed and fixed through previously described volar ulnar approach.
  - All other fractures are approached through the "FCR" or Henry exposure.

- Release the BR when radial column is involved.
- Do not open the volar wrist capsule when reducing the articular fragment.
  - This leads to radiocarpal instability and significant postoperative stiffness.
- Reduction and fixation sequence depends on the fracture location and size.
  - The largest and least comminuted fragments are reduced first.
  - The remaining fracture fragments are subsequently reduced.
- K-wires assist in the initial reduction and can be driven out the back of the wrist if they interfere with the placement of plate.
- Bone graft, or a bone graft substitute, may be needed to fill the metaphyseal defect.
- With relatively large fracture fragments, a precontoured plate is applied.
  - There is no superior plate or plating system.
  - All of the newer distal radius plates offer locking screw fixation and variable angle placement.
  - With comminuted fractures, or osteoporotic bone, there is little difference in the distal locking screws versus locking pegs. Both function to buttress the articular surface and provide a modest degree of rotational stability, especially in the coronal plane.
- Stabilizing the distal fragment first, followed by fixation to the radius metadiaphysis, aids in restoring the volar tilt in dorsally angulated extra-articular fractures.
  - This does not apply to volar shearing fractures.
- Verify that the distal screws or pins are not intra-articular.
  - This is best viewed on the lateral X-ray, with the wrist elevated on roll towels forming a 10- to 15-degree angle with the table, so that the fluoroscopic beam is tangential to the wrist joint in PA and lateral projection.
  - Do not be confused by the radial styloid screw, which often appears to be intra-articular.
  - 45-Degree pronation oblique view visualizes the subchondral bone and reveals the fixation screw penetration.
- Verify that the diaphyseal screws are of the correct length.
  - Long screws that penetrate the dorsal cortex by more than 1 to 2 mm will irritate the extensor tendons.
  - The "dorsal horizon view" is an additional view for detecting screw dorsal cortex penetration, which involves hyperflexion of the wrist and aiming of the image intensifier beam along the long axis of the radius (Fig. 11-6).

Fragment-Specific Fixation

- Indicated for complex intra-articular fractures.
- Individual fracture fragments are fixed through multiple smaller incisions.
- Fracture fragments are fixed with miniscrews, 2.0-mm miniplates, or 2.0-mm pin plates.
- The radial styloid fragment is fixed first, followed by the volar and/or dorsal fragments.
- The rigidity of the construct depends on placing implants in orthogonal positions (Fig. 11-7).

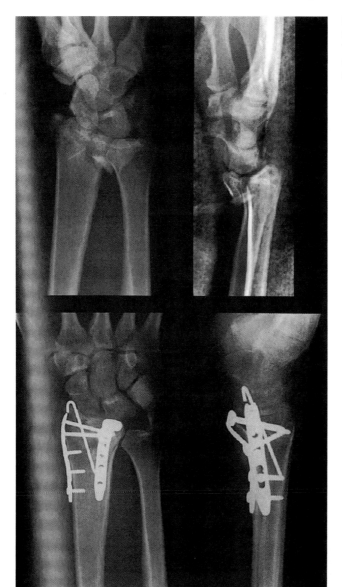

Figure 11-7 I Example of fragment-specific fixation used for a distal radius fracture. The volar implant supports the intermediate column fracture, while the radial implant supports the lateral column.

- Bone graft or bone graft substitutes may be necessary to provide additional buttress to the subchondral bone.
- Fragment-specific fixation for volar ulnar fracture fragments.
  - Larger plates often fail to capture the volar ulnar fracture fragments, resulting in delayed radiocarpal dislocations.
  - These fracture fragments are best managed with "wire-form" or hook plate fragment-specific fixation (Fig. 11-8).

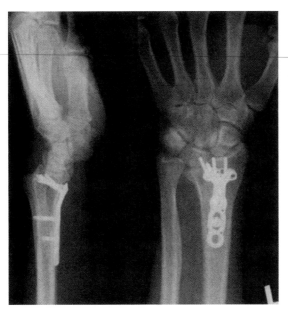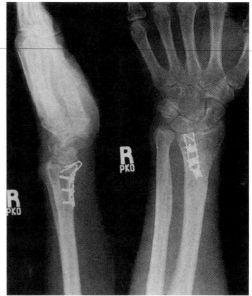

Figure 11-8 | After failed fixation of the volar medial corner fracture (**left** X-rays), the plate was removed, the fracture reduced, and definitive fixation performed with wire-form fixation (**right** X-rays).

Dorsal Plate Fixation

- Indicated for complex intra-articular fractures, with lunate die-punch fractures or dorsal ulnar fractures that do not reduce with closed manipulation or volar manipulation.
- Lunate facet approached through the fourth compartment, with incision over 4 to 5 compartment interval.
- Fracture fragments are fixed with miniscrews, 2.0-mm miniplates, or 2.0-mm pin plates.
- The radial styloid fragment is fixed first, followed by dorsal fragments.
- The rigidity of the construct is increased by placing the radial styloid plate 90 degrees to the volar and/or dorsal implants (Fig. 11-9).

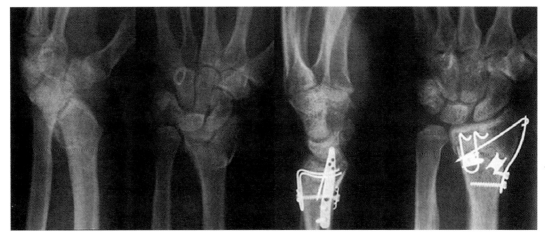

Figure 11-9 | A dorsal depressed die-punch fracture could not be adequately reduced from volar exposure. The dorsal fracture was approached, reduced, and transfixed through the dorsal 4 to 5 interval.

TIP

Fixation Technique for Comminuted Dorsal Rim Fractures of the Distal Radius

E. J. Harvey

Pathophysiology

- Some fractures of the distal radius are extremely difficult to reduce and obtain stable internal fixation.[1]
- Dorsal rim fractures are common, and the comminuted distal rim fracture is a fracture that is beyond the scope of most fixation techniques.
- Certain methods of fixation have been advocated in the past.
  - External fixation does not allow anatomic reduction but is a better option than a subluxated carpus.
  - Internal bridge plating, as popularized by Ruch and Hanel,[2] was associated with minimal complications and was proven to have superior fixation properties when compared with external fixation in later biomechanical studies. The advantage of obtaining a reduced carpus is offset by the relative temporary immobilization of the wrist in a flat neutral position with attendant scarring. Hanel et al.[3] looked at 912 consecutive patients who underwent operative treatment of distal radius fractures. Of these, 140 patients (15%) with 144 fractures were treated with a dorsally placed distraction plate. The authors could not identify any particular fracture pattern that was an absolute indication for distraction plating but did comment that it should be used instead of external fixation at any time.
- Often, the bridge plate does not provide a substantial benefit for this articular fracture.
  - Fragment-specific fixation and volar and dorsal locking plates allow fixation of almost all distal radius fractures.
  - The only specific fracture that may need internal distraction-type fixation is the very distal fracture dislocation pattern with no intact dorsal rim, as this fracture type allows dorsal dislocation if standard fixation devices are used (Figs. 11-10 and 11-11).

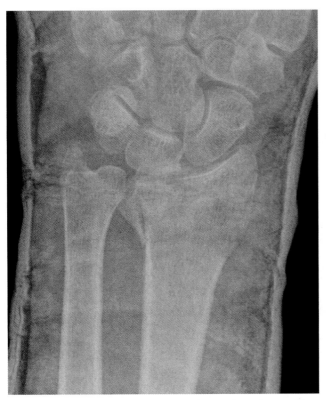

Figure 11-10 | Comminuted distal radius fracture in a 55-year-old male.

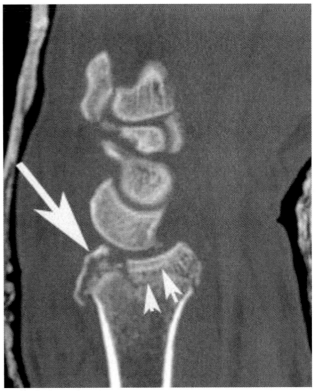

Figure 11-11 | Sagittal CT scan image of patient depicted in Figure 11-10 showing dorsal and volar comminution. *Large arrow* shows dorsal rim comminution. *Arrowheads* show impacted lunate facet.

- Spanning plate approaches require compliant patients. In our experience, if patients do not comply and miss follow-up evaluations, broken plates or other complications can result in a wrist fusion. This led to the search for a solution that would be more patient behavior independent.

Solution

Use of a dorsal plate that blocks dorsal subluxation but allows volar flexion seems to be a better method of fixing and maintaining reduction of these fractures.[1]

Technique

- Fixation progresses as with any complicated distal radius fracture—without traction or temporary external fixation.
- Volar plates may be used as an initial step, if necessary, as a buttress plate to bring anatomic reduction to the volar cortex (Fig. 11-12).

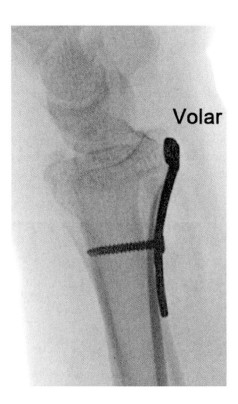

Figure 11-12 I Volar buttress plate provisionally holding volar surface of distal radius. This plate is initially inserted with only a proximal screw so that manipulation of the reduction does not result in volar subluxation of the distal radius and further comminution.

- This may require several K-wires, open reduction of both volar and dorsal surfaces, and the use of multiple plates (Figs. 11-13 and 11-14).

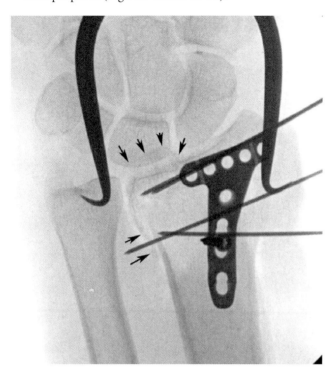

Figure 11-13 I Single metaphyseal screw provisionally securing volar buttress plate supplemented with K-wires. Note the *arrows* depicting impacted lunate facet and displaced DRUJ.

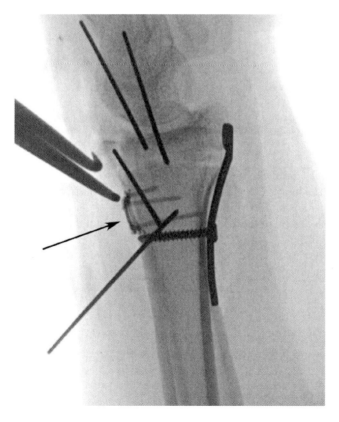

Figure 11-14 I Application of a small dorsoulnar plate (*arrow*) after reduction of the lunate and DRUJ. This plate is intended for the DRUJ reduction to maintain length of the dorsal cortex. It is not needed for all dorsal rim subluxation pattern fractures.

- Only proximal, metadiaphyseal screws are used initially, and then the distal screws are added with the final reduction to lock the distal fragment.
- On the dorsal side in particular, care should be taken to avoid further injury to the wrist capsule, as its attachment to the multiple dorsal rim pieces is important. If the capsular attachments remain mainly intact, it is a reduction aid when the extra-capsular dorsal plate is put in place. This allows

for reduction and maintenance of the dorsal rim in an anatomic position. A Pi-plate (Synthes) distal radius implant is used in an unconventional manner through a standard 3 to 4 interval. It is placed dorsally, over the first carpal row without contouring. The sidepieces that are perpendicular to the radius can be removed particularly for small wrists (Fig. 11-15).

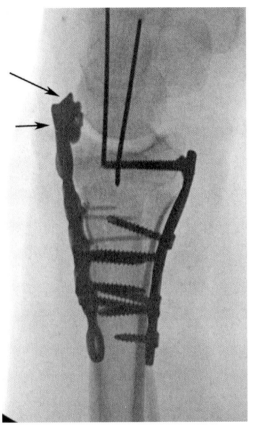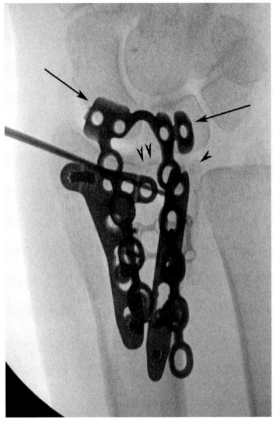

Figure 11-15 I Lateral and AP images demonstrating final reduction. *Arrows* show where the side pieces have been removed from the edges of the Pi-plate. *Arrowheads* show reduction of the lunate facet. Note also that the provisional oblique position of the volar buttress plate seen in Figure 11-13 has been altered prior to the insertion of two subsequent locking screws in the radial styloid and the most proximal hole of the plate.

- No screws are placed distally to the radiocarpal articulation, but the first carpal row and the intact soft tissue on the dorsum of the wrist permit reduction. Obviously, a block to dorsiflexion is present, but palmar flexion is permitted and encouraged.
- The final step is placement of the locking screw(s) if possible in the volar plate for the distal fragment (Fig. 11-15).
- Rehabilitation takes place like that for any distal radius screw treated with rigid fixation. The only difference is planned hardware removal at 6 months of the Pi-plate at least.

References

1. Martineau PA, Berry GK, Harvey EJ. Plating for distal radius fractures. *Hand Clin.* 2010;26(1):61–69. doi:10.1016/j.hcl.2009.08.002.
2. Richard MJ, Katolik LI, Hanel DP, et al. Distraction plating for the treatment of highly comminuted distal radius fractures in elderly patients. *J Hand Surg Am.* 2012;37(5):948–956. doi:10.1016/j.jhsa.2012.02.034.
3. Hanel DP, Ruhlman SD, Katolik LI, et al. Complications associated with distraction plate fixation of wrist fractures. *Hand Clin.* 2010;26:237–243.

Distal Radioulnar Joint

- With reconstruction of the intermediate column, specifically the sigmoid notch, DRUJ instability is rarely an issue.
- Restoration of anatomic mediolateral translation of the radius fracture also restores appropriate tension on the distal oblique bundle of the interosseous ligament, which can restore DRUJ stability even in the presence of TFCC tear.
- If the sigmoid notch and radial metaphysis fractures are accurately reduced and fixed, there is no relationship between the ulnar styloid fracture size and instability.
- If after radius reduction DRUJ instability persists, ensure that tendons, the triangular fibrocartilage complex (TFCC), or even the ulnar neurovascular bundles are not interposed between the ulnar head and radius.
- Arthroscopy (dry scope) will determine the integrity and location of injury to TFCC.
- If the sigmoid notch is reduced, and the TFCC is in continuity with radius and the DRUJ remains unstable, then consider fixation of ulnar styloid fragment and attached soft tissues.
- Easiest exposure of the ulnar head and styloid is through an incision placed along the subcutaneous border of the ulna while the elbow is flexed 90+ degrees and the forearm is in maximum supination.
    - By using blunt dissecting from proximal to distal, the dorsal cutaneous branch of the ulnar nerve is retracted distally and the fracture line will become obvious.
    - Once the fracture line is identified, the soft tissue dissection is complete.
    - Manipulate and reduce the fracture with a dental pick and secure the fracture with a K-wire and tension band.

Soft Tissue Injuries Associated with Wrist Fractures

- Nerve injuries: median or ulnar.
- Contusion, hematoma, and swelling following wrist fractures can cause median and ulnar nerve dysfunction.
- It may be impossible to distinguish between direct median nerve injury and nerve compression due to increased carpal tunnel pressure.
    - Best method is clinical examination and to correlate prereduction and postreduction examination.
- Prevention
    - Avoid splinting the wrist in flexion and ulnar deviation.
    - Avoid narrow retractors when reducing fractures and applying volar plates.
- Treatment
    - Acute contusion—reduce the fracture, and clear the carpal tunnel of all bone fragments.
    - Progressive sensory loss—urgent carpal tunnel release and fracture reduction.
        - If this occurs after reduction, return to OR for carpal tunnel release.
- Nerve injury: radial sensory
    - Most commonly occurs from direct injury from pin placement.
    - Prevention:
        - Place fixator pins on interval between ECRL and ECRB in the forearm.
        - Expose radial column fractures with longitudinal skin incisions and blunt dissection down the dorsal retinaculum, and elevate soft tissue in the plane between the retinaculum and overlying soft tissues.
- Compartment syndrome
    - This has been reported in the setting of closed reduction and circumferential casting.
    - Treatment—remove cast, decompress the forearm, and reduce and fix fracture.
- Complex regional pain syndrome
    - Prospective studies report much higher incidence than retrospective studies.
    - Frequently associated with untreated compression, neuropathy, and immobilization of the wrist in flexion.
    - Treatment
        - Avoid splinting in wrist flexion.
        - Recognize and decompress nerve injury.

- ▪ Minimize immobilization.
- ▪ Institute immediate hand therapy, with active motion, desensitization, edema management, and graded motor imagery.
    - ▪ Consider involvement of a pain specialist, neuropathic pain medication, and interventional nerve blocks.
- Tendon injury: rupture
    - Flexor and extensor tendon ruptures have been reported with both volar and dorsal plates, resulting from prominent screws and prominent plate edges.
        - ▪ Can occur months after fracture healing
        - ▪ Best prevented with attention to detail as described above
    - Patient education in the development of tendons "grinding."
    - Most surprising case is the EPL rupture that occurs after healing of minimally displaced fractures.
        - ▪ There is an apparent stenosis of the third dorsal compartment.
    - Treatment—remove offending structures, decompress tendon compartments, and repair tendon ruptures with grafts or transfers.
- Hand/wrist/forearm stiffness
    - Very little hand stiffness reported in recent literature compared to past.
    - Previously reported as a result of swelling, wrist flexion splinting, and cast constriction.
    - Presently, the greatest difficulty is in restoring supination (may take up to 1 year).

Postoperative Care of Wrist Fractures

- Immobilize wrist in slight extension (never in flexion).
- The first goal in the immediate postoperative recovery is avoidance of finger stiffness. Start "six-pack" exercises in recovery room.
- The most common limitation after distal radius fracture fixation is loss of supination
- In uncomplicated distal radius fractures with rigid internal fixation, stable distal radioulnar joint, and a reliable patient, consider applying a short arm splint and begin early active forearm rotation exercises with a removable brace in the 2 weeks following surgery.
- If the intermediate column is repaired, especially in fractures involving the sigmoid notch, or there is evidence of DRUJ instability in neutral or pronation, consider stabilizing the forearm in supination in a long arm splint for first 2 weeks as it provides protection while maximizing supination.
- At the 2-week visit, unstable fracture progresses from long arm cast to splint to nothing, as fracture heals (usually 4 to 8 weeks).
- Strengthening is started after regaining digit and forearm motion and evidence of fracture healing.
- DRUJ is usually the last to resolve and may take several months.

In Memoriam: Sarah C. Pettrone M.D.

The original coauthor of this chapter, Sarah C. Pettrone M.D., sadly passed away after a courageous battle with cancer in 2014. After completing her fellowship at the University of Washington, she joined her father's practice in Northern Virginia as a hand surgeon. She was an avid marathon runner, volunteered as a soccer and basketball coach for the Special Olympics, and participated in multiple medical missions to Bhutan, Ethiopia, and Honduras. She is sadly missed, and this chapter is dedicated in her memory.

Section 4
Pelvis/ Acetabulum

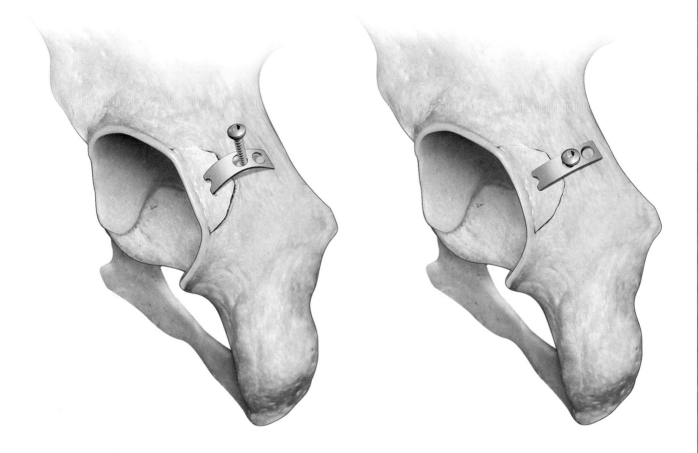

Chapter 12
Pelvic Ring Injuries

STEVEN M. CHERNEY

PETER A. COLE

BRYCE A. CUNNINGHAM

ANTHONY J. DUGARTE

JONATHAN EASTMAN

JASON M. EVANS

MICHAEL J. GARDNER

GARIN HECHT

JUSTIN F. LUCAS

RAYMOND D. WRIGHT JR

MILTON LEE (CHIP) ROUTT JR

Sterile Instruments/Equipment

- Large and small pointed bone reduction clamps (Weber clamps)
- Assorted pelvic reduction clamps
- Universal manipulator (femoral distractor)
- Handheld plate bender
- Implants
  - Extra long 3.5-mm screws
  - Extra long 4.5-mm screws
  - Extra long 7.0-mm cannulated screws, partially and fully threaded, washers
  - 5.0- and 4.0-mm Schanz pins
  - 3.5-mm pelvic reconstruction plates
  - Large external fixator
- K-wires and wire driver/drill

Patient Positioning

For additional details, see the Chapter 1.
- Supine position
  - Radiolucent table.
  - Use a clean sheet, folded into thirds, as a patient pelvic lifting and positioning device.
    - Assure that the folded sheet is wide enough to be positioned under the patient from the low lumbar level to the upper third of the thigh when placed transversely across the table.
    - This folded sheet remains beneath the patient and should be without any wrinkles that could cause skin injury.

- Once on the OR table, the folded sheet is then used to elevate the patient's pelvis from the table several inches.
  - A bump consisting of two-folded and stacked OR blankets, again folded into thirds, is placed posterior to the patient's pelvis and centered on the dorsal sacral area extending distally to the proximal thigh.
  - This double-stacked blanket bump elevates the supine patient from the table to allow iliosacral screws to be inserted easily without interference from the OR table.
- Avoid patient tilting on the bump.
  - An obliquely oriented patient frustrates and complicates accurate imaging during the surgery.
- If traction is desired, an apparatus can be fashioned out of a pipe bender to be affixed to the end of the operating table.
  - This can be draped into the sterile field using an impervious stockinette.
- Thorough patient prep is essential, since multiply injured patients routinely have had insufficient inhospital hygiene.
  - Take time to remove dirt and debris prior to the sterile preparation.
  - Shave the perineal hair and cleanse the skin and genitals with isopropyl alcohol or similar antiseptic agent.
  - Isolate the perineum as necessary from the planned operative field with plastic adhesive drapes.
  - Utilize Mastisol or other skin adherent prior to applying the isolation drapes in order to create a secure seal that may otherwise be violated during the prep.
    - These should be placed posteriorly enough to allow unobstructed access to the iliosacral screw starting point, but not be stuck to the OR table or folded on itself allowing a puddle of prep solution to form.
  - Drape widely, including the entire abdomen from the xyphoid process to the base of the penis or mons pubis to allow for placement of retrograde superior ramus screw, if necessary.
  - Prepare and drape both flanks for iliosacral screws, even if the preoperative plan only calls for unilateral insertion.
- This positioning and draping allows access to perform iliosacral screw insertions, open reduction of sacroiliac joint dislocations through an anterior approach, symphyseal and anterior ring open procedures, acetabular fractures through an ilioinguinal approach, and femoral head fixation using the Smith-Petersen exposure.
- A Pfannenstiel approach is used for symphyseal disruptions.
  - Avoid placing the incision in the intertriginous area of a pannus as this can be fungal infected and a difficult area for successful wound healing.
  - Incision is approximately 2 cm cranial to the palpable superior aspect of the symphysis.
  - Visualization of the superior ramus is enhanced by incomplete anteromedial elevation of the rectus abdominis insertion from the anterior aspect of the pubis without a tenotomy.
  - Use an appropriate sized malleable retractor for retraction of the bladder and avoid deep placement of the retractor.
- Prone position
  - Radiolucent table.
  - Double-rolled OR blankets used for chest rolls.
  - Position each arm such that the shoulders are slightly forward flexed and slightly abducted and the elbows are flexed with forearms supported and the ulnar nerve unencumbered (Fig. 12-1).
    - Special articulated arm supports make this physiological positioning easy.

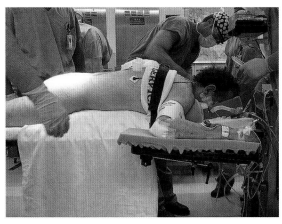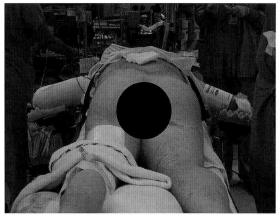

Figure 12-1 The prone positioning process is done sequentially and carefully. The face and neck are positioned anatomically and without pressure points. If a cervical collar is indicated for the patient, it is removed once prone and sandbags are applied during surgery. A cervical collar left on with the patient in the prone position risks chin necrosis. The chest rolls suspend the abdomen allowing normal anesthetic ventilation routines. The sheets are smoothed to avoid wrinkles and potential skin injury. The shoulders are slightly abducted, forward flexed, and internally rotated. The elbows are also slightly flexed and placed on padded articulated forearm supports. Blue foam can be used as padding, but the solid side should be exposed to the extremity (as seen on the left patient) rather than the "egg crate" side (as seen on the right side patient) to avoid pressure points. If the upper extremity has been splinted due to injury, the upper extremity positioning is adjusted accordingly, or in some situations, the splint is removed during surgery if the reduction is stable without a splint while under anesthesia. The splint is reapplied after surgery and radiographs assure no changes. The male patient's genitals should hang freely. The urinary catheter tubing is located anterior to the uninjured thigh-hip region and padded to avoid skin problems. The catheter-drainage tubing junction should be accessible for irrigation if necessary. The uninjured lower extremity is slightly flexed at the hip due to the chest roll suspension, and the knee is flexed slightly, while the leg-ankle-foot are supported on a pillow. The uninjured limb is padded anteriorly and taped securely. A sequential compression device may be applied, but the air hoses should be located remote from the bone or nerve prominent areas.

- A rolled egg crate foam pad under the anterior aspect of the shoulders prevents excessive shoulder sag and keeps the arm from abutting the OR table.
- Thoroughly shave, then cleanse with isopropyl alcohol, and then isolate the perineum with plastic adhesive drapes prior to prepping.
  - Mastisol or other skin adherent seals the barrier drapes well but avoid overapplication of the adherent onto the operative field.
- A laparotomy drape with a plastic bag is used, with the operative leg placed through the opening, and scissors are used to enlarge the opening to provide access for the posterior approach.
  - This is again sealed with iodine-impregnated adhesive strips after marking the proposed incision.

Reduction and Implant Techniques

- *Circumferential pelvic antishock sheeting (CPAS)*
  - Quickly decreases the pelvic volume and stabilizes the bony pelvis and the hematoma.
  - A hospital sheet is folded into thirds centered between the iliac crests and greater trochanters secured with towel clamps (Fig. 12-2).

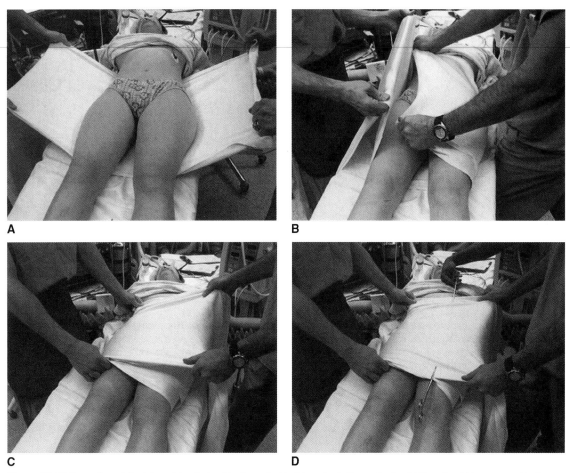

Figure 12-2 I Circumferential pelvic antishock sheeting is applied in this patient. The patient's clothing should be removed before application. The sheet is positioned beneath the patient's pelvis smoothly **(A)**. The ends of the sheet are crossed in an overlapping manner anteriorly **(B)** and are pulled taut **(C)**. Clamps secure the smooth and snug sheet **(D)**. (From Routt ML Jr, Falicov A, Woodhouse E, et al. Circumferential pelvic antishock sheeting: a temporary resuscitation aid. *J Orthop Trauma.* 2002;16:45–48, with permission.)

- Portals can be cut into the sheet for vascular access or placement of external fixator pins or percutaneous screws (Fig. 12-3).

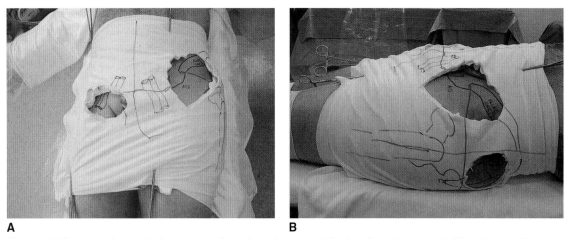

Figure 12-3 I Anterior view of the femoral vascular and anterior external fixation pin working portals **(A)** and lateral view demonstrating the iliosacral and antegrade ramus screw portals **(B)**. Working portals cut in the CPAS do not diminish the sheet function, yet allow pelvic angiography, simple anterior pelvic external frame application, or percutaneous screw fixation to proceed while the sheet maintains the reduction. (Adapted from Gardner MJ, Osgood G, Molnar R, et al. Percutaneous pelvic fixation using working portals in a circumferential pelvic antishock sheet. *J Orthop Trauma.* 2009;23:668–674, with permission.)

- *External fixation*
  - Anticipate the direction of deformity correction when planning the pin insertion site and skin incisions to minimize the skin tension and avoid the need for relaxing skin incision after the reduction maneuvers.
    - Insert a K-wire percutaneously aimed parallel with the center of the bone pathway from the anterior inferior iliac spine (AIIS) to the posterior ilium using the obturator oblique outlet view (Fig. 12-4).

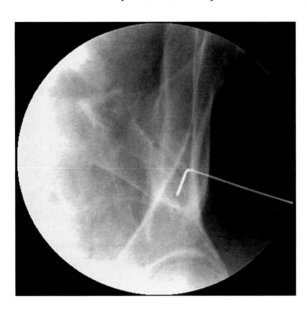

Figure 12-4 I An obturator oblique outlet view is used to obtain a starting point for supra-acetabular external fixation pins.

  - When the K-wire is on bone, bend wire 90 degrees several centimeters above the skin to allow simple C-arm imaging.
  - When tip of the wire is in the desired position, cut the bent portion and advance the K-wire using a wire driver into the AIIS several centimeters.
  - Incise the skin around the wire in the direction of the deformity correction.
  - Overdrill the K-wire with a cannulated drill and remove both the wire and the drill.
  - Insert 5.0-mm Schanz pin by hand.
    - Pin often needs to be at least 250 mm long.
  - Confirm trajectory using the obturator inlet (the pin remains between the tables) (Fig. 12-5) and the iliac oblique (the pin is cranial to the greater sciatic notch).

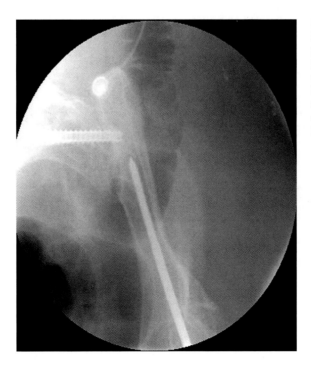

Figure 12-5 I This obturator inlet combination image reveals the osseous pathway for screw or pin insertion from the AIIS toward the posterior ilium between the iliac cortical tables. The pin is applied cranial to the greater sciatic notch and should not be too deep within the ilium that iliosacral screws are obstructed. These pins should also be applied so that antegrade ramus screws can be inserted beneath them, if necessary.

- A similar technique can be used to insert screws from the AIIS to the posterior superior iliac spine (PSIS).
- When placing reduction pins in the AIIS, a universal manipulator can be used as a pelvic compressor or distractor.
  - The advantage of using AIIS pins is that the angle of the pins relative to each other can be locked when using the distractor arms, effectively increasing the posterior closing effect of the pins.
- Alternatively, a surgical sponge can be used around each pin to achieve a provisional reduction, and then the sponges are clamped together at the midline to hold the reduction while the carbon rods and pin/bar clamps are applied (Fig. 12-6).

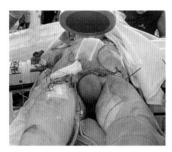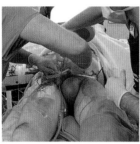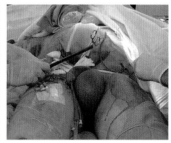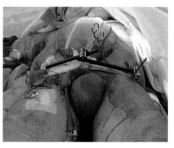

Figure 12-6 ▌ After the anterior pelvic pins are inserted, two individual surgical sponges are lashed around the pins and gathered centrally. The pins are then manipulated to achieve the needed compressive closed reduction and the overlapping sponges are clamped together. The reduction is maintained as the frame is built above the sponges. Once the frame is assembled and tightened, the sponges and clamp are released.

- This technique is much simpler and cheaper than using a manipulative device.
- The sponges do not obstruct the frame assembly as a manipulative device does.
- For external fixation frames mounted on AIIS pins that will be retained definitively, a cranial starting point and a caudally directed pin will facilitate patient mobilization and upright positioning by allowing slightly more hip flexion before the frame impinges on the thigh (Fig. 12-7).

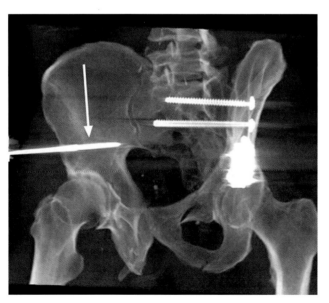

Figure 12-7 ▌ The right-sided iliac oblique view confirms the pin depth and obliquity. The pin is inserted beginning at the cranial aspect of the AIIS between the iliac cortical tables and is aimed to end just cranial to the greater sciatic notch (*arrow*). This small amount of pin "flexion" allows improved hip flexion and therefore eases sitting and patient mobility.

Routt 1: Quadrangular Anterior Pelvic External Fixation

Milton Lee (Chip) Routt Jr.
Bryce A. Cunningham
Steven M. Cherney

Pathophysiology

Anterior pelvic external fixation devices are used to stabilize acute pelvic ring disruptions. These devices are commonly simple frame constructs that are positioned to allow abdominal excursion and patient mobilization to the sitting position. Unfortunately, most anterior pelvic external frame constructs obstruct anterior pelvic and lower abdominal surgical access as shown in Figure 12-8.

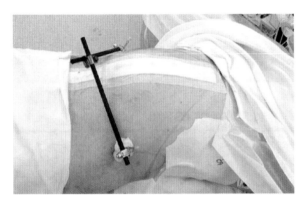

Figure 12-8 ∥ This anterior pelvic external fixation device was removed by the general surgeon because it obstructed anterior abdominal access during the laparotomy.

Delaying application of the frame until after abdominal operations or procedures risks ongoing pelvic-related hemorrhage. Removing the anterior frame allows unobstructed surgical access to perform open anterior pelvic, genitourinary, and lower abdominal operations but destabilizes the pelvic ring injury and risks losing the prior reduction.

Solution

If a routine anterior pelvic external frame construct is maintaining a satisfactory pelvic reduction but is obstructing anterior pelvic surgical access, it can be replaced by a quadrangular frame design without losing the reduction.

Technique

- In order to maintain the obstructing frame's reduction, the surgeon places a cotton sponge snugly around the iliac pins on each side and then clamps the sponge ends together.
  - The taut sponges maintain the reduction as the pin/bar clamps and bars are then removed (Fig. 12-9).

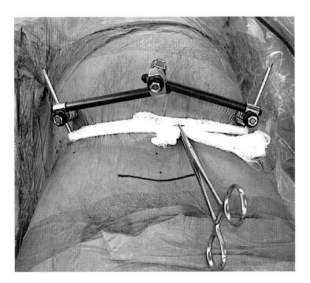

Figure 12-9 ∥ Two sponges are tightly wrapped around the iliac pins, and then their ends are clamped to maintain the pelvic compression.

- The pin to bar clamps, bars, and bar to bar clamp can then be removed without losing the reduction.
- The quadrangular frame is then applied to the iliac pins and positioned to maintain the overall pelvic reduction while allowing the surgeon unobstructed access to the anterior pelvis for open reduction and internal fixation (Fig. 12-10).

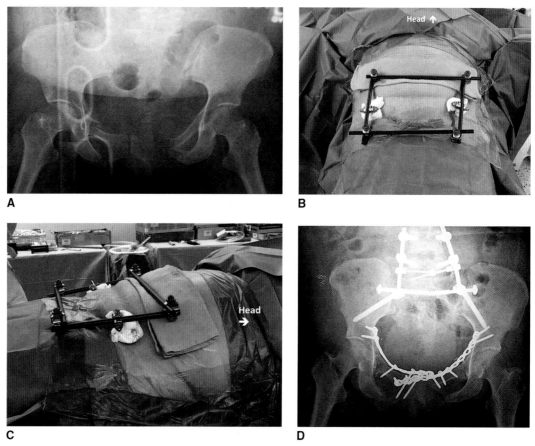

Figure 12-10 ▌ **A–D:** In this patient, a Pfannenstiel exposure was planned to treat her complex anterior pelvic fractures. Her initial anterior pelvic frame was applied during the resuscitation phase of her presentation and provided an acceptable pelvic reduction. Without the frame, her pelvic fracture displacements and deformities were excessive and would have complicated the operative repair. The intraoperative clinical photographs show the quadrangular frame that was exchanged for her initial device. The quadrangular frame was attached to the two iliac pins and positioned for unobstructed anterior pelvic surgical access. If a laparotomy had been needed, the upper transverse bar would have been selectively removed.

- After the operation is completed if the frame is needed for pelvic stability, it can be converted back to a simple anterior frame construct. However, if the pelvis is sufficiently stabilized by the surgery, then the iliac pins and frame are removed.

- *Pubic symphyseal plating*
  - The skin, local soft tissues, and rectus abdominis muscles assist in the reduction of the symphysis widening by providing a leverage point for Hohmann retractors.
    - The points of the retractors are placed just lateral to each pubic tubercle and posterior to the rectus insertions.

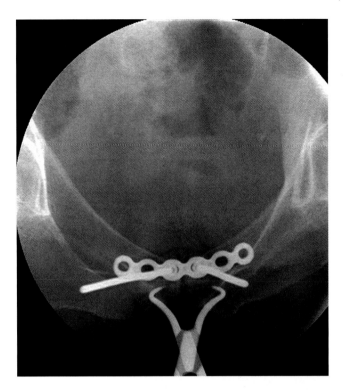

Figure 12-11 ▌ A small reduction clamp was applied to the pubic tubercles bilaterally to maintain the symphyseal reduction while the plate was attached. Clamp application into the obturator foramen is essentially never necessary although historically advocated.

- ▪ Alternatively, pointed reduction clamps may be used to reduce the pubic symphysis (Fig. 12-11).
- ● A straight six- to eight-hole 3.5-mm reconstruction plate is easily contoured to fit well and provides reliable symphyseal fixation.
- ● Place a slight prebend in the center and again just medial to both peripheral holes so that the peripheral screws can be directed toward the inferomedial symphyseal areas. This improves fixation by allowing triangulation of implants and allows for longer screws (Fig. 12-12).

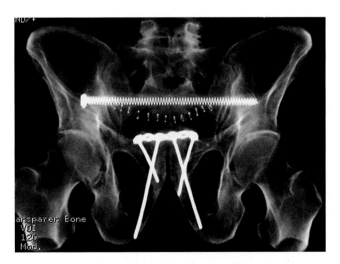

Figure 12-12 ▌ Long central hole medullary screws are bilaterally directed toward the ischium to improve fixation. The peripheral screws are directed toward the inferomedial symphyseal arcuate areas to triangulate each side of the symphyseal fixation construct.

- ● The plate can be used to assist with the reduction of slight residual symphyseal widening.
  - ▪ Predrill a hole on each ramus adjacent to the subchondral surface with the screw aimed slightly away from the midline.
  - ▪ Elevate the cartilage cap for direct visualization of the subchondral surface to ensure precise screw positioning.
  - ▪ Place the screws through the central two holes and sequentially tighten them, alternating from one to the other.
    - ● As the screw heads are tightened and contact the plate, the plate functions to reduce the disrupted symphysis.

- ▪ Be cognizant when using this technique that small inaccuracies in predrilled hole locations near the midline are magnified at the ends of the plate, potentially leading to a plate being off of the bone laterally.
- Transsymphyseal screws through the plate are used when routine screw placement fails due to poor bone quality, fracture comminution, or other issues (Fig. 12-13).

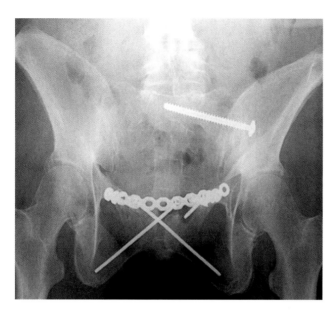

Figure 12-13 ▮ This patient was injured in an equestrian accident and had routine symphyseal plating. Three days after surgery, the routine plate fixation failed and was revised successfully to this construct using an anteriorly located and longer symphyseal plate with transsymphyseal screw fixation.

- Transsymphyseal retrograde ramus screws can be used to stabilize disruptions of the symphysis when it is desirable to have as little exposed surface implants as possible, such as in treatment of open pelvic disruptions (Fig. 12-14).

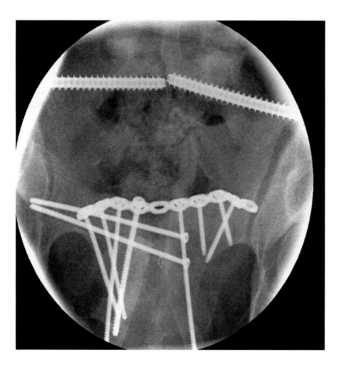

Figure 12-14 ▮ This patient developed early routine symphyseal plate fixation failure due to a deep anterior pelvic infection. The failed implants were removed, the wound was debrided, and the symphysis reduced and stabilized using this plating technique with supplemental transsymphyseal medullary ramus screws.

- Heavy, nonabsorbable suture may also be used to stabilize the symphysis in children or in open fractures to minimize the foreign body load.

- This is not as biomechanically sound and should be augmented with posterior fixation in most cases (Fig. 12-15).

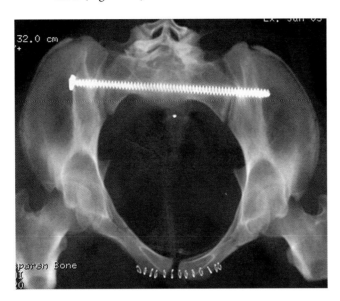

Figure 12-15 | This 14-year-old female had an unstable pelvic ring disruption due to an automobile crash. Her complete symphysis pubis disruption was treated with open reduction, and then suture fixation through parasymphyseal anterior to posterior bone tunnels was done.

- Unstable and displaced posterior pelvic injuries are often best treated with open reduction; however, review of the CT scan may reveal a corresponding sacral crush injury significant enough to preclude a good reduction read through an anterior approach (Fig. 12-16).

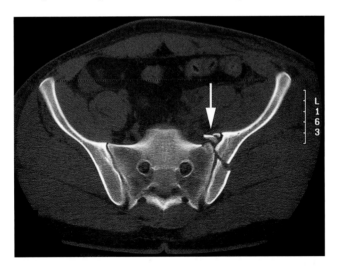

Figure 12-16 | This patient had a crescent fracture dislocation with significant ventral sacral impaction (arrow). This must be accounted for when considering the available reduction assessments through an anterior approach.

- This also creates a problem when trying to position clamps to obtain and hold the reduction, as the clamp in the sacrum will inevitably be in a comminuted fracture zone with little stable cortical bone available for the clamp.

TIP

The Pelvic Bridge

Peter A. Cole
Anthony J. Dugarte

Pathoanatomy

Fractures involving the anterior pelvic ring, specifically those with rami fractures, may require anterior fixation to allow for immediate weight-bearing or increased stability and comfort. External fixators have been used for this purpose, but are often associated with substantial morbidity that includes pin loosening, pin tract infection, and patient dissatisfaction.

Solution

Use of an anterior subcutaneous minimally invasive fixation technique or the anterior pelvis provides an alternative to external fixation and may be associated with improved patient comfort and fewer complications.

Technique

This technique provides fixation across the anterior pelvis, inserted percutaneously, and allowing fixation into the iliac crest and parasymphyseal region.

Implant(s): An occipital cervical plate-rod construct can be placed unilaterally or bilaterally. Its advantages include the following:

- Spans the injured anterior pelvis from the iliac wing to the contralateral pubic tubercle.
- Construct is passed subcutaneously, superficial to the external oblique fascia:
  - Parallels the course of the inguinal ligament and thus maintains a safe location from the critical neurovascular structures
  - Minimizes risk of impingement to lateral femoral cutaneous nerve (LFCN), femoral nerve, femoral artery, femoral vein, and spermatic cord/round ligament
- When compared to the InFix (another anterior internal pelvic fixator concept), the pelvic bridge has several advantages:
  - Parallels static inguinal ligament in an anterior location therefore maintaining a safe profile
  - Mitigates risk of LFCN impalement and compression
  - Biomechanically superior with more points of fixation into the pubic region as well as ilium
  - Allows for multiple multiplanar points of fixation
  - Stabilizes fractured pubis or rami, which serve as key insertions for muscles, allowing for greater comfort during mobilization
  - Does not interfere with abdominal cavity
  - More familiar and superficial landmarks for surgeons

Indications

- Can be used as a substitute for anterior pelvic external fixation
- Unstable anterior pelvic injuries
- Definitive management certain fracture patterns
- Promotion of early mobilization
- Obese patients with anterior pelvic lesions

Contraindications

- Dissociation of the iliac crest
- Open injury with peritoneal contamination
- Degloving over the iliac crest
- Hemodynamically unstable patients
- Isolated pubic disruption (recommend ORIF)
- Should not be used as sole management for anterior and posterior injuries/instability
- Untested in children <12 years old

Preoperative Planning

- Review pertinent imaging to determine operative plan (Fig. 12-17).
  - Assess adequacy of bone tunnels in both the iliac crests and parasymphyseal pubic rami.
  - Use a pelvic model to draw fracture lines and plan hardware positioning.

Patient Positioning

- Patient supine on radiolucent table.
- Elevate sacrum with midline bolster if iliosacral screws are to be used for posterior lesion.
  - Place patient's arms at <90 degrees of abduction, secured on arm boards.
  - Shave pubic hair and isolate the groin with an occlusive dressing. Prep and drape from the lower ribs to the proximal thigh.
  - C-arm imaging capacity, perpendicular to the table for pelvic AP, inlet, outlet and Judet views.

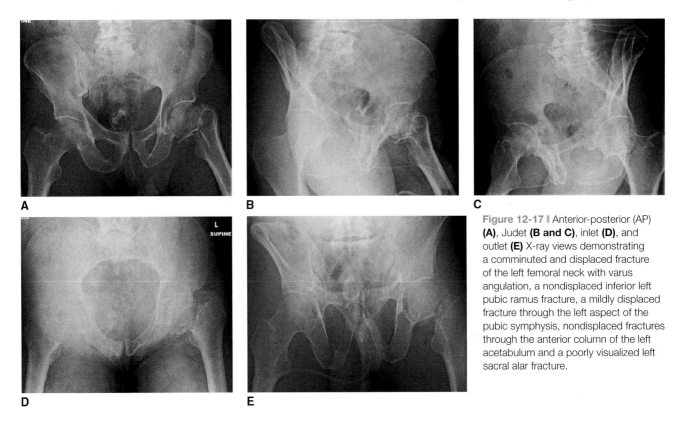

A

B

C

D

E

Figure 12-17 | Anterior-posterior (AP) **(A)**, Judet **(B and C)**, inlet **(D)**, and outlet **(E)** X-ray views demonstrating a comminuted and displaced fracture of the left femoral neck with varus angulation, a nondisplaced inferior left pubic ramus fracture, a mildly displaced fracture through the left aspect of the pubic symphysis, nondisplaced fractures through the anterior column of the left acetabulum and a poorly visualized left sacral alar fracture.

Approach

- Make lateral incision over ASIS (Fig. 12-18), extending posteriorly along the crest for 5 cm.
  - Dissect down to external oblique fascia.
  - Dissect and expose iliac crest to reveal a fixation point for plate-rod construct.

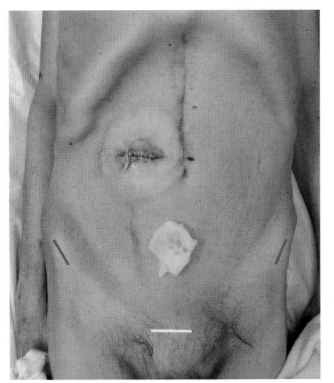

Figure 12-18 | In a cadaver demonstration, incisions are placed over both anterior-superior iliac spines (ASIS, *blue*), as well as a Pfannenstiel-type incision over the pubic symphysis (*yellow*).

- In the midline, use a horizontal, 6- to 8-cm Pfannenstiel incision (Fig. 12-18), centered over the pubic symphysis.
  - Use cautery or scalpel to dissect down to the rectus abdominis fascia.
  - Make a vertical incision in the linea alba.
  - Identify the pubic symphysis and tubercles.
  - Next, use a periosteal elevator or Cobb elevator to establish a subcutaneous tunnel, superficial to the inguinal ligament.

Contouring the Construct
- We use the following spinal instrumentation as an off-label use (Fig. 12-19):
  - Synthes (DePuy-Synthes, Westchester, PA) occipital cervical plate-rod construct from spinal fusion system (4.0-mm diameter rod)
  - Synthes Synapse System polyaxial screws (4.5 mm)
  - Cross-links

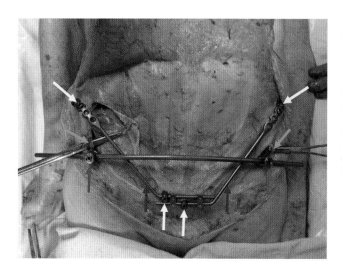

Figure 12-19 ▌Cadaveric specimen shows the proximity of another variety of internal pelvic fixation device (*blue arrow*), its 2 points of pelvic fixation (*red arrows*), and the proximity of each pedicle screw to the lateral femoral cutaneous nerve (LFCN, *green arrows*). The pelvic bridge bilateral, plate-rod construct (*purple arrows*) follows the course of the inguinal ligament, a static structure, and renders 4 different points of fixation (*yellow arrows*) in this case. The LFCN (*green arrows*) is undisturbed by the pelvic bridge.

- Contour the plate with a gentle curve to accommodate the iliac crest.
- Where the plate meets the rod, place approximately a 25-degree bend perpendicular to the plate in a caudal direction.
- At the pubic tubercle, a second bend is made so the rod courses parallel to the symphysis.
  - This bend is about 60 degrees, allowing for the rod to border the anterior-superior border of the superior pubic tubercles.
- Ensure the contour is safely superficial to the inguinal ligament such that there is no chance of compressing underlying neurovasculature.
- The rod should not place any posterior compression on the inguinal ligament if it follows a vector from the ASIS to the pubis.
- It is possible that the construct will need to be adjusted to ensure best fit.

Passing the Plate-rod Construct
- Insert the rod and pass from lateral to medial, superficial to the inguinal ligament (Fig. 12-20).
- Assess the plate contour on the iliac crest.
- Provisional screw placement is established at the iliac crest. A pelvic reduction can be performed before finalizing rod position over the tubercles and deploying pedicle screws.
  - Fluoroscopy may further assist in determining the adequacy of the contour.

Reduction
- Reduction usually consists of simple manual compression of iliac crests when the pelvic bridge is being used to augment a pelvis that is stable (or stabilized) posteriorly
  - If control for rotation and vertical translation are needed, Schanz pins can be inserted either into the crest, posterior to the plate, or in the supra-acetabular corridor using a small ancillary incision.
    - These pins can be used as joysticks to control the hemipelves to further assist in reduction.
  - A distal femoral traction pin can be used to augment reduction of the hemipelvis as well.

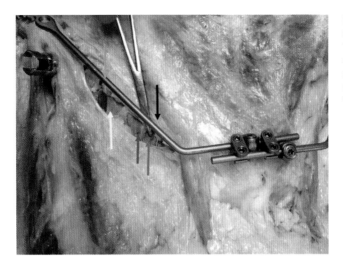

Figure 12-20 ▌ The superficial positioning of the pelvic bridge (*green arrow*) relative to the inguinal ligament (*black arrow*) maintains a safe distance from the underlying neurovascular bundle. The femoral nerve (*yellow arrow*), artery (*red arrow*), and/or vein (*blue arrow*) are depicted.

Fixation to the Ilium

- Place a single large fragment titanium screw through the plate into the iliac crest; this allows rotation (pivot) of the construct for optimal placement on the both the crest and symphysis.
- The trajectory is down the iliac crest into the anterior column and is similar to the Schanz pin placement for application of an iliac crest-based external fixator, except not as posterior in the gluteus medius tubercle.
  - Use oblique and rollover views of the iliac crest for assistance (Fig. 12-21).
  - Usually, a 15-degree external rollover view from an outlet position is ideal to assess.
  - The drill resistance can provide feedback for appropriate intraosseous position; 50 to 100 mm screws are typical.

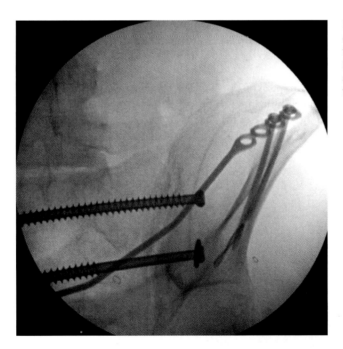

Figure 12-21 ▌ Intraoperative C-arm image demonstrates the medial and caudad trajectory of two 4.5-locking bolts into the left iliac crest. Either a large fragment titanium screw or a locking screw designed for femoral nails can be used.

Unilateral Anterior Construct

- Insert 4.5-mm polyaxial pedicle screws into the pubic tubercle (Fig. 12-22), in line with the rod construct, and then lock to the rod with a locking cap.
  - Trajectory of these screws mimics those used to secure a plate into the pubic symphysis; however, with extension arms off the rod, multiplanar pedicle screws can be deployed when needed such as in osteoporotic bone.

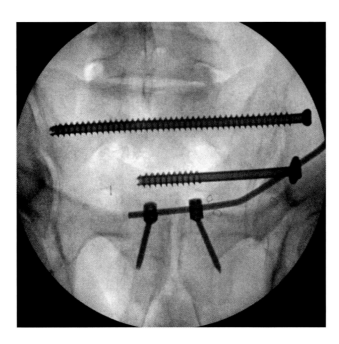

Figure 12-22 ▌ Intraoperative C-arm image shows the trajectory of 4.0-pedicle screws into each pubic tubercle to capture the rod.

Bilateral Anterior Construct

- Apply a plate-rod construct to the contralateral iliac crest and pass subcutaneously as previously described.
- Each rod requires a minimum of 1 polyaxial screw inserted on the contralateral pubic tubercle; 2 screws on each side of the symphysis provide a stronger construct.
- Overcrowding of polyaxial screws may occur.
  - This is remedied by inserting subsequent screws off-axis (Fig. 12-23).

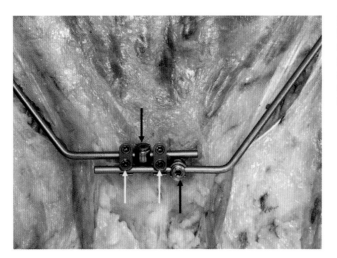

Figure 12-23 ▌ Bilateral construct of the pelvic bridge shown in a cadaveric specimen. Note the option for multiplanar placement of the pedicle screws (*black arrow*) in each pubic tubercle. Stability is greatly enhanced by rod connectors (*yellow arrows*).

- When fixation about the symphysis is achieved, 2 or 3 additional cortical screws can be inserted into the iliac crest if needed.
  - Two screws typically provide adequate fixation (Fig. 12-24).

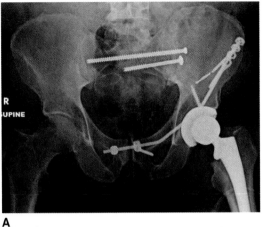

A

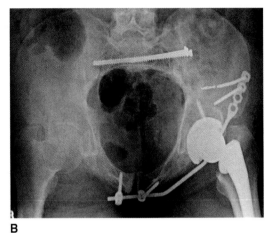

B

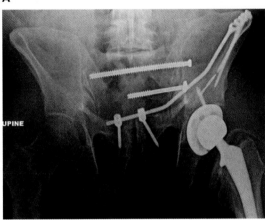

C

Figure 12-24 ▌ Postoperative AP **(A)**, inlet **(B)**, and outlet **(C)** X-ray views demonstrating stable positioning of the unilateral pelvic bridge.

References

1. Kim WY, Hearn TC, Seleem O, et al. Effect of pin location on stability of pelvic external fixation. *Clin Orthop Relat Res.* 1999;361:237–244.
2. Hiesterman TG, Hill BW, Cole PA. A percutaneous method of subcutaneous fixation for the anterior pelvic ring, the pelvic bridge. *Clin Orthop Relat Res.* 2012;470:2116–2123.
3. Kuttner M, Klaiber A, Lorenz T, et al. Der subkutane ventral Fixateur interne (SVFI) am Becken. *Unfallchirurg.* 2009;112:661–669.
4. Hesse D, Kandmir U, Solberg B, et al. Femoral nerve palsy after pelvic fracture treated with INFIX: a case series. *J Orthop Trauma.* 2015;29:138–143.
5. Vaidya R, Colen R, Vigdorchik J, et al. Treatment of unstable pelvic ring injuries with an internal anterior fixator and posterior fixation: initial clinical series. *J Orthop Trauma.* 2012;26:1–8.

- *Iliosacral screws*
  - Critical evaluation of the morphology of the upper sacral segments is imperative to proper screw positioning.
  - The space available for a screw can be determined using the axial images at the level of the upper sacral nerve root tunnel.

- ■ The "safe zone" is measured from the anterior portion of the upper sacral segment's tunnel to the anterior cortex of the sacrum (Fig. 12-25).

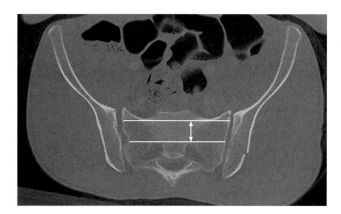

Figure 12-25 ▌ Preoperative planning for iliosacral screws using axial CT allows for safe zone determination (*double arrow*).

- ● It should also be determined if the screw can be safely oriented as a "sacral-style" screw.
- ● Some patients have substantial safe zones and pathology that permits screws to be directed across the midline up to or through the contralateral sacroiliac joint and ilium (transiliac-transsacral screws) (Fig. 12-26).

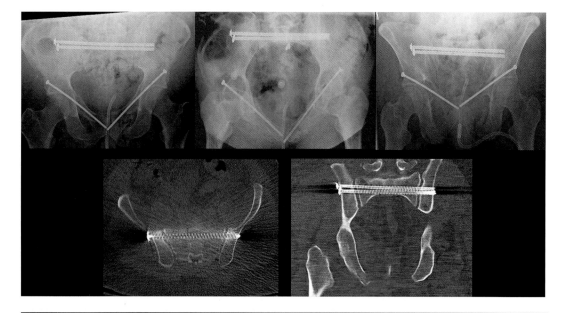

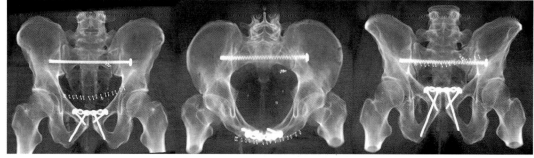

Figure 12-26 ▌ Transiliac-transsacral screws are used to stabilize the bilateral posterior pelvic injuries. Long screws up to 180- to 190-mm lengths are necessary for these applications.

- ■ Usually, this requires a screw length >170 mm, and the longer screws may only be available with larger diameters.
  - ● This may impact the ability to place these screws in narrow safe zones.

Preoperative Planning of Transiliac-Transsacral Screw Placement With Standard Computed Tomography Imaging

Justin F. Lucas
Jonathan G. Eastman

Pathoanatomy

Percutaneous stabilization of posterior pelvic ring injuries allows for reliable and effective fixation of pelvic fractures without the associated morbidity of an open procedure. The size of each patient's S1 and S2 osseous fixation pathways are incredibly variable. A thorough understanding of patient specific anatomy combined with methodical preoperative planning is important for the safe insertion of transiliac-transsacral screws. Incomplete assessment of pelvic anatomy including unrecognized sacral dysmorphism may result in aberrant screw placement and associated neurovascular injury. Screw placement too anteriorly may breach the cortex of the sacral ala. A posterior and inferiorly placed screw can violate the sacral neuroforaminal tunnel.

Solution

Numerous imaging modalities and postacquisition processing methods exist but are not widely accessible or cost-effective. Standard computed tomography (CT) data including axial and sagittal plane reformatted images can be used to preoperatively plan for accurate screw placement. In addition to an accurate reduction, correct intraoperative fluoroscopic assessment of osseous landmarks and correct technical execution must occur for safe percutaneous screw fixation. The technique outlined below aids in preoperative planning for transiliac-transsacral screw placement by allowing the arrow cursor to mimic the position of the screw as it traverses the posterior pelvis.

Technique

- Assess axial plane CT imaging at the desired level of screw placement for the presence of an osseous fixation pathway amenable to transiliac-transsacral screw fixation.
- Draw two parallel transverse lines extending from the ilium, through the sacrum, and traversing the contralateral sacral ala and ilium. One line should be posterior to the anterior sacral cortex, and the other line should be anterior to the sacral neuroforaminal tunnel. The distance between the two lines should measure at least the diameter of the screw to be used (Fig. 12-27).

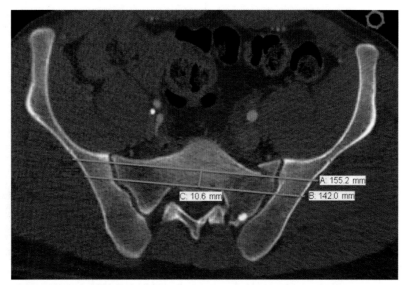

Figure 12-27 | Axial CT scan at the level of the S1 body. The potential intraosseous pathway has been outlined and measured to be 10.6 mm (C). Potential screw lengths can also be estimated (A, 155 mm; B, 142 mm).

- The size of the available osseous fixation pathway visualized on the axial imaging can vary depending on the amount of lumbosacral lordosis or kyphosis.[1] Without specialized reformatting, the sagittal plane reformations demonstrate the variability present and can verify the presence of a viable pathway (Fig. 12-28).

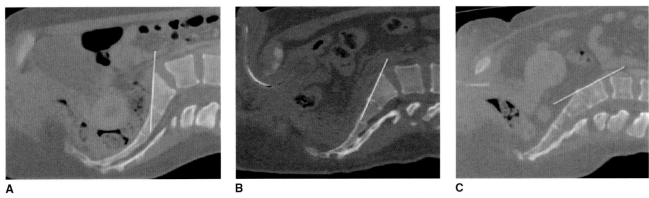

A   **B**   **C**

Figure 12-28 I Midline sagittal CT reconstruction images of uninjured pelvic rings demonstrating the amount of variability in the posterior pelvis. Note how the amount of lordosis decreases from **(A–C)**. The nonreformatted axial CT images of these sacral bodies would display notably different appearing osseous fixation pathways due to the amount of the sacral body that would appear in the serial images.

- Using the measurement or ruler tool, draw a line similar in size to the cursor arrow measuring approximately 7 to 8 mm (Fig. 12-29). This is consistent with the diameter of commonly used implants. The overall magnification of the image may need to be changed to ensure the appropriate size. Once obtained, the magnification must not be changed.

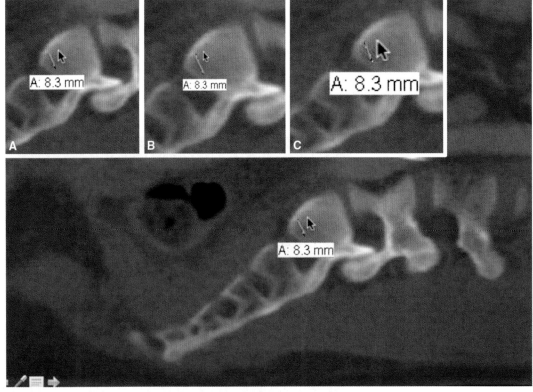

Figure 12-29 I Sagittal CT reconstruction with measurement line drawn to approximate implant diameter in relation to cursor height. **A:** Appropriate amount of magnification with the *arrow* approximately 8.3 mm in size. **B:** Overmagnification with *cursor arrow* appearing smaller than the appropriate reference of 8.3 mm resulting in overestimation of a safe screw path. **C:** Undermagnification with *cursor arrow* appearing larger than the appropriate reference of 8.3 mm resulting in underestimation of a safe screw path.

- To use the cursor arrow to mimic the path of a transiliac-transsacral screw, begin at the level of the sacral neuroforaminal tunnel of the uninjured side or the side with the least amount of displacement.
- Place the cursor in the ideal screw location: posterior to the anterior sacral cortex, anterior and superior to the neuroforaminal tunnel, and caudal to the superior cortex of the superior sacral body and neuroforaminal tunnel. Without moving the cursor scroll, the sagittal images toward the ipsilateral ilium. Next, scroll in the opposite direction past the ipsilateral sacral neuroforaminal tunnel, into and across the sacral body, through the contralateral neuroforaminal tunnel zone and ala, and into the contralateral ilium (Fig. 12-30).

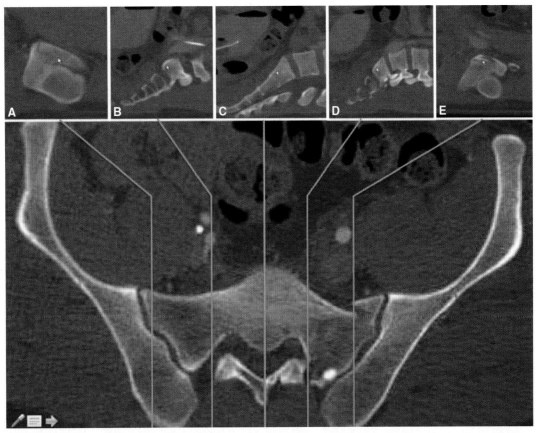

Figure 12-30 ▌ Sagittal CT images of the *cursor arrow* mimicking the initial transiliac-transsacral screw in a caudal anterior position within the osseous fixation pathway. Isolated images at **(A)** right sacral ala/sacroiliac joint, **(B)** right neuroforaminal tunnel, **(C)** midline sacral body, **(D)** left neuroforaminal tunnel, and **(E)** left sacral ala/sacroiliac joint. The cursor remains intraosseous throughout, and a transiliac-transsacral screw can be placed safely in this osseous corridor. The location of each sagittal CT image is referenced on the axial image by corresponding *blue lines*.

- If the cursor remains intraosseous throughout the entire process, it can be confirmed that there is an osseous corridor large enough to accommodate transiliac-transsacral screw fixation at that level.
- If the cursor becomes extraosseous at some point, attempts are made to reposition the cursor into a more optimal position and the process is repeated.
- If multiple screws are to be placed at the same level, repeat the process with the cursor in a new location (Fig. 12-31). For two screws, the initial screw is typically in a low and anterior position. The second screw is just superior and posterior to the initial screw.
- One limitation to this technique results from malpositioning of the patient during acquisition of CT imaging. If the patient is notably off-axis in relation to the axial plane, the osseous fixation pathway may appear too oblique and a screw path may seem not to exist when a screw path is available.

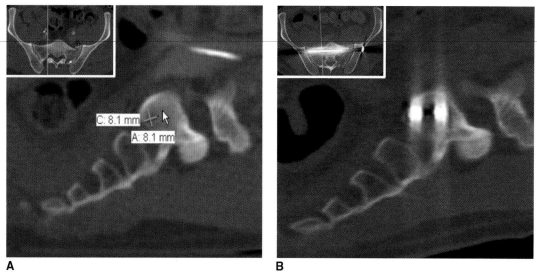

A   **B**

Figure 12-31 ‖ **A:** Sagittal CT image using scaled measurement lines in addition to *cursor arrow* to assess space for multiple screws. **B:** Sagittal CT images obtained postoperatively demonstrating safe placement of two transiliac-transsacral screws. Inset images demonstrate location of sagittal plane reformat in relation to axial image.

Reference

1. McAndrew CM, Merriman DJ, Gardner MJ, et al. Standardized posterior pelvic imaging: use of CT inlet and CT outlet for evaluation and management of pelvic ring injuries. *J Orthop Trauma*. 2014;28(12):665–673.

- Distal femoral traction (10 to 15 lb) is helpful to improve the reduction of many posterior pelvic ring deformities.
- Flexion/extension and internal/external rotation deformities can be manually addressed or reduced with the aid of an external fixator or pelvic manipulator attached to Schanz pins placed in each ilium.
  - For this method to be maximally effective, an intact hemipelvis is required.
- After reduction, three views are used to guide safe iliosacral screws: pelvic inlet, pelvic outlet, and true lateral sacral views (Fig. 12-32).

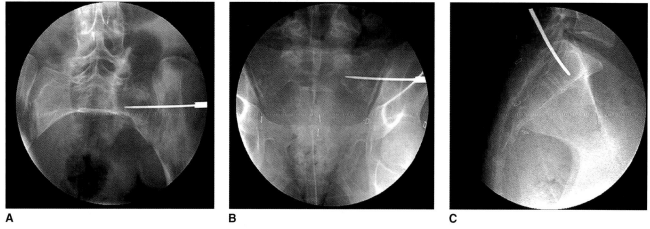

A   **B**   **C**

Figure 12-32 ‖ The initial upper sacral segment iliosacral screw is positioned low and anterior to allow simple subsequent screw insertions if needed. A guide wire is drilled to the lateral aspect of the sacral neural tunnel as seen on the inlet **(A)** and outlet **(B)** images. The true lateral image **(C)** is then assessed to assure that the wire tip is cranial to the neural tunnel, posterior to the anterior vertebral cortical limit, and appropriately directed before it is inserted further. On the true lateral sacral image after reduction, the iliac cortical densities are superimposed and reveal the alar slope for most nondysmorphic sacral ala. The upper sacral neural tunnels are also well seen on this image.

- If bowel gas or contrast is obstructing, slight additional C-arm obliquity can be used to clarify the field of vision (Fig. 12-33).

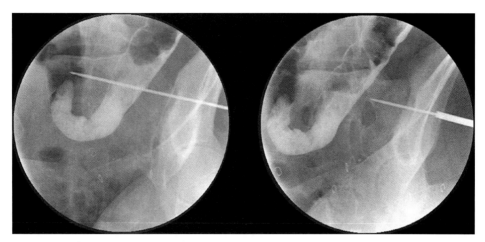

Figure 12-33 I In this patient, evaluative bowel contrast agents were administered prior to transfer. The loop of contrasted bowel obstructs routine outlet imaging of the upper sacral segment specifically at the neural tunnel exit or foramen. By simply rolling the C-arm intensifier slightly to an obturator oblique outlet combination image, the ventral foramen and guide wire tip are well seen.

- Prior to prepping, obtain pelvic inlet and pelvic outlet views and mark the position of the C-arm with tape on the C-arm and/or on the floor.
  - This sets the appropriate angles and the views remain consistent and easily reproducible as long as the OR table height stays constant.
- There are many subtleties to the inlet view.
  - Some upper sacral segments are fairly linear with the anterior borders of S1–S3 superimposing to form a clear cortical density at the same inlet tilt.
  - Other sacra have significant kyphosis through these levels, and determining which segment's cortical border is imaged can be difficult.
  - This can be anticipated by viewing the lateral scout image from the CT scan, from which the level of maximum kyphosis and the approximate tilt for the correct inlet view can be estimated.
- The radiographic "indentations" of the dysmorphic upper sacral segment must be clearly visualized on the pelvic inlet view prior to placing the screws (Fig. 12-34).

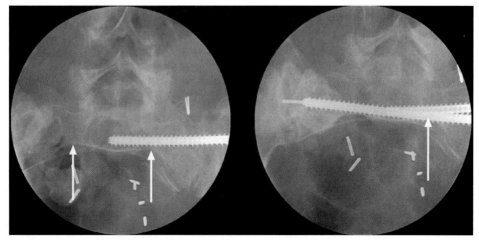

Figure 12-34 I On the pelvic inlet fluoroscopic image, this dysmorphic upper sacral segment's anterior cortical indentations represent the alar cortical limits (*arrows*). The second sacral segment screw direction and location obstruct these upper sacral important cortical markers, so the upper segment screws should be inserted initially in dysmorphic patients.

- These indentations represent the anterior cortical limit of the upper segment.
- These will be obstructed by a second sacral segment screw and make safe placement challenging. Therefore, the upper screw should be placed first.
  - Starting point.
    - The entry point in the skin is different for a sacroiliac-style screw compared to a sacral-style screw.
    - It is helpful to obtain both the inlet and outlet views and draw a line perpendicular to the beam with each view (parallel to the receiver of the C-arm) and draw them on the surgical field for reference.
    - The anterior-posterior plane is adjusted from the pelvic inlet view, and the cranial/caudal plane is adjusted based on the pelvic outlet view.
    - Intersecting lines drawn from the ASIS perpendicular to the floor and along the axis of the femur create quadrants as visual cues to appropriate skin starting position.
    - The correct skin entry point is often in the posterior and cranial quadrants (Fig. 12-35).

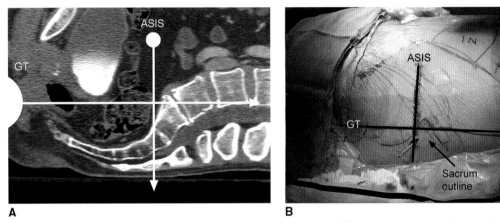

A   **B**

Figure 12-35 | A: Approximate palpable bony anatomy overlying a sagittal CT scan demonstrating their relationships. **B:** Skin surface markings using palpable bony landmarks: the anterior-superior iliac spine (ASIS) and greater trochanter (*GT*) help to guide initial pin insertion position.

- In addition to these, obtain an inlet view and insert a 0.062-inch K-wire into the skin in the proposed path of screw insertion so that the tip of the wire is along an imaginary line drawn between the center points of the faces of the C-arm.
- Once satisfied with the wire position on this view, check the pelvic outlet view.
  - Commonly, this places the cranial aspect of the symphysis at the level of the second sacral segment.
  - If the pin position is excellent on the pelvic outlet view, the skin can then be incised parallel to the axis that requires slight correction.
  - Be sure to incise the tensor fascia lata in order to create a single soft tissue tunnel for repeated instrument insertion; otherwise, several punctures in the deep fascia can prevent reliably finding the same starting point.
- Insert the guide wire sleeve over the K-wire, and hold the guide steady on the lateral ilium while exchanging the K-wire for the 2-mm threaded guide wire.
- Secure the 2-mm guide wire to the drill with a Jacob's chuck.
- The insertion point can be adjusted slightly by translating the pin and guide in the desired direction.
- For maximal control of direction of the wire, use the nondominant hand placed securely on the OR table, underneath the drill similar to a camera's stabilizing tripod.
  - Rest the driver on this forearm just proximal to the wrist.
  - This provides a stable "tripod" to maintain direction of insertion and also provides the ability to make small corrections with flexion and extension of the wrist.
- The guide wire can then be advanced if both the starting point and the trajectory are perfect.
- Alternatively, advance the guide wire several millimeters into the ilium without entering the SI joint space to anchor the pin.

- The cannulated drill can be inserted and oscillated to just past the tip of the pin, and small corrections can be made with the drill.
- The aim can also be slightly redirected by removing the drill and placing a guide wire into the hole at one edge of the drilled hole and then tapped forward into the cancellous bone.
- The drill is then reinserted over this guide wire and is slowly advanced forward to etch out one side of the hole and effectively alter the trajectory.
- The true lateral sacral view should superimpose the iliac cortical densities (ICDs) and greater sciatic notches, which mark the sacral ala in nondysmorphic sacra, and is confirmed on preoperative CT scans.
  - If the guide wire or screw is:
    - Caudal and posterior to the ICD when at the level of the lateral edge of the upper sacral nerve root tunnel and
    - Cranial and anterior to the nerve root tunnel, the screw is safely contained within the bone (Fig. 12-36).

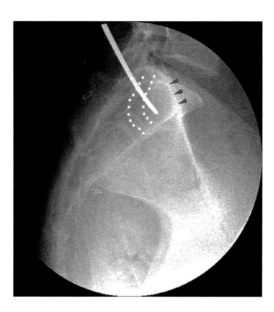

Figure 12-36 I This true sacral lateral fluoroscopic view is taken with the guide wire just lateral to the nerve root tunnel. On this view, the wire is seen posterior and caudal to the superimposed iliac cortical densities (*arrowheads*), and cranial and anterior to the nerve root tunnel (*dotted line*), indicating safe position. (Adapted from Farrell ED, Gardner MJ, Krieg JC, et al. The upper sacral nerve root tunnel: an anatomic and clinical study. *J Orthop Trauma.* 2009;23:333–339, with permission.)

- Obtain an AP view with a 20-degree rollover, to image down the ilium and confirm the washer is fully seated and not intruded through the cortex (Fig. 12-37).

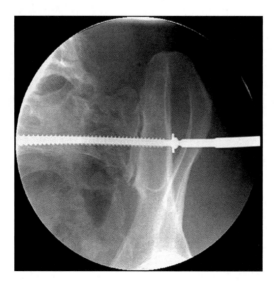

Figure 12-37 I This view "down the ilium," obtained by approximately 20 degrees of C-arm roll over, images the washer as it is fully seated.

Transiliac-Transsacral Screw Shuttling for Closed Reduction and Percutaneous Stabilization of Bilateral Posterior Pelvic Ring Injuries

Garin Hecht
Jonathan G. Eastman

Pathoanatomy

Bilateral posterior pelvic ring injuries, ranging from sacral fractures, sacroiliac joint fracture dislocations, and sacroiliac joint dislocations, vary in severity and can be challenging to treat.

Solution

With each hemipelvis being mobile, a common sequence in the treatment algorithm is to stabilize one hemipelvis first in order to create a stable posterior segment. The hemipelvis with the least amount of displacement or with the less complicated reduction is usually chosen first. Once that reduction is successfully completed the other hemipelvis can then be manipulated back onto the stable base. Often, this is aided with the use of multiplanar Schanz pins, other percutaneous instruments, and an external fixator or universal distractor aligned in the appropriate force vector. Once reductions are obtained, stability is commonly provided with iliosacral or transiliac-transsacral screws depending on multiple factors including but not limited to injury severity, bone quality, available osseous fixation pathways, anticipated patient compliance, and surgeon preference.

The technique of using transiliac-transsacral style screw in at least one sacral segment is useful for sequentially stabilizing bilateral posterior pelvic ring injuries. Once the first hemipelvis is reduced, it is stabilized with at least one transiliac-transsacral style screw. Once the contralateral hemipelvis is successfully reduced, the cannulated screw construct is then used to help provide temporary stability and then final fixation. This allows for successful stabilization of bilateral injuries along with the benefits of percutaneous fixation.

Technique

- A 43-year-old male involved in a motorcycle collision sustaining a complex pelvic ring injury including complete symphysis disruption, bilateral superior rami fractures, incomplete left sacroiliac joint disruption, and complete right sacroiliac joint disruption (Fig. 12-38).

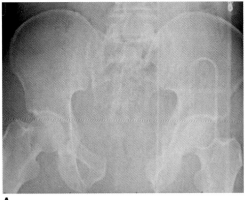
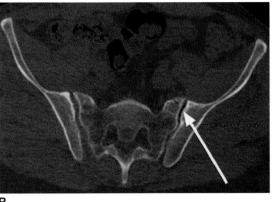

A   B

Figure 12-38 | **A:** Injury AP pelvis demonstrating symphysis pubis disruption and bilateral posterior pelvic ring injuries. **B:** Axial CT imaging obtained in pelvic binder demonstrating a complete right sacroiliac joint injury and incomplete left sacroiliac joint injury. Note the air present (*yellow arrow*) in the anterior left sacroiliac joint, which may be associated with a ligamentous injury.

- The left hemipelvis is closed reduced using multiplanar Schanz pins and then stabilized with an S1 iliosacral style screw and then an S2 transiliac-transsacral style screw in standard fashion. Note that the guide wire is left inside the transiliac-transsacral screw for later advancement into the contralateral ilium. Note too that no washer is placed on the S2 screw in anticipation of future screw removal (Fig. 12-39).

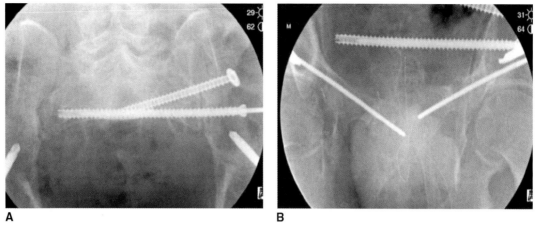

Figure 12-39 | A: Intraoperative fluoroscopic inlet view demonstrating left sacroiliac joint reduction and stabilization with S1 iliosacral and initial temporary S2 transiliac-transsacral screw. **B:** Corresponding intraoperative fluoroscopic outlet view. Note there is no washer present and the guide wire remains inside the S2 screw.

● The anterior pelvic ring injury is reduced and temporarily secured. After anterior ring reduction, the right sacroiliac joint remained incompletely reduced. The right hemipelvis reduction is completed with the use of multiplanar Schanz pins as well as percutaneous manipulation with a ball-spiked pusher. Once reduction is obtained, the guide wire from the previously placed transiliac-transsacral screw is then advanced across the sacroiliac joint and out the contralateral ilium (Fig. 12-40).

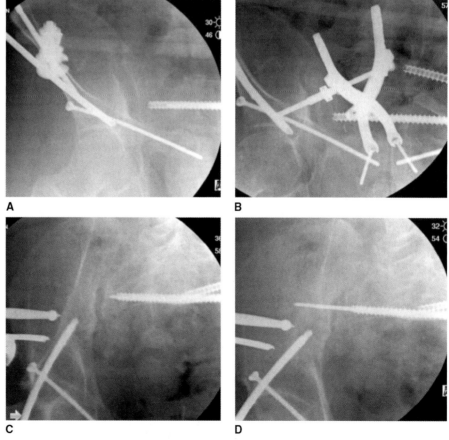

Figure 12-40 | Intraoperative fluoroscopic outlet view demonstrating residual displacement of the right sacroiliac joint before **(A)** and after **(B)** reduction of the symphysis pubis. Some persistent displacement is visualized in the caudal right sacroiliac joint. **C:** Intraoperative fluoroscopic obturator inlet oblique view demonstrating incomplete reduction of the right sacroiliac joint. A percutaneous ball-spike pusher is placed percutaneously and positioned for anticipated reduction. **D:** Using the ball-spike pusher and multiplanar Schanz pins, the right sacroiliac joint is completely reduced and the previously placed 3.2-mm guide wire is driven through the provisional S2 transsacral screw, across the SI joint and out the right ilium to stabilize the provisional reduction.

- The large caliber 3.2-mm guide wire provides adequate temporary stability to help maintain reduction until definitive implants can be placed. If needed, additional temporary wires can be placed percutaneously from the other side. Alternatively, if the osseous fixation pathways are large enough, two transiliac-transsacral style screws can be used and two points of fixation can be obtained with two wires.
- An AP with a 20- to 25-degree rollover fluoroscopic view is obtained and a wire is placed onto the ilium adjacent to the prior screw marking the cortex. Once appropriate view is identified, the profile of the ilium is noted and the AP rollback view is obtained focusing on the contralateral ilium is obtained. This allows for accurate screw length measurement and helps prevent washer intrusion on the lateral iliac cortex[1] (Fig. 12-41).

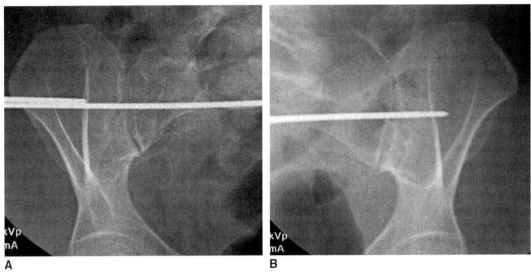

A   **B**

Figure 12-41 I Intraoperative fluoroscopic AP with ipsilateral 20- to 25-degree rollover **(A)** and contralateral rollback **(B)** views can be used to accurately measure the length of the anticipated transiliac-transsacral screw length and avoid washer intrusion on the lateral cortex of the ilium.[1] The second guide wire is placed onto the cortex immediately adjacent to the first. The fluoroscopic profile of the ilium on the AP rollover view **(A)** is noted and is specific to that point of the ilium. The contralateral view is obtained by having the C-arm roll back until a similar iliac wing profile view is obtained **(B)**, and the wire is advanced out the contralateral cortex. Note that a different patient imaging was used to show this step with a cleaner image.

- Once screw length is confirmed, the guide wire is advanced out of the ilium and tamped through the soft tissues and until the guide wire is palpable through the skin.
- A 1-cm incision is made over the guide wire, and the screw with washer is placed over the guide wire proceeding toward the previously placed screw.
- The new screw is advanced through the ilium and the sacroiliac joint until reaching the previously placed screw. At this point, the initial screw is then slowly removed as the new screw is slowly advanced (Fig. 12-42).

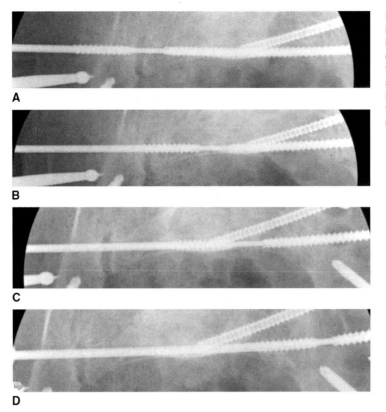

Figure 12-42 I A–D: Sequential intraoperative fluoroscopic inlet views demonstrating insertion of the right-sided S2 transiliac-transsacral screw and safe shuttling across the established S2 corridor as the provisional left transiliac-transsacral screw is removed simultaneously.

- This simultaneous sequence allows maintenance of the bilateral reduction as well as keeping the guide wire centered in the previous path. If the screw was not present, the wire would be free in the prior screw path. It could easily become eccentric, and the screw could potentially diverge from the prior screw path and create a larger footprint leading to suboptimal screw purchase as well as endangering neurovascular structures.
- The new screw is fully tightened (Fig. 12-43).

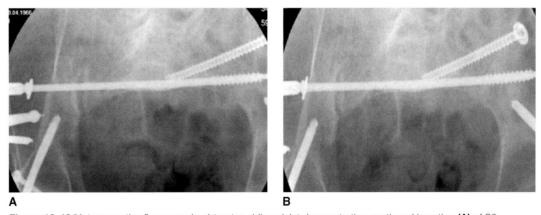

Figure 12-43 I Intraoperative fluoroscopic obturator oblique inlet demonstrating continued insertion **(A)** of S2 transiliac-transsacral screw with final tightening **(B)** with no intrusion of the lateral cortex. The right sacroiliac joint reduction has been maintained satisfactorily.

- Both posterior ring reductions are secure. Additional definitive posterior and anterior fixation is placed as needed and as the osseous anatomy allows (Fig. 12-44).

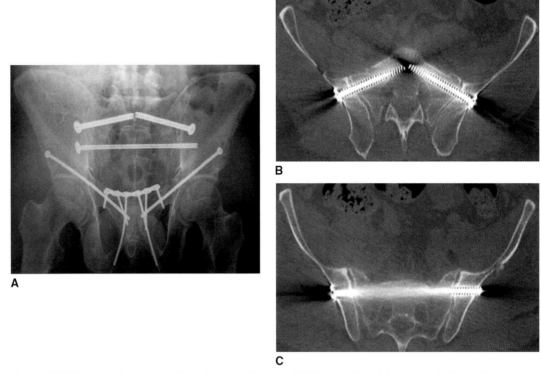

Figure 12-44 ▮ Immediate postoperative outlet view **(A)** and axial CT scans **(B and C)** demonstrating final fixation construct with safe S1 and S2 implant position and appropriate reduction and stabilization of the bilateral sacroiliac joint injuries.

Technique Notes

- No washer is placed on the initial transiliac-transsacral style screw. Enough stability is present, but no washer is left to retrieve once the screw is removed.
- The C-arm is able to remain on the same side as when the initial screws are placed. This saves operative time by not having to reverse the operative field setup. It also decreases radiation exposure as no fluoroscopic views are needed to localize and obtain the appropriate starting site and entry vectors for the screw if it were being placed in standard fashion starting from that contralateral side.

Reference

1. Firoozabadi R, Oldenburg F, Krieg J, et al. Prevention of iliosacral screw intrusion through the lateral iliac cortex. *Tech Orthop.* 2015;30(1):57–60.

- Sacral dysmorphism
  - It is critical to recognize the presence of sacral dysmorphism, as well as preoperatively plan when placing an iliosacral screw into a dysmorphic sacrum.[1]
  - One feature of sacral dysmorphism is a greater upslope of the sacral ala.
    - This can be screened using the lateral scout view of the CT scan (Fig. 12-45).

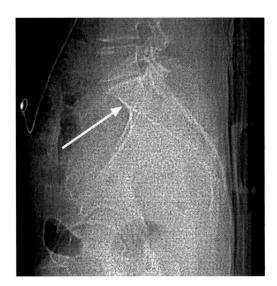

Figure 12-45 ❚ This lateral CT scout view demonstrates the marked upslope of the sacral ala associated with sacral dysmorphism (*arrow*).

- ▪ This often narrows the safe zone for screw placement and changes the obliquity (Fig. 12-46).
  - • The upper sacral segment screw generally needs to be angled more caudal to cranial and more posterior to anterior.
  - • This usually precludes a transiliac-transsacral–type screw in the upper sacral segment.
  - • When the guide wire is at the level of the sacral nerve root tunnel on the outlet view, the true lateral sacral view may demonstrate the wire anterior to the ICDs.
    - ▪ This may still be a safe screw, as dictated by the preoperative plan, as the ICDs are not collinear with the anterior sacral ala, and cannot be used as an indicator for the anterior sacral ala on the true lateral sacral view.

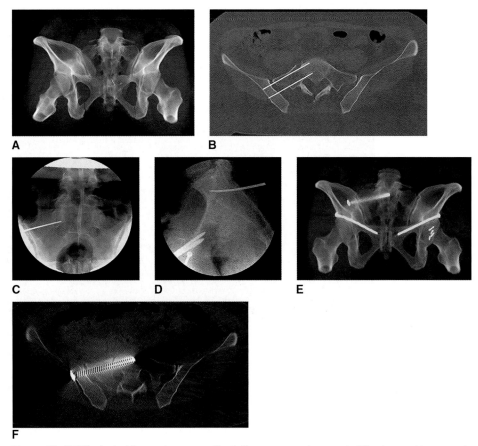

Figure 12-46 ❚ The typical iliosacral screw position in the upper sacral segment of the dysmorphic sacrum is more oblique, from caudal to cranial and posterior to anterior on the pelvic outlet and inlet views, respectively.

▪ When an oblique screw is necessary in a dysmorphic sacrum, often, this results in suboptimal fixation in the sacral body.
  ● A second segment screw is often desirable to reinforce the construct (Fig. 12-47).

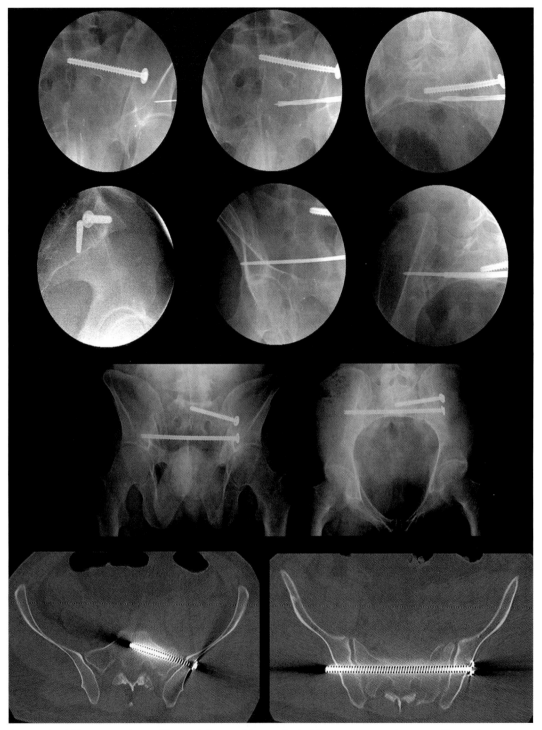

Figure 12-47 ▌In many patients with sacral dysmorphism, a short oblique upper sacral segment iliosacral screw is not relied upon as the sole implant for posterior pelvic fixation. The second sacral segment is typically larger in sacral dysmorphism and offers a good opportunity for fixation augmentation.

Removing Washers from Iliosacral Screws

Peter A. Cole
Anthony J. Dugarte

Pathoanatomy

Advancements in pelvic ring fixation have led to increased popularity of percutaneous iliosacral (IS) screw placement. These screws are often augmented with washers to augment and distribute compressive forces and minimize cortical penetration. Removal of the washers often leads to unnecessary operative and fluoroscopic time, soft tissue trauma, and frustration due to bone and scar tissue ingrowth.

Solution

A C-arm and a Kocher clamp can be used as a safe and reliable method to quickly remove retained washers (Fig. 12-48).

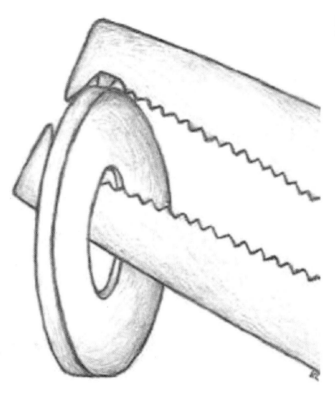

Figure 12-48 | Illustration of the Kocher Clamp jaws engaged with the washer.

Technique

- Patient positioning and imaging:
  - Patient is supine on a radiolucent table.
  - With C-arm, obtain inlet and outlet pelvic images.
- Approach and cannulated screw removal:
  - With fluoroscopic assistance, make a stab incision and direct a 2.7-mm guide wire into the head of the cannulated screw (Figs. 12-49 and 12-50).

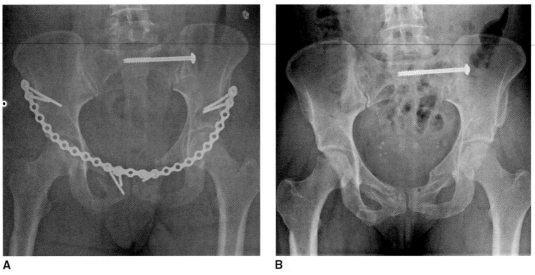

Figure 12-49 I A: Anterior-posterior (AP) film demonstrating initial management consisting of ORIF of anterior pelvic ring with LISS fixator technique and left IS screw fixation of pelvic ring injury. **B:** Anterior-posterior film demonstrating healed left zone 2 sacral fracture and parasymphyseal fractures and retained IS screw after removal of LISS anterior plate.

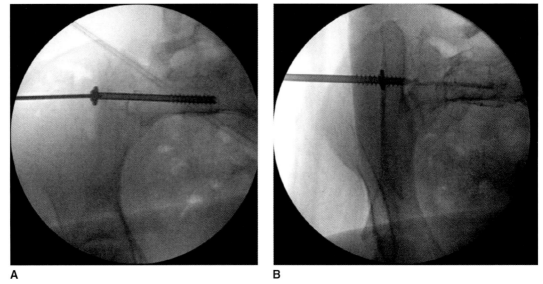

Figure 12-50 I A: Intraoperative fluoroscopy demonstrating the 2.7-mm guide wire used to identify the trajectory for the cannulated screwdriver **(B)**.

- Ensure the cannulated screwdriver is well seated by tapping the handle with a mallet.
- If the screw simply turns in bone, use a 0.25-inch osteotome to free up bone overgrowth and fibrous membrane.
- After screw removal, shift focus to retained washer.
- Retained washer removal
  - First, insert Kocher clamp in stab incision under C-arm imaging.
  - Next, use the C-arm to obtain inlet and outlet pelvic views to ensure the Kocher blades are guided through the washer (Fig. 12-51A).
  - Retract Kocher slightly, open the jaws perpendicular to the plain of the C-arm image, and then tilt your hand and the Kocher approximately 10 degrees caudal (Fig. 12-51B).
  - Again, advance the Kocher until the washer is within the grasp of the forceps (Fig. 12-51C).
  - Clamp the forceps and withdraw the Kocher (Fig. 12-51D).

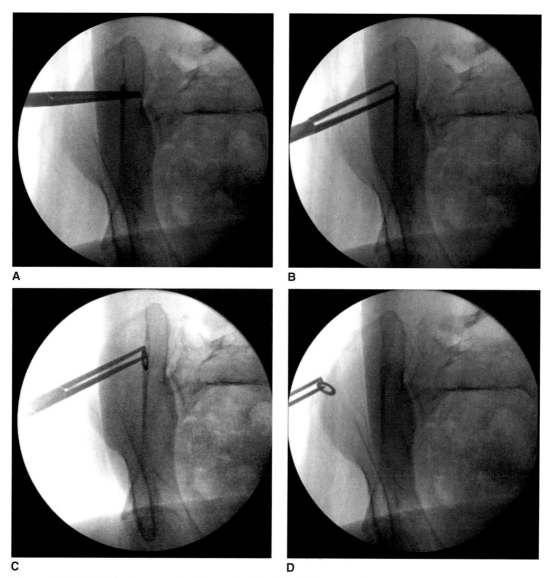

Figure 12-51 I A: Under fluoroscopic guidance, the tips of the Kocher are advanced through the washer. **B:** The Kocher is retracted just over the edge of the washer, angled approximately 10 to 15 degrees, the jaws are opened, and a single limb of the clamp is readvanced through the washer. **C:** The forceps are clamped around the washer, and **(D)** it is retrieved.

References

1. Matta JM, Saucedo T. Internal fixation of pelvic ring fractures. *Clin Orthop Relat Res.* 1989;242:83–97.
2. Routt ML Jr, Nork SE, Mills WJ. Percutaneous fixation of pelvic ring disruptions. *Clin Orthop Relat Res.* 2000;375:15–29.
3. Hinsche AF, Giannoudis PV, Smith RM. Fluoroscopy-based multiplanar image guidance for insertion of sacroiliac screws. *Clin Orthop Relat Res.* 2002;395:135–144.

- *Reduction and fixation of iliac crest fractures*
  - The fracture fragment can be held with a small pointed reduction clamp through small drill holes in the crest, or with a Farabeuf clamp.
  - Screw path drilling is facilitated by placing a Hohmann retractor over the posterior iliac crest and predrilling the glide hole, to avoid penetrating the lateral ilium with the screw.
  - Drill so that the drill path can be seen just under the inner table, and then reduce the fracture.
  - A 2.5-mm drill is then used to complete the drilling.
    - A calibrated drill allows for direct measurement and quick exchange with the appropriate screw.

- Often, the ilium fracture fragment is displaced in extension and external rotation due to the pull of the abductor and tensor muscle origins.
  - To counteract this force, use of a small fragment plate as a tension band along the inner table, with supplemental intertable screws creates a mechanically sound construct (Fig. 12-52).

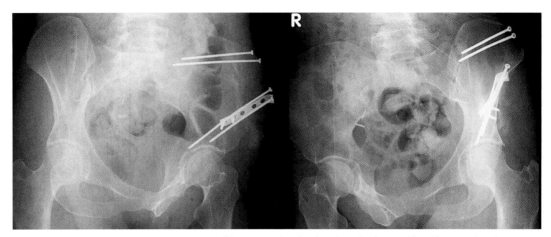

Figure 12-52 I In this iliac crest fracture, a small fragment plate is placed on the inner table with an antitension function. This is supplemented with intertable lag screws.

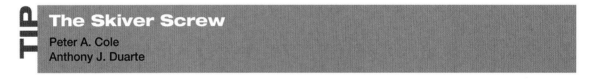

TIP: The Skiver Screw

Peter A. Cole
Anthony J. Duarte

Pathoanatomy

Achieving stability with intraosseous fixation of curved, flat bones is challenging.

Solution

To address this issue, we developed the Skiver Screw technique as an alternative to traditional plate and screw fixation. This bone-"air"-bone screw uses an in-out-in technique and has been effective for both iliac crest and scapula fractures.

Technique

Indications
- Fractures of curved, flat bones
  - Isolated, comminuted iliac wing fractures (Fig. 12-53)
  - Fractures of the ilium associated with acetabular injuries during access to the lateral window
  - Scapula fractures

Patient Positioning
- Supine

Approach
- Approach to iliac fossa
  - An incision is made along the iliac crest extending to the intermuscular interval between external oblique (medial) and tensor fascia lata/gluteus medius (lateral) (Fig. 12-54).
  - Next, a subiliacus approach is developed to the sacroiliac joint and pelvic brim to expose the fracture site.

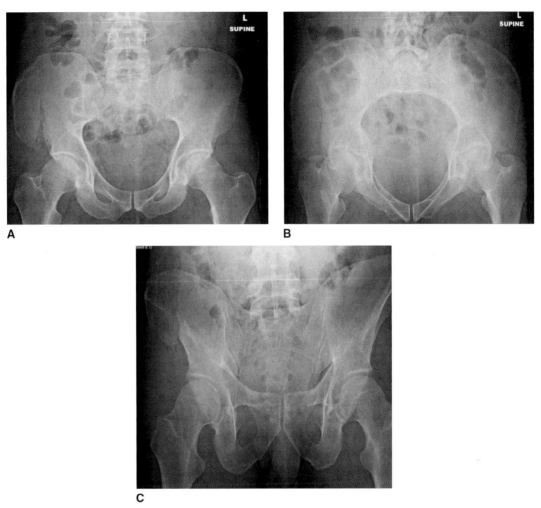

Figure 12-53 I (A) Anterior-posterior (AP), **(B)** inlet, and **(C)** outlet images demonstrating a fracture involving the right iliac wing with over 1 cm displacement.

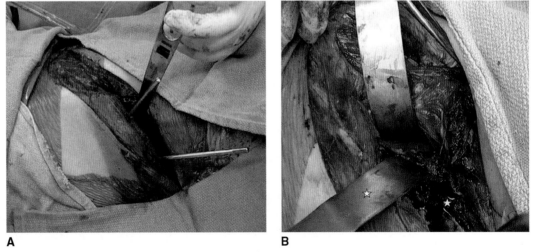

Figure 12-54 I A: Incision for lateral window to access iliac fossa. **B:** Malleable (*white star*) superior to iliacus muscle (*yellow star*).

Reduction and Fixation

- After accounting for iliac/column fragment rotational displacement, pointed bone tenaculums are used to reduce the fracture. Traction (for acetabular fractures) and a Schanz pin in the anterior column or ilium may be helpful aids.
- After fracture reduction is achieved, cortical screws are directed from the iliac crest with an anterior-posterior or lateral-medial method.
  - Both directions can use an in-out-in technique starting at iliac wing.
  - The drill bit and screw exit the crest inside the iliac fossa, traverse the concavity, and reenter the cortex on the far side of the concavity (Fig. 12-55).

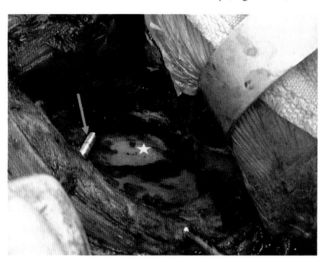

Figure 12-55 I **A:** Drill bit and screw (*blue arrow*) exit the ilium and skive along the iliac fossa (*yellow star*).

  - Since the angle is quite acute, there is a tendency for drill bit and screw to skive across fossa without reentering curved bone once it has exited the second cortex of the proximal crest segment.
  - To address this issue, a Cobb elevator (or curved gouge) can be used to block the bit and direct it to reenter ilium in the desired site opposite the fracture.
  - Use this same technique to pass the screw.
    - A tap may also be helpful in cutting threads in the bone at the site of screw reentry.
- Multiple screws can be used in a similar fashion and placed anywhere along the length of the ilium (Fig. 12-56).
- Countersink screwheads to avoid prominence at the iliac crest.
- Use a combination of inlet and outlet, Judet, and 15 degrees rollover fluoroscopic views to assess screw length and insertion vectors.

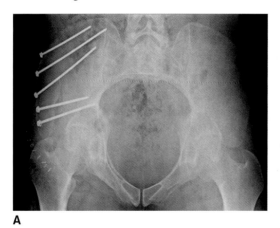
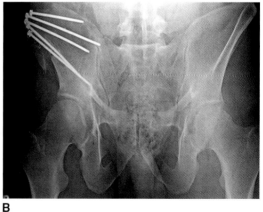

A   B

Figure 12-56 I **(A)** Inlet and **(B)** outlet postoperative X-rays demonstrating 5 sequential 3.5-mm cortical screws with washers along the inner table of the pelvis, advancing into the posterior column.

Reference

1. Cole PA, Jamil M, Jacobson AR, et al. The skiver screw: a useful fixation technique for iliac wing fractures. *J Orthop Trauma.* 2015;29(7):e231–e234.

- *Sacroiliac joint ORIF*
  - During an anterior open reduction with plate fixation of the SI joint, a screw placed into the sacrum is facilitated by drilling with the joint unreduced so there is direct visualization of the cartilage of the joint so that it is parallel (Fig. 12-57).

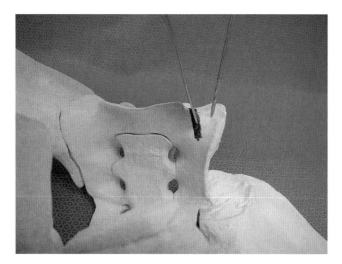

Figure 12-57 I During open reduction of the SI joint from an anterior approach, the sacral screw path should be drilled prior to joint reduction to maximize the accuracy. The *blue mark* indicates the approximate path of the L5 nerve root.

  - This screw should exit posterolaterally from the dorsal sacrum due to the kyphosis of the sacrum, at approximately the S3 level (Fig. 12-58).

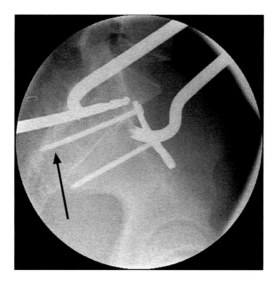

Figure 12-58 I The sacral screw inclination typically exits dorsally around the S3 level (*arrow*).

  - For SI joint clamp application through an anterior approach, a small incision is made in the tensor fascia lata origin, and a clamp tine is passed deep to the muscle along the outer table of the posterior ilium.
  - The anterior second tine is placed on the sacral ala, lateral to the L5 sacral nerve root (Fig. 12-59).

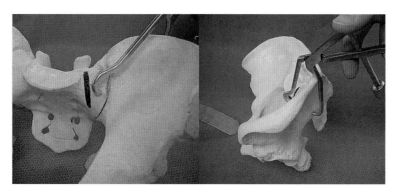

Figure 12-59 I Clamp application for open reduction of the SI joint from an anterior approach. The *blue mark* indicates the approximate path of the L5 nerve root.

- *Antegrade superior ramus/anterior column screw.*
    - The starting point is generally along the gluteus medius pillar and first identified on the pelvic inlet view.
    - The guide wire position on the obturator oblique outlet view demonstrates the cranial/caudal trajectory and position of the drill and screw, but its anterior-posterior position can be inferred by observing its relationship to the lateral ilium cortical stripe—an anterior position will be medial to the stripe and a posterior pin will be lateral to the stripe (Fig. 12-60).

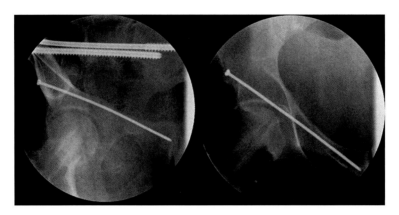

Figure 12-60 I Ramus screw position is visualized on the obturator outlet view (*left*) and the inlet view (*right*).

- Finding the starting point for repeated instrumentation insertion is facilitated by completely incising the fascia of the tensor fascia lata once the appropriate starting position has been achieved.
    - This helps create one soft tissue tract for the repeated insertion of the guide pin, drill, and screw.
- After drilling the gliding hole, remove the 3.5-mm drill and use the blunt end of a guide pin to feel the superior pubic ramus anteriorly and superiorly all the way to the fracture site.
    - This can help determine if the current path remains contained in bone.
    - Oscillating a 2.5-drill will allow the drill bit to "bounce" off the cortex and deform to remain intraosseous, rather than penetrating cortex.
- Drill until final resistance of the far cortex is met, remove the drill, and place the guide wire for direct measurement of screw length.
- Careful attention when obtaining the starting point will help when trying to seat the final screw.
    - The original image of the starting point should be saved and later referred to when seating the screw.
    - The screw head should rest at the same level as the tip of the guide wire, which should mark the lateral ilium.
- *Retrograde superior ramus screw*
    - Start with a 0.062-inch K-wire and check the starting point on the pelvic inlet view of the symphysis and the obturator oblique views (Fig. 12-61).

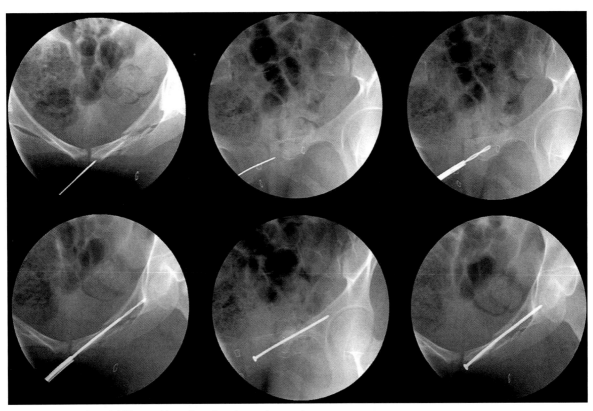

Figure 12-61 | Progression of drilling and insertion of a retrograde superior ramus screw.

- A cranial and anterior screw or drill position risks penetrating the cortex in the pectineal gutter.
- A caudal screw that is too anterior will penetrate the hip joint, whereas a screw just as caudal that is more posterior may stay intraosseous.
- Place a 3.5-mm drill sleeve over the K-wire and exchange for the drill after pushing the drill guide into symphyseal cartilage to maintain its position.
- Attempt inserting the screw long enough to penetrate the lateral ilium, and leave several screw threads proud to facilitate removal, should the screw break and removal is necessary.
- Drill with the 3.5-mm drill to fracture line to create a glide hole to facilitate finding the hole with the 2.5-mm drill and screw percutaneously.
- Drill the remainder of the tract with a 2.5-mm-long calibrated drill.
- Direct measurement can be made by subtracting the length of the drill guide from the reading on the calibrated drill.
- If planning on placing a ramus screw in addition to an AIIS frame, the AIIS pins should be placed more cranially to prevent the Schanz pin from blocking the path of the ramus screw (Fig. 12-62).
  - Placing the superior ramus screw first decreases the chance of error.

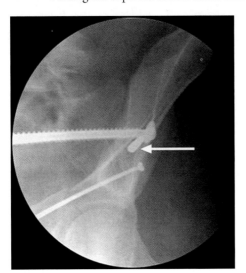

Figure 12-62 | In this case, the AIIS pin was placed initially and was intentionally placed superiorly (arrow), so as not to interfere with the subsequent superior ramus screw.

Retrograde-Antegrade-Retrograde Screw Insertion for Superior Ramus Fracture Stabilization

Justin F. Lucas
Jonathan G. Eastman

Pathoanatomy

Instability of the anterior component of unstable pelvic ring injuries may be treated by percutaneous fixation, which is an alternative to open procedures.

Solution

Fixation of the superior pubic ramus allows for maintenance of anterior ring reduction and increased overall pelvic ring stability. Intramedullary implants can be inserted percutaneously in an antegrade or retrograde fashion. The small segment of intact bone present in parasymphyseal fractures makes retrograde screw insertion favorable biomechanically.

Several patient-related factors can make primary retrograde superior ramus screw insertion difficult or unsafe. Some factors include the following:

- Soft tissue prominence from the presence of obese thighs
- The proximity of patient's external genitalia (Fig. 12-63)
- The unique curvilinear superior ramus osseous corridor of each patient

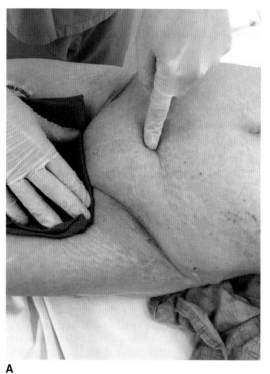
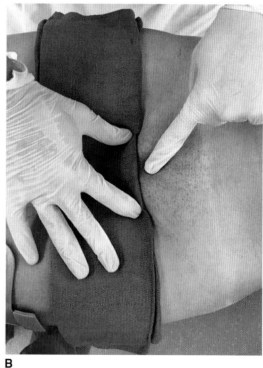

A   **B**

Figure 12-63 I Intraoperative photographs demonstrating the variable distance from the pubic symphysis to the superior part of the external genitalia. The blue towel is placed directly on the superior aspect of the external genitalia, and the superior symphysis pubis is palpated. Note the significant difference between an elderly patient **(A)** and a younger patient **(B)** and how the proximity of the external genitalia could impede obtaining the correct starting point for a retrograde superior ramus screw.

When one or several of these factors are present, it can be difficult to achieve the appropriate screw starting site and pathway for drill insertion as well as the desired screw trajectory.

If the ideal trajectory or path cannot be obtained during initial attempts at standard retrograde drilling, a secondary technique that may be effective is to use a bent-tipped 2.0-mm Kirschner wire to redirect the intraosseous path.[1] The wire is used in an analogous fashion as a curved ball-tipped guide wire is used for intramedullary femoral nailing. The prebent 2.0-mm wire can be passed by positioning the bend in the appropriate direction and by gently, manually advancing the wire with small taps of a mallet into a new and more acceptable location. A cannulated drill bit can then be used to drill the new path. Screw insertion of the guide wire proceeds in the usual fashion.

There are a few clinical situations in which the bent-tip Kirschner wire technique will not allow an appropriate correction. The technique described and illustrated here is a way to safely stabilize an unstable ramus component of a pelvic ring injury with a cannulated retrograde intramedullary implant in the situation where proximity of external anatomy, presence of abundant thigh soft tissue, or irregular osseous anatomy prevents direct retrograde screw insertion.

Technique

- Although pelvic ring injuries are highly variable, a typical treatment algorithm will include supine positioning and reduction using closed, percutaneous, or open techniques.
- Once a reduction is obtained, percutaneous stabilization of the posterior pelvic ring can be performed. The surgical technique as well as the number and size of implants used are based on injury pattern, bone quality, available osseous fixation pathways, anticipated patient compliance, and surgeon preference.
- Once the posterior pelvic ring is stabilized, the stability of the anterior ring is reassessed.
  - This is performed using an inlet view specific to the patients' anterior pelvic ring morphology and application of a lateral compressive force of 10 to 15 lb (Fig. 12-64).
  - If instability remains, percutaneous fixation of the superior pubic ramus is performed.

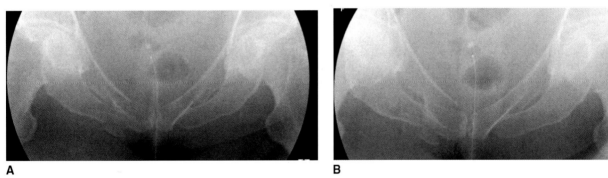

A **B**

Figure 12-64 | Intraoperative fluoroscopic inlet view of an unstable anterior component of a pelvic ring injury without **(A)** and with **(B)** 15 lb of lateral compressive load. Note the significant residual displacement of the anterior pelvic ring through the right superior ramus fracture.

- Obtain the appropriate intraoperative fluoroscopic images of the affected hemipelvis including pelvic inlet and combined obturator oblique outlet views.
- Percutaneously place a 1.6-mm Kirschner wire to achieve the appropriate retrograde starting site on both views.
  - Once correct, oscillate the wire into bone 1 cm and make a 1-cm oblique skin incision around the wire (Fig. 12-65).

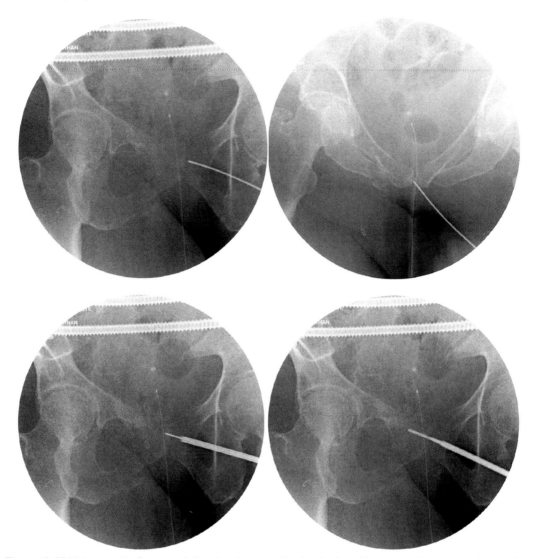

Figure 12-65 I Intraoperative fluoroscopic imaging demonstrating localization of the appropriate starting site on inlet (*top right*) and combined obturator oblique outlet (*top left*) views using a 1.6-mm Kirschner wire. Placement of drill sleeve over the Kirschner wire to maintain the entry site (*bottom left*) with subsequent wire removal and placement of a 3.2-mm noncannulated drill (*bottom right*).

- Note that in order to place a retrograde implant, the surgeon is standing on the contralateral side to the fracture and the C-arm is ipsilateral.
- Assess the size of patients' osseous fixation pathway.
  - Typically, the intraosseous space above the acetabulum as seen on the combined obturator oblique outlet image and the isthmic section of the diaphyseal ramus dictates the size of implant possible.
  - In Figure 12-65, the size of the osseous fixation pathway present can only accommodate a 4.5-mm implant.
- If a 4.5-mm screw is planned, a soft tissue guide is placed over the wire followed by wire removal and insertion of a solid 3.2-mm drill.
- If a 7.0-mm screw is used, a cannulated 4.5-mm drill (often used for iliosacral screws) can be used and placed directly over the wire.
  - Care must be taken to obtain and maintain the appropriate starting site.
  - With small parasymphyseal segments, an entry site too anterior can risk drilling out the anterior cortex and ultimately jeopardizing the stability of the implant.
  - The drill is advanced using oscillation, confirming maintenance of an intraosseous pathway in the appropriate trajectory by visualization with alternating images.
  - The drill is advanced to the superomedial aspect of the acetabulum (Fig. 12-65).
- If a satisfactory trajectory for safe drill and screw passage cannot be obtained (Fig. 12-66), and the secondary 2.0-mm bent-tip Kirschner wire technique is also unsuccessful (Fig. 12-67), remove the wire proceed as below.

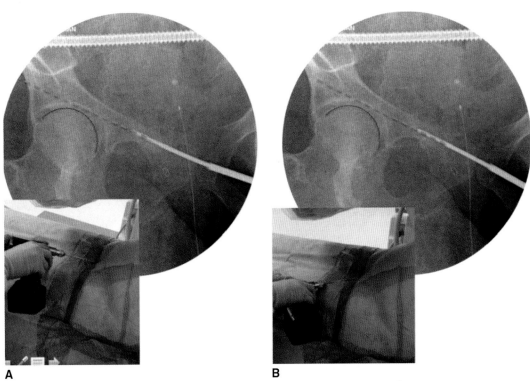

Figure 12-66 I Intraoperative fluoroscopic obturator oblique outlet view demonstrating the approximate drill path (*blue dashed line*) in relation to femoral head (*red line*) and acetabulum after initial insertion of drill (**A**: **upper left** image) without significant interference from soft tissues (**A**: **lower left**, inset photo). After caudal repositioning of the hand and drill (**B**: **upper right** image) the desired drill path is not attainable due to obstruction from soft tissues of the thigh (inset photo, **B**: **lower right**). Note how the thigh prevents any further caudal positioning of the hand and drill. The new drill path (*blue dash*) will still violate the femoral head (*red line*) and acetabulum if advanced further.

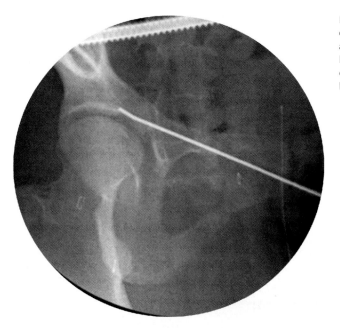

Figure 12-67 I Intraoperative fluoroscopic obturator oblique outlet view demonstrating attempted use of the 2.0-mm bent-tip Kirschner wire technique. Note the wire cannot be positioned into a new acceptable location superior to the acetabulum.

- Using the same fluoroscopic views, place a 1.6-mm Kirschner wire at the appropriate starting site for antegrade screw insertion.
- Insert the wire into bone and make a 1-cm skin incision around the wire. Use the appropriate drill to obtain a new entry site.
  - A 3.2-mm cannulated drill bit is used if a 4.5-mm screw is anticipated, or a cannulated 4.5-mm drill bit is used if a 7.0-mm screw is to be inserted (Fig. 12-68). Note that if a 4.5-mm screw is going to be used, do not use a 4.5-mm drill for this entry site. Doing so will create a glide hole, and the screw will have no purchase once placed in retrograde fashion.

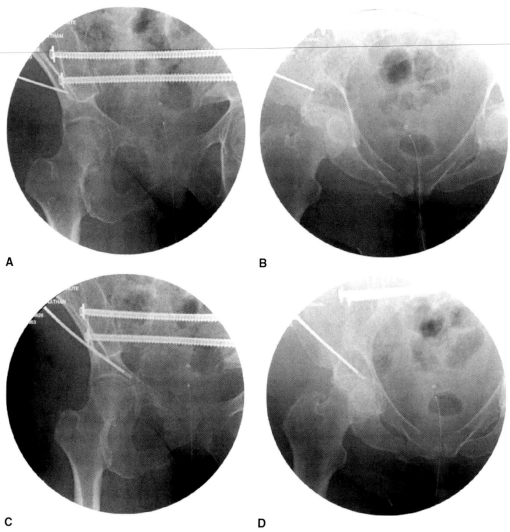

A

B

C

D

Figure 12-68 I Antegrade drilling for retrograde screw insertion. The starting site is obtained on both the combined obturator oblique outlet (**A**, *upper left*) and inlet (**B**, *upper right*) views with a 1.6-mm Kirschner wire. Once appropriately positioned, the wire is inserted into bone and a 3.2-mm cannulated drill is placed over the wire to enter the osseous fixation pathway. This is advanced to the level of the acetabular dome on the combined obturator oblique outlet (**C**) and inlet (**D**) views.

- Advance the drill through the osseous corridor aiming at the initial retrograde starting site until at or near the superomedial aspect of the acetabulum (Fig. 12-68).
  - Note the change in the operating room setup so that the surgeon is now ipsilateral and C-arm is contralateral to the side of the fracture (Fig. 12-69).

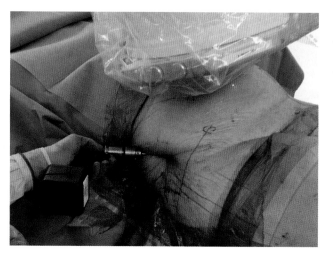

Figure 12-69 I Intraoperative photograph demonstrating appropriate drill positioning for an antegrade pathway without the interference of anterior thighs and external soft tissues.

- Remove the drill and replace with a 2.0-mm bent-tip Kirschner wire. Pass the wire in antegrade fashion with redirection as needed toward the retrograde starting site (Fig. 12-70).

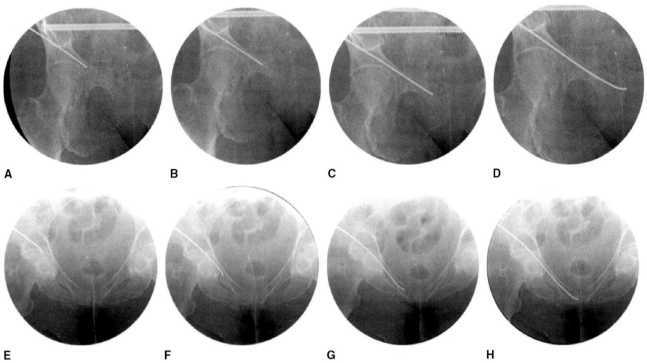

A   **B**   **C**   **D**

E   **F**   **G**   **H**

Figure 12-70 ▌ Intraoperative fluoroscopic views demonstrating sequential advancement of the bent-tip 2.0-mm Kirschner wire on both the obturator oblique outlet view **(A–D)** and pelvic inlet view **(E–H)** paired images (i.e., A–E, B–F, C–G, and D–H). Note the turning and advancement of the wire into the appropriate position at the retrograde starting site.

- Measure length of anticipated screw using a subtraction technique with another wire of identical length (Fig. 12-71) or the appropriate calibrated depth measurement gauge.

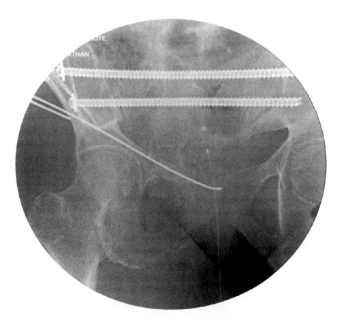

Figure 12-71 ▌ Intraoperative fluoroscopic obturator oblique outlet view demonstrating measuring of anticipated antegrade screw length using an identical length Kirschner wire and subtraction technique. Note the new wire is positioned at the caudal aspect to avoid inaccurate screw length measurement.

- Advance the wire out of the prior, retrograde insertion starting site and retrieve the wire from the initial skin incision using a small clamp or the appropriate screw measurement guide (Fig. 12-72) to prevent damage to surrounding soft tissues.

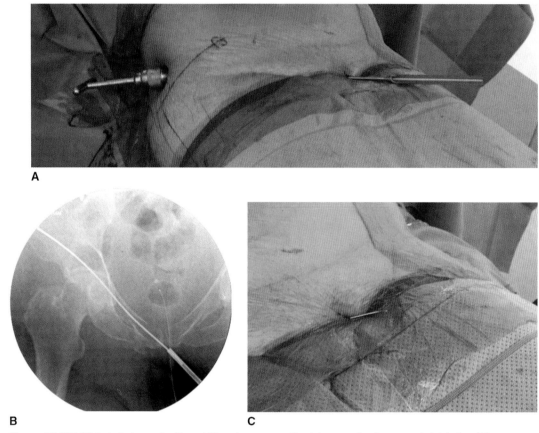

Figure 12-72 | Clinical photographs **(A and C)** and corresponding intraoperative fluoroscopic inlet view **(B)** demonstrating a T-handle chuck for wire advancement and the cannulated screw length measurement guide used as a tool to retrieve the bent-tip Kirschner wire. Once the wire is inserted into the depth measurement guide, it is advanced and then retrieved safely through the preexisting incision without surrounding soft tissue injury **(C)**.

- Insert the appropriate length screw over the wire in a retrograde direction (Fig. 12-73) with fluoroscopic assistance and tighten appropriately (Fig. 12-74).

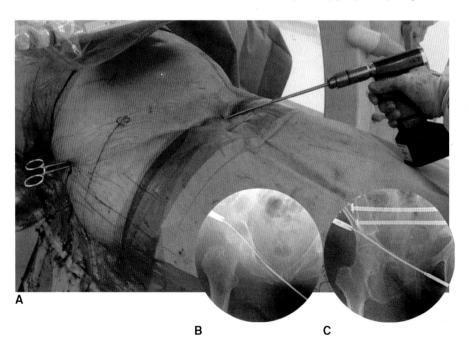

Figure 12-73 | Clinical photograph **(A)** and corresponding fluoroscopic inlet view **(B)** and obturator oblique outlet view **(C)** demonstrating percutaneous placement of clamp on the Kirschner wire to prevent unintentional wire advancement during retrograde screw insertion.

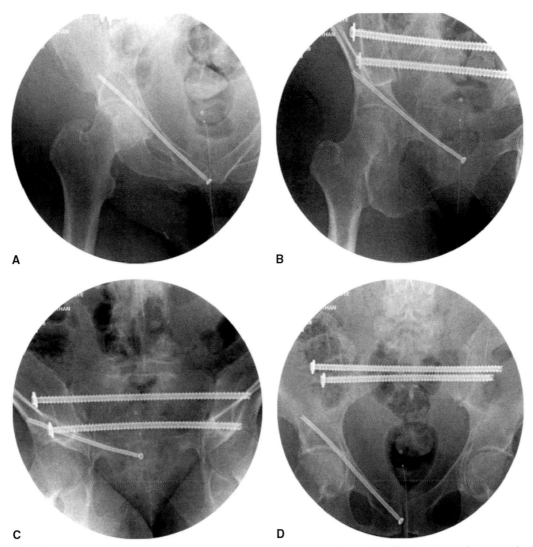

Figure 12-74 | Final fluoroscopic images of retrograde superior ramus screw successfully placed utilizing a retrograde-antegrade-retrograde technique as seen on the inlet **(A)**, combined obturator oblique outlet **(B)**, outlet **(C)**, and AP pelvis view **(D)**. Note the improved and extra-articular position of the screw on the combined obturator oblique outlet view **(B)**.

- Note, for this technique, a cannulated 4.5-, 5.5-, 6.5-, or 7.0-mm screw can be used.
- Wounds are irrigated and closed in standard fashion.

Reference

1. Scolaro JA, Routt ML. Intraosseous correction of misdirected cannulated screws and fracture malalignment using a bent tip 2.0 mm guide wire: technique and indications. *Arch Orthop Trauma Surg.* 2013;133(7):883–887.

Intramedullary Reduction of Superior Ramus Fractures to Facilitate Medullary Screw Insertion

Raymond D. Wright Jr.

Pathophysiology

A pelvic ring fracture with superior pubic ramus displacement that precludes medullary ramus screw insertion.

Solution

Perform an intramedullary reduction maneuver to provide for sufficient reduction to allow medullary ramus screw insertion. Many displaced superior pubic rami can be reduced with this technique after the posterior ring has been reduced or if there is no posterior pelvic ring displacement.

Technique

Sterile Instruments and Equipment:

- 3.5-mm drill
- 3.5-mm drill sleeve × 110 mm in length
- 2.0-mm Kirchner wires
- Implants:
  - 6.5-/7.3-mm cannulated screw set
  - Long 4.5-mm screws
  - Long 3.5-mm screws

Patient Positioning

- Supine position allows for retrograde and antegrade insertion of drills/implants into superior ramus.
- Radiolucent table.
- Use a sheet folded into thirds as a drawsheet.
- If antegrade ramus screw is planned, C-arm is placed on opposite side of to the fractured ramus.
- If retrograde ramus screw is planned, C-arm may be placed on the same or opposite side of the fractured ramus.

Illustrative Case #1

- A 34-year-old male involved in a motor vehicle crash with a right femoral shaft fracture treated with a retrograde medullary nail and a left bicondylar tibial plateau fracture treated with closed reduction and a knee-spanning external fixator.
  - Additionally, he has a pelvic ring fracture that includes a left complete sacroiliac joint injury, a right incomplete sacroiliac joint injury, and a left displaced superior ramus fracture (Fig. 12-75).
  - In order to assist in this patient's resuscitative effort, a percutaneous technique is employed to achieve pelvic stability.

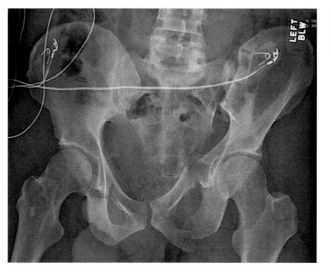

Figure 12-75 AP radiograph demonstrates complete left SI joint injury, incomplete right SI joint injury, and a left superior and inferior ramus fracture.

- The patient undergoes routine imaging including CT scan. Five volume-rendered reconstructions are created to simulate AP, inlet, outlet, and Judet views of the pelvis. These images demonstrate displacement of the superior ramus that may preclude medullary screw placement (Fig. 12-76).

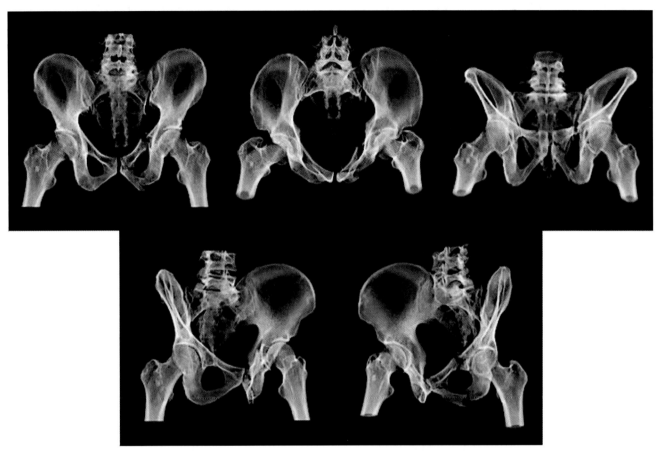

Figure 12-76 ▌ AP, inlet, outlet, and Judet oblique views of the injury generated from the CT scan data characterize the pelvic ring fracture.

- The left superior ramus fracture is segmental has an intercalary segment with an intact soft tissue hinge at the level of the symphysis pubis. This fracture pattern is ideal for a medullary reduction tactic. The three-dimensional reconstructions of the axial CT scan more clearly demonstrate this fracture morphology (Fig. 12-77).

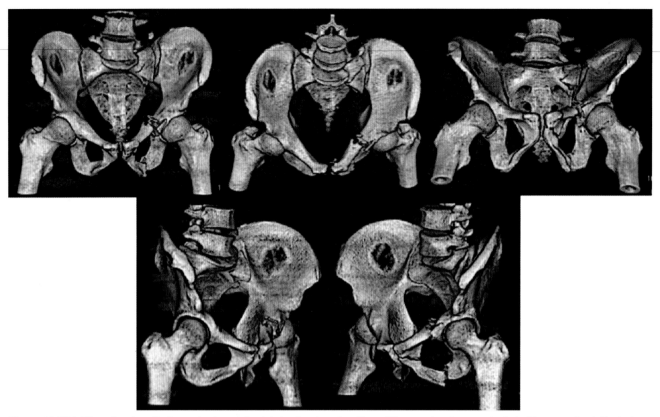

Figure 12-77 I Although not routinely required as part pelvic fracture imaging, these 3D reconstructions are included to more clearly illustrate the ramus fracture morphology. The left superior ramus fracture is segmental with an intact soft tissue hinge medially at the level of the symphysis pubis.

- The patient is placed supine on a midline lumbosacral bolster. Traction is maintained for the left lower extremity through a distal femoral traction pin, and approximately 15 lb of weight is applied to a rope. The posterior portion of the pelvis is reduced and secured on both sides.
- A retrograde insertion point is established with a 2.0-mm wire using inlet and obturator oblique outlet views. Once the starting point has been established, a 3.5-mm drill is passed through a 3.5-mm drill sleeve to the level of the fracture (Fig. 12-78). When the 3.5-mm drill is advanced in a retrograde fashion, it must be placed out of the way of the definitive antegrade screw. Therefore, the surgeon needs to be aware of the radiographic limits of safety in the superior ramus.

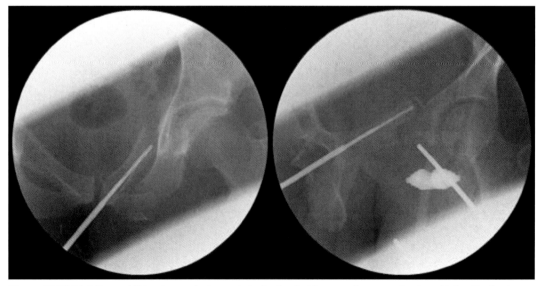

Figure 12-78 I A 3.5-mm drill is advanced retrograde to the level of the superior ramus fracture. Notice the fracture displacement would preclude successful advancement of a medullary superior ramus screw.

- Once the drill is advanced to the level of the fracture, the drill is disengaged from the drill bit. The drill and drill sleeve are then used to lever the 3.5-mm drill bit to achieve an accurate reduction of the superior ramus (Fig. 12-79).

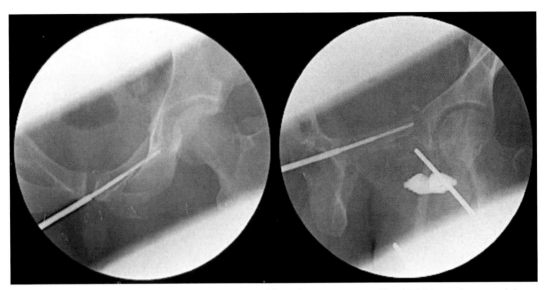

Figure 12-79 I The 3.5-mm drill bit has been disengaged from the power source. The drill bit is used as a medullary reduction tool by manipulating is through the 3.5-mm drill sleeve. Notice the 3.5-mm drill bit is placed in the anterior and cranial aspect of the superior ramus in anticipation of definitive antegrade fixation.

- The 3.5-mm drill bit is then exchanged for a 2.8-mm drill-tipped guide pin. The pin is passed by hand through the 3.5-mm drill sleeve. A mallet is then used to gently advance the guide pin just beyond the fracture and docked into the stable segment to maintain a provisional reduction (Fig. 12-80).

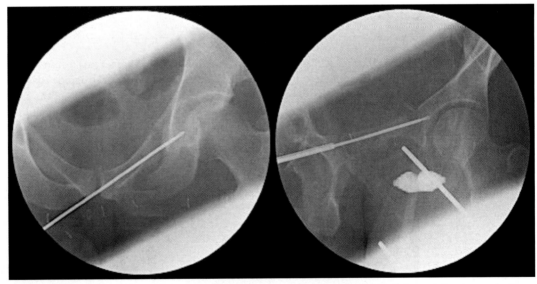

Figure 12-80 I The 3.5-mm drill bit is exchanged for a 2.8-mm guide pin. The guide pin is carefully advanced with a mallet just beyond the fracture. Provisional accurate reduction is maintained.

- Alternatively, a second pin or K-wire can be placed adjacent to the reduction drill bit and inserted to the proximal fragment to maintain reduction, taking care not to penetrate the hip joint (Fig. 12-81).

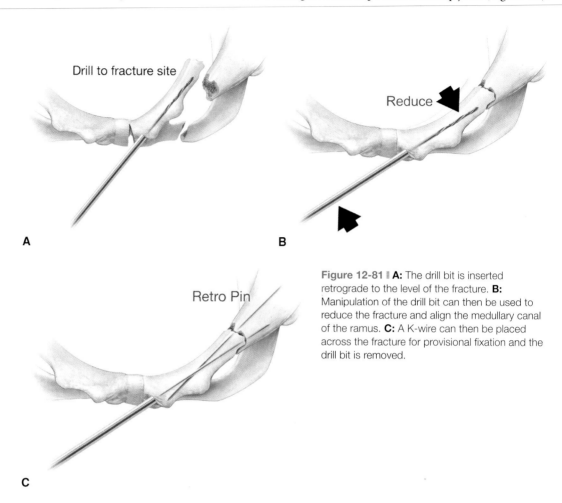

Figure 12-81 I **A:** The drill bit is inserted retrograde to the level of the fracture. **B:** Manipulation of the drill bit can then be used to reduce the fracture and align the medullary canal of the ramus. **C:** A K-wire can then be placed across the fracture for provisional fixation and the drill bit is removed.

- Once the reduction is achieved and provisionally maintained, a 3.5-mm drill is advanced antegrade on inlet and obturator oblique outlet views. Just as with the retrograde advancement, a 2.0-mm wire is used to obtain an osseous starting point. The 3.5-mm drill bit replaces the 2.0-mm wire. The antegrade trajectory must be posterior to the 2.8-mm guide pin that is maintaining reduction (Fig. 12-82).

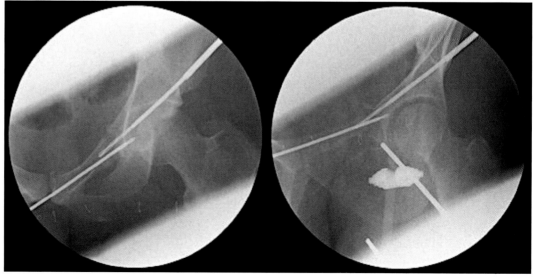

Figure 12-82 I A 3.5-mm drill bit is advanced in antegrade fashion. Notice the antegrade drill is closely approximated to the posterior cortical limit of the superior ramus on the inlet view.

- The 3.5-mm drill bit is advanced to establish an appropriate trajectory and is inserted to its maximal depth through a 3.5 × 110-mm drill sleeve. The 3.5-mm drill bit is then exchanged for a drill-tipped 2.8-mm guide pin. The guide pin is advanced to the pubic tubercle and the depth measured (Fig. 12-83).

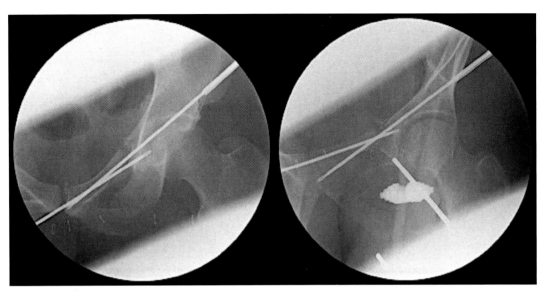

Figure 12-83 I The 3.5-mm drill is exchanged for a 2.8-mm drill-tipped guide pin. The guide pin is advanced to the pubis tubercle and its depth measured.

- The 2.8-mm guide pin is then over drilled with a 5.0-mm cannulated drill to create a pilot hole for a 4.5-mm screw. Once the pilot hole is drilled, the 2.8-mm guide pin is withdrawn and a 4.5-mm solid cortical screw is inserted (Fig. 12-84). Alternatively, a cannulated screw may be placed over the 2.8-mm guide pin if the osseous corridor will accept and contain it.

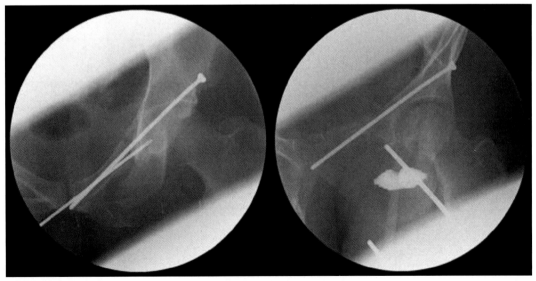

Figure 12-84 I A 4.5-mm cortical screw is inserted and the 2.8-mm provisional fixation is removed.

- Once the definitive medullary ramus screw is inserted, the retrograde provisional guide pin can be removed. Reduction is maintained in the patient's final radiographs (Fig. 12-85).

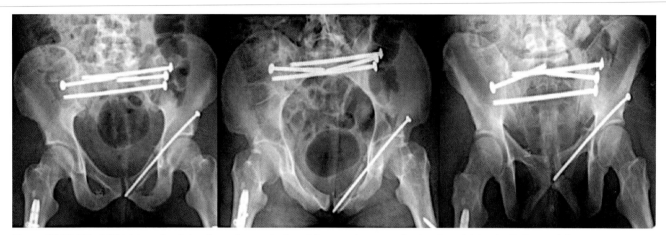

Figure 12-85 I Final AP, inlet, and outlet radiographs—reduction of the superior ramus fracture is maintained with the medullary ramus screw.

Illustrative Case #2

This second case example demonstrates that the provisional and definitive fixation can be inserted in retrograde fashion so long as the osseous corridor is large enough to safely accept and contain both.

- A 78-year-old is involved in a tractor rollover injury resulting in a pelvic ring disruption. He had an unstable pelvis by physical exam, and radiographs and CT scan demonstrated a right complete transforaminal sacral fracture and ipsilateral pubic root injury in the superior ramus. The AP injury radiograph is shown below (Fig. 12-86).

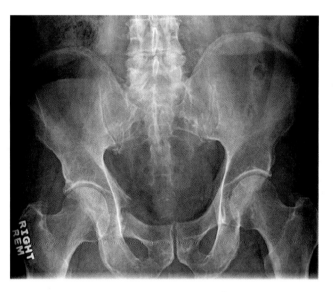

Figure 12-86 I AP injury radiograph. The displaced right superior ramus is easily visualized. Medullary ramus fixation could not be safely contained with this ramus displacement. There is no deformity through the sacral fracture—an intact soft tissue hinge is present at the level of the symphysis pubis.

- The AP, inlet, outlet, and Judet oblique views of this injury are demonstrated below (Fig. 12-87).

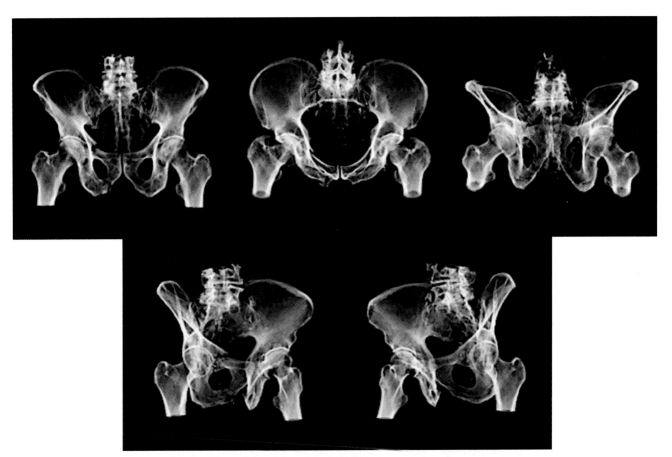

Figure 12-87 I AP, inlet, outlet, and Judet oblique views of the pelvic ring injury.

- The patient is placed supine on a lumbosacral bolster. There is no deformity through the posterior pelvic ring on this patient, and therefore, the anterior portion of the pelvic ring may be secured either before or after posterior fixation.
- A retrograde starting point is obtained on inlet and obturator oblique outlet views with a 2.0-mm wire. This provisional starting point is more anterior and cranial than the starting point for the definitive retrograde ramus screw (Fig. 12-88).

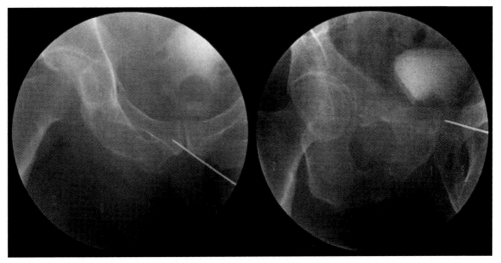

Figure 12-88 I A retrograde starting point is obtained to place a medullary reducing aid. Notice the starting point is somewhat more anterior and cranial than the starting point for a definitive retrograde ramus screw. The displacement through this ramus fracture precludes safe intraosseous placement of a medullary ramus screw.

- A 3.5-mm drill bit is then inserted in retrograde fashion to the level of the fractured pubic root. The 3.5-mm drill is then used to manipulate the fracture into a position of accurate reduction so as to pass a medullary ramus screw (Fig. 12-89).

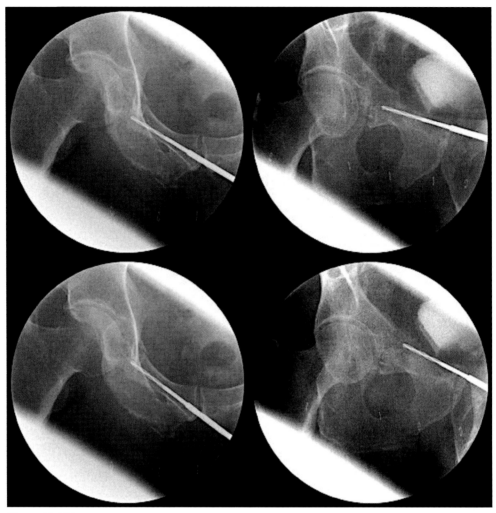

Figure 12-89 I The 3.5-mm drill bit is advanced retrograde to the level of the fracture. The drill bit is manipulated through the drill sleeve to achieve an accurate reduction of the right superior ramus fracture.

- Once the ramus is reduced, the 3.5-mm drill is replaced with a 2.8-mm guide pin and advanced gently with a mallet into the stable segment. The reduction is maintained with the guide pin, while a 3.5-mm drill bit is advanced retrograde in a position more suitable for a definitive screw (Fig. 12-90).

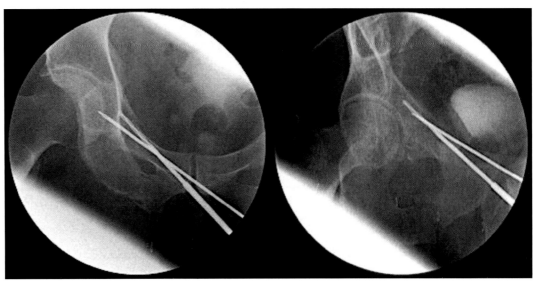

Figure 12-90 I The reduction is maintained with a 2.8-mm guide pin, while a 3.5-mm drill is advanced retrograde. The 3.5-mm drill is advanced such that it closely approximates the posterior cortical limit of the superior ramus on the inlet view.

- The 3.5-mm drill is removed and a 2.8-mm guide pin is inserted to the supra-acetabular region (Fig. 12-91). The depth is measured and a screw inserted. Since the osseous corridor is large in this patient, a 7.3-mm cannulated screw was inserted over the 2.8-mm guide pin (Fig. 12-92). Smaller screws may be used as in the previous case example depending on the patient's anterior pelvic osseous morphology.

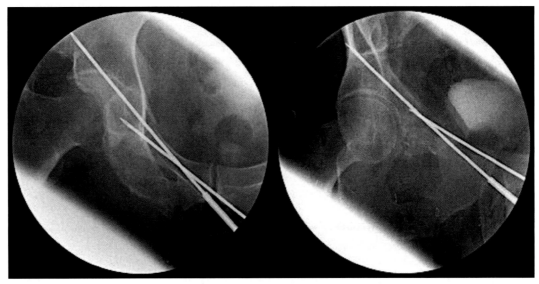

Figure 12-91 I The 3.5-mm drill is replaced by a 2.8-mm drill-tipped guide pin and advanced to the supra-acetabular region.

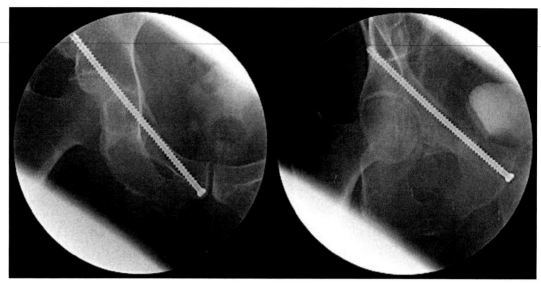

Figure 12-92 I A 7.3-mm cannulated screw is placed over the 2.8-mm guide pin. The provisional fixation is removed, and the reduction is maintained.

- The final patient radiographs demonstrate maintenance of reduction and symmetry of the pelvis bilaterally (Fig. 12-93).

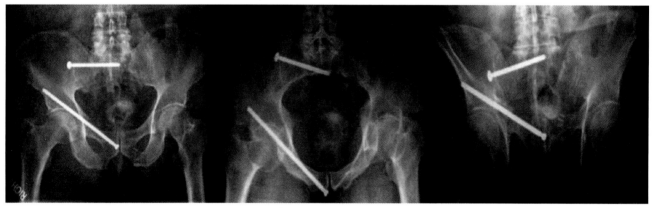

Figure 12-93 I Final AP, inlet, and outlet radiographs demonstrate adequate reduction.

References

1. Routt ML Jr, Simonian PT, Agnew SG, et al. Radiographic recognition of the sacral alar slope for optimal placement of iliosacral screws: a cadaveric and clinical study. *J Orthop Trauma*. 1996;10:171–177.
2. Routt ML Jr, Simonian PT, Grujic L. The retrograde medullary superior pubic ramus screw for the treatment of anterior pelvic ring disruptions: a new technique. *J Orthop Trauma*. 1995;9(1):35–44.

Reference

1. Routt ML Jr, Simonian PT, Agnew SG, et al. Radiographic recognition of the sacral alar slope for optimal placement of iliosacral screws: a cadaveric and clinical study. *J Orthop Trauma*. 1996;10:171–177.

Chapter 13
Acetabular Fractures

JONATHAN G. EASTMAN

REZA FIROOZABADI

MOTASEM REFAAT

ZACHARY V. ROBERTS

MILTON LEE (CHIP) ROUTT JR

Sterile Instruments/Equipment

- Large and small pointed bone reduction clamps (Weber clamps)
- Assorted pelvic reduction clamps
- Femoral distractor
- Plate bender
- Implants
  - Long 3.5-mm screws
  - Long 4.5-mm screws
  - Long 7.0-mm cannulated screws
  - Minifragment screws for free ostcochondral fragments
  - 3.5-mm reconstruction plates
- K-wires and wire driver/drill

Patient Positioning

(For additional details, see the Chapter 1.)
Prone

- Radiolucent table.
- Chest rolls are made from two blankets folded into thirds without wrinkles.
  - Gel rolls are not radiolucent.
- Prep the leg free, clean and scrub the perineum with alcohol, and drape out with plastic adhesive drapes prior to the Betadine prep.
- After prepping, towel out the surgical field and drape.

Supine

- Radiolucent table.
- Two blanket bolster under the sacrum to allow access for iliosacral screw placement if needed.
- Prep down to the table, from the genitalia to the xiphoid process. Include the lower rib cage in surgical field.

Surgical Approaches

Kocher-Langenbeck

- The Kocher-Langenbeck approach is the most common approach used for treating acetabular fractures involving the posterior wall and column.
- Incision comprises an oblique limb from the posterior superior iliac spine (PSIS) to the greater trochanter and a vertical limb that continues distally over the lateral aspect of the femur.

- The vertical limb is made first by incising the skin and subcutaneous fat to identify the fascia of the iliotibial (IT) band.
  - The IT band is then incised longitudinally from distal to proximal until fibers of the gluteus maximus are encountered at the level of the greater trochanter.
- The oblique limb of the incision is then begun at the cranial portion of the vertical limb and continued in a direction toward the PSIS.
  - The fascia overlying the gluteus maximus is identified and incised, and the muscle fibers are split bluntly.
  - The orientation of the oblique limb should parallel the gluteus maximus muscle fibers, allowing this muscle to be split more easily.
- The superior gluteal neurovascular bundle and its major branches can be identified by palpation in the interval between the gluteus medius and the gluteus maximus and should be preserved if possible.
- Identify the sciatic nerve dorsal to the quadratus femoris.
  - Displaced fracture fragments will often distort or disrupt the anatomy of the piriformis, gemelli, and obturator internus tendon, making identification of the sciatic nerve difficult in this traumatized zone.
- With the sciatic nerve identified, debride the trochanteric bursa.
- Identify and tenotomize the piriformis and obturator internus.
  - Place a retention suture in these tendons for later repair.
- Follow the obturator internus tendon to the lesser sciatic notch.
- With the knee flexed, retract the obturator internus tendon and sciatic nerve.
- Debride the injured superior and inferior gemelli muscles from the lateral ischium.
- The caudal portion of the gluteus minimus is often significantly damaged and should be debrided back to the level of the caudal branch of the superior gluteal neurovascular bundle.
  - This debridement will improve exposure to the supra-acetabular region of the ilium.
  - This can also minimize the risk of postoperative heterotopic ossification development.[1]

Ilioinguinal approach

- The surface landmarks for the incision are the pubic symphysis, anterior superior iliac spine (ASIS), and the iliac crest.
- The incision begins 1 to 2 cm cranial to the pubic symphysis, extends toward the ASIS, and follows the iliac crest to the level of the gluteus medius pillar, where it continues cranially for several centimeters.
- Identify the fascia along the length of the incision; also identify and preserve the spermatic cord/round ligament and external inguinal ring.
- Which window is opened first is a matter of preference.
  - Important considerations include the location of major fracture components; whether certain windows are needed to visualize, clean, clamp, or apply fixation to fracture components; and, finally, anticipated bleeding issues.
- The iliac window is frequently associated with significant fracture bleeding upon exposure (particularly when there is iliac wing comminution), and often, this bleeding is controlled only by fracture reduction.
  - Thus, if the middle or Stoppa windows are needed for the reduction or fixation, it is reasonable to expose them first.
- The fracture often must be cleaned to obtain anatomic reduction; however, this should be the last step of the exposure.
  - Debridement of clot from fracture planes tends to produce bleeding from the cancellous surfaces, which often can only be controlled by fracture reduction.
  - Thus, be ready to implement the reduction and fixation plan immediately after cleaning the fracture to avoid excessive bleeding.

Iliac window

- The common insertion of the abdominal obliques joins the origins of the tensor fascia lata and gluteus medius at the lateral edge of the iliac crest.
  - This tendinous structure should be divided from ASIS to the gluteus medius pillar, leaving the abductor origin intact on the ilium.
- The gluteus medius pillar roughly marks the equator of the pelvic ring (in the supine position).
  - Roughly at this landmark, the exposure may either be continued posteriorly along the iliac crest or extended cranially, splitting the fibers of the external oblique muscle.
  - If the latter is performed, the transversus abdominis and internal obliques are released from their insertion using electrocautery, working from the inner table of the iliac crest outward.

- Elevate the iliacus from the iliac fossa subperiosteally.
- Bleeding is often encountered from the nutrient vessel that enters the ilium just lateral to the pelvic brim and anterior to the sacroiliac joint.
  - Bone wax may help provide hemostasis for bleeding associated with this nutrient foramen.
  - Fractures in this region can also bleed vigorously.

Middle window

- The external oblique fascia is incised from the ASIS to a point 1 cm cranial to the external inguinal ring and reflected inferiorly to identify the inguinal ligament.
- The internal oblique and transversus abdominis insertions on the inguinal ligament are incised along the length of the ligament with a 1-mm cuff to facilitate repair.
  - This will expose the iliopectineal fascia, which needs to be carefully dissected and incised to open the middle window and allow mobilization of the iliac vessels and iliacus muscle.
- The iliopectineal fascia is an oblique fascial structure that spans the superior ramus and the inguinal ligament anteriorly.
  - It becomes confluent with the periosteum of the ilium as it courses dorsally along the pelvic brim to the sacroiliac joint.
  - It separates the lacuna vasorum containing the iliac vessels, lymphatics, and pectineus origin from the lacuna musculorum containing the iliopsoas and femoral nerve.
- Adequate release of the iliopectineal fascia increases the utility of the iliac and Stoppa windows.
  - The intact iliopectineal fascia will limit medial retraction of the iliacus while working in the iliac window and anterolateral retraction of the iliac vessels while working in the Stoppa window.

Stoppa window

- Use of this window requires the surgeon to stand on the opposite side of the patient than the side of injury and provides access to the quadrilateral surface, the upper surface of the superior ramus, and the pubic symphysis.
- The fascia between the rectus abdominis muscles is divided longitudinally in the midline.
- Frequently, one or both rectus abdominis muscles may be avulsed from their insertion on the pubis.
  - If not, 2 to 3 cm of the insertion can be elevated from the anterior surface of the pubis to increase exposure.
  - As long as the distal insertion is left intact, it can be repaired easily to the contralateral side without tension.
- Malleable retractors are used to retract the bladder.
- The periosteum overlying the superior ramus is incised, and dissection proceeds medial to lateral in a subperiosteal fashion.
- Retropubic vascular anastomoses between the superficial and deep iliac vascular systems are common and should be identified, ligated, and divided in a controlled manner, if present.
- The obturator neurovascular bundle is tethered distally by the obturator membrane and thus limits the caudal extent of the Stoppa window's exposure.
- The upper extend of the Stoppa window merges with the medial extent of the middle window after the iliopectineal fascia insertion is released from the pelvic brim.

Fracture Assessment Tips

- According to the system developed by Emile Letournel, acetabular fractures are classified by fracture morphology and location into elementary or associated fracture patterns.
- Collectively understanding the fracture morphology and the behavior of its component fragments is vital to developing and executing a successful operative plan.
- The pelvis fractures along predictable fault planes, producing several commonly recurring fracture fragments.
  - Fragment displacement is often asymmetric along the fracture plane, being tethered at one edge by intact soft tissues that act as a point of rotation or hinge between the two fragments.
  - These soft tissue hinges are helpful in that they can allow a strategically placed clamp to compress the entire fracture surface, despite its relatively large area.
  - Likewise, indirect reduction of a secondary fragment may be accomplished upon reduction of the primary fragment, if intact soft tissues span the two.

Reduction and Fixation Techniques

The Posterior Wall Fragment

- It is the most common elementary acetabular fracture pattern but has extremely variable morphology.
- It may be caused by axial load applied through an intact femur (Fig. 13-1), as in a posterior hip fracture dislocation, or it may be caused by avulsion mechanism in associated patterns (Fig. 13-2) where there is significant medial displacement of the femoral head relative to the posterior wall of the acetabulum.

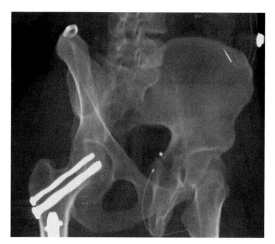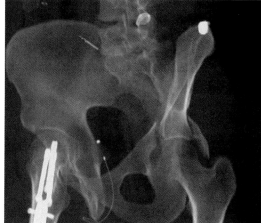

Figure 13-1 ▮ The posterior wall component of this associated transverse and posterior wall acetabular fracture demonstrates the type of fracture that is "pushed off" by the femoral head during axial load, with tension failure of the caudal labrum and an intact cranial labrum.

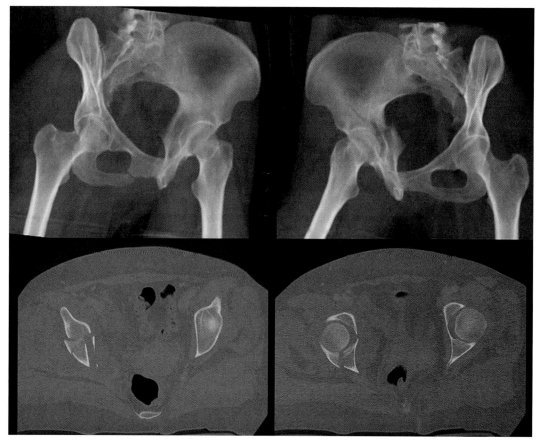

Figure 13-2 ▮ "Avulsion" posterior wall. In addition to having an incomplete anterior column component, this associated both-column acetabular fracture has a large posterior wall fracture component. In this type of posterior wall fracture, the fragment is avulsed from the intact ilium as the femoral head dislocates medially. The labrum and capsule are typically intact; however, the stability of the hip joint should be assessed after repair of the column components to determine the need for reduction and fixation of this posterior wall fragment.

- Posterior wall fracture fragments typically have an intact labral attachment.
  - In fractures with a single dominant wall fragment produced by an axial force, this attachment is typically cranial, allowing the fragment to displace primarily by rotation around this tethered point (Fig. 13-3).

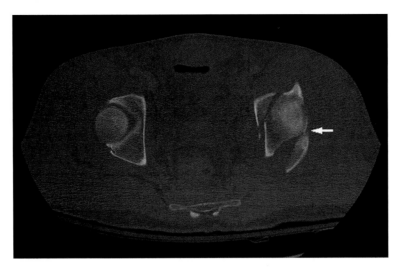

Figure 13-3 I The CT scan demonstrates rotatory displacement of a "pushed-off" posterior wall fragment (*arrow*) around an intact cranial labrum.

- Comminuted posterior wall fractures produced by axial force may have both cranial and caudal labral attachments, allowing the fragments to rotate open similar to a saloon door.
  - Avulsion posterior wall fractures are usually found to have an intact labrum and a capsule.
- Marginal impaction is frequently present and can occur on the intact portion of the acetabulum or on the fractured wall (Fig. 13-4).

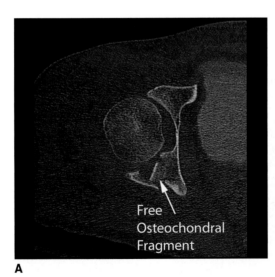
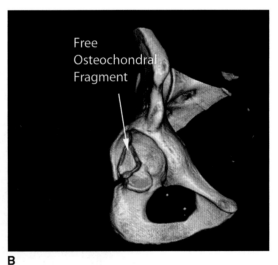

A   **B**

Figure 13-4 I Preoperative axial **(A)** and 3D **(B)** CT scans demonstrating marginal impaction.

- Impacted articular segments should be reduced to the femoral head and their cancellous defects bone grafted (Fig. 13-5).

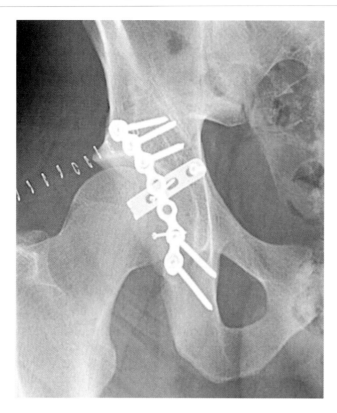

Figure 13-5 I Spring plate and minifragment screws deployed for peripheral posterior wall acetabular fracture.

- Minifragment intraosseous screws may be useful for stabilization of these small osteochondral fragments (Fig. 13-6).

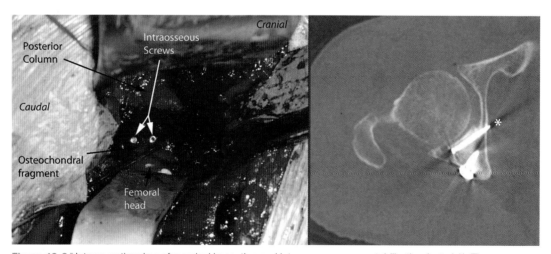

Figure 13-6 I Intraoperative view of marginal impaction and intraosseous screw stabilization (*asterisk*). The postoperative CT scan demonstrates the reduction and position of the screw.

- In addition, the femoral head may cause impaction of the cancellous fracture bed, which will result in an imperfect fit between the cancellous portions of the fracture fragments during reduction if not disimpacted.

- Balanced buttress plate(s) are the mainstay of posterior wall fracture fixation (Fig. 13-7).
  - A seven- or eight-hole undercontoured 3.5 reconstruction plate is usually sufficient for this application, depending on the cranial extend of the fracture.

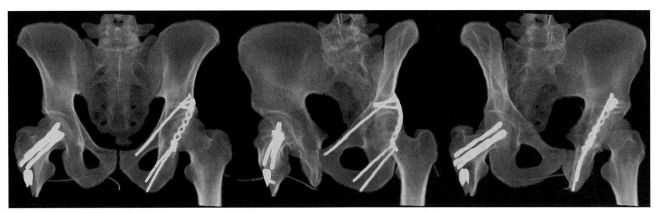

Figure 13-7 ▌ The posterior wall component of this associated transverse and posterior wall fracture is fixed with a balanced, slightly undercontoured buttress plate. This implant is usually a seven- or eight-hole reconstruction plate and is the mainstay for posterior wall acetabular fractures. This plate also functions to stabilize the posterior column portion of the transverse fracture.

Fixation Plate Contouring and Application for Posterior Wall Acetabular Fracture

Reza Firoozabadi
Milton L. Chip Routt Jr

Pathoanatomy

Failure of posterior wall acetabular fracture fixation is usually due to misapplication of the supporting plate. Secure plate fixation for posterior wall acetabular fracture patterns depends on the fracture pattern, the cortical surface of the fragment, the quality of reduction, and the plate contouring and application details.

Solution

Slight undercontouring of the supporting plate provides improved contact and compression to the fracture fragment's cortical surface thereby improving stability. The plate is best positioned on the fracture fragment midway between the posterior wall edge and the medial extent of the fracture. As the fixation screws are tightened, the plate compresses the fracture fragment.

Technique

- First, the posterior wall fracture fragment is accurately reduced and temporarily held with extra-articular K-wires.
  - The temporary reduction wires must be positioned so as not to obstruct the ideal position for eventual plate application.
- For most posterior wall fractures, a seven- or eight-hole, 3.5-mm pelvic reconstruction plate is selected.
  - The plate is first slightly undercontoured relative to the posterior wall fragment's cortical surface osteology using handheld bending pliers.
- Next, identify the peripheral edge of the posterior wall, the medial extent of the fracture, and the midpoint between these two limits from the cephalad to the caudad edges of the fracture (Fig. 13-8).
  - The pathway of these midpoints is where the plate will be located in order to provide balanced fixation.
  - In larger posterior wall fractures, two plates should be utilized, one on the peripheral edge and one on the medial edge to provide additional stability.
- The periosteum and other remaining soft tissues must be removed from the cortical surface of the fracture fragment along this planned plate location site.

- Next, the undercontoured plate is inserted and grossly aligned with the planned location site and then secured with an appropriate length screw placed through the second hole from the bottom (Figs. 13-8 and 13-9).
  - Prior to completely tightening the screw, the plate's contour and position can be fine-tuned so as to obtain an optimal position, balanced between the wall's edge and the medial fracture line.

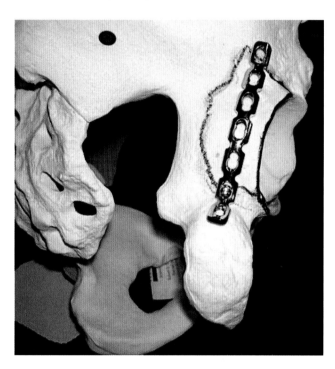

Figure 13-8 I The malleable reconstruction plate is adjusted so that it is located midway between the labral edge and medial fracture line and then secured with a screw in the second from the bottom hole. Prior to tightening the screw, the plate can be adjusted medially or laterally.

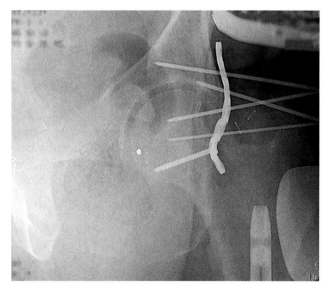

Figure 13-9 I The intraoperative obturator oblique image demonstrates the temporary fixation wires and the slight undercontouring of the plate.

- Once the proper plate location is achieved, a plate screw is inserted in the screw hole located just above the acetabular dome.
  - Because of the slight undercontouring of the plate, the depth assessment for the screw may be several millimeters too long. The surgeon can either apply the screw recognizing that it will eventually be exchanged for a shorter screw once the fixation construct is completed, or the distance between the undercontoured plate and the cortical surface can be subtracted from the screw length (Fig. 13-10).

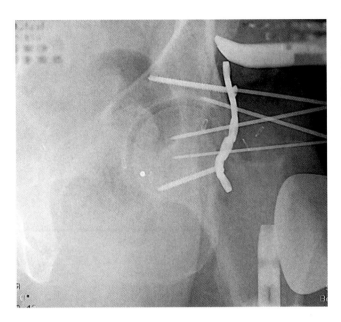

Figure 13-10 ‖ The screw in the second from the top hole has been inserted but not yet completely tightened. The undercontoured plate has not yet been applied onto the cortical surface of the fracture fragment.

- Tightening the screw first causes the slightly undercontoured plate to be slowly compressed against the cortical surface of the posterior wall fracture fragment. Further screw tightening then causes the plate to compresses the posterior wall cancellous fracture surfaces together using the femoral head as a template for the articular surface of the fracture fragment (Fig. 13-11).

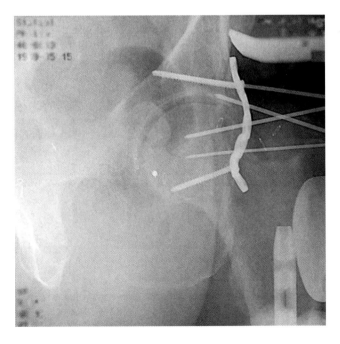

Figure 13-11 ‖ As the screw is tightened, the plate is compressed against the cortical bone. Further tightening causes compression at the fracture surface.

- The caudal screw is then directed toward the ischial tuberosity and the cranial screw is inserted last. The wires are then removed and the stability provided by the plate is assessed using a dental probe.
  - If the fixation construct is stable, the posterior wall fracture fragment will have no movement. If the posterior wall fracture fragment can be moved beneath the plate, then the applied plate does not have an intimate fit with the cortical surface of the wall fracture fragment and must be better contoured to provide stable fixation (Fig. 13-12).

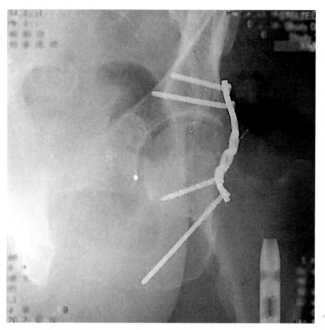 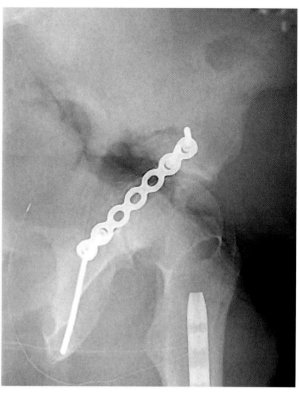

Figure 13-12 I (Obturator oblique and iliac oblique images) The remaining screws above and below the joint have been filled, the wires removed, and the fracture stability assured. The iliac oblique image demonstrates that the plate screws are extra-articular.

- Stiff, nonmalleable plates should not be utilized. If a stiff plate is used, this technique will be compromised due to the inability of the plate to contour and capture the wall fragment, especially in osteopenic bone (Fig. 13-13).

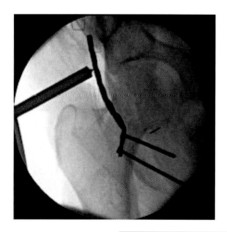 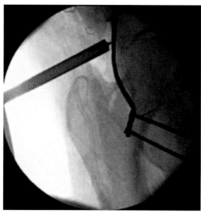

Figure 13-13 I In this example, the plate has been secured using two caudal screws and then a spiked pusher is used to apply the slightly undercontoured plate onto the bone prior to inserting the screw.

Spring Plate

- A "spring plate" can be used for peripheral posterior wall fractures that are incompletely captured by the buttress reconstruction plate.
  - This implant is fashioned from a three-hole one-third tubular plate and should be placed underneath the buttress plate.

- To make a hook plate, the end hole of the one-third tubular plate should be flattened and bent 90 degrees through the hole of the single-hole side of the plate.
- Once bent, a section of the bent hole should be cut out to fashion two prongs (Fig. 13-14).
- The spring plate is applied with the prongs set in bone on the peripheral edge of the posterior wall fragment.
- Avoid placing the prongs in soft tissues or labrum, as this may result in erosion of the femoral head.

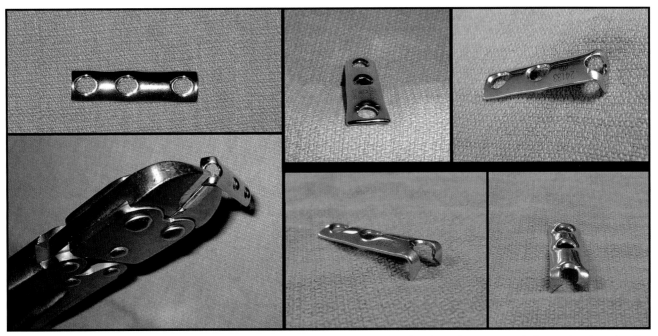

Figure 13-14 I A spring plate can be fabricated from a standard three-hole one-third tubular plate using two sets of pliers and a wire cutter. To begin, flatten the single-hole end of the plate and bend it to 90 degrees as shown. The size and location of the fracture fragment will determine the depth of the tines, which can be varied based on how much of the residual plate is removed.

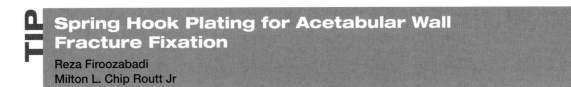

TIP

Spring Hook Plating for Acetabular Wall Fracture Fixation

Reza Firoozabadi
Milton L. Chip Routt Jr

Pathoanatomy

Certain acetabular posterior and anterior wall fracture fragments located on the far edges of the joint are very difficult to stabilize effectively using standard malleable plating techniques.

Solution

Special plates can be fashioned with small sharp peripheral hooks. The hooks can be applied onto the cortical surfaces of small fracture fragments to fix them securely. Compression can be added to the fracture with proper plate contouring and screw insertion sequencing.

Technique

- Spring hook plates (SHP) are usually fashioned using a standard 3-holed one-third tubular plate. These plates have several special features that make them useful for this application.
  - First, the three holes are not spaced uniformly. Two of the holes are located on one end of the plate, and the third hole is located on the opposite end. That third hole will be used to form the hooks so that the middle hole will be located farther away from the joint for later fixation.
  - To fashion the SHP, the one-third tubular plate curvature is first flattened using either a mallet or with a plate press (Fig. 13-15).

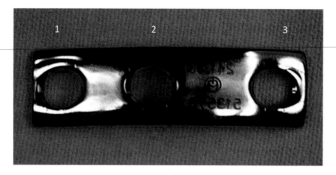

Figure 13-15 I The three-holed one-third tubular plate has been flattened. The #1 and #2 holes are located more closely together on one end of the plate, while the #3 hole is located on the opposite end.

- In order to apply compression at the fracture surfaces, the plate must be "overcontoured" relative to the cortical surface that it will be placed upon. This plate contouring is performed between the plate holes using a handheld bender (Fig. 13-16).

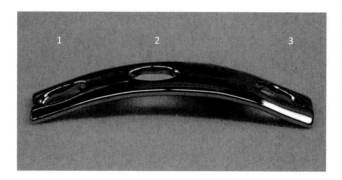

Figure 13-16 I The plate is "overcontoured" relative to the cortical surface that it will be placed upon. This prebending allows the plate hooks to apply compression at the fracture surface as the plate deforms elastically to fit the cortical surface.

- Then the #3 hole is then cut with a wire or pin cutters yielding two tines that will later be folded toward the plate's convexity forming two hooks.
  - The depth of the cut into the third hole determines the length of the tines and the obliquity of the cut determines their widths.
  - A shallow and flatter cut into the hole leaves a longer and wider tine, while a deep and oblique cut into the hole leaves a shorter and thinner tine. In some fractures, it is helpful for fixation if the tines are of different lengths so the appropriate sized hooks can be formed (Fig. 13-17).

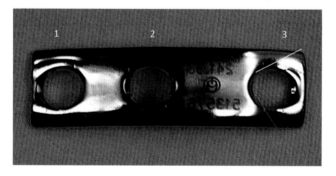

Figure 13-17 I The location and obliquity of the *yellow line* cut would produce a longer and thinner tine than that of the *red line*. Usually, the cuts are made symmetrically so the tines are of equal length and width.

- Once the #3 hole has been cut away, the tines are bent to form hooks. The hooks must not be too long in order to avoid penetration through the fracture fragment.
  - The initial flattening of the one-third tubular plate separates the hook tips. If the plate remains unflattened, the hook tips will converge due to the one-third tubular shape of the plate.
- The SHP is applied onto the peripheral fragments before other fixation plates are placed. The peripheral fracture fragment is first reduced and temporarily stabilized with a small diameter wire, dental pick, or other technique.
  - The tines are located onto the cortical surface of the peripheral acetabular wall fracture fragment avoiding the labrum.
  - The plate is then secured to the bone using an extra-articular screw placed through the #2 hole. As the screw is tightened, the overcontoured plate will begin to flatten as the opposite medial end of the plate slides away from the joint (Fig. 13-18).

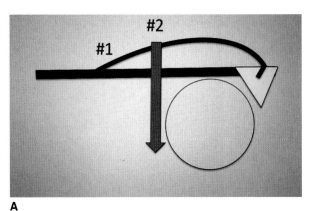

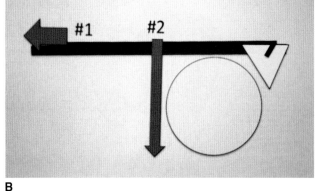

A   **B**

Figure 13-18 I A: The SHP is shown in *black* and is overcontoured relative to the *blue* cortical bone surface. The hooks of the SHP are engaged in the cortical bone of the peripheral wall fracture fragment. The *red arrow* in the #2 hole represents an extra-articular screw that has not been tightened. **B:** The #2 screw has been tightened, and the plate has deformed to fit the cortical surface. The plate moved medially away from the joint as the screw was tightened transferring compression to the fracture surface.

- If the medial end of the plate is not allowed to slide due to bone, soft tissue, or other obstructions, then the technique fails because then the hook end of the plate will displace laterally causing disengagement of the hooks as the plate slides laterally.
  - Once the #2 screw is inserted and tightened and the SHP has compressed the fracture, the #1 hole is filled with an extra-articular screw to prevent rotational displacement of the plate around the #2 screw.
- For most posterior wall acetabular fractures, the SHP should be reinforced with a standard malleable pelvic reconstruction plate. This is because of the SHP's flexibility. The reinforcing plate should be located over (superficial to) the peripheral portion of the SHP and posterior wall fracture (Figs. 13-19 and 13-20).

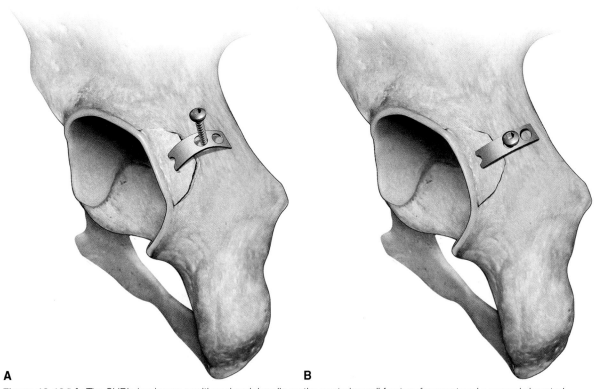

A   **B**

Figure 13-19 I A: The SHP's hooks are positioned peripherally on the posterior wall fracture fragment and a screw is inserted eccentrically. **B:** As the screw is tightened, the fragment is compressed into its anatomical bed.

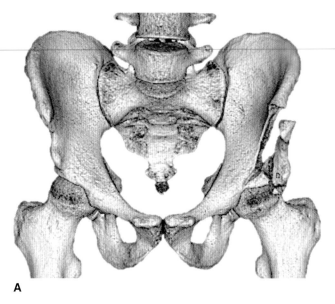

A

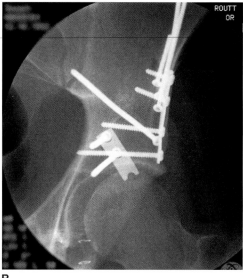

B

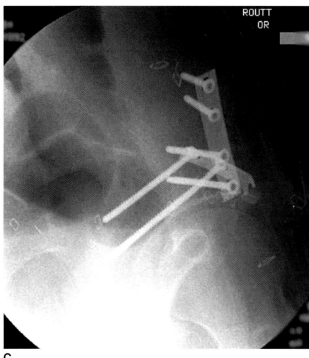

C

Figure 13-20 ▮ **A:** The 3D-reconstructed image shows the comminuted fracture including the small anterior wall articular fragment. **B and C:** Intraoperative fluoroscopy images demonstrate the SHP technique used to stabilize the anterior wall fracture fragment.

In summary, for the SHP to function:

1. The hooks must capture the cortical surface of the peripheral fragment.
2. The hooks must not be located on the labrum or capsule to prevent the hooks damaging the femoral head.
3. The plate must be slightly overcontoured relative to the cortical surface to which it is being applied.
4. The #2 screw is inserted first to properly deform the plate so the hooks can compress the fracture surface as the plate deforms and slides medially.
5. The medial side of the plate must be unobstructed as the #2 screw is tightened so that the plate can slide medially as it flattens to fit the cortical surface.
6. Assure that the hooks cannot penetrate through the fragment and damage the femoral head.
7. The #1 screw is inserted last to prevent rotational instability of the plate.
8. Reinforcing plates must be located properly to function effectively.

Universal Distractor

- With the leg prepped free, the universal distractor can be also used to improve access to the joint for extraction of intra-articular fracture debris (Fig. 13-21).

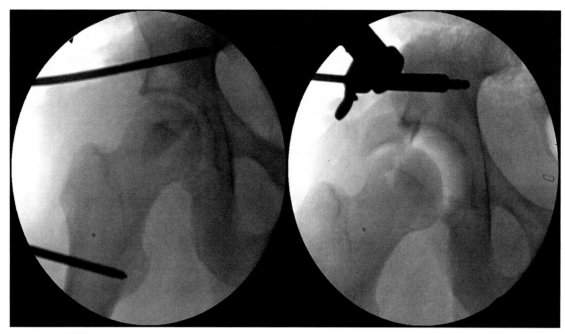

Figure 13-21 I The universal distractor may be used to improve visualization of the hip joint while extracting fracture debris. Make sure the threaded bar is oriented to provide a lateral and caudal distraction vector that roughly parallels the femoral neck.

Intraoperative Distractor Pin Placement during Acetabular Fracture Fixation without Fluoroscopic Assistance

Motasem Refaat
Jonathan G. Eastman

Pathoanatomy

Some acetabular fractures may require hip joint distraction for the removal of intra-articular debris or visualization of reduction.

Solutions

To perform such distraction, femoral traction can be accomplished manually, using a small caliber distal femoral traction pin and Kirschner wire bow, a larger caliber larger proximal femoral Steinmann or Schanz pin, or through the use of a traction table. Another option is to use an AO Universal Distractor (Synthes, Paoli, PA). This is commonly applied when a Kocher-Langenbeck approach is used and has been described previously.[1]

When using a universal distractor with two Schanz pins, one Schanz pin is placed bicortically or unicortically (deep) into the ilium just superior and anterior to the greater sciatic notch. Care is taken to protect the superior gluteal neurovascular bundle. The second Schanz pin is placed into the proximal femur at or above the level of the lesser trochanter. This location minimizes the iatrogenic creation of a stress riser. To verify this location, intraoperative fluoroscopy is used commonly. Combining the evaluation and assessment of preoperative CT scans with intraoperative correlation of osseous landmarks, a Schanz pin can be placed into this desired location without the need for fluoroscopy. The technique as described below leads to safe pin placement with decreased operative time, blood loss, and radiation exposure.

Technique

- Evaluation of preoperative coronal CT reformations allows direct measurement of the distance between the tip of the greater trochanter and the level of the lesser trochanter. The anticipated intraoperative measurement to ensure a pin location proximal to the lesser trochanter is made (Fig. 13-22). Commonly, this is typically about 6 cm.

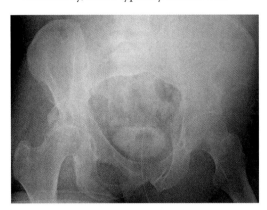

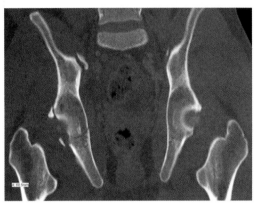

Figure 13-22 | Preoperative AP pelvis radiograph and coronal reformatted CT image of a patient with a transverse posterior wall acetabular fracture. Measurement tool from the PACS system is used to measure the distance from the tip of the greater trochanter to the lesser trochanter (*lower image*, A: 60.5 mm). A Schanz pin placed at or <6 cm from the tip of the greater trochanter will be in a safe position above the lesser trochanter.

- In either prone or lateral position, a standard Kocher-Langenbeck exposure is performed and deep dissection exposes the retroacetabular surface.
- The hip is kept in an extended position with the knee flexed at or past 90 degrees. The sciatic nerve is identified and protected appropriately.
- The gluteus medius pillar Schanz pin can be located superior and anterior to the greater sciatic notch out of the way of anticipated clamps or implants.
- Using a soft tissue guide, a 3.5-mm drill bit is used to predrill the path for the 5-mm Schanz pin. An appropriate length partially threaded Schanz pin is then inserted into the gluteus medius pillar with care taken to protect the superior gluteal neurovascular bundle.
- The tip of the greater trochanter is palpated (Fig. 13-23).

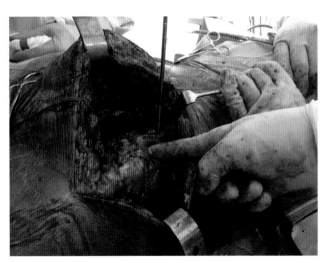

Figure 13-23 | Intraoperative clinical photograph demonstrating direct palpation of the tip of the greater trochanter.

- A ruler is used to measure 6 cm from the tip of the greater trochanter aiming distally down the midline of the femur (Fig. 13-24). This marks the safe starting point at or above the level of the lesser trochanter.

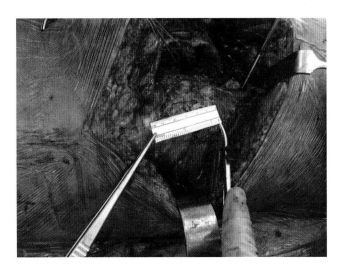

Figure 13-24 I Intraoperative clinical photograph depicting utilization of a precut paper ruler to measure 6 cm extending distally from the tip of the greater trochanter distally in the midline of the femur.

- The surgeon can palpate the alignment of the limb and aim appropriately caudal or cranial to ensure a transverse pin path. A 3.5-mm drill is used to create the path and the Schanz pin is then placed (Fig. 13-25). The pin is placed either bicortically or deeply unicortical depending on the anticipated amount and duration of force needed.

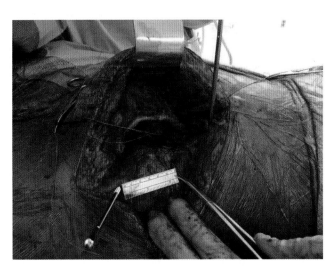

Figure 13-25 I Intraoperative clinical photograph demonstrating placement of a 5-mm Schanz pin 6 cm distal from the tip of the greater trochanter at the level of the lesser trochanter.

- The universal distractor is then applied to each pin in standard fashion, used and removed once the procedure is completed (Fig. 13-26).

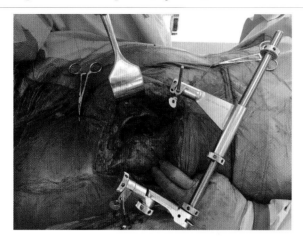

Figure 13-26 I Intraoperative clinical photograph demonstrating universal distractor placement. Note the threaded bar position, which is out of the view of the hip joint as well as the correct lateral and caudal vector of distraction.

- Schanz pin placement can be verified at any time if needed intraoperatively but will also be apparent on postoperative imaging (Fig. 13-27).

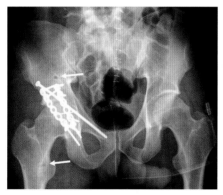
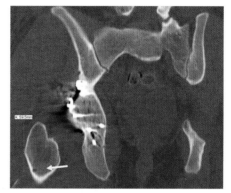

Figure 13-27 I Postoperative AP pelvis radiograph and coronal reformatted CT image radiograph demonstrating safe placement of Schanz pin in posterior column and in the femur 6 cm distal to the tip of the greater trochanter and just proximal to the lesser trochanter (*yellow arrows*).

The Caudal Segment of a Transverse Fracture

- The transverse acetabular fracture pattern is an elementary acetabular fracture that occurs when a single fracture plane divides the acetabulum into cranial and caudal fragments (Fig. 13-28).

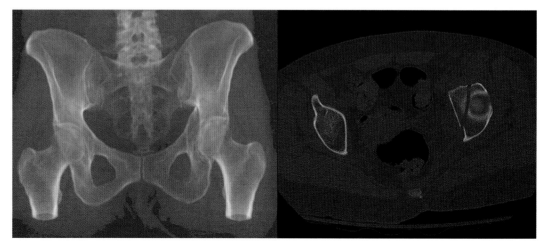

Figure 13-28 I The caudal segment of this transtectal transverse acetabular fracture is shown in *red*. Note the disruption in both the iliopectineal and ilioischial lines on the AP radiograph.

- By definition, this fracture plane must traverse the anatomical areas of the anterior and posterior columns, as well as the areas of the anterior and posterior walls. This can be confusing since there are also fracture patterns named after these anatomical areas.
- The transverse acetabular fracture disrupts the pelvic ring and can occur in conjunction with sacral fractures, sacroiliac joint injuries, or disruptions to the pubic symphysis. Look carefully for these associated injuries.
- The caudal segment is usually the unstable component of the transverse acetabular fracture pattern and typically displaces medially.
  - Often, the caudal segment displacement has a rotational component and is "hinged" either anteriorly or posteriorly by intact soft tissues.
  - The location of maximal displacement usually determines the surgical approach required for reduction.
- The caudal segment of the transverse acetabular fracture should behave as a unit during reduction efforts and can often be accurately reduced with strategic clamp placement.
- It can be difficult to assess the reduction intraoperatively since direct visualization of both columns simultaneously is not possible without extensile or combined simultaneous approaches.
- The surgical approach is decided based on the anatomic column that needs to be visualized intraoperatively, which most often is determined by the region of maximal displacement but may occasionally be determined by the need to clean comminution from the primary fracture plane (Fig. 13-29).

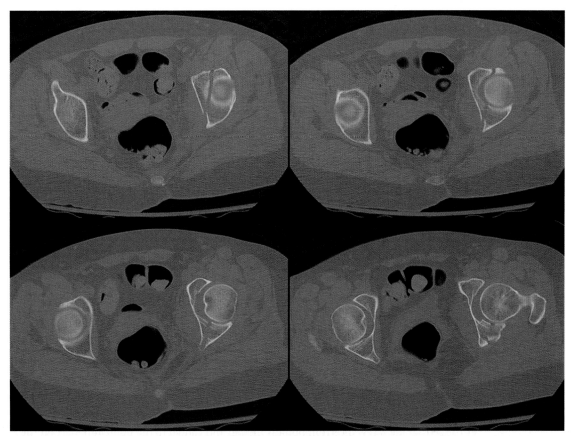

Figure 13-29 | Use the CT to plan the surgical approach for transverse fractures. The column that requires direct visualization (usually the most displaced) determines the approach. While the displacement of this transtectal transverse fracture is fairly symmetric, there is comminution in the area of the posterior wall (*magenta*) that will prevent an anatomic articular reduction if it is not addressed. The ideal approach for this fracture is a prone Kocher-Langenbeck approach.

- The medullary superior ramus screw is a useful implant to stabilize displaced pubic root fractures whether they occur in the context of a pelvic ring injury or the anterior column component of an acetabular fracture (Fig. 13-30).

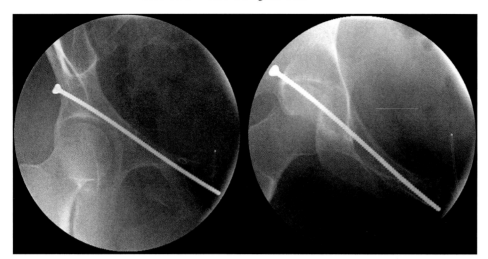

Figure 13-30 ▌ Medullary superior ramus screw. These screws can be inserted antegrade or retrograde using the obturator outlet (*left*) and inlet (*right*) fluoroscopic views. The superior ramus is a triangular tube of bone oriented roughly 45 degrees oblique to the coronal plane. To remain safe, the screw trajectory should course through the largest area of the medullary canal, which is cranial and posterior (shown). Use blunt rather than self-tapping screws, and overdrill the starting point to make screw insertion easier.

- This implant is applicable in patients who have sufficient anatomy in the anterior supra-acetabular area to accommodate the screw and can be inserted with the patient supine or prone, and in an antegrade or retrograde direction, depending on patient anatomy (Fig. 13-31).

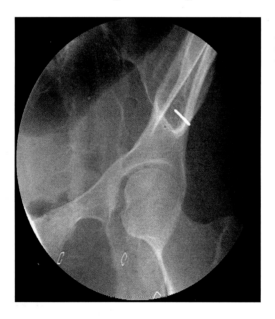

Figure 13-31 ▌ This patient's superior ramus is narrow and undulating, which makes antegrade medullary fixation difficult. However, this parasymphyseal ramus fracture would be appropriate for a shorter retrograde screw.

- The fluoroscopic views used during superior pubic ramus screw insertion are the obturator oblique and the inlet.
- The starting point for an antegrade screw is 1 to 2 cm cranial to the acetabulum on the gluteus medius pillar.
- The retrograde screw insertion point is medial and caudal to the pubic tubercle, on the anterior edge of the pubic symphysis.
- The near cortex is overdrilled to allow easier screw insertion.
- The ideal screw trajectory is central to high on the obturator oblique view and posterior on the inlet view.
- A 3.5-mm screw is most commonly used and is often sufficient; however, a 4.5-mm screw can be used when the surgeon desires and the patient's anatomy will accommodate the larger screw.
- Options for plate fixation of the anterior portion of the anterior column require an ilioinguinal approach and have been discussed in the section "The Anterior Column Fragment."
- Reduction of the displaced posterior portion of the caudal segment is accomplished most often with direct visualization through a prone Kocher-Langenbeck approach.

- A modified Weber clamp (or two) placed through drill holes in the ilium and ischium is usually sufficient.
- A 4- or 5-mm Shantz pin in the ischial tuberosity may be used to help correct rotational deformity but should be remotely placed from anticipated fixation sites.
- The anterior portion of the caudal segment may be accessed for palpation or clamp application through the greater sciatic notch.
- There is frequently not enough room to palpate the anterior reduction after application of a clamp through the greater sciatic notch (Fig. 13-32).

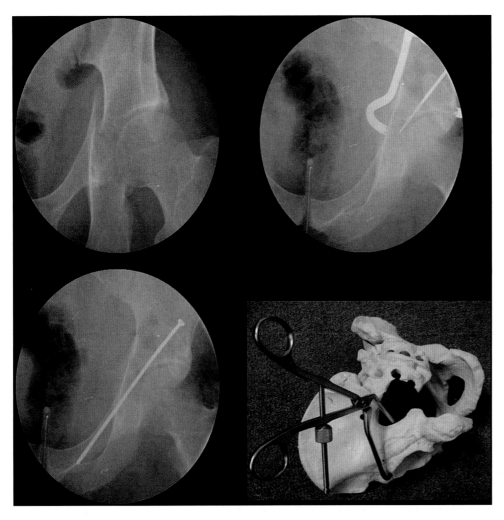

Figure 13-32 | The transverse portion of the associated transverse and posterior wall fracture is cleaned and then clamped as shown. A portion of the obturator internus muscle origin must be elevated subperiosteally and the knee must be flexed to allow application of this clamp. A medullary superior ramus screw maintains the reduction of the anterior column portion after clamp removal.

- An associated posterior wall fracture allows an articular reduction read in addition to cortical and radiographic assessments.
  - When working from the posterior approach, clamp and reduce and fix the anterior column first.
- Plate fixation for the posterior portion of the caudal segment is similar to that of the posterior column fragment, which is described in the section "The Posterior Column Fragment."
  - If there is an associated posterior wall fracture, the caudal segment should be reduced and stabilized first with the posterior wall fragment displaced, as this allows visualization of the articular surface from which one can further assess the quality of the caudal segment reduction.
- Malreductions occur usually in the column opposite the surgical approach, and there are several reasons that may explain this issue.
  - First, the surgeon is unable to directly visualize the reduction of the opposite column and may incorrectly interpret intraoperative radiographs.
  - Second, insufficient cleaning of the unvisualized portion of the fracture can result in the inability to effect an accurate reduction.

- Third, fixation options for the opposite column are limited, and inadequate fixation may result in early displacement.
- Finally, undercontoured implants on the posterior column can displace the anterior column if it is unfixed and its periosteal hinge is insufficient.

The Posterior Column Fragment

- The posterior column fragment occurs in the elementary posterior column fracture pattern and also in several associated fracture patterns to include the anterior column plus posterior hemitransverse, associated both-column, and the T-shaped fracture patterns.
- The posterior column fragment is produced by a fracture that traverses the obturator ring, divides the acetabulum into anterior and posterior halves, and exits cranially and posteriorly into the greater sciatic notch.
  - The exit point in the greater notch is variable, as is the obturator ring exit point (Fig. 13-33).

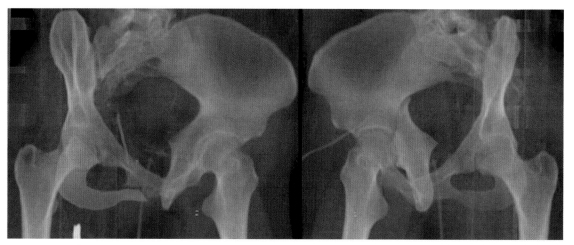

Figure 13-33 | These Judet views define the posterior column fragment (*green*) in an elementary posterior column fracture. Note the posterior spike of bone created as the fracture enters the greater sciatic notch. Although the bone quality in this area is typically quite good, the spike tends to be plastically deformed and may not be reliable for assessing the articular reduction.

- Displacement of the posterior column fragment is maintained in part by deforming muscular forces, specifically the abductor group, hamstrings, and rectus femoris.
  - The posterior column thus assumes a medialized, flexed, and, occasionally, internally rotated position (Fig. 13-34).

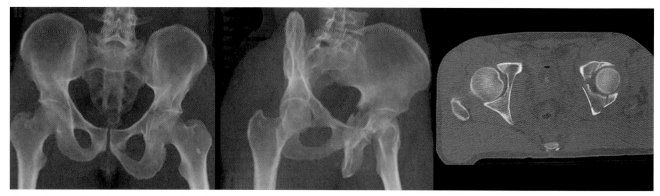

Figure 13-34 | This elementary posterior column fracture demonstrates flexion and internal rotation deformities. Note the asymmetry of the obturator foramina on the AP and the distraction at the greater sciatic notch on the iliac oblique. A Schantz pin applied in the ischial tuberosity may be useful to correct any residual malrotation that may be present after clamp application. Consider using a smaller 4.0-mm pin and make sure its location is compatible with both the reduction maneuver and the anticipated fixation strategy. When a large pin cavitates, it can negatively affect fixation options.

- The posterior capsule is usually in continuity between the femoral neck and the fractured posterior column fragment, resulting in the tendency for the femoral head to follow the displacement of this fragment.
- Fracture displacement in the region of the greater sciatic notch can result in an injury to the sciatic nerve and/or the superior gluteal neurovascular bundle.
- Fractures involving the posterior column frequently produce a "spike" of bone that remains on the posterior column fragment as the fracture plane exits the greater sciatic notch.
  - This "spike" is occasionally plastically deformed and may not be a reliable reduction read.
- Not all fractures involving the greater sciatic notch produce a posterior column fracture fragment.
  - For this fragment to occur, the fracture plane must divide the obturator ring.
- Long screws can be placed into the posterior column from the inner table of the ilium using the iliac window portion of an ilioinguinal exposure.
  - Typically, these screws are applied through or adjacent to a reconstruction plate, which acts as a washer to fortify the proximal screw purchase.
  - The iliac oblique and outlet fluoroscopic views are used to guide the placement of these screws (Fig. 13-35).

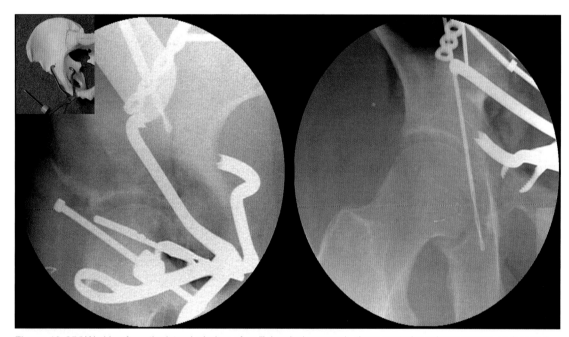

Figure 13-35 | Working from the lateral window of an ilioinguinal approach, these posterior column screws are inserted through the distal end of an eight-hole reconstruction plate using the iliac oblique and outlet fluoroscopic views. The trajectory is just posterior to the acetabulum and just lateral to the quadrilateral surface toward the medial aspect of the ischial tuberosity. The plate functions as a large washer, preventing the intrusion of the screw heads through the inner table of the ilium. The large clamp is applied through the Stoppa window, with one tine on the quadrilateral surface and the other over the pelvic brim near the psoas gutter. Axial CT images are used during preoperative planning to determine the appropriate vector for this clamp application.

  - The screw path should course from its starting point lateral to the pelvic brim and anterior to the sacroiliac joint to the medial aspect of the ischial tuberosity for maximal length.
  - Screws with a more lateral trajectory will exit on the dorsolateral surface of the ischium in the area of the posterior wall and will be shorter as a result.
  - For longer screws, the ideal path is just posterior to the acetabulum on the iliac oblique and adjacent to the quadrilateral surface on the outlet.
- Fixation of the posterior column fragment using the Kocher-Langenbeck approach most often is accomplished with reconstruction plates. Depending on the fracture morphology, one or two plates may be used to obtain stability of the posterior column (Fig. 13-36).
- Elementary posterior column fractures are usually associated with a labral tear that can obstruct the reduction.
  - If present, the torn labrum should be identified and its unstable portion repaired or debrided.

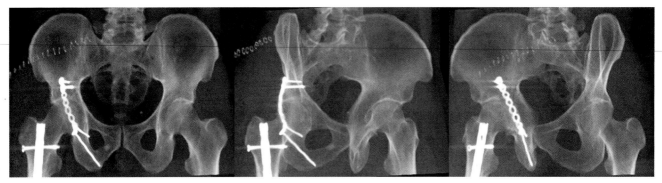

Figure 13-36 I This elementary posterior column fracture has been stabilized using a single appropriately contoured eight-hole reconstruction plate.

The Anterior Column Fragment

- Several variants of the anterior column fracture pattern have been described, differentiated by where the fracture plane exits the ilium.
  - The high fracture variant spans the iliac crest and inferior ischiopubic junction, traversing the iliac wing dorsal to the gluteus medius pillar, entering the acetabulum at its cranial margin.
  - The low fracture variant involves the area caudal to the anterior inferior iliac spine (AIIS) in the region of the psoas gutter or pubic root and traverses the acetabulum and obturator ring to exit the inferior ramus at the ischiopubic junction.
- Fractures involving the anterior column produce two common fracture fragments and can occur as an elementary anterior column fracture or as a component of associated fracture patterns (Fig. 13-37).

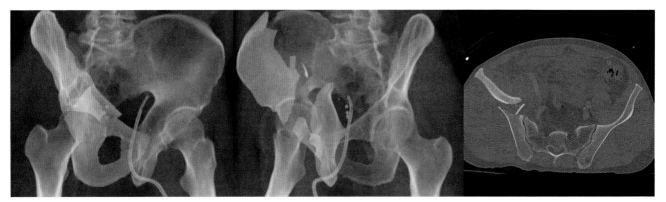

Figure 13-37 I This associated both-column acetabular fracture produced three dominant fragments: the anterior iliac fragment (*yellow*), the pubic fragment (*blue*), and the posterior column fragment (*green*). Additionally, there is comminution at the pelvic brim, noted on the iliac oblique and the axial image.

- The anterior iliac fragment occurs in fractures that have a high anterior column component and usually includes the anterior half of the ilium including the medius pillar, as well as a larger portion of the acetabular dome.
  - When present, it usually demonstrates multiplanar displacement, with an extension in the sagittal plane and concurrent rotation and medial translation in the coronal plane.
  - Often, the fracture runs obliquely between the inner and outer tables of the ilium, exiting the pelvic brim near the anterior margin of the sacroiliac joint and the outer table just dorsal to the gluteus medius pillar.
  - Comminution of the dense bone at the pelvic brim complicates the reduction since the unicortical portion of the iliac fossa is often plastically deformed.
- The pubic fragment is formed when a fracture involving the psoas gutter divides the caudal portion of the anterior column from its iliac portion.
  - If displaced, its hinge point is usually the pubic symphysis.

- Plastic deformity in the unicortical portion of the anterior iliac fragment can complicate the articular reduction since reduction of the iliac crest and upper portions of the inner table may not effect an accurate reduction of the articular surface.
  - Thus, the most accurate articular reduction is often obtained indirectly through extra-articular cortical reduction near the pelvic brim and quadrilateral surface. The relative density of the bone in this area makes it resistant to plastic deformation.
  - If this area is comminuted, reassembly of the comminuted fragments is often necessary to effect an accurate reconstruction of the joint surface.
- Occasionally, the iliac portion of the fracture will be incomplete at the crest and displacement at the joint will occur through plastic deformation along the iliac wing.
  - The incomplete fracture usually must be completed to achieve an accurate articular reduction, and residual plastic deformity in the iliac wing can be manifest as an imperfect reduction of the iliac crest despite anatomic reduction at the level of the pelvic brim (Fig. 13-38).

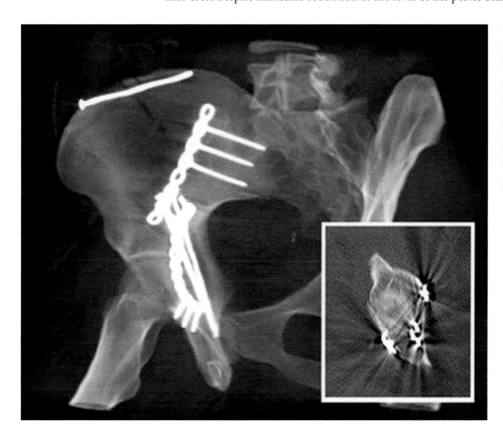

Figure 13-38 I This is the postoperative radiograph of the associated both-column fracture in Figure 13-37. The incomplete fracture of the anterior column was completed with an osteotome and reduced using a cortical read at the pelvic brim. Note that plastic deformation through the unicortical portion of the ilium causes an imperfect reduction at the iliac crest despite accurate restoration of the articular surface.

- Secure fixation of the iliac fracture requires fixation both at the crest and at the brim.
- Reduction of the anterior iliac fragment requires traction, lateralization at the level of the pelvic brim, and rotation in the coronal plane.
  - Often, a clamp at the iliac crest is helpful in stabilizing a fragment cranially, allowing the fragment to be abducted, flexed, and internally rotated around this point.
- A buttress plate along the pelvic brim is very useful in stabilizing the caudal aspect of the iliac fracture.
  - A seven- or eight-hole plate is most often used.
  - The proximal and posterior screws gain purchase in the posterior iliac crest and angle medially paralleling the sacroiliac joint.
  - Distal fixation is available with screws into the cortical bone of the greater sciatic notch (consider undersizing these screws as the density of the bone in this area tends to cause the screw head to strip before it is fully seated) or with longer screws into the posterior column.

- If long posterior column screws are planned, do not twist the plate to match the contour of the iliac fossa, as doing so will interfere with the ability to aim longer screws along the quadrilateral surface into the ischium. (Posterior column screws are described in the section "The Posterior Column Fragment.")
  - Alternatively, an opportunity for screw fixation at the pelvic brim exists in the "tube" of bone between the AIIS and the PSIS.
    - The fluoroscopic views used for insertion of this screw are the obturator outlet, the obturator inlet, and the iliac oblique.
    - The starting point is located on the obturator outlet view, while the screw trajectory is followed on the other views (Fig. 13-39).

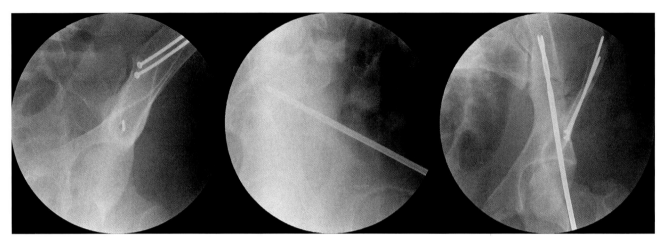

Figure 13-39 I One opportunity for medullary fixation at the level of the pelvic brim is the conduit between AIIS and PSIS. The starting point is identified using an obturator outlet view (*left*). Use the iliac oblique view (*center*) to aim cranial to the acetabulum and the greater sciatic notch and the obturator inlet view (*right*) to guide the trajectory between the inner and outer tables. It is important to consider the need for superior ramus screws and adjust the starting point appropriately. The screw shown will likely obstruct the path of an antegrade superior ramus screw (see *left*).

- The intrapelvic plate is applied through the Stoppa window and is useful for stabilizing low anterior column fractures but is most useful for buttressing the posterior column and quadrilateral surface in fractures involving both the anterior and posterior columns.
  - This is usually a 10-hole reconstruction plate.
  - It should have a slight undercontoured bend to accommodate the quadrilateral surface and should be twisted anteriorly through the anterior four holes to allow easier screw insertion into the superior ramus.
  - The posterior three holes should be overreamed with a 3.5-mm drill to allow increased angulation of the screw in the plate.
  - If long posterior column screws are planned, make sure to evaluate the location of the plate relative to the posterior column screw trajectory, which usually courses adjacent to the second and third holes.
  - The obturator inlet is useful for checking the length of the posterior screws (Fig. 13-40).

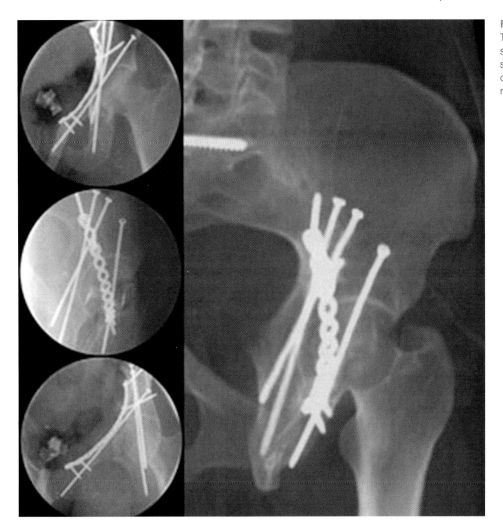

Figure 13-40 Intrapelvic plate. This 10-hole reconstruction plate spans the posterior column and the superior ramus. Note the trajectory of the posterior column screws relative to the plate.

TIP

Details for Intrapelvic Plate Contouring and Application

Reza Firoozabadi
Milton L. "Chip" Routt Jr

Pathoanatomy

The posterior column component (PCC) of an associated both-column acetabular (ABCA) fracture has a variety of presentations. Most consist of a large portion of the quadrilateral surface and are medially displaced, and the sagittal fracture plane usually exits the greater sciatic notch (GSN) (Fig. 13-41).

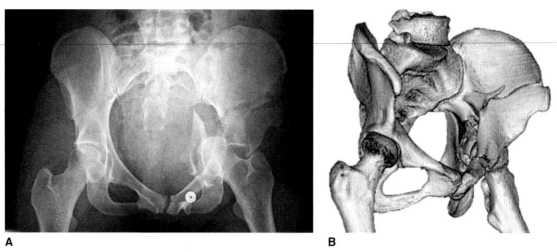

A   **B**

Figure 13-41 ▌**A, B:** The plain pelvic radiograph reveals the medially displaced PCC of this ABCA fracture. The intact stable iliac fragment adjacent to the GSN and the PCC are both noted after closed reduction on the 3D iliac oblique reconstructed image.

- Open reduction and internal fixation using the ilioinguinal middle (vascular) surgical exposure allow access to the PCC sagittal fracture plane for removing debris and clot and for certain clamp applications.
- The intrapelvic surgical interval allows the surgeon direct visualization of the fracture at the GSN and the ability to apply a buttressing plate spanning from the intact ilium to the pubis and beyond.
- If the intrapelvic plate is poorly contoured or mistakenly located, it can harm the surrounding neurovascular structures and fail to stabilize the fracture.

Solution

Careful preoperative planning allows the surgeon to understand the most effective plate locations and fixation techniques. Proper contouring, sculpting, location, and application of an intrapelvic plate improve the safety, function, and durability of the fixation construct.

Technique

- For most adult patients, a straight 10- to 12-hole 3.5-mm pelvic reconstruction plate will completely span from the stable iliac fragment cranial and proximal to the GSN to the parasymphyseal pubis.
  - To function as desired, the plate must be in direct contact with the upper quadrilateral surface and posterior pubic ramus cortical surfaces. The plate should be "overcontoured" prior to insertion so that compression occurs as it is applied to the bone (Fig. 13-42).

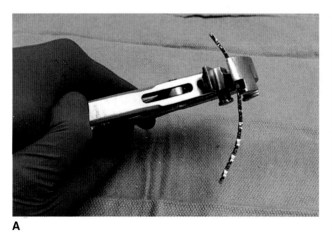
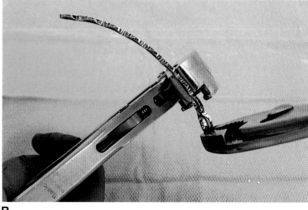

A   **B**

Figure 13-42 ▌**A:** Overcontouring of the plate improves the cortical contract and therefore the supporting function of the implant when applied properly. **B:** Twisting the plate medially improves the cortical fit and simplifies screw insertions in the parasymphyseal region.

- It is easiest if the surgeon sights the anticipated plate location along the PCC and pubic ramus after reduction. The initial screw hole at the intact stable ilium is best drilled independently prior to inserting the plate (Fig. 13-43).

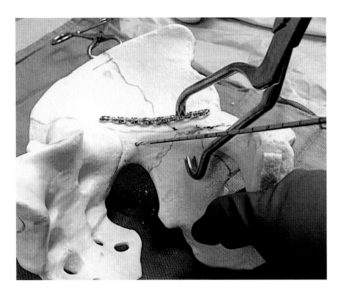

Figure 13-43 I With the anterior column fracture fragment already reduced and stabilized, the PCC has been reduced and clamped to both the anterior column fracture fragment and the stable ilium. The surgeon has planned the ideal plate location along the quadrilateral surface and posterior pubic ramus cortical surfaces. The initial drill hole is located and its depth assessed without the plate in the wound.

- The overcontoured plate is then introduced into the wound and attached to the stable ilium with an appropriate length screw. As the screw is tightened, the plate location is adjusted along the PCC and the pubic ramus cortical surfaces (Fig. 13-44).

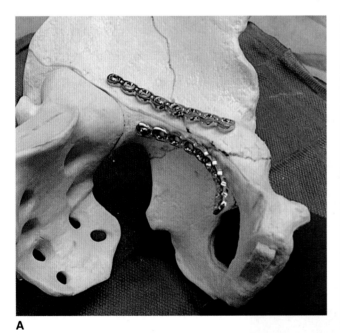

A

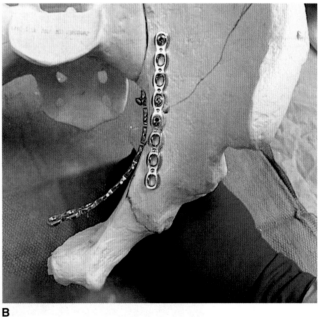

B

Figure 13-44 I A: The pelvis is viewed obliquely as the surgeon would see the intrapelvic plate application. As the screw is tightened, the flexion-extension of the plate is fine-tuned. B: The inlet view demonstrates the plate overcontouring. The initial screw is prominent due to its oblique direction through the plate hole. That hole can be obliquely sculpted with a 3.5-mm drill prior to insertion if desired.

- The overcontoured plate is clamped to the parasymphyseal fragment so that it is firmly applied to the cortical surfaces (Fig. 13-45).

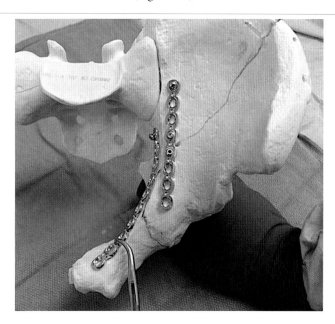

Figure 13-45 ▌ The plate has an intimate fit as the tenaculum clamp positions it onto the bone. The clamp is removed once the parasymphyseal screws are inserted.

- The PCC can be further stabilized using lag screws inserted from the pelvic brim into the PCC (Fig. 13-46).

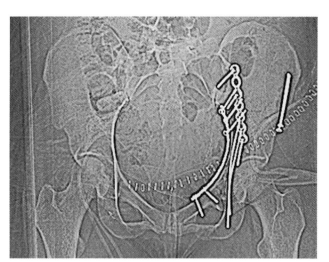

Figure 13-46 ▌ The postoperative image shows the final construct. "Overcontouring" the intrapelvic plate, drilling the initial hole independently at the stable ilium, and obliquely sculpting the initial plate hole are all performed prior to inserting the plate. Adjusting the plate location to fit the cortical surfaces improves the insertion safety, function, and durability of the implant. Lag screws further stabilize the PCC. These are located posterior to the hip and are inserted via the lateral surgical interval directed from the pelvic brim to the ischium.

The Independent Dome Fragment

- Frequently, the acetabular dome is displaced as a separate fragment (Fig. 13-47).

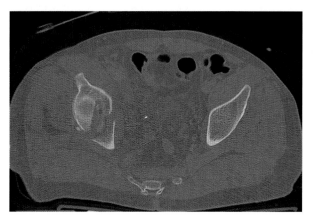

Figure 13-47 ▌ Dome fragment. This elementary posterior column fracture has comminution in the area of the acetabular dome. This fragment must be reduced anatomically or it will prevent reduction of the posterior column. These osteochondral fragments should be supported with bone graft if there is an adjacent cancellous impaction present.

- This fragment is commonly seen in the posterior wall, posterior column, transverse plus posterior wall, and T-shaped fractures.
- It is important to accurately reduce this fragment, not only because of its location within the weight-bearing surface of the acetabulum but also because malreduction of this fragment frequently prevents accurate reassembly of the remainder of the joint.
  - In effect, the malreduced dome fragment prevents an accurate reduction of the column or wall pieces.
- When displacement of this fragment occurs, it often occurs through impacted or compacted cancellous bone, and when the articular surface is realigned, a cancellous void remains.
  - The void should be assessed, and it should be filled with some form of structural bone graft if it renders the independent fragment unstable.

Reference

1. Rath EMS, Russell GV, Washington WJ, et al. Gluteus minimus necrotic muscle debridement diminishes heterotopic ossification after acetabular fracture fixation. *Injury.* 2002;33:751–756.

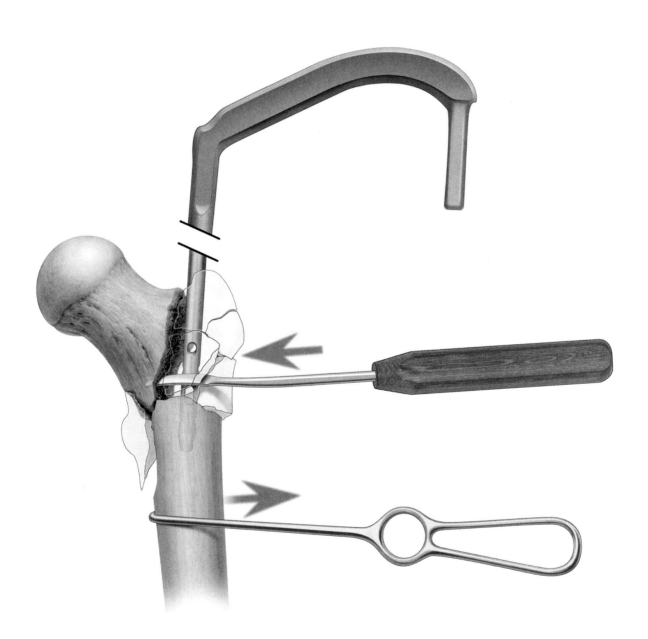

Chapter 14
Femoral Head Fractures

MILTON LEE (CHIP) ROUTT JR
RAYMOND D. WRIGHT JR

Sterile Instruments/Equipment

- Deep retractors
- Large nonabsorbable suture for rectus femoris and capsular tagging
- Free needles for postfixation rectus femoris and capsular repair
- Dental picks
- Large and small pointed bone reduction clamps ("Weber clamps")
- Implants:
  - 2.0- or 2.4-mm screws
- K-wires and wire driver/drill

Patient Positioning

- Supine on a radiolucent table.
- A padded bump, 3 inches thick and 12 inches wide, is placed in the midline of the patient, from the midlumbar spine caudal to the perineum.
- The entire ipsilateral lower extremity is circumferentially prepped and draped to allow manipulation of the operative limb.
- The C-arm is placed on the contralateral side of the operative extremity.

Surgical Approach

- The caudal limb of the Smith Petersen approach allows optimal exposure. Alternatively, the modification of the Smith Petersen approach as described by Hueter can be used.
- The skin incision is from the palpable anterior superior iliac spine, distally approximately 15 to 20 cm, in line with the lateral border of the patella (Fig. 14-1).

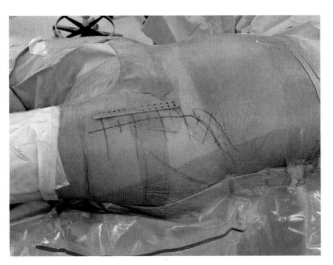

Figure 14-1 ▌ Skin incision for a femoral head fracture from the ASIS, in line with the lateral patellar border.

- Use blunt dissection to avoid injury to the lateral femoral cutaneous nerve.
- After developing the superficial muscular interval between the sartorius and the tensor fascia lata, a tenotomy of the common tendon of the rectus femoris is performed (Figs. 14-2 and 14-3).

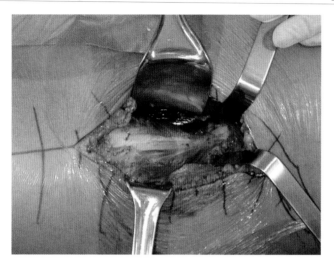

Figure 14-2 | Deep to the tensor fascia lata/sartorius interval, the origin of the rectus femoris is exposed.

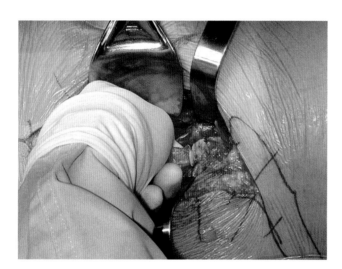

Figure 14-3 | The rectus femoris origin is incised just distal to the anterior inferior iliac spine.

- Sutures are placed in the distal portion for caudal retraction of the tendon and later tendon repair (Fig. 14-4).

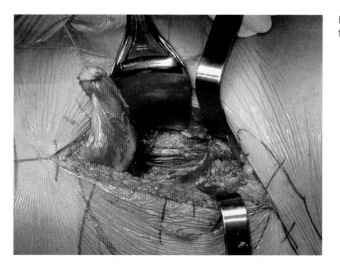

Figure 14-4 | The rectus femoris tendon is tagged and retracted distally.

- Create a short proximal stump in order to keep it out of the surgical field.
- Debride the iliocapsularis muscle.
  - This is a lateral outcropping of the iliopsoas muscle that overlies the hip joint capsule.
  - It is of variable size and may be a nidus for the postoperative ectopic bone formation.
- Retract the iliopsoas medially.
- Create a T-shaped capsulotomy.
  - Transverse limb should be cranial and lateral (e.g., parallel) to the labrum to avoid injuring the capsular perforating blood vessels (Figs. 14-5 and 14-6).

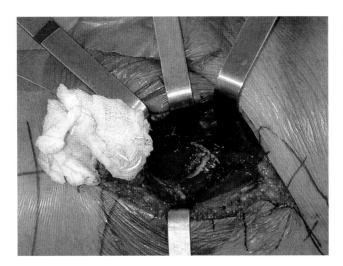

Figure 14-5 | Retraction of the iliopsoas exposes the anterior hip capsule, and an oblique T-shaped capsulotomy is marked.

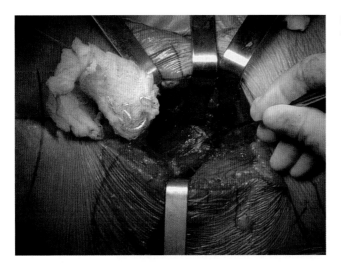

Figure 14-6 | The capsulotomy is completed.

- Avoid incising the labrum with the transverse limb of the capsulotomy.
  - Making an accurate capsulotomy is critical to avoid damaging both the blood supply and labrum. To ensure an accurate capsulotomy, place a K-wire in the femoral head and another into the intertrochanteric ridge.

- Confirm the wire locations on fluoroscopy. The line between the two wires estimates the longitudinal limb of the capsulotomy and the proximal wire helps estimate the relative position of the vertical limb (Fig. 14-7).

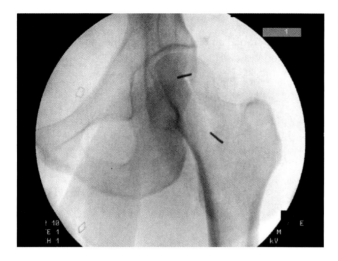

Figure 14-7 ▌ K-wires are placed in the planned trajectory for the longitudinal limb of the capsulotomy and confirmed on fluoroscopy to ensure accurate capsulotomy location. The proximal wire can be used to confirm location of the proximal T limbs as well.

- The femoral head is then gently dislocated anteriorly for complete visualization (Fig. 14-8).
  - Axial traction, hip extension, adduction, and external rotation.
  - Bone hook may be used very cautiously on the caudal aspect of the femoral neck to assist dislocation.
  - Place leg in figure of 4 position.

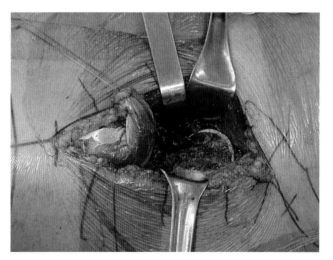

Figure 14-8 ▌ Anterior dislocation of the femoral head allows complete exposure of the fracture surfaces.

Reduction and Fixation Techniques

- Reduction of the femoral head fragment must be performed using the chondral fracture margins to assess an anatomical fracture reduction.
- The free femoral head fragment(s) may be predrilled on the sterile back table prior to dislocation of the hip and fracture reduction (Fig. 14-9).

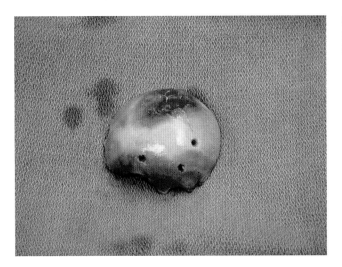

Figure 14-9 | The fracture fragment is prepared on the back table, with strategically placed 2.0-mm glide holes.

- Reduction is maintained provisionally with K-wires (Fig. 14-10).

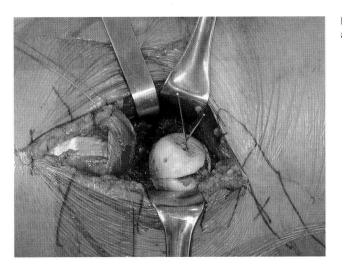

Figure 14-10 | The fracture is reduced anatomically and stabilized provisionally.

- Two or three 2.0- or 2.4-mm countersunk lag screws are used for fixation for the major fragment(s).
- Examine the acetabulum critically for osseous and chondral debris.
- Reduce the hip expeditiously and check the range of motion and stability under fluoroscopy, especially when an ipsilateral posterior wall acetabular fracture is present (Fig. 14-11).

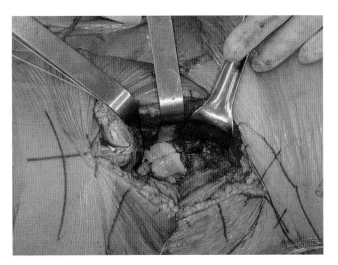

Figure 14-11 | Following screw fixation, the femoral head is reduced into the acetabulum.

- Close the capsule completely (Fig. 14-12).
- Repair the rectus femoris tendon using the previously placed suture as a core suture.
    - Augment the repair with size 0 resorbable sutures in the paratenon (Figs. 14-13 and 14-14).

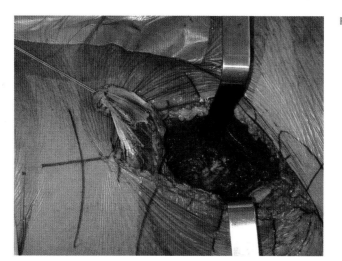

Figure 14-12 I The capsulotomy is repaired.

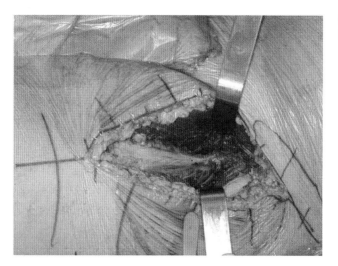

Figure 14-13 I The rectus tendon is then repaired.

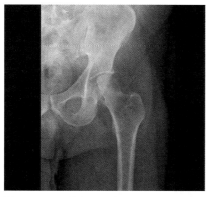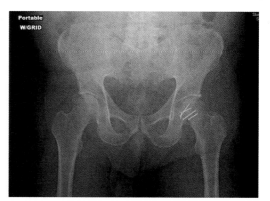

Figure 14-14 I Injury and postoperative radiographs demonstrating fixation of a comminuted femoral head fracture with multiple buried 2.0- and 2.4-mm screws.

Chapter 15
Femoral Neck Fractures

MARK R. ADAMS

JASON M. EVANS

REZA FIROOZABADI

MICHAEL F. GITHENS

ANNA N. MILLER

MICHAEL S. SIRKIN

BRANDON J. YUAN

Sterile Instruments/Equipment

- 2.5- or 4.0-mm Schanz pins for use as joysticks in the femoral head/neck fragment
- Large pointed reduction forceps
  - Modified (straightened) tines for engagement in drill holes
- Small pointed reduction forceps
  - Modified (straightened) tines for engagement in drill holes
- Small fragment drill to assess for the vascularity following reduction
- 5.0-mm Schanz pins for rotational control of distal (shaft) fragment
- 5/64 inch (2.0-mm) K-wire for use as a distal traction pin with a tensioned traction bow
- Implants
  - Sliding hip screw and side plate device or similar fixed angle implant for unstable fracture patterns (e.g., Garden III/IV)
  - 6.5-, 7.0-, or 7.3-mm fully threaded and partially threaded screws for stable patterns (e.g., Garden I/II) and select subcapital fractures.
  - Reconstruction and/or minifragment plates for provisional stabilization of anteromedial femoral neck in comminuted fractures.
  - Bone graft for comminution.

Positioning

- Supine on radiolucent table with C-arm from opposite side of the table.
- A small rolled towel bump under the injured hip allows for lateral imaging of hip.
  - A bump may not be necessary, as long as fluoroscopic visualization on a cross-table lateral is possible.
- Elevate the operative lower extremity on the leg ramp.
  - This relaxes the hip flexors and minimizes deforming forces.
  - To increase the hip flexion and offset muscular forces, a radiolucent tibial nailing triangle may be placed under the knee.
- Isolate the perineum from the operative site with an exclusionary drape.
- Sterilely prepare and drape the entire leg circumferentially for maximum control during reduction.
- Sterile skeletal traction using table attachment or dedicated fracture table may facilitate reduction.

343

Reduction and Fixation Techniques

- Consider obtaining a CT scan to understand location and degree of comminution.
  - If there is circumferential comminution, the benefit of an open reduction may be obviated. In this situation, consider planning for closed or percutaneous methods of reduction.
- Closed reduction attempt by Ledbetter or other femoral neck fracture reduction maneuver.
  - Hip flexion, external rotation, and abduction followed by gentle traction with hip in flexion.
  - Subsequent hip extension and internal rotation may result in an anatomic-appearing reduction on fluoroscopy.
  - However, this frequently underestimates the amount of residual displacement that is found upon direct visualization following capsulotomy.
- Closed reduction reserved for subcapital fractures primarily, especially in the geriatric population, or those with circumferential comminution where an open reduction will be of limited value.
- Percutaneous methods can be used to fine-tune a closed reduction.
  - Gentle distal femoral skeletal traction can maintain length and alignment (Fig. 15-1).

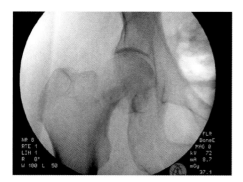
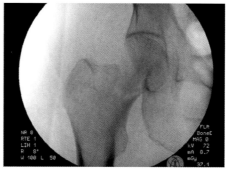

Figure 15-1 Closed manipulative reduction and gentle skeletal traction may be effective in restoring length and alignment.

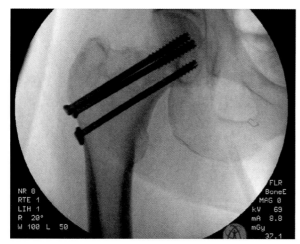

- A shoulder hook placed over the calcar can be used to effect coronal and sagittal plane alignment (Fig. 15-2).

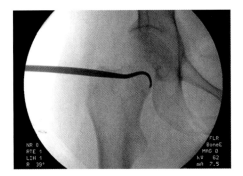
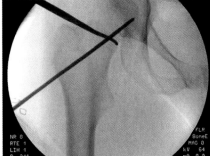

Figure 15-2 | Percutaneous application of a shoulder hook is used to improve a closed reduction before implant placement.

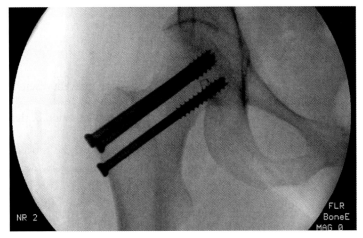

- A spiked pusher percutaneously applied directly anteriorly can be very effective in correcting an apex anterior deformity and restore normal version (Fig. 15-3).

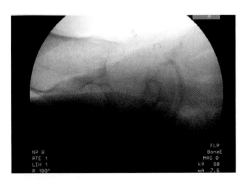
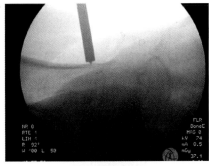

Figure 15-3 | Percutaneous reduction of an apex anterior (extension) deformity using an anterior spiked pusher restores normal femoral anteversion.

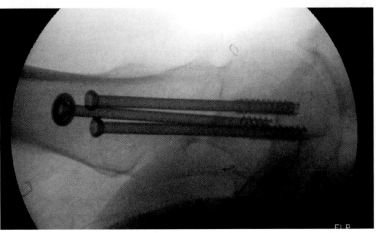

- If closed reduction is deemed acceptable (preferably anatomical on orthogonal and oblique views), consider percutaneous fixation with a decompressive capsulotomy to release the hematoma and to decrease intracapsular pressure, potentially decreasing the avascular necrosis risk.

- An anterior capsulotomy can be performed utilizing a small laterally based skin incision, with a scalpel blade advanced proximally along the anterior femoral neck.
- C-arm localization is helpful (Fig. 15-4).

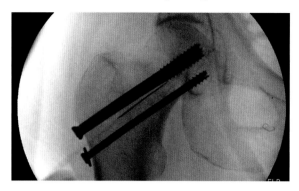

Figure 15-4 ▮ Fluoroscopic image of a percutaneous capsulotomy being performed with a disposable scalpel.

- Consider using a disposable scalpel, with the blade integrated into the handle, to prevent disengagement of blade from knife handle, in the stout soft tissues.
- Either an anterolateral or an anterior approach can be useful for visualization and reduction of the femoral neck fracture.
    - If a Watson-Jones (anterolateral) approach is used, reduction and implant placement can proceed through the same incision.
        - However, visualization of the neck fracture and soft tissue retraction is more difficult with a Watson-Jones than with an anterior approach.
- A modified Smith-Petersen (Hueter) approach allows excellent visualization of the anterior femoral neck for reduction and clamp placement (Fig. 15-5).

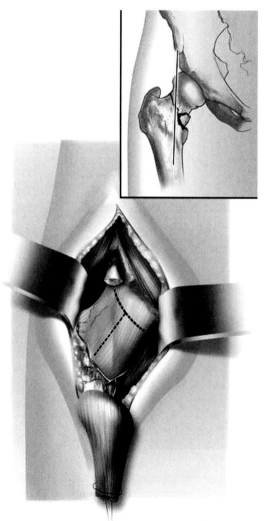

Figure 15-5 ▮ These illustrations of a right hip anterior exposure demonstrate the retraction of the sartorius and the iliopsoas muscles medially and the lateral retraction of the tensor fascia lata muscle. The rectus femoris tenotomy is shown, and the planned oblique T-shaped capsulotomy is indicated by the *dotted lines*. (Adapted from Molnar RB, Routt ML. Open reduction of intracapsular hip fractures using a modified Smith-Petersen surgical exposure. *J Orthop Trauma*. 2007;21(7):490–494, with permission.)

- A second, small lateral approach is necessary for implant placement if an anterior approach is used.
- Additional exposure can be achieved by
  - Detaching the rectus femoris tendon origin
  - Flexion of the hip by placing a triangle under the leg to relax the rectus, psoas, and sartorius muscles (Fig. 15-6).

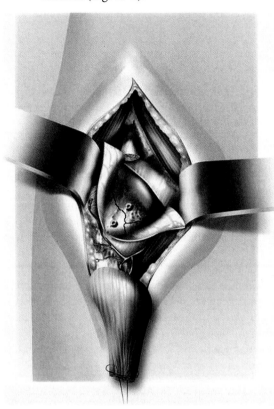

Figure 15-6 I The anterior hip capsulotomy has been made, preserving the local vascular anatomy and the anterior labrum. The manipulative reduction screws are shown. (Adapted from Molnar RB, Routt ML. Open reduction of intracapsular hip fractures using a modified Smith-Petersen surgical exposure. *J Orthop Trauma.* 2007;21(7):490–494, with permission.)

- Sharp elevation of iliocapsularis may minimize development of heterotopic ossification rather than blunt removal with an elevator.
- Make a T-shaped capsulotomy, beginning initially distally on the femoral neck and incising proximally to the acetabular labrum to create the vertical limb.
  - The transverse (oblique) limb of the capsulotomy can be made either parallel to the intertrochanteric line (along the base of the femoral neck) or parallel to the labrum (while avoiding labral injury).
  - Care must be taken to avoid extension of the superior limb of a basilar capsulotomy as the main trunk of the blood supply is at risk in this location.
  - The location of the fracture and the associated comminution typically determines the type and location of the capsular extensions.
  - In significantly displaced patters, application of traction prior to the capsular incision will aid in placement of an accurate capsulotomy (Fig. 15-7).
  - Additionally, K-wires can be placed in the proximal and distal segments and checked under fluoroscopy to confirm accurate capsular incisions. The line between the two wires estimates the longitudinal limb of the capsulotomy, and wire location helps estimate the relative position of the vertical limb (Fig. 15-7).

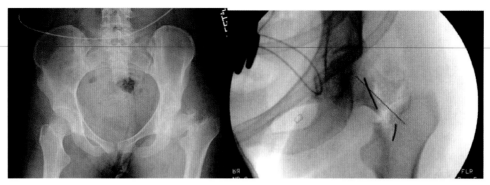

Figure 15-7 I An AP pelvis radiograph demonstrates a displaced femoral neck fracture. Intraoperative fluoroscopy shows gross fragment realignment with gentle traction prior to making the capsulotomy. Additionally, K-wires placed in the anticipated capsulotomy trajectory indicate that the planned capsulotomy is suboptimal. Using the location of the wires as a guide, a more accurate capsulotomy is made along the femoral neck.

- Place heavy nonabsorbable sutures in each corner of the capsule to allow for retraction and to facilitate reapproximation for repair later.
- Avoid placing Hohmann retractors around the superior (and inferior) portion(s) of the femoral neck after the capsulotomy has been made, as their tips lever against the posterior femoral neck.
  - This may interfere with the primary blood supply to the femoral head, which enters the capsule posterosuperiorly.
  - Instead use large Sofield- or Hibbs-type retractors for exposure.
- A small (2.0- or 2.5-mm) drill hole can be made at the femoral head/neck junction for use as a docking site for clamp application and to assess for femoral head vascularity.
- A 2.5- or 4.0-mm Schanz pin placed in the femoral head as a joystick is also a helpful reduction aid for directly manipulating the proximal fragment, which is frequently rotationally displaced.
- Large pointed reduction forceps can be modified (one tine straightened) for more effective reduction control (Fig. 15-8).

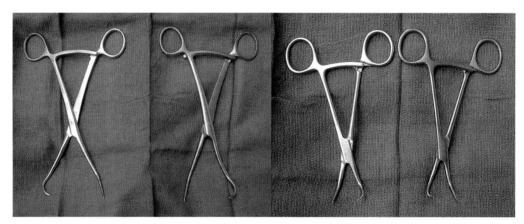

Figure 15-8 I "Modified" large Weber (left) and small Weber (right) clamps, with one tine straightened, are useful for femoral neck clamp reductions using unicortical drill holes through an anterior approach.

- The most consistent cortical reduction assessment is both anteriorly and inferiorly (both should be visualized), with comminution most frequently found posteriorly.
  - Even when anterior and inferior neck fracture margins appear anatomic, an extension deformity may exist due to posterior comminution resulting in fracture extension (retroversion).
    - This is best assessed with a cross-table lateral radiograph with the x-ray beam orthogonal to the long axis of the femoral neck, and not the long axis of the femoral shaft.
- An extension deformity may be avoided by placement of an anterior bone clamp.
  - However, the bone available for clamp application is limited, and when clamps are placed anteriorly, the result may be an apex posterior angular malreduction (i.e., neck anteversion and flexion), particularly in patients with anterior or inferior comminution.
  - To avoid this, place the tines of the clamp as deeply into the femoral head or medial femoral neck as possible, so the tines are near the neutral axis/center of rotation.
  - Alternatively, a Farabeuf clamp can be applied to screws strategically placed into the head and neck.

- The longer lever arm of the screws may afford a more even distribution of the compression, especially if the screws are inserted slightly off an orthogonal axis.
  - The disadvantage is that the clamp is large and will obstruct further access to the reduction through the relatively surgical small window.
- A curved tine of a large Weber clamp can be placed laterally on the greater trochanter, cranial to the proposed insertion site of the definitive fixation construct, especially in Pauwels' type III fracture patterns.
- Particular emphasis should be placed on obtaining an anatomic reduction of the inferior/medial spike in basicervical or vertical femoral neck fractures to improve the overall stability of the construct and diminish the likelihood of late translation/displacement.
- Multiple large-diameter (2.0/2.4-mm) K-wires are placed to provisionally hold the reduction. These should be placed strategically as to not impede final implant application.
- If comminution exists anterior and inferiorly, a 2.4-mm straight plate or 2.7-mm reconstruction plate can be contoured and placed anteroinferiorly for additional stability and maintenance of neck length prior to definitive fixation of the femoral neck (Figs. 15-9 and 15-10).

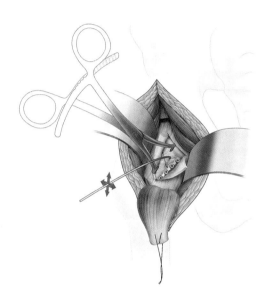

Figure 15-9 Effective femoral neck fracture reduction maneuvers through an anterior approach include manipulative Steinmann pin joysticks, clamp placement through unicortical drill holes, and provisional reconstruction plates.

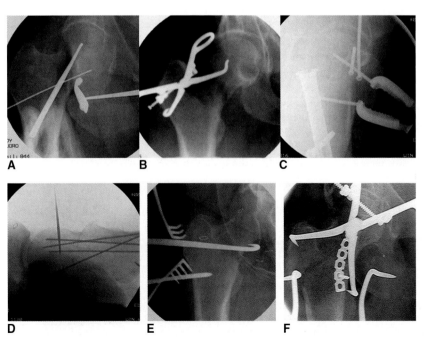

Figure 15-10 Reduction aids. **A:** Shoulder hook in femoral head and an intracapsular small Hohmann retractor at inferior femoral neck spike. **B:** Large modified large pointed bone reduction (i.e., Weber) clamp from femoral head to greater trochanter. **C:** Farabeuf clamp with 3.5-mm screws. **D:** 2.5-mm Schanz pin as anterior joystick in femoral head/neck; provisional K-wires stabilizing the neck fracture. **E:** Shoulder hook around the inferior neck spike. **F:** Provisional (or definitive) anterior/inferior 2.4- or 2.7-mm reconstruction plate and large pointed bone reduction clamp from inferior neck to greater trochanter.

Interior Buttress Plate for Comminution of the Caudal Femoral Neck

Mark R. Adams
Michael S. Sirkin

Pathoanatomy

- Vertical femoral neck fractures (Fig. 15-11) typically fail in tension at the cranial neck and in compression at the caudal neck.
- The compression side often has associated comminution (Fig. 15-12).

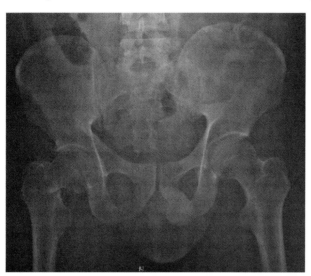

Figure 15-11 | AP pelvis radiograph demonstrating a displaced right femoral neck fracture.

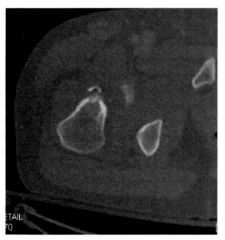
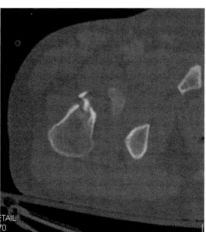
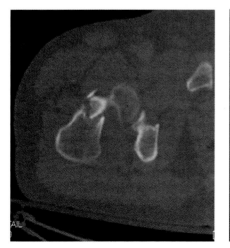
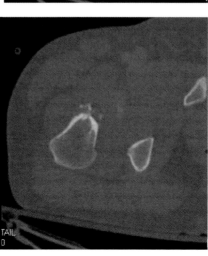

Figure 15-12 | Axial CT images though the inferior femoral neck demonstrating comminution of the caudal neck.

Solution

- A buttress plate placed caudally on the compression side can add mechanical stability, helping to resist varus deformity and shortening (Fig. 15-13).

Technique

- A Smith-Petersen approach is necessary to gain access to the caudal/medial femoral neck.
- An open reduction of the fracture is performed.
- This will permit sufficient stability to access the inferomedial femoral neck with hip flexion and external rotation.
- The operating surgeon may benefit from standing on the contralateral side for plate fixation.
- If the comminution is extensive and precludes direct cortical contact with an anatomic reduction, a tricortical graft can be fashioned to fill the defect.
- A varus malreduction should not be accepted; slight valgus may be preferable to a perfectly anatomic reduction, particularly if the patient is elderly, if bone quality is poor, or if superior comminution exists.

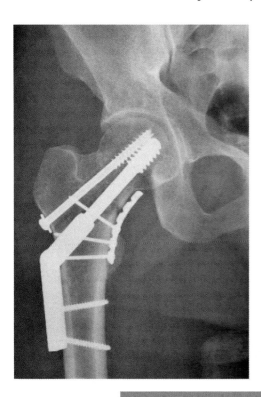
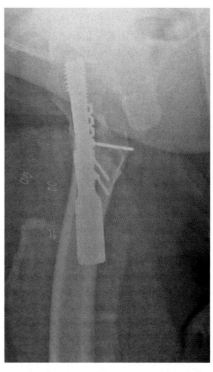

Figure 15-13 ▌AP and lateral hip radiographs demonstrating a femoral neck status post open reduction and internal fixation with a partially threaded 7.3 cannulated screw, a sliding hip screw, and a nonheat annealed 2.7 reconstruction plate at the caudal neck. Note that the plate acts solely to buttress the inferior neck and the absence of screws in this region. This will allow unimpeded sliding of the hip screws with resulting impaction/compression of the femoral neck fracture.

Fixation Constructs

Unstable Patterns (Displaced Fractures and Any High Pauwels' Angle Fracture) and Basicervical Patterns

- A fixed angle sliding hip screw device is the optimal implant for unstable fracture patterns.
- Manufacturers' designs differ in regard to the type of lagging device. Newer designs include a blade rather than screw, which offers several potential advantages including less rotational forces exerted on the proximal segment with terminal insertion as compared to a screw.
- Use of the blade rather than a screw in comminuted and particularly unstable patterns may prevent loss of reduction with device insertion.
- The guidewire for the sliding hip screw device is placed in perfect center-center position in the femoral head to achieve a tip-apex distance <25 mm.
  - When placing this guidewire, it is critical that the guide is perfectly flush with the lateral femoral cortex. If it is not, a deformity will be introduced when the side plate is fixed to the lateral cortex.
  - If a valgus deformity occurs upon insertion of the side plate, switching to a lower angle implant will help alleviate this. If a varus deformity occurs, insertion of a higher-angle side plate is advised.

- An antirotation screw is placed cranial to the sliding hip screw for rotational control.
  - This screw can be placed before or after the lagging device is placed. If placed before, definitive implant position must be considered.
  - This screw should be parallel to the sliding hip screw to allow controlled fracture collapse.
  - The preferred implant is a cannulated partially threaded 6.5- or 7.0-mm screw +/− a washer.
- If the greater trochanter is also fractured, a trochanteric stabilizing plate must be added to the construct to prevent uncontrolled collapse.

Stable Subcapital and Transcervical Patterns (Valgus Impacted, Nondisplaced Fractures with a Low Pauwels' Angle)

- Most common fixation constructs consist of 6.5- to 7.3-mm cannulated screws (three, sometimes four) in various configurations (Fig. 15-14).
- Some manufacturers' screws have larger-diameter screw cannulations, allowing for stiffer guidewires, which are easier to control.
  - This often facilitates accurate screw placement as the trajectories of these stiffer guidewires are better controlled than those of smaller and more flexible guidewires.
- The starting point for screws should be above the level of the lesser trochanter to minimize the possibility of iatrogenic subtrochanteric fracture due to a stress riser effect.
  - This region typically correlates with the metaphyseal flare, just distal to the vastus lateralis ridge.
  - If a triangular configuration is used, a single screw should form the inferior apex of the triangle to minimize the risk of secondary subtrochanteric fracture.
- Screws should be placed to optimize compression across the fracture site.
- Screw spread should be maximized, placed as peripherally as possible within the femoral neck, to allow for stable fixation.
  - Placement of the inferior screw within 3 mm of the medial cortical bone of the femoral neck may help to minimize inferior displacement of the femoral head.
  - Placement of a screw within 3 mm of the posterior cortex of the femoral neck may help to minimize posterior translation and retroversion of the femoral head.
  - For subcapital and transcervical fractures, the inferior screw should be supported both at the lateral cortex and at the most medial aspect of the portion of the femoral neck that is attached to the shaft component.
    - This position effectively supports the screw along a large portion of its overall length and reduces cantilever "bending" failure of the construct.
    - More cephalad screws do not achieve this mechanical benefit.

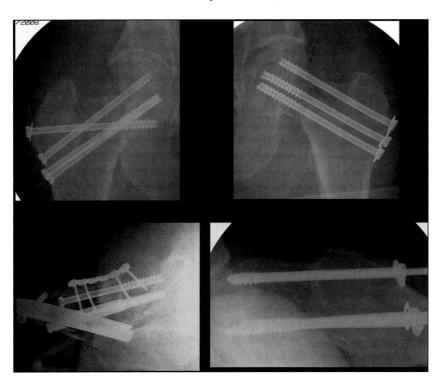

Figure 15-14 I Typical implant constructs for femoral neck fractures. Attention should be paid to maximizing the spread of the screws within the femoral neck.

- Consideration should be given to avoidance of screw placement in the posterosuperior quadrant of the neck and head, as this is the primary area of vascular perfusion into the femoral head.
  - The posterior screw can be placed at the midcranial aspect or centrally (when viewed sagittally), or placed at the most cranial portion of the neck (Fig. 15-15).

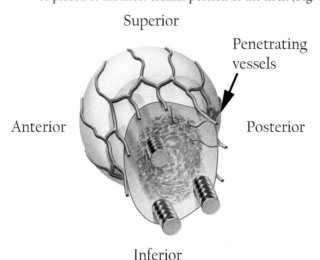

Superior

Penetrating vessels

Anterior

Posterior

Inferior

Figure 15-15 ▌ Avoidance of screw placement in the posterosuperior quadrant (*upper right* in figure) minimizes risk to the perforating vascular supply to the femoral head.

- When placing screws to obtain compression, insert the anterior/superior screw first, as it is least likely to create a deformity by compressing across a comminuted fracture zone.

TIP

Precise Percutaneous Placement of Cannulated Screws for Femoral Neck Fractures

Brandon J. Yuan
Reza Firoozabadi
Anna N. Miller

Pathoanatomy

The guidewires for the 7.0 or 7.3 cannulated screws create a significant hole that can lead to a stress riser and an increased risk of lateral cortex fracture if multiple holes are drilled. Additionally, the wires are more difficult to redirect than drill bits if their trajectory needs to be changed.

Solution

Instead of using the larger-diameter guide pins for cannulated screws, the use of small K-wires will increase the precision of screw placement and optimize screw trajectories.

Technique

- The patient is positioned supine on a flat radiolucent table.
  - The ipsilateral flank and hemipelvis is supported with a folded blanket. This elevates the injured proximal femur to allow for lateral fluoroscopic imaging without interference from the contralateral femur or hemipelvis (Fig. 15-16).

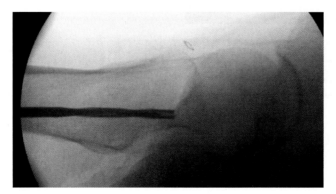

Figure 15-16 ▌ Lateral fluoroscopic image obtained during percutaneous screw fixation of the femoral neck in the supine position. Note the visualization of the posterior femoral neck.

- The ipsilateral lower extremity is elevated on a foam ramp or stack of folded blankets to allow for approximately 20 degrees of hip flexion.
- The C-arm is positioned on the contralateral side of the patient and oriented obliquely at a 55-degree angle to the long axis of the body to allow for the lateral fluoroscopic image to be perpendicular to the axis of the femoral neck (Fig. 15-17). The injured lower extremity including the hip is then prepped and draped into the surgical field.

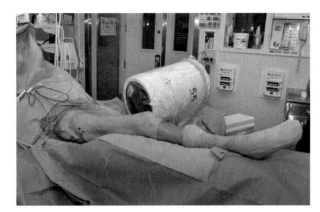

Figure 15-17 I Supine position with C-arm positioned for lateral fluoroscopic image.

- Three partially threaded screws are planned to be placed across the femoral neck fracture in either a triangular configuration or a modified inverted triangular configuration.
  - In the modified inverted triangle, the posterosuperior screw is positioned in a slightly more inferior position to avoid perforation of the femoral neck in this location given the immediate proximity of the lateral retinacular vessels (Fig. 15-18). Alternatively, a triangular configuration can be utilized. Theoretically, the triangle configuration can result in higher subtrochanteric femur fracture rates if multiple cortical perforations are performed.

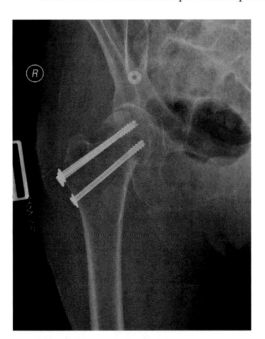

Figure 15-18 I Valgus impacted femoral neck fracture treated with percutaneous screw fixation. Note the spread of the screws on the lateral cortex and the inverted triangle configuration.

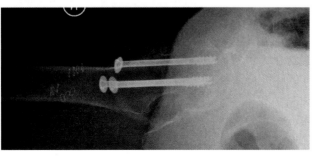

- After a satisfactory reduction is obtained through either an open or a closed method, the appropriate starting point for the inferior screw is obtained.
  - This is first performed with a 0.062 inch K-wire, which allows for minimal trauma to the overlying soft tissues as fine adjustments are made to obtain the appropriate starting point and trajectory vector on both the anteroposterior (AP) and lateral fluoroscopic images (Fig. 15-19).

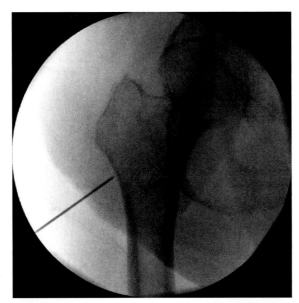

Figure 15-19 ‖ AP and lateral fluoroscopic view demonstrating the appropriate starting point obtained with the 0.062 inch wire.

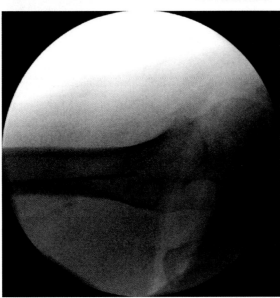

- The K-wire insertion track and lateral cortical pilot hole are significantly smaller than the traditional aperture created by a 2.8- or 3.2-mm guidewire. If the trajectory of the K-wire is not appropriate, an additional K-wire can be placed in the appropriate start site. However, the use of a larger guidewire places multiple larger holes in the proximal femur if the appropriate start site is not obtained initially. Once the appropriate start site and trajectory have been obtained, the K-wire is then advanced into the lateral cortex of the femur for no more than 3 to 5 mm.

● Using an 11-blade, the skin and iliotibial band are incised longitudinally to allow for subsequent passage of the cannulated drill, screw, and washer. A cannulated 3.2- or 4.5-mm drill is then passed over the top of 0.062 inch K-wire down to the lateral cortex of the femur. The cannulated drill is then advanced on oscillate mode through the lateral cortex of the femur and over the end of the K-wire (Fig. 15-20).

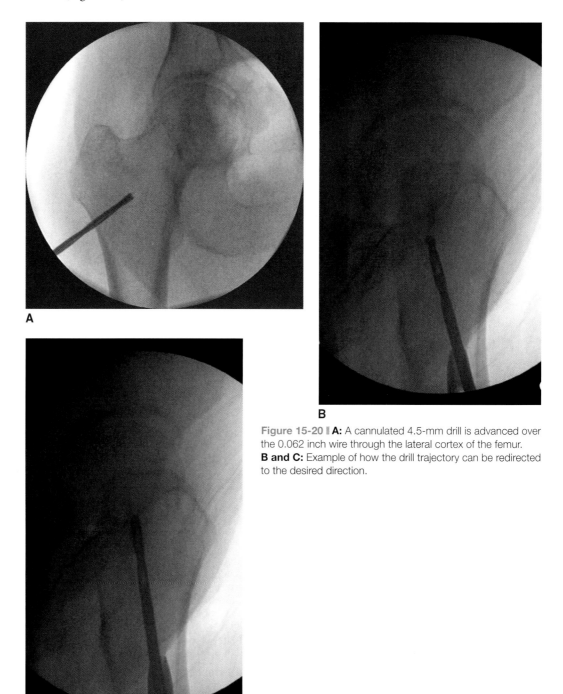

Figure 15-20 I A: A cannulated 4.5-mm drill is advanced over the 0.062 inch wire through the lateral cortex of the femur. **B and C:** Example of how the drill trajectory can be redirected to the desired direction.

● Use of a 4.5-mm drill instead of the standard 2.8- or 3.2-mm guidewire has two major advantages. The 4.5-mm drill is stiffer than the 0.062 inch K-wire or the larger guidewires, and thus small adjustments to the vector of the drill may be made as it is advanced into and across the femoral neck, afforded by its increased rigidity. This allows for very precise placement of the subsequent guidewire and cannulated screw.

- Secondly, advancing the 4.5-mm drill on oscillate allows the surgeon to feel if the cortex of the femoral neck is encountered prior to drilling through it, thus reducing the risk of subsequent placement of an "in-out-in" screw. Care should be taken to not make excessive corrections with the cannulated drill, as a large aperture can be created in the lateral femoral cortex.
  - Larger corrections should be made in the most lateral aspect of the pathway.
- Once the 4.5-mm drill has been advanced into the femoral neck to the level of the fracture, the drill is exchanged for the appropriate-sized threaded guidewire (2.8 or 3.2 mm), which is then advanced into the femoral head (Fig. 15-21).

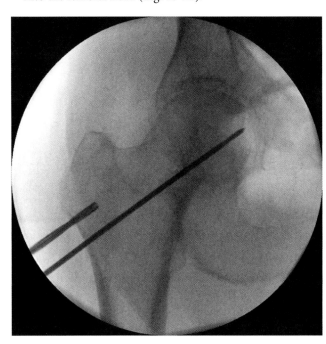

Figure 15-21 ‖ The 4.5-mm drill is exchanged for the appropriately sized guidewire for a large cannulated screw and advanced to the subchondral bone.

- The procedure is repeated for the posterosuperior and anterosuperior screw positions (Fig. 15-22).
- If cortical perforation of the femoral neck is suspected, the osseous pathway can be inspected with a 2.0-mm guidewire with a small bend in it. This is similar to the method of palpating the pathway for a spinal pedicle screw with a ball-tipped guidewire. Alternatively, the entire path of the screw can be predrilled with a 4.5-mm drill and the blunt end of the guidewire can be placed along the pathway to determine if the pathway has violated the cortex. This is especially important for the osseous pathway in the posterosuperior femoral neck.

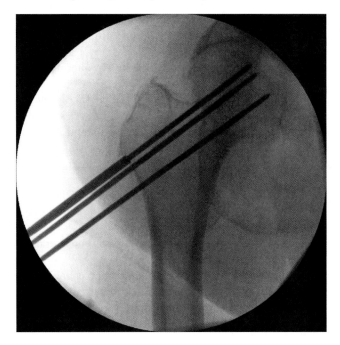

Figure 15-22 ‖ The process is repeated for the posterosuperior and anterosuperior screw positions.

- Each guidewire is measured, and the appropriate length screws are placed. For most incompletely reduced fractures, the initial screws are placed inferiorly and the anterosuperior screw is placed last (Fig. 15-23).

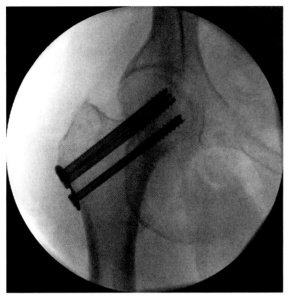
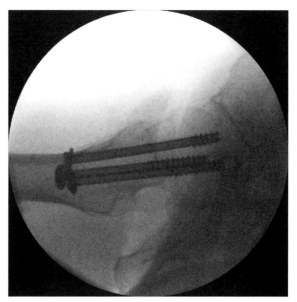

Figure 15-23 ▮ The anterosuperior screw is placed last to compress the anterior cortical surface, which typically fractures in tension and is noncomminuted.

- As the femoral neck typically displaces with apex anterior angulation, the anterior cortex fails in tension and is typically not comminuted. This allows for final anatomic compression through the anterosuperior screw if the remainder of the fracture has been stabilized first. The authors prefer to use partially threaded screws to ensure compression across the fracture. If severe comminution is present, fully threaded screws may be considered.
- Washers have been shown to increase compression and fracture stability and are used routinely in cases of compromised bone quality.

Intertrochanteric Osteotomy (Fig. 15-24)

- All patients with femoral neck fractures should be informed of the risks of nonunion, malunion, and avascular necrosis, in addition to standard surgical risks.
- In the event of a nonunion, a valgus intertrochanteric osteotomy is a reliable procedure to obtain healing.
- Any rotational or sagittal plane deformity can be corrected by altering the plane of the intertrochanteric osteotomy.
- Using preoperative templating, the appropriately sized wedge can be determined that will allow for conversion of the vertical fracture line/nonunion to achieve an orientation roughly parallel to the joint reaction forces; for optimal healing, this angle is ideally about 25 degrees from the horizontal.
- Blade entry point must be at least 15 mm above the osteotomy site to avoid communication of the blade entry site with the osteotomy during reduction and compression, thereby losing fixation strength.
- Guidewires are placed above the planned blade entry point across the base of the piriformis fossa.
- First, osteotomy cut is made parallel to the planned blade entry path, usually perpendicular to the femoral shaft, at the top level of the lesser trochanter.
    - Check flexion and extension as well as rotation (anteversion) on lateral fluoroscopic view.
    - Correct any rotation prior to second cut.
- Use K-wires to measure and determine the appropriate version change, if needed.
    - After chisel, seat the blade 8 to 10 mm proud to allow lateralization of shaft.
    - After the blade is seated, place unicortical screw distally.

- Use osteotomes to keep proximal plate 8 to 10 mm off of the femoral shaft distal to osteotomy. With the distalmost aspect of the plate abutting the bone, create a triangular space between the lateral cortex and the plate.
  - Osteotomy site should be in increased valgus relative to the final anticipated correction at this point.
  - Insert and tighten the most proximal screw in the distal fragment, removing the osteotomes.
  - This pulls the bone to the plate, hinging off of the distal unicortical screw, while correcting the tilt, and achieves strong compression across the osteotomy, by using the principle of bone length/plate length mismatch.

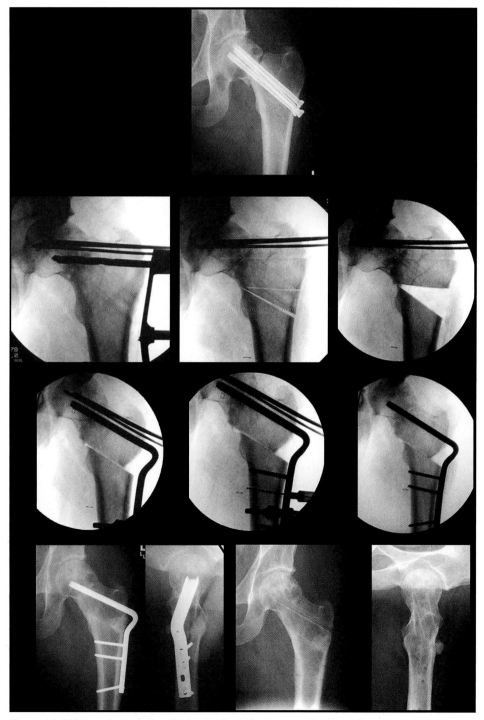

Figure 15-24 I Stepwise technique for intertrochanteric osteotomy for femoral neck nonunion.

Chapter 16
Intertrochanteric Femur Fractures

MICHAEL J. GARDNER
ZACHARY V. ROBERTS

Sterile Instruments/Equipment

- Radiolucent OR table with traction device or fracture table
- 5.0-mm Schanz pins for manipulative joysticks
- Large pointed bone reduction clamps (Weber clamps)
- Ball-spike pushers
- Shoulder hook/bone hook
- K-wires and wire driver/drill
- Reamers
- Implants: depending on the fracture pattern and consistent with the preoperative plan
  - Intramedullary nail (trochanteric cephalomedullary nail)
  - Screw-side plate device (dynamic hip screw or similar)
  - Blade plate (95-degree angle)

Patient Positioning

- Supine on a radiolucent table with attachment for sterile traction (see Femur Fracture Positioning) or supine on a fracture table.
- Positioning is largely a matter of the surgeon's preference, with each having advantages and disadvantages.
  - For some fractures and in some patients, the use of a fracture table offers predictable indirect reduction and intraoperative imaging and reduces the need for an assistant.
  - However, with unstable fracture patterns, the use of a fracture table tends to accentuate deformity in the sagittal plane (usually apex posterior angulation) and posterior translation of the distal fragment(s).
  - Some patients have contralateral hip arthrosis and contractures that prevent adequate abduction and flexion to allow quality lateral intraoperative imaging.
  - The use of a fracture table has also been implicated in a number of complications to include compartmental syndrome of the contralateral limb, pudendal nerve dysfunction, and perineal skin breakdown.
  - Finally, the use of a fracture table requires the presence of a skilled unscrubbed assistant to make intraoperative changes in limb position or traction.
  - Prepping the leg free on a flat radiolucent table allows the surgeon unencumbered access to limb position and eliminates complications caused by traction against a perineal post.
  - The use of a flat radiolucent table often avoids posterior displacement of the distal fracture fragment as is commonly seen with fracture tables, since the thigh is supported and can be elevated on rolled sterile towels (towel bump).
  - However, imaging the hip intraoperatively can be more challenging with intertrochanteric fractures than with other proximal femur fractures.

Imaging Tips

- When using the radiolucent flat top table, place a bolster under the ipsilateral sacrum and torso to roll the patient away from the surgeon about 10 to 15 degrees and flex the hip 10 to 15 degrees when the operative limb is placed on a leg ramp.
  - This allows for cross-table lateral hip imaging.
  - Avoid too large a hip/pelvic bolster so that the cross-table lateral of the hip does not demonstrate "relative" neck-shaft retroversion.
- To adequately image the hip, the C-arm must mirror these positioning modifications.
  - The position of the C-arm should be individualized to obtain a true AP image of the hip, with a small crescent of lesser trochanter visible.
    - Often, a straight vertical C-arm position with patient bumped up 10 to 15 degrees will offset the anteversion and will give a true AP of the hip (Fig. 16-1).
    - However, some C-arm rollback may better simulate an AP image.

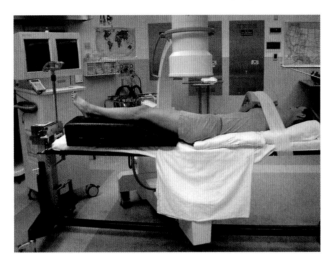

Figure 16-1 | Patient positioning and fluoroscopic setup for AP view for intertrochanteric fracture treatment.

- To obtain a lateral, roll the unit all the way back so that the beam is flat on the floor (Fig. 16-2).

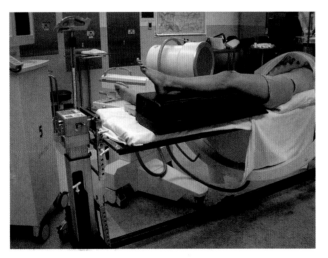

Figure 16-2 | Fluoroscope position for obtaining a lateral view.

- This view should be perpendicular to the "long" axis of the femoral neck (i.e., ~45 degrees relative to the longitudinal axis of the OR table).
- There should be no significant "retroversion/anteversion" visible on the image if the fracture is reduced and the leg is internally rotated to match the normal anteversion.
  - Since the patient is on a bump, the contralateral hip should be out of the C-arm image as it is posterior to the imaged hip.
  - In obese individuals, a C-arm position just above the horizontal will prevent extremity and hip radiographic overlap.

■ If the cross-table lateral shows the femoral neck in "retroversion," the patient's ipsilateral hemipelvis may be elevated too far and relatively "internally rotated."

■ Excessive internal rotation of the pelvis and attached proximal femoral fragment will make the lateral radiograph difficult to obtain.

● This may require the intraoperative placement of a clamp or Schanz pin to help control and externally rotate the proximal fragment(s).

● Alternatively, a smaller bump/bolster can be used.

Implant and Reduction Techniques

● A sliding hip screw with a two- to four-hole side plate is one of the two implants of choice for most intertrochanteric hip fractures.

● Two-hole side plates are usually sufficient for basicervical femoral neck fractures and stable two-part intertrochanteric fracture patterns.

● This implant is less expensive than most intramedullary devices. It can be applied through a lateral approach to the proximal femur, by elevation of the proximal vastus lateralis.

● Intertrochanteric fracture "stability" is a topic of debate and depends on a number of factors, including the displacement, integrity of the lateral cortex, the presence of significant posteromedial comminution, involvement of the subtrochanteric area of the femur, and the fracture pattern, especially the orientation of the primary fracture plane (standard or reversed obliquity).

■ A trochanteric stabilizing side plate should be added if a separate greater trochanteric fragment is noted intraoperatively.

● Intramedullary devices are indicated for unstable fracture patterns, reversed obliquity patterns, or pathological fractures, including severe osteoporosis.

Reduction Techniques

● Often, a satisfactory closed reduction can be achieved by application of traction and limb positioning alone.

● If an adequate closed reduction cannot be obtained, multiple percutaneous methods may be deployed.

● A flexion deformity may be corrected by pushing the proximal segment down with a percutaneously inserted 2.5-mm Schanz pin or spiked pusher from a direct anterior position.

● A percutaneously inserted bone hook placed anteriorly and around the calcar can be used to correct deformity and maintain the reduction (Fig. 16-3).

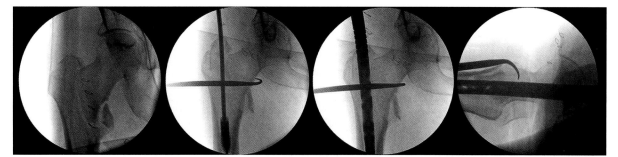

Figure 16-3 I A bone hook can be used to reduce the proximal fragment prior to reaming.

● A lateral percutaneously inserted spiked pusher on the distal segment can be used in concert with a bone hook over the medial femoral neck for control of both the proximal and distal segment.

● Alternatively, 5.0-mm Schanz pins may be placed into the proximal segment, the distal segment, or both for greater control.

■ Schanz pins should be placed thoughtfully so as not to interfere with the chosen definitive implant.

■ If a Schanz pin is placed in the distal segment, it should be bicortical for manipulation. If using an IM nail, it will have to be backed out to a unicortical position for guidewire and nail passage.

Shoehorn Reduction of Flexion Deformity in Pertrochanteric Fractures

Michael J. Gardner

Pathoanatomy

Commonly, a sagittal plane deformity exists in pertrochanteric fractures, which often involves either flexion or extension and/or anterior or posterior translation (Figs. 16-4 and 16-5). These deformities are critical to reduce to obtain maximal inherent bone stability to "protect" the fixation and minimize implant stresses to reduce the risk of fixation failure.

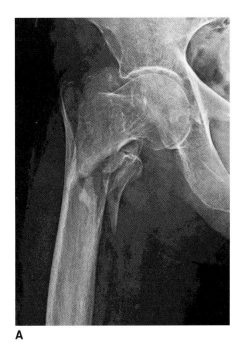

A

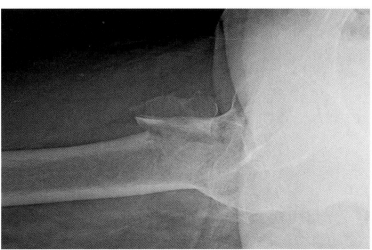

Figure 16-4 I Comminuted proximal femur in a geriatric patient **(A)** with extension deformity (the proximal fragment is flexed relative to the shaft fragment) **(B)**.

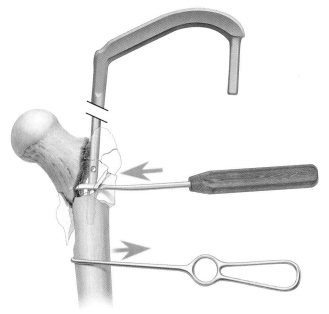

B

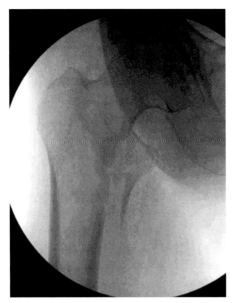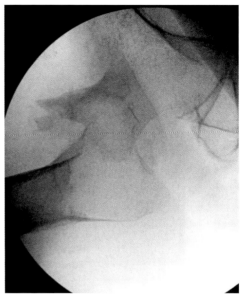

Figure 16-5 ▍ Fracture table traction allows for restoration of the neck-shaft angle in the coronal plane, but significant translation and angulation remain in the sagittal plane.

Solution

An anteriorly based, fluoroscopically positioned Hohmann retractor can be used to correct an extension/posterior translation deformity.

Technique

- The patient is placed supine on a fracture table. Traction is applied and fluoroscopic images obtained. Figure 16-5 shows posterior translation of the femoral shaft with some extension through the fracture.
- On an AP fluoroscopic view, an incision is marked that is in line with the intertrochanteric fracture line. A longitudinal 2-cm incision is made, and the fascia is subsequently incised.
- After blunt dissection, a pointed Hohmann retractor is inserted with the tip angled proximally and advanced distal to the proximal fragment until it rests on the proximal extent of the distal fragment. A lateral view is obtained (Fig. 16-6).

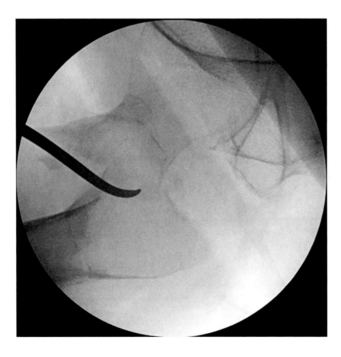

Figure 16-6 ▍ The tip of the Hohmann is advanced proximally at an angle until it reaches the proximal edge of the distal fragment.

- The tip of the Hohmann is advanced proximally at an angle until it reaches the proximal edge of the distal fragment (Fig. 16-7).

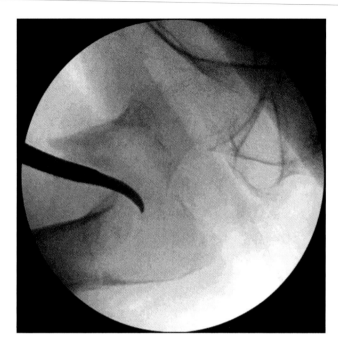

Figure 16-7 I The Hohmann is then rotated 180 degrees so that the tip is pointing posteriorly.

- The Hohmann is then rotated 180 degrees so that the tip is pointing posteriorly (Fig. 16-7).
- The Hohmann is then angled proximally, using it as a lever, or "shoehorn," to restore the sagittal plane alignment of the two main fracture fragments (Figs. 16-8 and 16-9).

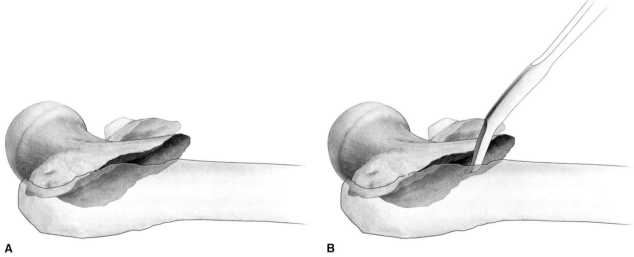

A   B

Figure 16-8 I Shoehorn maneuver for reduction of intertrochanteric fractures (A–E).

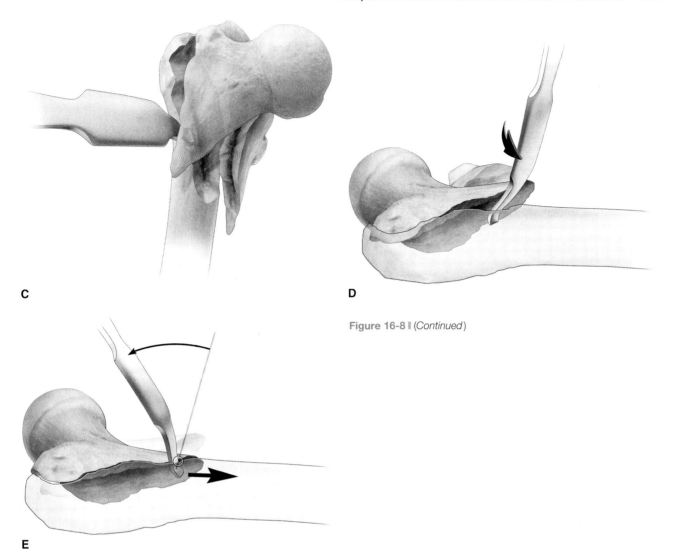

C

D

Figure 16-8 I (*Continued*)

E

Figure 16-9 I The Hohmann is then angled proximally, using it as a lever, or "shoehorn," to restore the sagittal plane alignment of the two main fracture fragments.

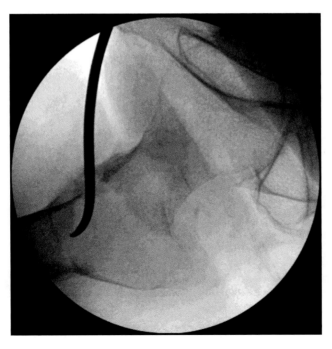

- An anterior view can then be obtained, and the shoehorn can be retained while the nail path is prepared and the nail is inserted (Figs. 16-10 and 16-11).

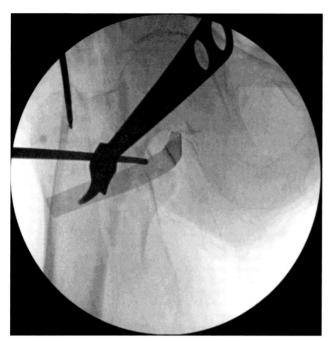

Figure 16-10 | An anterior view can then be obtained, and the shoehorn can be retained while the nail path is inserted.

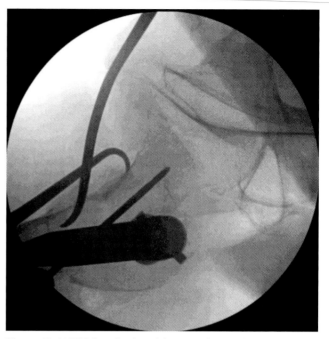

Figure 16-11 | While reduction of the posterior translation and extension are maintained with a Hohmann, a bone hook also has been inserted through a lateral incision to assist in the reduction of the coronal and sagittal plane deformities. Note the tip of the Hohmann positioned anterior to the nail path. The bone hook helps to "extend" the head and neck fragment while simultaneously correcting coronal plane deformity. Only after an acceptable reduction has been obtained in both coronal and sagittal planes is the nail path initiated with insertion of the guide pin. The reduction is maintained during nail insertion and then the cephalomedullary guide pin is inserted for the lag screw or blade.

- Final reduction after cephalomedullary nail stabilization is shown in Figure 16-12. Note restoration of neck-shaft angles and translation in both the sagittal and coronal planes.

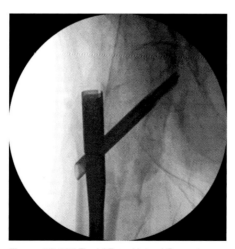
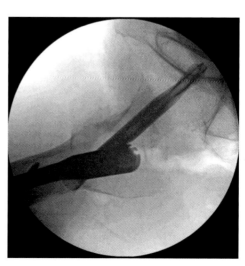

Figure 16-12 | Final AP and lateral C-arm images.

Reduction of Intussuscepted Varus Pertrochanteric Fractures

Michael J. Gardner

Pathoanatomy

Geriatric pertrochanteric fractures can present with a variety of fracture fragments and associated deformities (Fig. 16-13). This often includes varus intussusception of the head/neck fragment (Fig. 16-14), which is an inherently unstable position and is also very difficult to reduce. Correcting this deformity, restoring anatomy, and applying stable fixation provides the best chance to maintain reduction until healing so as to maximize functional outcome.

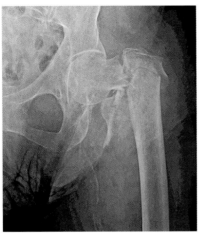 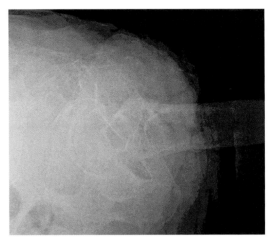

Figure 16-13 | Injury radiographs of an 82-year-old female with a complex pertrochanteric femur fracture, including a basicervical head/neck fracture fragment, greater trochanteric fracture, and lesser trochanteric fracture.

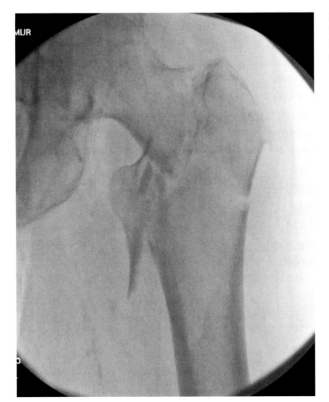

Figure 16-14 | After fracture table traction, the basicervical head/neck fragment remains in varus and intussuscepted, despite slight overdistraction.

Solution

Using meticulously placed percutaneous and intraosseous reduction instruments, this deformity can be corrected and maintained during intramedullary nail placement.

- While traction is maintained, a bone hook is inserted percutaneously, through a small lateral incision at the subtrochanteric level. This hook is advanced through the IT band and vastus lateralis and anterior to the femur.
  - The hook is then rotated 90 degrees to provide a lateralizing force on the femoral shaft component. This reduces the intussusception (into the intertrochanteric region) of the head/neck fragment by lateralizing the shaft relative to the femoral head and neck (Fig. 16-15).

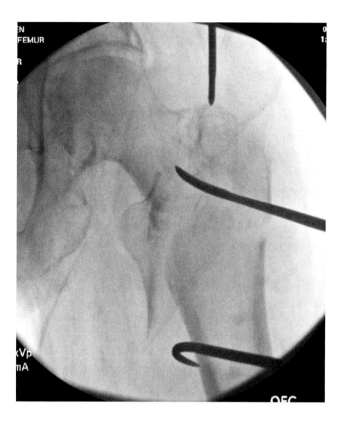

Figure 16-15 I Using a percutaneously placed hook, the diaphyseal segment can be lateralized while a percutaneously placed elevator can be placed through the fracture site into the intraosseous region of the femoral neck, realigning the medial femoral neck and calcar.

- An elevator is introduced through a second percutaneous incision at the basicervical/intertrochanteric region.
  - The elevator is advanced into the fracture and used to push medially on the inferior neck. As the femoral head is "stabilized" by the acetabulum and hip capsule, this force produces a rotational moment on the head/neck fragment, rotating it out of varus and realigning the medial neck and calcar (Fig. 16-15).
- While the forces and reduction are maintained, insertion of the IM nail guide pin is initiated (Fig. 16-15).
- Alternatively, the reduced head and neck fragment can be maintained by insertion of several large K-wires (~2.4 mm) through the greater trochanteric fragment into the head. Care must be taken to place these anteriorly and posteriorly to the intended path of the femoral nail and the cephalomedullary implant (screw or blade).
  - When positioned correctly, these K-wires act as "slalom gates" through which the nail should pass easily.
- Reduction of the fracture must be maintained while creating the nail path and during nail insertion (Figs. 16-16 and 16-17).

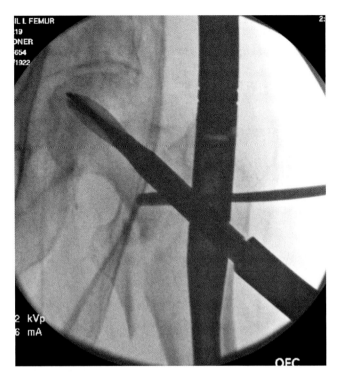

Figure 16-16 ▌ The elevator can be maintained anterior to the nail during insertion to maintain the reduced position of the head and neck fragment. Lateralization of the shaft is maintained by the bone hook, which is not seen on this C-arm image.

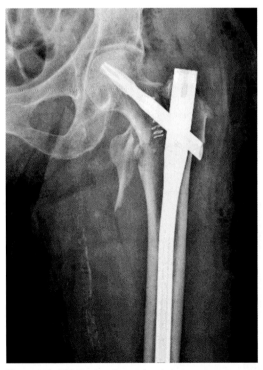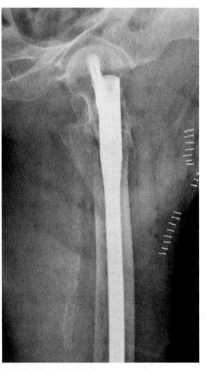

Figure 16-17 ▌ Final radiographs demonstrate an acceptable reduction.

- In thinner individuals, a displaced fracture that cannot be reduced by the above techniques may be clamped percutaneously.
- Larger patients and young patients with high-energy injuries will often require an open reduction (Figs. 16-18 and 16-19).
  - Orient clamp to allow passage of the reamers and subsequent nail and femoral head element.

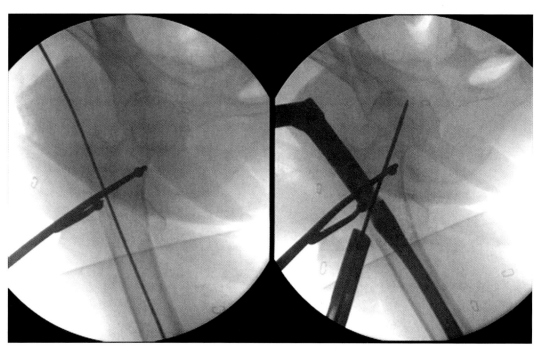

Figure 16-18 I A long cephalomedullary nail was chosen to treat this three-part intertrochanteric femur fracture predominately because of the patient's marked osteoporosis. A percutaneous clamp was used to reduce the fracture prior to its fixation. Placement of the clamp should consider the path of the cephalomedullary screw/blade.

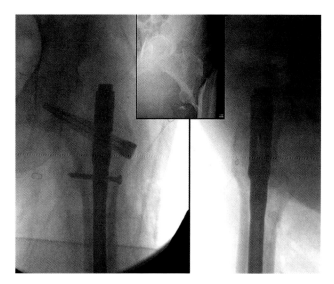

Figure 16-19 I This cephalomedullary nail entry portal (piriformis) was chosen to spare the lateral cortex of the proximal segment, which allows the greater trochanter to resist varus displacement. This fracture required an open reduction prior to medullary nail insertion.

- Alternatively, depending on the fracture, place the clamp obliquely or more toward the coronal plane (Fig. 16-20).

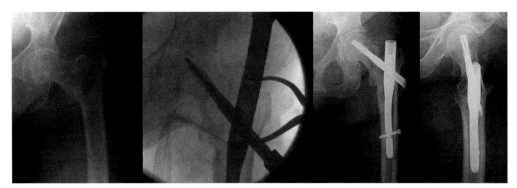

Figure 16-20 | Careful placement of a clamp in the coronal plane may help resist/correct varus deformity but should be positioned carefully so it does not interfere with cephalomedullary instrumentation.

Sliding Hip Screw Technique

- The proximal femur is exposed using a lateral approach.
- Localize the incision fluoroscopically with an extracutaneous guide pin running parallel with the center of the femoral neck to determine its "intersection point" over the lateral thigh.
  - The proximal extent of the incision is generally at the level of the lesser trochanter.
- If the femoral neck portion of the fracture is rotationally unstable, in addition to the guide pin used for screw placement, consider multiple additional larger-diameter (2.0-mm) K-wires or pins to control torsional forces associated with reaming/tapping/screw insertion.
  - One pin may be replaced with an antirotational 5.0, 4.5, or 3.5 lag screw (Fig. 16-21).

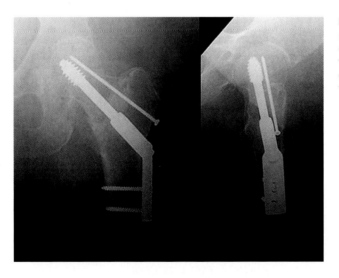

Figure 16-21 | Placement of a screw-side plate device with an "antirotational" 3.5 cortical lag screw. A 3.5-mm gliding hole was created in the lateral femoral cortex/ greater trochanter with a 2.5-mm pilot hole for the femoral neck/head.

Intramedullary Devices

- Most intramedullary devices are designed to treat the intertrochanteric fractures common to a geriatric population.
- Thus, they have a relatively large proximal nail diameter to accommodate the cephalomedullary screw or blade.

- Obtain a reduction prior to reaming the canal, and maintain the reduction during reaming.
  - The starting point in the proximal segment should be collinear with the proximal geometry and anticipated path of the nail.
- When reaming, avoid eccentric reamer passage, which may occur in comminuted and malreduced fractures.
  - Eccentric reaming often leads to thinning of the distal-posterior and proximal-lateral portions of the proximal fragment (due to its flexion/abduction if unreduced).
  - A ring clamp (e.g., the handle of a large Kocher clamp) placed over the guidewire and reamer shaft can be used to guide the entry path of each reamer by applying an anteromedially directed force.
    - This can help control the entry position and path of each reamer as it enters and transits the proximal fragment.[1]
- The tip apex distance remains important for intramedullary devices.
  - The nail and the proximal targeting jig can obscure the trajectory of the cephalomedullary guide pin, making optimal placement difficult (Figs. 16-22 and 16-23).

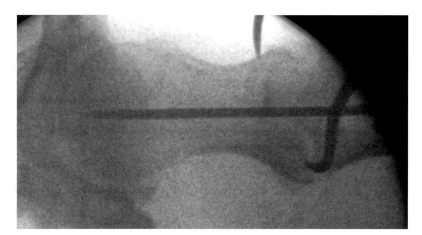

Figure 16-22 I Positioning the base of the C-arm toward the patient's feet, so that it approximates 45 degrees to the long axis of the patient, will orient the beam perpendicularly to the femoral neck and will allow better imaging of the femoral head in the cross-table lateral view.

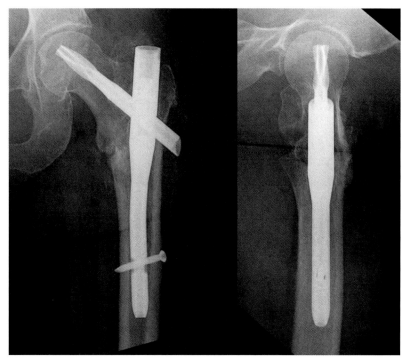

Figure 16-23 I Final images demonstrating the optimal femoral head implant position.

- If a long intramedullary nail is used, the knee should be imaged on the lateral view as the nail is inserted.
  - Mismatch between the curvature of the nail and femur may occur in the elderly and can lead to either anterior cortical perforation or extrusion of the nail beyond the anterior cortex of the distal femur.
  - When recognized, this may be avoided by selecting an implant with a smaller radius of curvature or modifying the implant using a bending device to match its curvature to that of the patient's femur (Fig. 16-24).
- A long nail ending at or above the metaphyseal flare leaves the patient at risk of a distal peri-implant fracture. Ending the nail at the level of the distal femoral physeal scar minimizes this risk.

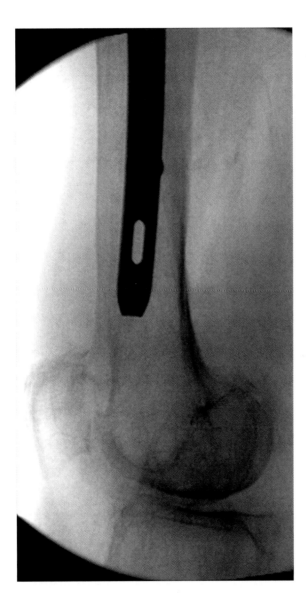

Figure 16-24 ∥ A lateral view of the knee should be assessed to ensure that the nail does not penetrate the anterior femoral cortex.

Reference

1. Palm H, Jacobsen S, Sonne-Holm S, et al. Integrity of the lateral femoral wall in intertrochanteric hip fractures: an important predictor of a reoperation. *J Bone Joint Surg Am.* 2007;89:470–475.

Section 6
Femur

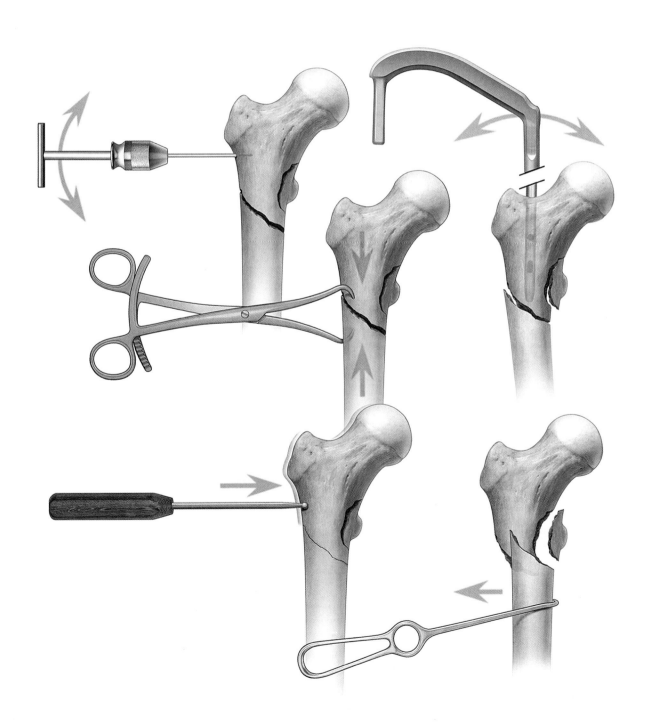

Chapter 17
Subtrochanteric Femur Fractures

MICHAEL J. GARDNER

ROBERT A. HYMES

CONOR KLEWENO

MATTHEW P. SULLIVAN

Sterile Instruments/Equipment

- On-table traction or fracture table
- 5.0-mm Schanz pins for manipulative joysticks
- Large pointed bone reduction clamps (Weber clamps)
- Serrated bone reduction clamps
- Femoral distractor
- Ball-spike pushers
- Shoulder hook/bone hook
- 2.7-mm reconstruction plate
- K-wires and wire driver/drill
- Reamers
- Implants
  - Intramedullary nail
    - Reconstruction or cephalomedullary
    - Greater trochanteric versus piriformis design
  - Proximal femoral locking plate
  - Blade plate

Positioning

Supine on a radiolucent table

- Bump under the ipsilateral hemipelvis and torso.
- Move the patient as far as possible to the table's edge so that the buttock is partially overhanging the edge of the table, particularly if a piriformis nail is being planned.
  - Improves access for nail insertion
  - Confirm ability to obtain adequate intraoperative AP and lateral images prior to prepping and draping.
- Skeletal traction through a distal femoral pin is useful in restoring the fracture length.
  - Limb elevated on radiolucent foam ramp or triangular wedge
  - Assists in reducing fracture and matching flexion of distal fragment to proximal fragment's flexion deformity

Lateral on a radiolucent table

- Facilitates reduction by allowing the surgeon to flex the leg to correct the flexion deformity and takes advantage of gravity to reduce abduction deformity

- Easy access to entire femur for percutaneous or open reduction strategies
- Axillary roll
- Blanket rolls to support the torso
- Arm of a universal arm holder
- Down leg padded and surrounded by folded blankets
- Nothing between the legs
- C-arm in from the patient's anterior

Surgical Approaches for Open Treatment

- Standard lateral approach to proximal femur.
- Incise iliotibial band.
- Elevate vastus lateralis origin from vastus ridge; identify perforating vessels.
- Selective approaches for clamp placements or joysticks.

Reduction and Implant Techniques

- The most common deforming forces are flexion, abduction, and external rotation of the proximal fragment due to tendon insertions and muscular forces (Fig. 17-1).

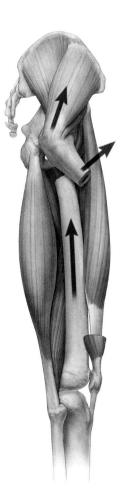 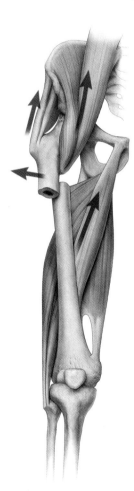

Figure 17-1 ▌ The primary forces that must be counteracted with reduction maneuvers in subtrochanteric fractures are flexion, abduction, and external rotation of the proximal fragment.

- Two main reduction methods can be used separately or in combination.
  - Reducing the distal fragment to the proximal fragment without manipulating the proximal fragment.
    - This requires matching the flexion, external rotation, and variable abduction with concomitant traction.
    - Easiest to achieve in the lateral position.

Antegrade Femoral Intramedullary Nailing in the Lateral Position without a Traction Table

Matthew P. Sullivan
Conor P. Kleweno

Pathoanatomy

Supine nailing of the femoral shaft can be difficult in a variety of settings. These include the following:

- Obesity
- Piriformis entry (vs. trochanteric entry)
- Subtrochanteric (and proximal femoral shaft) fractures associated with flexion of the proximal fragment

Solutions

Use of the lateral position in femoral nailing has several benefits, which address many of these difficulties.

- Obtaining the starting point (particularly the piriformis starting point) in patients in the lateral position can be significantly less challenging than in the supine position. The torso naturally laterally flexes (down toward the floor) in the lateral position thus presenting the proximal lateral femur. In addition, the patient's torso can be forward flexed slightly and the operative leg adducted—both make access to the proximal femur less obstructed.
- In particular, obtaining the entry portal in obese patients with a large soft tissue envelope is considerably easier compared to supine nailing. Gravity flattens out the soft tissues and allows excessive adipose tissue to "fall away" from the insertion site.
- The operative leg can be flexed easily to assist in the closed reduction for proximal diaphyseal and subtrochanteric fractures.
- When properly positioned with the pelvis perpendicular to the floor, accurate restoration of anatomic femoral rotation of comminuted or segmental fractures anecdotally appears to be easier than supine nailing. The reason is that in the lateral position, the legs are simply positioned next to each other (with the operative hip slightly flexed to separate the distal femurs for imaging) when placing distal interlocking screws. Thus, one does not need to rotate the operative leg for obtaining perfect circles.

Technique

Lateral femoral nailing can be performed using a fracture table or a radiolucent flat-top table. For surgeons accustomed to supine nailing on flat top tables, the major challenges are

- The surgeon's comfort with the patient's less familiar orientation
- The positioning of the fluoroscope and the interpretation of the lateral fluoroscopic view
- The tendency for distal femoral fractures to "fall into" valgus when using a fracture table and traction

Lateral nailing is advantageous for

- Subtrochanteric femur fracture patterns
- Obesity

Relative contraindications

- Concomitant injuries in which lateral positioning is unfavorable (e.g., flail chest, contralateral transtectal transverse acetabular fracture, unstable spinal fractures, etc.)
- Concomitant procedures where access to medial distal thigh or medial leg is required (e.g., vascular procedures, medial femoral condyle injuries)

Prior to positioning

- Obtain comparative length and rotational assessments of the uninjured side. These should be done with standard techniques used for all treatment of femoral shaft fractures to assess for native length, alignment, and rotation: lesser trochanter profile, femoral neck version, trochanteric crossover, and femoral length measurement.

Positioning Tips (see Chapter 1 also)

- Flat top radiolucent table
- Two rolled blanket bolsters—each made of two hospital blankets tightly rolled and taped or a "bean bag"
- "Axillary" roll (high chest roll to protect the axilla)
- Rolled blanket bolsters are positioned adjacent to the torso, anteriorly and posteriorly, from buttock to chest. These are tightly rolled "in reverse," into the drawsheet in order to prevent them from dislodging during surgery.
  - Although a subtle technical point, two blankets are used in succession to prepare the rolled blanket bolsters. The first blanket needs to be rolled and taped independently and the second blanket rolled over the first one and then taped separately. This creates a much more rigid bolster compared to simply rolling both blankets together at the same time.
- Folded blankets are placed anteriorly to the dependent (down) lower extremity to create a stable surface for the operative leg when it is placed in the flexed position on top of the normal dependent (down) limb.
  - The critical feature of this folded blanket surface is that it allows the operative limb to rest in a slightly adducted position easing access to the greater trochanter.
- Minimal or no padding should be placed between the legs so that the operative (up) leg can adduct. Foam wedges or padding between the legs abducts the operative leg, thus negating the advantage of lateral position for access to the proximal femoral entry site.
- Sterile draping can be performed creating a wide sterile field with access to the posterior and medial buttock when compared to supine positioning.
  - With supine positioning, the patient's buttock hangs over the edge of the table to improve access to the posterior buttock, posterosuperior to the greater trochanter.
- A distal femoral traction pin can be used with sterile rope and weights hung off the end of the bed over a table support or a lateral table attachment (to accommodate a flexed hip) (Fig. 17-2).
- Drapes are protected from the traction bow with sterile folded towels.

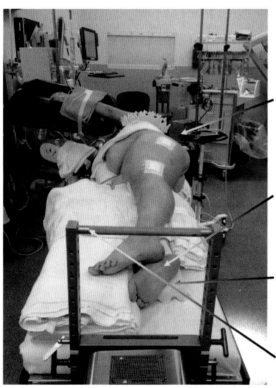

A. The pelvis is positioned perfectly perpendicular to the floor

B. The down extremity is extended and work on the operative limb is performed anterior to the down limb

C. Foam protecting the peroneal nerve

D. As an option (although not always necessary), distal femoral traction weights can be hung over a spine frame or lateral table attachment

Figure 17-2 | A: To assist in restoring accurate femoral rotation, the pelvis should be positioned perfectly lateral and perpendicular to the floor. **B:** The dependent ("down"/uninjured) extremity is extended to allow for unimpeded lateral fluoroscopic imaging of the distal femur, particularly important for placing distal interlocking bolts. **C:** All sites of nerve compression are padded. **D:** Distal femoral traction weights are hung over a table's frame or a lateral attachment.

- Leg positioning: The dependent ("down") extremity (nonoperative leg) is placed in a relatively extended hip position. This allows for the operative limb ("up hip") to be flexed compared with the dependent limb (Fig. 17-3). This is important for two reasons:
  - It separates the femoral shafts to facilitate lateral imaging in the distal femur.
  - It assists with indirect reduction given that the proximal femoral segment will be flexed due to the psoas.

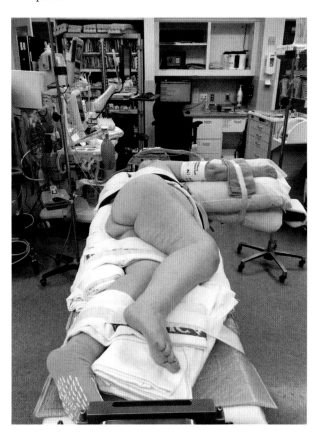

Figure 17-3 | Notice the relative position of the operative ("up") extremity compared to the dependent ("down") extremity. It is slightly forward flexed at the hip in order to facilitate lateral imaging of the distal femur as well as reducing the distal fracture segment toward the proximal femur, which tends to be in a flexed position from the deforming forces of the hip flexors. Additionally, the stable surface created by folded blankets anterior to the dependent limb allows for some adduction of the operative extremity. This facilitates access to the piriformis entry site.

Imaging

- Fluoroscopic imaging of proximal femur (both AP and lateral) is unimpeded and provides excellent radiographic views of the femoral neck (Fig. 17-4). The notion that imaging is more difficult in the lateral position is a misconception.

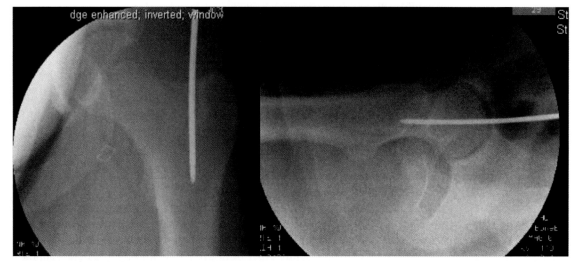

Figure 17-4 | AP and lateral fluoroscopic images of the proximal femur demonstrating unobstructed views allowing for rapid acquisition of the piriformis starting point. The lateral view is obtained with a 15- to 20-degree C-arm rollover. Note the excellent image quality.

- The lateral neck view is obtained by bringing the C-arm base in perpendicular to the table, and then rolling over 15 to 20 degrees (Fig. 17-5). In addition, the C-arm can be positioned into 10 to 15 degrees of "inlet" to help "shoot down" the femoral neck if desired.

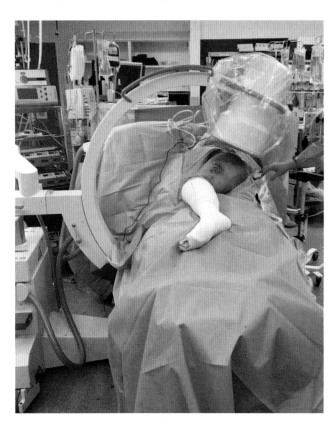

Figure 17-5 I C-arm position for obtaining lateral images. C-arm base is brought in perpendicular to the table and the beam is rolled over 15 to 20 degrees.

- The AP image is obtained by rolling the C-arm under the table so that the beam is parallel to the floor and orthogonal to the flexed femur (Fig. 17-6).

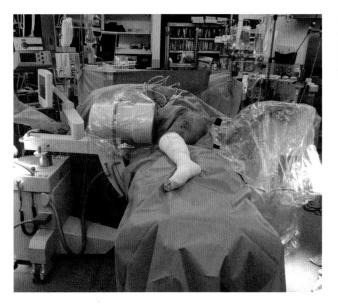

Figure 17-6 I C-arm position for obtaining an AP image. C-arm base is brought in perpendicular to the femur (i.e., the beam is angled distally such that it is perpendicular to the flexed proximal femur).

- In the lateral position, there is an expected valgus deformity (sagging) of the distal fracture segment. This is easily corrected with a towel bump placed proximally between the thighs (not shown). This simple technique often perfectly reduces the fracture in the coronal plane.
- The remainder of the procedure is performed in a similar fashion to that of supine antegrade femoral nailing.

- Reducing the proximal fragment to the distal fragment without manipulating the distal fragment.
  - This is accomplished by controlling the proximal fragment either directly (open technique) or percutaneously with joysticks, reduction clamps, or other devices.
  - In this scenario, the deforming forces on the proximal fragment are counteracted by adducting, extending, and internally rotating the proximal fragment.
  - This is difficult to correct with traction alone.
- Limb alignment and fracture reduction must be maintained during reaming and implant placement so as to assure a concentric nail position, while maintaining fracture reduction.
- When placing a trochanteric entry nail with cephalomedullary fixation (i.e., reconstruction screws), the starting point should be slightly more anterior and medial than is typical for treating a shaft fracture.
- When placing a reconstruction nail with planned cephalomedullary fixation via a piriformis entry, the starting point should be slightly more anterior to allow reconstruction screws to be placed centrally in the femoral head.
- The primary advantage of a piriformis entry is the insertion of the nail in line with the anatomic axis of the femur. This reduces the chance of introducing a varus malreduction with nail insertion. This occurs commonly with trochanteric entry nails with too lateral a starting point.
- If the fracture pattern has proximal extension into the trochanteric region, a piriformis start should be avoided.
- A properly placed starting point is critical for obtaining and maintaining an acceptable reduction. This starting point is variable and based on the specific implant used. Adequate AP and lateral intraoperative imaging is necessary to confirm perfect entry point placement.
  - Occasionally, attempts at translating the reamers medially will displace fracture fragments medially instead of reaming medial bone.
  - When reaming with the patient supine, after each reamer is removed, the guidewire will tend to rest in the posterolateral aspect of the reamer track due to guidewire's trajectory, gravity, and flexion/abduction of the proximal fragment.
    - This will cause each successive reamer pass in the proximal fragment to occur more and more laterally and posteriorly if this is not addressed and counteracted (Fig. 17-7).

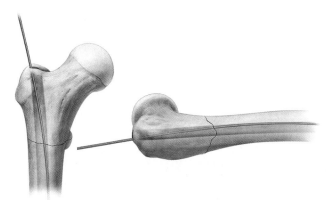

Figure 17-7 I Gravity and soft tissue forces will tend to position the guidewire laterally (*left*) and posteriorly (*right*). If not corrected, this may cause eccentric reaming of the entry portal with each successive reamer pass.

■ Use the ring of a clamp or other instrument to medialize the wire during reaming, thus preventing eccentric reaming of the starting portal.
■ Each reamer can be passed through the clamp ring without requiring its removal until guidewire exchange or nail placement (Fig. 17-8).

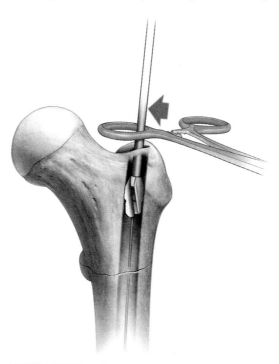

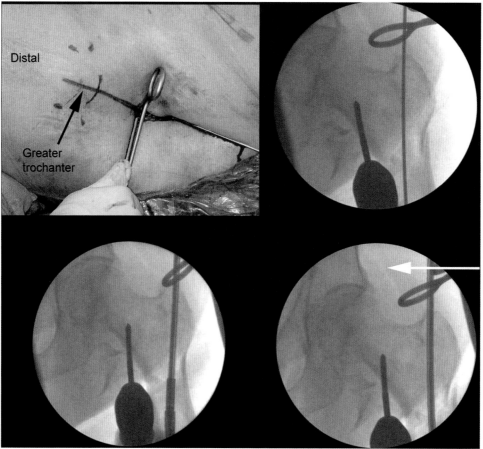

Figure 17-8 ▌ Placing the ring of a clamp over the guidewire and reamer shaft allows for medialization to avoid eccentric starting point reaming. The large amount of possible reamer shaft excursion is evident with medialization in this example (*lower right*).

- Alternatively, when an intact lateral cortex is present, a small plate may be placed laterally within the starting portal to force an improved and more medial reaming path as progressively larger reamers are used (Fig. 17-9).

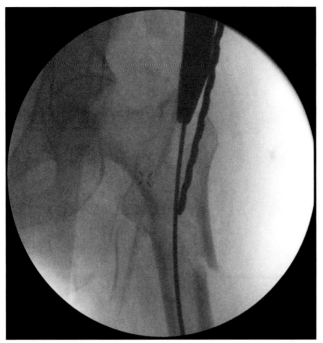

Figure 17-9 ▍If varus deformity results after fully seating the nail, this may be due in part to an excessively lateralized reamer track in the proximal segment. This can be corrected by repeat reaming with a plate placed along the tract to preferentially ream the medial bone of the entry point.

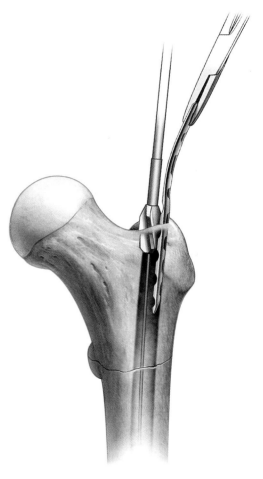

- Place a bone reduction clamp open across fracture under direct visualization prior to reaming for nail placement (Fig. 17-10).

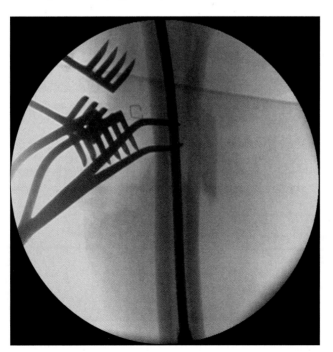

Figure 17-10 ▍A small incision that allows for subtrochanteric clamp placement is effective in stabilizing the fracture reduction during the nailing procedure.

- Place clamps in a position so as not to interfere with the nail jig during nail insertion and proximal screw insertion.
- If the fracture is more proximal, pointed reduction clamps can be placed from the greater trochanter to the shaft to obtain and maintain reduction during reaming and nail insertion (Fig. 17-11).

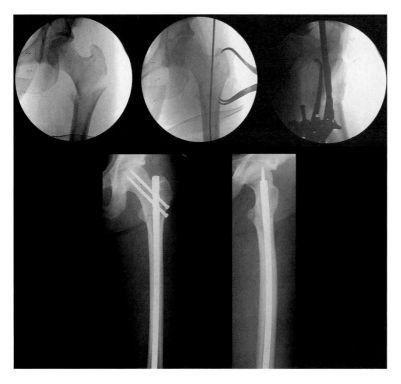

Figure 17-11 ‖ Clamps may be placed from the greater trochanter to the shaft to reduce the varus deformity. A unicortical hole in the lateral cortex of the distal fragment may be required for Weber clamp application.

- Alternatively, a Schanz pin may be placed from lateral to medial, posterior to the path of the nail, to joystick of the proximal fragment (Fig. 17-12).

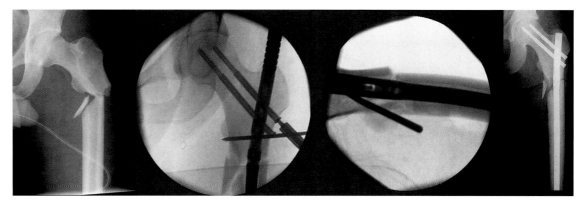

Figure 17-12 ‖ In this subtrochanteric fracture, a Steinmann pin was placed laterally, posterior to the path of the nail, for use as a manipulative joystick. Note that the starting portal was a bit more anterior than optimal, resulting in a reduction in slight extension.

- When the distal fracture orientation is more in the sagittal plane, a linear bone reduction clamp may achieve the correct fracture reducing force vectors (Fig. 17-13).

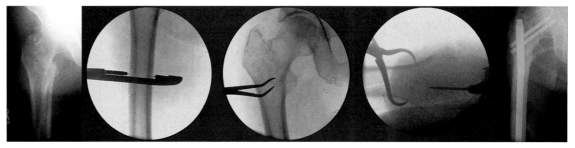

Figure 17-13 ‖ In this example, the fracture spiraled distally, and the distal fracture was more in the sagittal plane. A linear reduction clamp, with standard clamps proximally, allows for establishment of correct force vectors resulting in an anatomic reduction.

- It is critical to reduce and provisionally stabilize the flexion deformity of the proximal fragment.[1]
  - Place a Schanz pin percutaneously from anterior to posterior.
  - Place a towel or laparotomy sponge on the external part of the pin and use it to pull distally, reducing the flexion.
  - It is important to use the contralateral intact femur so as to match limb length and rotation.
  - Clamp the sponge or towel distally to a fixed object or drapes to maintain the reduction and to avoid interference with fluoroscopy (Figs. 17-14 and 17-15).

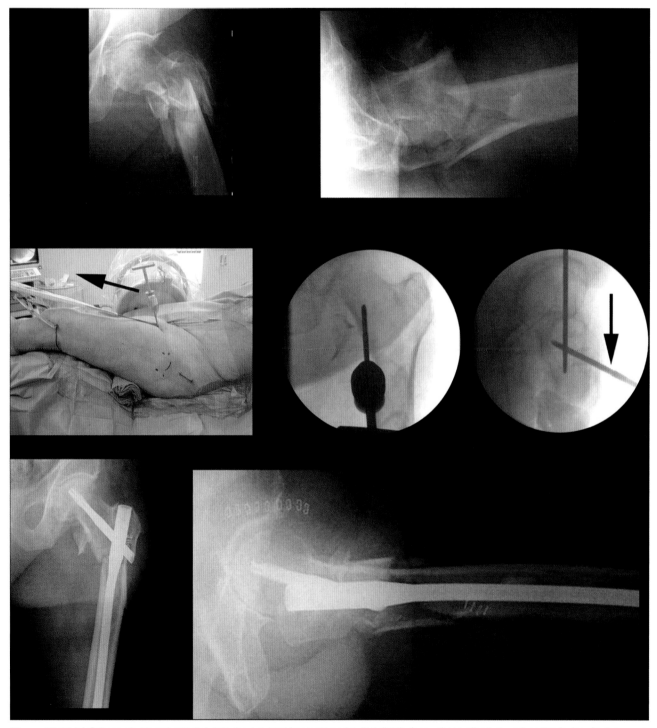

Figure 17-14 | A Schanz pin placed anteriorly into the proximal fragment and pulled distally (*arrows*) can effectively reduce the flexion displacement.

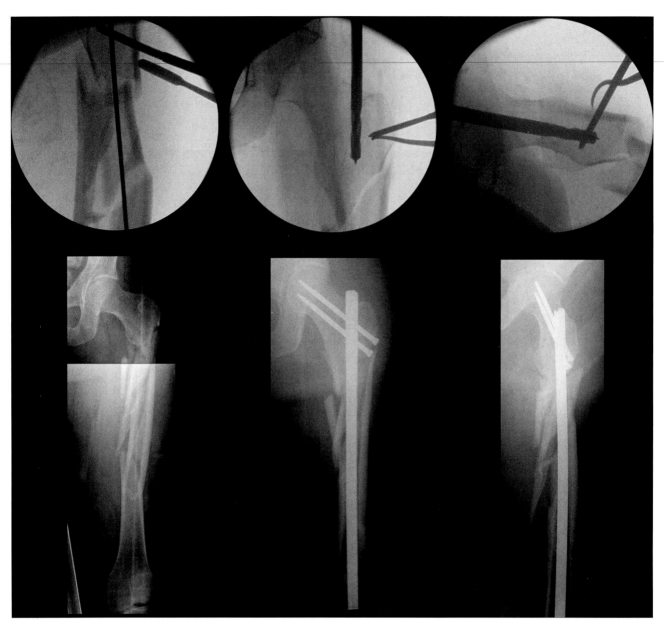

Figure 17-15 I Another case example using an anterolateral Schanz pin for multiplanar control of the proximal fracture fragment.

- Eccentric reaming in the proximal medial cortex of the distal fragment (or the distal medial cortex of the proximal fragment) may also lead to varus alignment or translational deformity, especially in fractures with medial comminution.

● Following provisional reduction, a bone hook may be placed through the comminution to ensure reamers are appropriately lateralized in the distal fragment so that they maintain contact with the lateral endosteal cortex (Fig. 17-16).

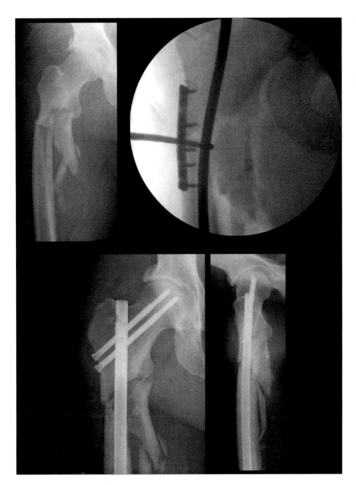

Figure 17-16 ‖ A bone hook can be placed in the comminution and used to manipulate laterally in the distal fragment to prevent eccentric reaming. A provisional plate was also used laterally in this case.

- Percutaneously inserted spiked pushers placed anteriorly and laterally (or a single one placed anterolaterally) can correct both coronal and sagittal plane malreductions (Fig. 17-17).

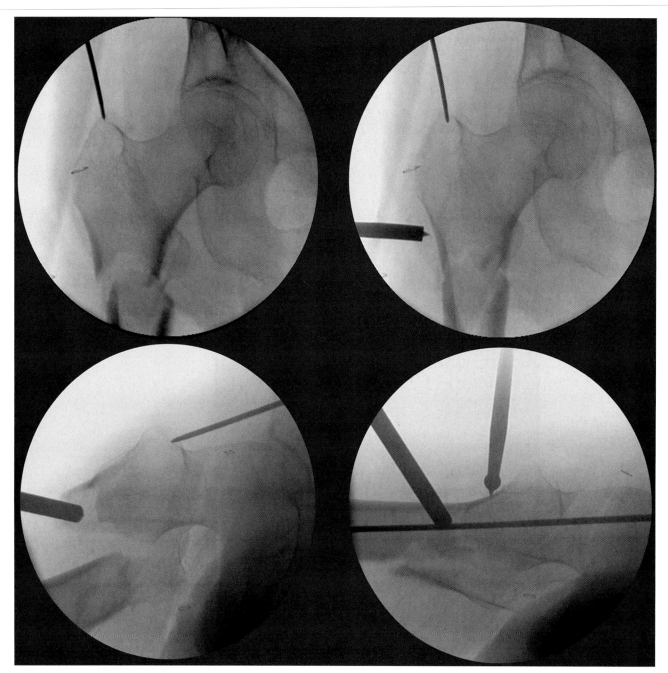

Figure 17-17 I Spiked pushers can be inserted through small incisions to improve fracture reductions. It is important to consider multiple planes of deformity. In this case, the initial laterally placed spiked pusher reduced the coronal plane deformity (*upper right*), but the lateral view demonstrated that the fracture was unreduced in the sagittal plane (*lower left*). This was corrected with an additional spiked pusher inserted anteriorly (*lower right*).

- A bone hook placed around the distal fragment, in combination with a spiked pusher on the proximal fragment, can be used to reduce fractures with predominantly coronal plane translational deformities (Fig. 17-18).

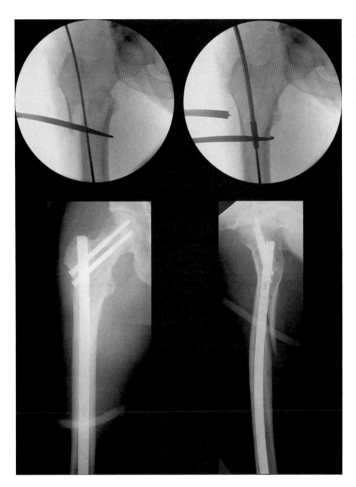

Figure 17-18 | A hook may be placed through a small incision to lateralize the distal fragment. A spike pusher on the lateral cortex of the proximal fragment can assist in minimizing the eccentric endosteal reaming, coronal plane translation, and varus.

- With adequate radiographic views and attention to the correctly placed starting point, nails may be used to reduce fractures indirectly.
  - If the entry portal and nail path matches precisely the nail geometry, the subtrochanteric fracture will reduce indirectly.
- This technique should rarely be relied upon as the sole reduction maneuver (Figs. 17-19 and 17-20).

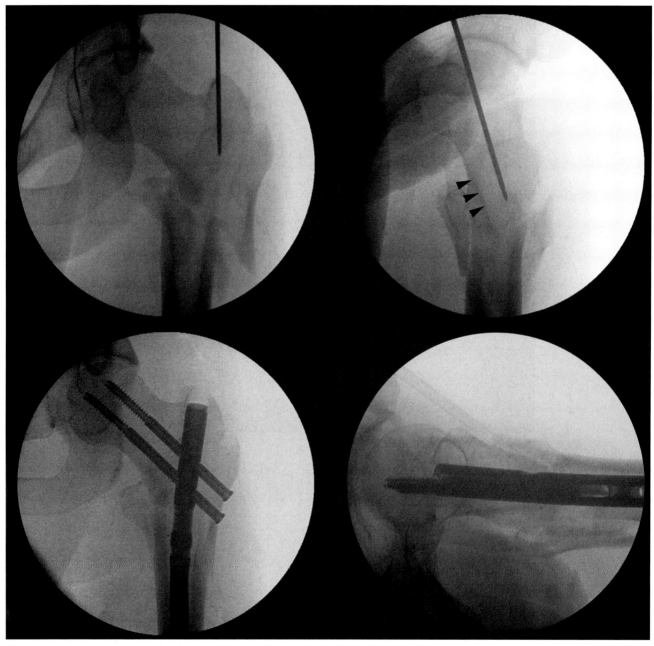

Figure 17-19 By understanding the deforming forces and the correct starting point, the nail can be used to reduce the fracture indirectly. On the lateral view, the guidewire should be collinear with the posterior corticated margin of the vastus ridge (*arrow heads* on *upper right* figure).

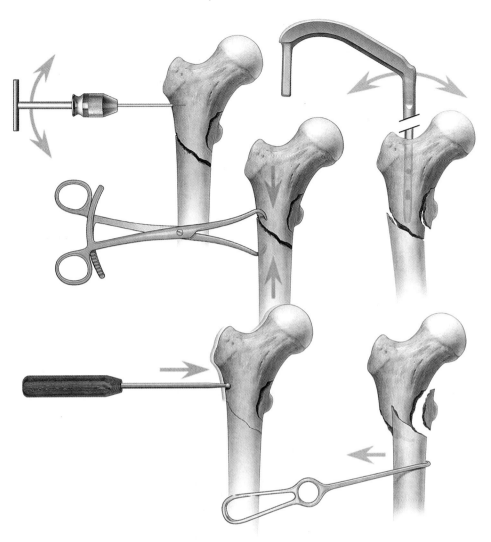

Figure 17-20 | Summary of various reduction maneuvers for subtrochanteric femur fractures. *Arrows* indicate force vectors of the reduction instruments.

Troubleshooting

- If varus malalignment results after a standard trochanteric starting point, a rongeur, awl, or other instrument may be used to remove additional bone medial to the initial starting portal.
  - This will prevent the nail from causing a varus fracture reduction by removing the contact point between the nail and the medial cortex of the reamer tract (Fig. 17-21).

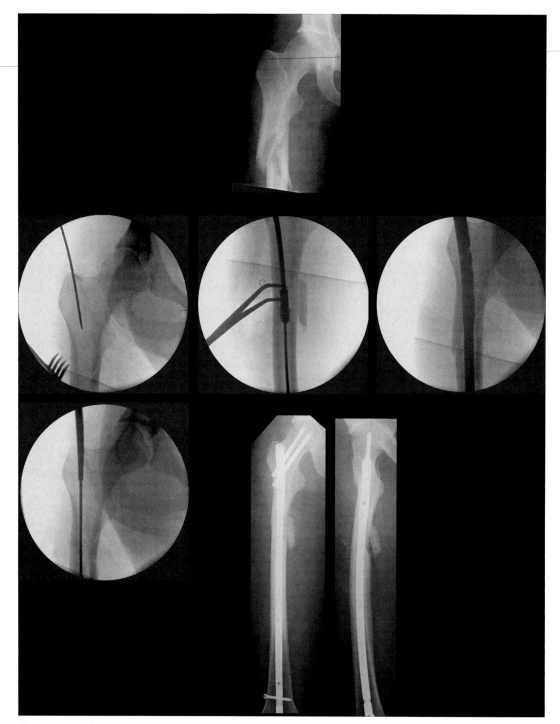

Figure 17-21 I Clinical example of a subtrochanteric femur fracture treated with a trochanteric entry nail. A small incision was made for clamp reduction, and the intramedullary canal was reamed with the fracture reduced anatomically. When the nail was seated, varus deformity was produced. The nail was removed, and additional cortical bone was removed from the medial edge of the starting portal. Deformity was subsequently improved.

- If this strategy fails, a medial blocking strategy can be deployed to redirect the nail in the proximal segment.
  - The nail is removed and a stout wire or drill bit is placed in the proximal segment just medial to the nail's desired path as a blocking device.
  - The blocking device is maintained throughout the entire case and may be replaced at the end of the case with an interlocking bolt from the nail set (Fig. 17-22).

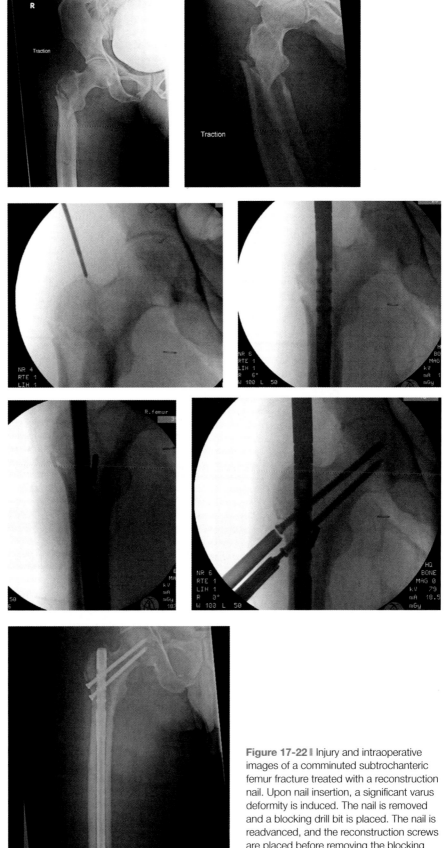

Figure 17-22 I Injury and intraoperative images of a comminuted subtrochanteric femur fracture treated with a reconstruction nail. Upon nail insertion, a significant varus deformity is induced. The nail is removed and a blocking drill bit is placed. The nail is readvanced, and the reconstruction screws are placed before removing the blocking device.

Treatment of Subtrochanteric Femoral Nonunion using Provisional Small Fragment Plate as Tension band for Deformity Correction and Stabilization with Femoral Nailing

Robert A. Hymes

Pathoanatomy

● Alignment of nonisthmic, stiff, hypertrophic nonunions is not corrected with this insertion of intramedullary nails.

Solution

● In the setting of stiff hypertrophic or oligotrophic nonunions with deformity, provisional correction of the deformity can be obtained and maintained using a small plate convex side of the deformity.

Technique

● In this example, a subtrochanteric nonunion occurred after treatment of the fracture with a proximal femoral locking plate. Figure 17-23A and B demonstrate a plated, subtrochanteric nonunion with a mild varus deformity.

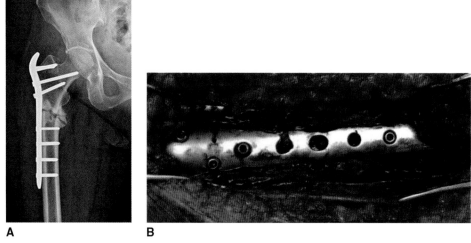

A   **B**

Figure 17-23 I A: Varus nonunion of femoral shaft fracture treated with proximal femoral locking plate. B: Intraoperative photograph of proximal femoral locking plate (PFLP).

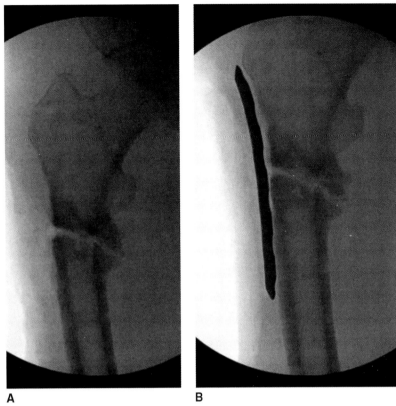

A   B

Figure 17-24 I A: Intraoperative fluoroscopy after PFLP removed. **B:** Small fragment plate contoured.

- After removal of the proximal femoral locking plate (Fig. 17-24A) and screws, a small fragment plate is contoured in valgus (Fig. 17-24B).
- The plate is applied on the lateral aspect of the proximal femur slightly anteriorly (Fig. 17-25).

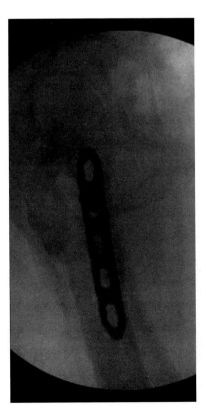

Figure 17-25 I Plate along anterior cortex of femur.

- It is fixed to the proximal head/neck fragment with two screws placed anteriorly so as to avoid the intended path of an IM nail (Fig. 17-26).
- The plate is tensioned with an articulated tensioning device for deformity correction and to obtain compression across the femoral nonunion (Fig. 17-26A and B).

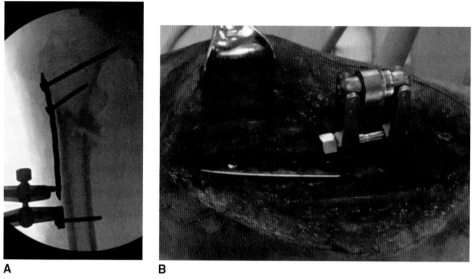

A   **B**

Figure 17-26 I A: Applying compression through the nonunion. **B:** Photograph of articulated tension device.

- Note that an anteriorly placed plate may assist in the correction of an extension deformity. The plate may also be placed posteriorly, just anterior to the linea aspera. Such a posterolateral application can also avoid the intramedullary canal and will aid in the correction of a concomitant flexion deformity.
- A Verbrugge plate holding clamp may also be useful in controlling the plate's alignment to the distal fragment.
- In this example, the implant is placed anteriorly to allow unencumbered intramedullary access of the guidewire, reamers, and nail (Fig. 17-27A–C).

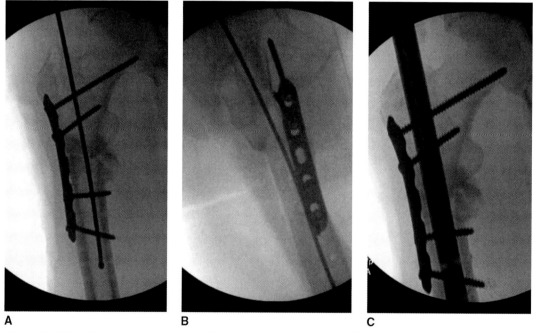

A   **B**   **C**

Figure 17-27 I A, B: Passing the guidewire with the nonunion compressed with a small fragment plate. **C:** The IM nail is inserted with the plate/screw construct in place.

- By targeting the screws away from the intramedullary canal, the tensioned plate can maintain the restored alignment and interfragmentary compression during the entire nailing and nail locking process.
- The plate may either be retained or removed prior to definitive closure (Fig. 17-28A and B).

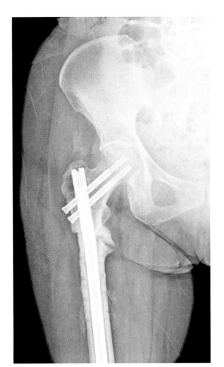

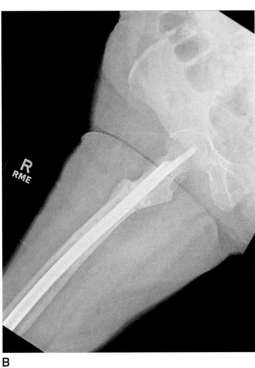

A

B

Figure 17-28 I **A, B:** Six-week follow-up showing early healing.

Reference

1. Browner BD. Pitfalls, errors, and complications in the use of locking Küntscher nails. *Clin Orthop Relat Res.* 1986;212:192–208.

Chapter 18
Femoral Shaft Fractures

DAVID P. BAREI

JONATHAN EASTMAN

JASON M. EVANS

ERIC D. FARRELL

REZA FIROOZABADI

STEPHEN A. KOTTMEIER

JAMES LEARNED

ADEN N. MALIK

Sterile Instruments/Equipment

- On-table traction
- Towel bumps
- Radiolucent triangle if retrograde nailing
- 5.0-mm Schanz pins for manipulative joysticks
- Femoral distractor
- Ball-spike pushers
- Shoulder hook/bone hook
- Large standard and modified Weber clamps
- Co-linear clamp
- Steinmann pins
- K-wires and wire driver/drill
- Reamers
- Implants
  - Intramedullary nail
    - Reconstruction versus condylomedullary
    - Retrograde versus antegrade
  - Large fragment locking or nonlocking plate

Patient Positioning

- Supine on fully radiolucent table, with a folded towel bump or bolster under the ipsilateral hip and flank, acknowledging spine injuries and stabilizing appropriately.
  - Bump can be one or two rolled blankets, but one is typically adequate.
  - If bump is too big, lateral imaging can be difficult.
- Position patient in a slight "C" position with shoulders centered on the table and the affected hip brought as far as possible to the side, preferably overhanging the edge of the table slightly to provide access to the starting point.
- A traction apparatus can be secured to the end of the table and draped into the sterile field (Fig. 18-1).

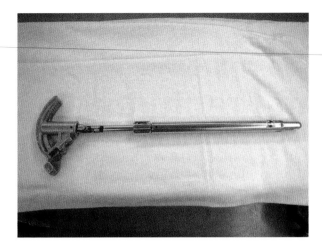

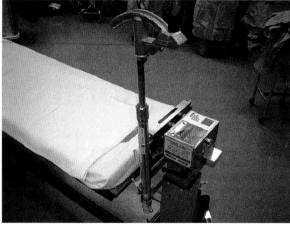

Figure 18-1 I A "traction post" fashioned from a pipe bender is applied to the end of the operating table to allow for an on-table axial lower extremity traction that is easily removable.

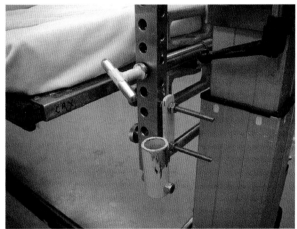

TIP

Sterile Skeletal Femoral Traction and Reduction Techniques

Eric D. Farrell

Pathoanatomy

An obstacle to sterile intraoperative skeletal traction can be the unavailability of a commercial traction device that can be attached to the OR table. Sterile skeletal traction is a useful technique to help obtain and maintain reduction during intramedullary nailing of many types of femur fractures as well as ORIF of femoral neck, pertrochanteric, and subtrochanteric fractures.

Solution

Adapting common operating room equipment to assemble a table-mounted traction apparatus and as surgical reduction aids.

Technique

Assemble the common operating room equipment:

- "Candy cane" leg holder and rail clamp (Fig. 18-2)
- OSI (Jackson) radiolucent flat-top OR table
- Generic traction pulley (Fig. 18-3)
- Kirschner wire bow or Steinmann pin bow (Fig. 18-4)
- Sterile rope or sterile Bovie cord if rope is unavailable
- 2.4 mm × 9 inch K-wire (as a substitute for an "S" hook) (Fig. 18-5A–C)
- 5.0 or 4.5 or 4.0 Schanz pins and the matching drill bits (with soft tissue protection sleeve[s])
- Blankets
- Sterile bolsters

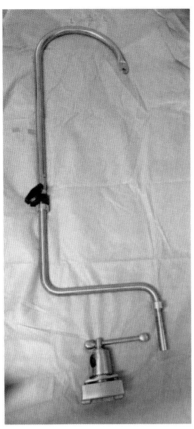

Figure 18-2 | Candy cane leg holder and rail clamp.

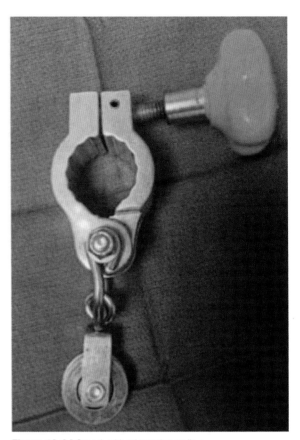

Figure 18-3 | Standard bed traction pulley.

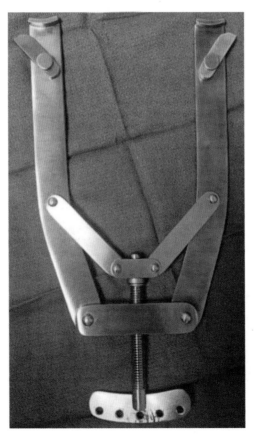

Figure 18-4 | Kirschner wire bow.

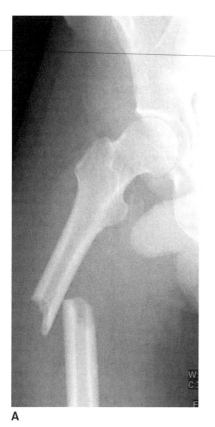

A

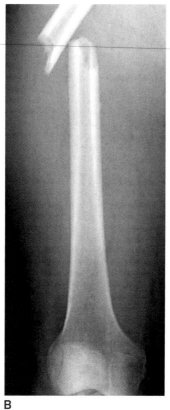

B

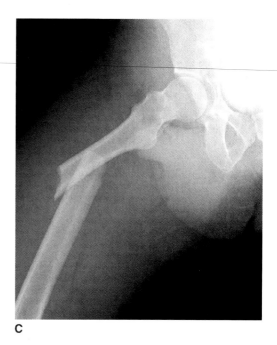

C

Figure 18-5 ▌ **A–C:** AP and lateral images of the right femur in a 54-year-old male with multiple injuries. This common operating room equipment was used in the treatment of this patient's closed right proximal third femur fracture.

- The patient is positioned supine on a flat-top OSI (Jackson) table with a bolster ("bump") under the affected limb's ischium/buttock/hemisacrum.
- The bolster is made by tightly rolling one blanket and then adding tape to secure the roll. If a greater diameter is desired, a towel or sheet may be added for obese patients (Fig. 18-6A–C).
- Maintain full spine precautions when necessary by extending the bolster along entire torso to the shoulder.

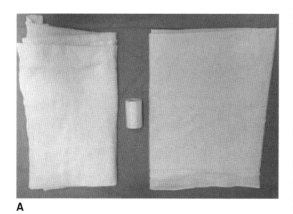

A

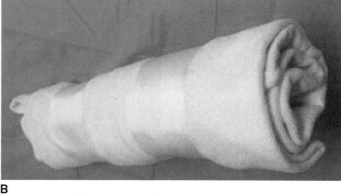

B

Figure 18-6 ▌ **A:** Blanket, tape, and sheet. **B:** One blanket roll. **C:** Blanket + sheet roll.

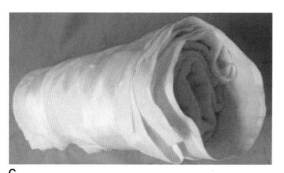

C

- Tip: The patient should be moved close to the lateral edge of the table so that the hip or trochanter is tangential to or protrudes slightly beyond the table's edge.
- Tip: For piriformis entry, place the bolster slightly more proximally and medially (under the ipsilateral hemisacrum) to permit access to the buttock soft tissues proximal to the piriformis fossa.
- Tip: If needed, C-arm imaging of the femoral entry site and of the femoral shaft can be checked to ensure high-quality AP and lateral images. Assemble the traction apparatus while anesthesia is induced.
- The candy cane leg holder is attached to the distal portion of the Jackson table's rail on the side opposite the fractured extremity.
- The height and rotation of the candy cane are adjusted as in Figure 18-7 so that the pulley is over the table, and then all clamps tightened firmly.

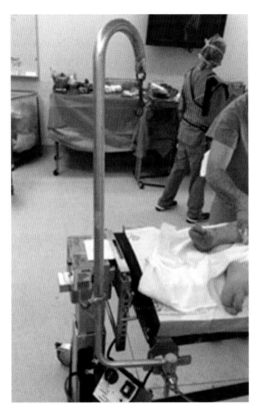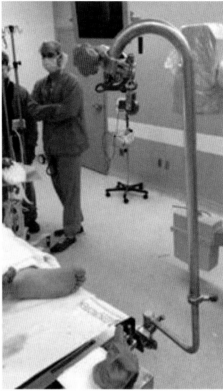

Figure 18-7 I "Candy cane" leg holder attached to left bed rail for right femur fracture. Traction pulley attached to top end of candy cane.

- A pulley is then added to the end of the candy cane. A hospital bed pulley/clamp can be used (as shown) or any pulley.
- Prior to prepping and draping, the right lower extremity is washed from toes to pelvis and right hindquarter with a hexachlorophene and alcohol prescrub and then rinsed with isopropyl alcohol and completely dried. A "U-drape" is applied to exclude the groin and perineum from the operating field.
- The extremity is then prepped and draped so that the limb is free circumferentially.
- A bump is placed under the knee, and a perfect lateral of the knee is obtained with fluoroscopy.
- A 5/64 inch (or 2 mm) K-wire is used as the traction pin, which is placed in the anterior-distal femur under fluoroscopic guidance. Avoid the central medullary canal so that traction can be maintained during IM nail placement, and the nail can be inserted posterior to the traction pin (Fig. 18-8).

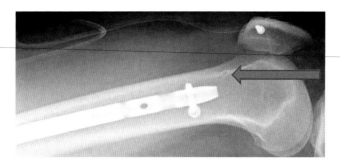

Figure 18-8 ‖ *Arrow* shows site of distal femoral traction pin used during nailing.

- The traction bow is then applied and attached to the traction rope or Bovie cord by creating a loop in the end of the sterile rope. The other end of the rope or cord is passed through the pulley to the circulating nurse who creates another loop and then applies the weight(s).
  - Tip: An "S" hook can be made by bending a 2.4-mm K-wire into an "S" with pliers.
- As the tension bow is being assembled, the C-arm can be brought to an AP of the fracture site, and an assistant can begin placing Schanz pins as reduction aids if needed.
- Schanz pins are placed percutaneously by first localizing the fracture site with fluoroscopy and then using a Freer to mark the entry site of the pin, which is approximately 4 cm from the fracture.
- A stab incision is made on the lateral thigh (through the IT band) over the entry site for the Schanz pin. A triple sleeve is inserted through the IT band to bone. The central trocar is replaced by a 3.5-mm drill bit (Fig. 18-9) inserted, and the posterior cortex of the femur is palpated with the drill tip. A 3.5-mm hole is drilled for a posterior unicortical pin or in the linea aspera. The pin should be placed out of the canal so as to not interfere with reamer or nail passage. A 5.0-mm Schanz pin is then inserted through the guide.
  - Tip: A smaller, 4.0- or 4.5-mm Schanz pin can also be used and may allow for less interference with the nail.

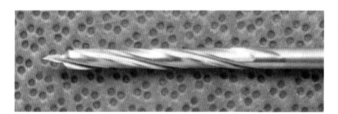

Figure 18-9 ‖ A pointed-tip drill bit allows for precise drill placement on curved, dense cortical bone surfaces.

- A second Schanz pin may be inserted into the second major bone fragment in a similar fashion.
- T-handled Jacob's chucks are affixed to the Schanz pins for control (Figs. 18-10 and 18-11).

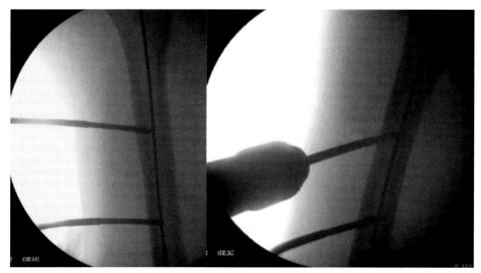

Figure 18-10 ‖ Unicortical Schanz pins used to facilitate and maintain fracture reduction.

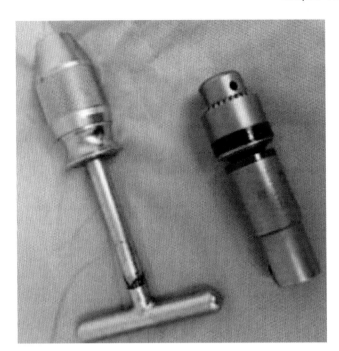

Figure 18-11 | *Left*, a T-handled Jacob's chuck. *Right*, a power tool Jacob's chuck attachment.

- Tip: A sterile towel roll may be of benefit when used to elevate a posteriorly displaced fracture fragment.
- Tip: Knee extension may also facilitate sagittal plane translation. A bolster placed under the calf will usually achieve sufficient knee extension.
- Tip: A Jacob's chuck can be used in place of a T-handled chuck, once the reduction is achieved.
- Once the fracture is reduced, traction can be reduced if length stable.
- Control of the Schanz pins should be maintained to prevent loss of reduction, especially during reaming.
- Occasionally a satisfactory reduction is achieved by traction alone (Fig. 18-12).

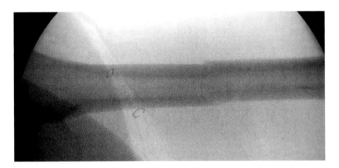

Figure 18-12 | A satisfactory reduction with traction alone.

Tips for accessing the entry site in obese patients:

- Use a "femur finder" to position a piriformis or trochanteric entry pin. These cannulated and curved awls assist in elastically bending pins around prominent trochanters and through voluminous obese soft tissues.

- Make the piriformis fossa or trochanter more accessible by adducting the proximal femoral fracture fragment. Place the lower leg and traction device in an adducted position and use the Schanz pin in the distal portion of the proximal fragment to adduct it maximally. This assists in the percutaneous insertion of the starting guide pin (Fig. 18-13).
- The entry incision for the guide pin should be proximal and posterior to the greater trochanter/piriformis fossa in order to be as coaxial as possible with the femoral intramedullary canal (Fig. 18-14).
- Once the optimal insertion site is attained, the proximal femur is opened with the cannulated opening drill bit or entry reamer. These are removed, and a ball-tipped guide rod is placed to the fracture. The fracture can now be reduced, and the guide pin is then advanced across the fracture and into a center-center position in the distal femoral metaphysis (Fig. 18-15).

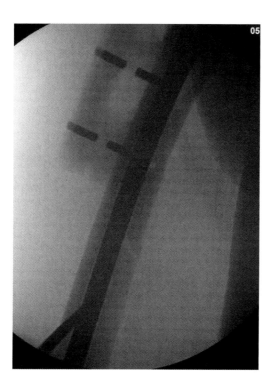

Figure 18-13 I After placement of the femoral IM nail, note the two posteriorly placed sites from the Schanz pins. The most distal Schanz pin remains in place unicortically.

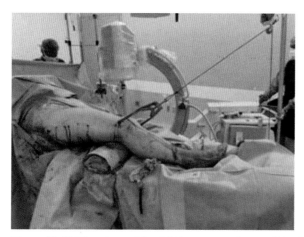
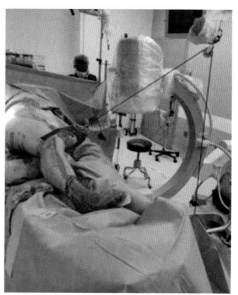

Figure 18-14 I Two views of the right lower extremity after IM nail insertion. The limb was managed with distal femoral traction on a flat-top radiolucent table.

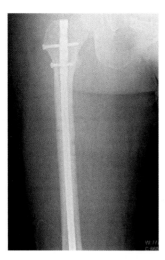
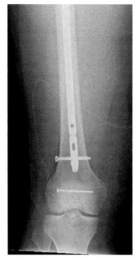
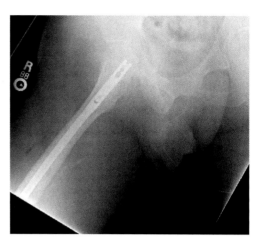

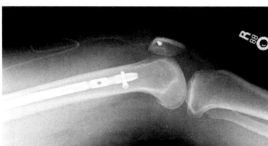

Figure 18-15 | Postoperative AP and lateral images after antegrade femoral nailing.

- A tensioned distal femoral traction pin (5/64-inch or 2.0-mm K-wire) is placed at the level of the superior pole of the patella as anteriorly as is possible to allow space to pass the guidewire/nail (Figs. 18-16 and 18-17).

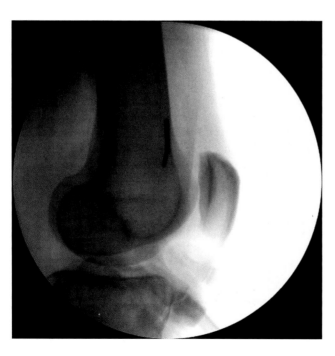

Figure 18-16 | A 2.0-mm smooth Steinmann pin is placed at the level of the superior pole of the patella, just posterior to the anterior-distal femoral cortex to allow for nail passage.

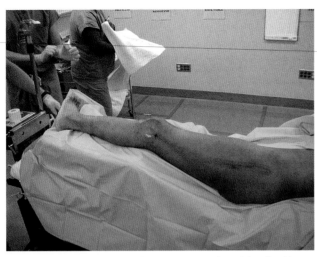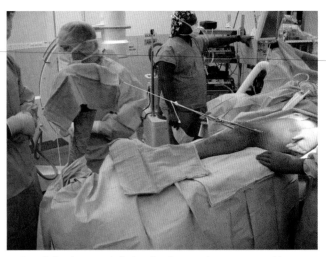

Figure 18-17 I With the traction post mounted, and the distal femoral traction pin in place, a sterile traction bow and rope are used to achieve traction. Weights are placed to hang from the rope distally off the traction post.

- Alternatively, use a femoral distractor to restore length prior to nailing.[1]
- Place a radiolucent foam ramp under the leg to elevate and assist with lateral imaging.
- Nailing without use of traction table has several advantages:
  - Ease of positioning in polytrauma patients
  - Simplified imaging
  - Access to opposite leg for comparison of length and rotational alignment
  - Circumferential access to the limb with unlimited ability to manipulate the leg to achieve reduction or starting point
  - Avoids pressure complications from perineal post
- For retrograde nailing, position supine on radiolucent flat-top table.
  - Position similar to above except the patient does not need to be positioned with the hip at off the edge of the table.
  - Do not tape the foam ramp down as it may be removed and replaced during the case to accommodate the radiolucent triangle as needed.
- Prior to prepping, place ramp under the contralateral limb and obtain comparison images to assist with rotational reduction.[2]
  - With C-arm in full lateral position (beam parallel to the floor), rotate the leg to obtain a perfect lateral view of the knee (superimposed posterior femoral condyles) and save the image.
  - While holding this exact limb rotation, rotate the C-arm up 90 degrees (beam perpendicular to the floor) and shoot AP image of the hip.
  - Center on the lesser trochanter, and magnify the lesser trochanter. Save this image.
  - Alternatively, while holding the same limb rotation, obtain a cross-table lateral image of the femoral neck (so that the neck's axis is co-linear with the proximal femoral diaphysis). This will correspond to the angle of femoral version (anteversion). Obtain the magnitude of this angular measurement from the C-arm's rotational orientation.
  - Use radiolucent ruler to accurately identify proper length (Fig. 18-18).

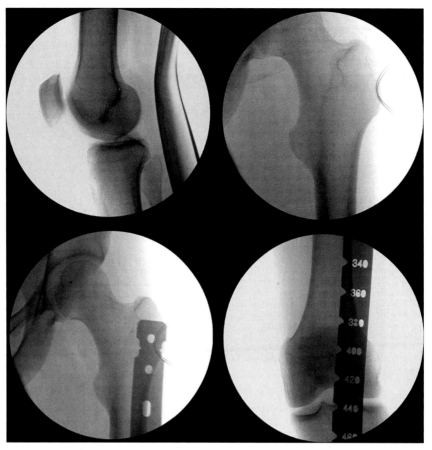

Figure 18-18 ‖ Contralateral fluoroscopic views are used to profile the lesser trochanter to ensure proper rotation of the fractured femur (*top row*). The uninjured limb is also used for length assessment (*bottom row*).

Implant and Reduction Techniques

- Percutaneous guides permit a small incision (3 to 4 cm) for nail insertion.
- Use a guidewire to locate piriformis fossa.
  - It is helpful to have the guidewire co-linear with the femoral shaft on both views (Fig. 18-19).
  - If the starting point is correct on both the AP and lateral views, but the wire's insertion angle is not optimal, a smaller cannulated drill can be used to "swallow" the guidewire (such as from the hip screw instrument set), and then the drill can be used to correct the insertion angle since it is stiffer and can provide a more controlled correction of angulation.

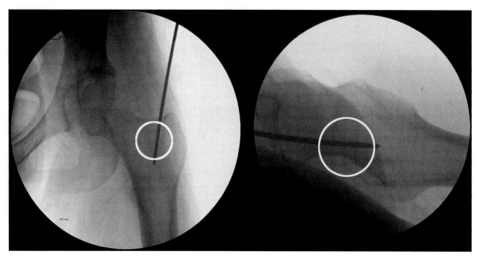

Figure 18-19 ‖ The piriformis fossa starting point is localized with a guide pin on the AP and lateral views.

- For proximal fractures, use the lateral view to assist with direction of drilling for the starting point.
  - The projection of the endosteal surface under the vastus tubercle on the C-arm can assist the surgeon in directing the guidewire. The drill/wire should be parallel to this endosteal surface (Fig. 18-20).

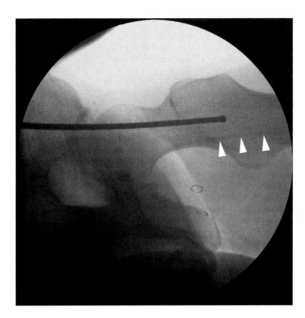

Figure 18-20 I The posterior aspect of the vastus ridge (*arrow heads*) can be visualized on the lateral view and can be used to guidewire insertion vector.

- An accurate starting point minimizes the proximal femoral stresses during nail insertion and can minimize iatrogenic fractures caused when the stiff nail is directed toward the medial, anterior, or posterior cortex.
- Trochanteric entry nails are helpful in obese patients to reduce radiation exposure, although special attention to the proper starting point is necessary to avoid varus malreduction, particularly in proximal fractures.
  - The proper starting point takes into account the degree of lateral bend built into the proximal portion of the trochanteric nail, as well as the radius of curvature of the nail. This varies by manufacturer and nail design.
  - The starting point should be just lateral to the vertical cortical density at the lateral margin of the piriformis fossa in most cases.
  - The guidewire should be directed toward a point in the center of the canal at the level of the lesser trochanter (Fig. 18-21).

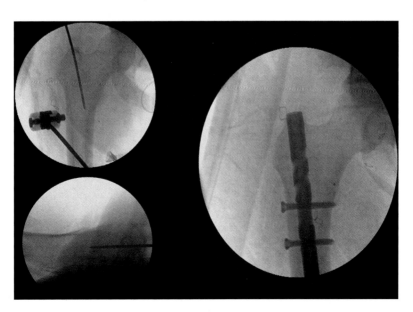

Figure 18-21 I The trochanteric starting point is generally just lateral to the piriformis fossa (*upper left*) and slightly anterior to the midline on the lateral view.

- The proper starting site for a retrograde femoral nail is the center of the intercondylar notch on an AP view and the anterior most point of Blumensaat's line on the lateral view.
- Retrograde nailing can be advantageous in specific situations:
  - When nailing ipsilateral femur and tibia fractures, the patient does not need to be repositioned
  - For very obese patients in whom a proximal starting point is difficult to obtain
  - In a polytraumatized patient for whom simultaneous upper extremity surgery is anticipated
  - For distal metaphyseal femur fractures and simple intra-articular distal femur fractures with metaphyseal extension
    - When retrograde nailing a fracture with a simple intercondylar split, clamp the fracture and place lag screws first, anticipating the nail location.
    - Screws should be placed anterior along the subchondral bone.
    - Additionally, a lag screw may be placed just posterior to the anticipated nail location (Fig. 18-22).

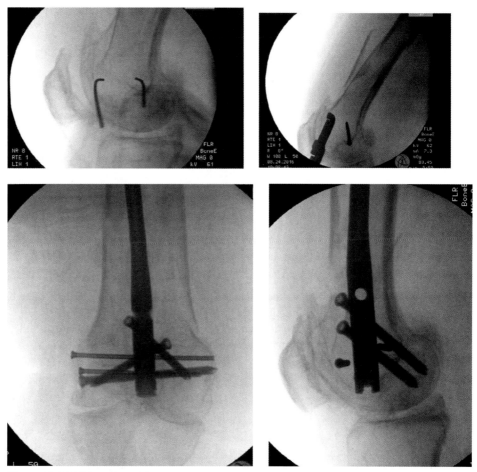

Figure 18-22 I AP and lateral fluoroscopic images demonstrating strategic lag screw placement to compress and stabilize a simple intra-articular split prior to retrograde IM nailing.

- A femoral distractor or external fixator can be used to obtain and maintain provisional reduction.
  - Pins must be placed strategically out of the way of the nail path.
  - Proximally, the pin can be placed just medial to the nail.

- Distally, the pin can be placed from anterior to posterior (unicortically or medial or lateral to the nail path) or from lateral to medial (typically posterior to the nail path in the linea aspera) (Fig. 18-23).

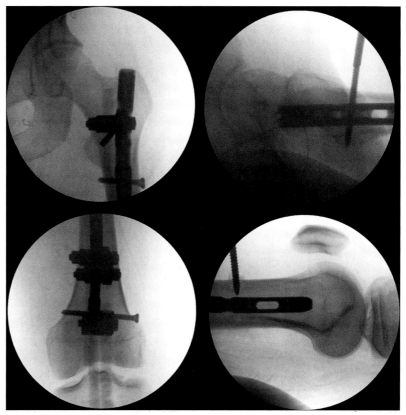

Figure 18-23 I When using an external fixator or femoral distractor, Schanz pins should be planned to avoid the nail path.

- If necessary, use percutaneously placed unicortical 5.0-mm Schanz half pins in each fragment to assist with reduction.
  - These can be placed unicortically to allow simultaneous manipulation and avoid interference during reaming (Fig. 18-24).

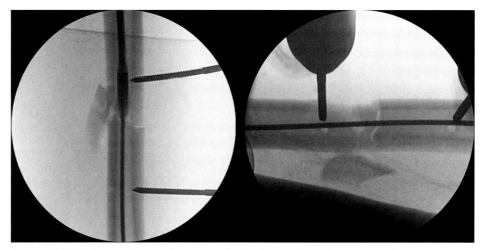

Figure 18-24 I Unicortical Schanz pins can be effective for provisional fracture reduction during guidewire placement and reaming. Self-drilling pins have a drill bit on the tip and are generally ineffective.

- Alternatively, a spiked pusher and shoulder or bone hook can be inserted percutaneously to obtain and hold reduction while reaming and inserting the nail (Fig. 18-25).

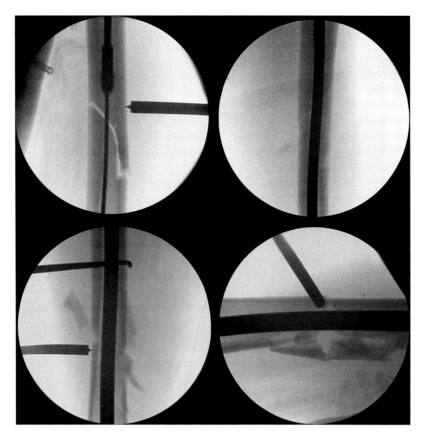

Figure 18-25 ‖ Two case examples using a ball-spike pusher (*upper row*) and a ball-spike pusher with a shoulder hook (*lower row*), both with an on-table skeletal traction, for femoral fracture reduction.

- For fractures with medial comminution, a provisional unicortical plate may be placed to realign the canal and not violate the medial soft tissue.
  - Additionally, the reamer will tend to displace medially and not ream the lateral endosteum if there is no cortex to contain it medially.
  - A bone hook can be placed around the reamer shaft to draw it laterally while reaming thus laterally, avoiding unintentional eccentric reaming and minimizing the risk of varus deformity upon seating of the nail (Fig. 18-26).

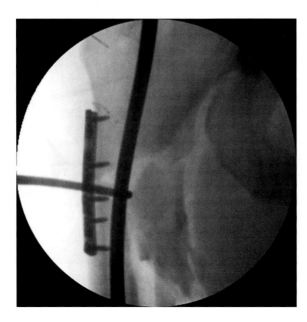

Figure 18-26 ‖ Using a provisional unicortical plate and a shoulder hook can assist in maintaining appropriate fracture reduction and reamer lateralization.

- Pass the guidewire so the ball tip is aimed at the medial tibial spine on an AP knee view.
  - A slight bend at the end of the wire prior to insertion facilitates its passage across the fracture.
    - This is also useful for making slight corrections in its distal placement by rotating the wire and then using slight mallet strikes to advance.
  - If the wire has been passed eccentrically in the distal segment, it can be difficult to redirect, as it tends to follow the previous path.
    - In this instance, a percutaneous K-wire can be strategically placed to "block" the incorrect path as it is withdrawn and reinserted (Fig. 18-27).

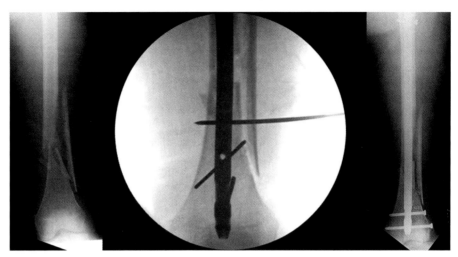

Figure 18-27 I Blocking Steinmann pins were used to direct the guidewire centrally in the distal fragment to maintain anatomic alignment.

- Verify on the lateral projection that the guidewire is posterior to the distal femoral traction pin.
- Occasionally, the nail will be blocked from final seating in the distal fragment by the traction pin.
  - Rather than removing or exchanging the traction pin, it is possible to retain the pin and pass the nail by impacting the nail against the wire, placing an intraosseous bend in the wire.
  - The nail can then be withdrawn slightly, and the traction pin rotated 90 degrees so that the "V"-shaped bend is now more anterior, allowing the nail to pass posterior to it (Fig. 18-28).

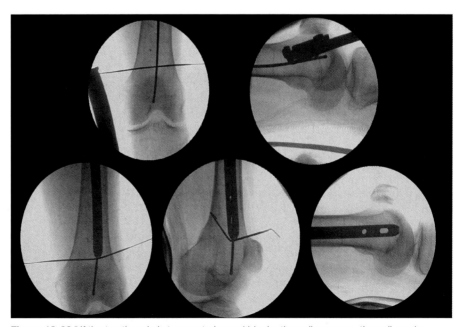

Figure 18-28 I If the traction pin is too posterior and blocks the nail passage, the nail can be impacted into the pin to create a bend, and the pin then rotated to allow the nail to pass.

Use a Retrograde Guidewire to Direct an Antegrade Femoral IM Nail

Stephen A. Kottmeier
Aden Malik

Pathoanatomy

Antegrade intramedullary nailing of infraisthmal distal femoral fractures may result in angular (or rotational) malalignment.

Solution

Placing an antegrade nail in the central portion of the distal femoral metaphysis/epiphysis is often a valuable way to avoid angular deformity (varus/valgus or flexion/extension).

Technique

There are a variety of methods that may be used to reduce the chance of an angular deformity when using a closed antegrade nailing technique for distal femoral fractures. These include the following:

- Selecting the proper entry portal
- Obtaining and maintaining fracture reduction during reaming and nail insertion
  - This may be assisted with percutaneous Schanz pins or bone clamps.
- Guiding the nail to the correct location with blocking ("Poller") screws
- Guiding the nail to the correct location with a retrograde guide pin or guidewire

The technique of using a retrograde guidewire to guide the nail to a more ideal location uses the standard retrograde nail entry site.

- This is initiated with a guide pin, which is inserted in the femoral intercondylar notch, in the midline on the AP radiograph, and at the anterior end of Blumensaat's line on the lateral image (Fig. 18-29).

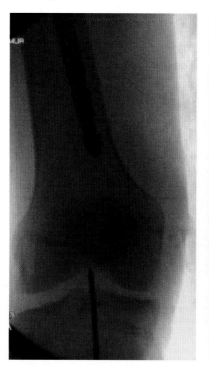
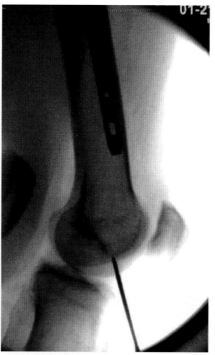

Figure 18-29 I AP and lateral images of the entry site for insertion of a retrograde guidewire.

- The guidewire's diameter should be less than approximately 3.5 to 4.0 mm so that it will enter the tip of the nail.
- If the antegrade nail has already been advanced into the distal femoral metaphysis over an antegrade guidewire, first withdraw the nail so that it is just beyond the fracture.
- Next, withdraw the antegrade guidewire and advance the distal guide pin into the tip of the nail, far enough to be secure (Fig. 18-30).

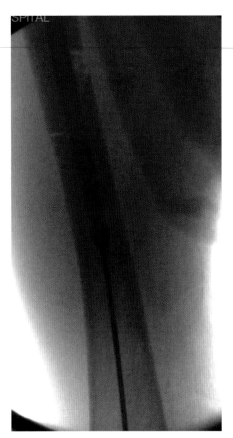
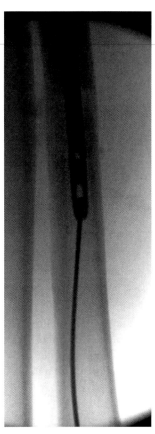

Figure 18-30 ▌ AP and lateral images of the retrograde guide pin's tip advanced into the end of the nail.

- If you do not have a guide pin of sufficient length, it may be exchanged for a second guidewire.
- Then advance the nail distally into its desired central position over the retrograde guide pin or guidewire (Fig. 18-31A and B).

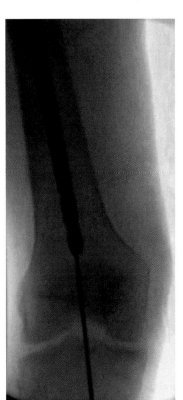
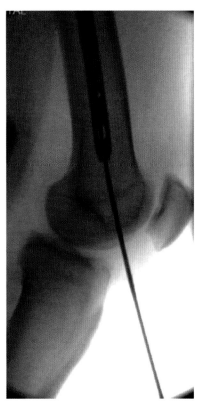

Figure 18-31 ▌ AP and lateral images showing that nail trajectory is maintained as nail in advanced into distal femoral meta-epiphysis.

- The nail should be placed into the denser bone of the distal femoral "epiphysis." Locking screws add stability, and at least one coronal plane screw should be placed before the wire is completely withdrawn.
- While this technique avoids placement of blocking screws for reduction, it permits their use if additional mechanical support is desired.
- Elderly patients frequently have an accentuated femoral bow relative to younger patients.
  - Most femoral nails on the market do not account for this increased bow and may extrude the anterior cortex whether placed antegrade or retrograde.
  - Plan for this by
    - Choosing a nail with a smaller radius of curvature (more bend)
    - Modifying the nail to increase the bend
    - Using a shorter straight nail
    - Using a starting point as anterior as feasible
- Check the lateral knee image prior to placing the distal interlocking screws.
  - The distal interlocking holes should be nearly perfect circles when the perfect knee lateral is seen, if the fracture has been reduced properly and the nail has been placed with neutral rotation.
  - When the perfect circles are not seen with a perfect lateral of the distal femur, the surgeon must determine if the fracture is malaligned or if the nail is malrotated.
- If the fracture was significantly comminuted, or in the presence of bilateral fractures, be critical of possible rotational malreductions.
  - Combining a lateral view of the knee (and nail) with the lateral view of the femoral neck will indicate the reconstructed anteversion and will ensure that no retroversion is present.
  - At the completion of the procedure, with the patient supine and with a level pelvis, flex the hips and knees simultaneously and compare the hip rotation bilaterally.
    - The total ROM should be symmetric in the absence of preoperative pathology.
  - If malrotation is a concern preoperatively, such as in segmentally comminuted fractures without good cortical apposition potential, it may be advisable to use only single interlocking screws in the proximal and distal fracture fragments.
    - If the fracture is later determined to be malrotated, it can be more easily corrected acutely by removal of the single distal interlock, derotation of the nail or fracture, and insertion of two new interlocks.
    - This technique helps to avoid a "snowman" or "planter's peanut" configuration of interlock holes, in which the new locking bolt site may be contiguous with the old hole, compromising purchase.
  - Changing the distal interlocking screw will more often allow for a native screw path, as the femoral condyles have a larger diameter compared to the proximal segment. For proximal fractures, the proximal segment is typically flexed, externally rotated, and abducted.
    - A spiked pusher placed through a stab incision can counter this displacement with a force directed posteromedially while reaming and seating the nail.[3]
  - Use as long a nail as possible.
    - The bending stress experienced by the most proximal distal interlock is inversely proportional to the distance of the bolt from the fracture site.
- For fractures with significant segmental comminution and wide displacement, stopping the reamer and manually pushing through the comminuted segment can prevent possible damage to soft tissue structures that may be displaced in the comminuted segment.

TIP

Percutaneous Removal of Incarcerated Cortical Fragments during Intramedullary Nailing

Jonathan Eastman
Reza Firoozabadi
David Barei

Pathoanatomy

When treating long bone fractures with varying degrees of comminution, it is possible for associated cortical bone fragments to become entrapped within the intramedullary canal (Fig. 18-32).

This can occur both in the proximal and/or the distal segments of the fracture and has the potential to obstruct passage of reamers and nails or create iatrogenic comminution. When a bone fragment

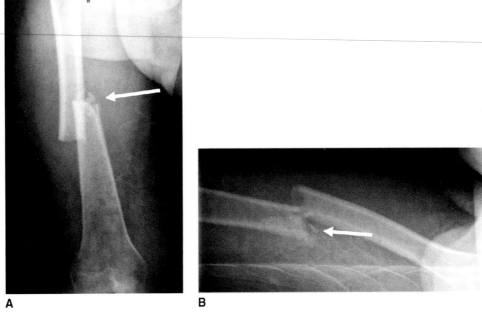

A   **B**

Figure 18-32 I Injury anteroposterior **(A)** and lateral **(B)** radiographs of the right femur demonstrating a diaphyseal femur fracture with local comminution at the fracture site (*white arrows*).

obstructs the medullary canal, retrieval, removal, or displacement of the fragment should be considered as forcing a guidewire, reamer, or nail past the fragment may drive the fragment deeper and more securely into the canal or metaphysis or create iatrogenic comminution. Commonly, these fragments can cause deformity by acting as an intramedullary blocking screw resulting in an eccentric location of the guidewire, reamer, and nail (Fig. 18-33).

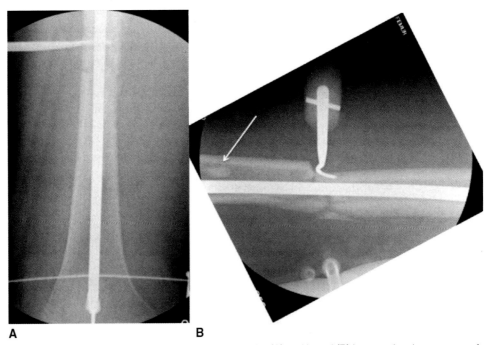

A   **B**

Figure 18-33 I Intraoperative fluoroscopic anteroposterior **(A)** and lateral **(B)** images showing passage of the reamer across the fracture. Note the deformity demonstrated on the lateral view caused by the reamer passing posterior to the incarcerated cortical fragment (*white arrow*) resulting in an extension deformity.

Solutions

Although the occurrence is relatively uncommon, the first key is to recognize the possibility or presence of an incarcerated fragment. Although opening the fracture for removal is always an option, preservation of the fracture hematoma and performing a "closed nailing" is the ideal outcome. Once detected, possible solutions may include the following.

- If the fragment is adjacent to the fracture, it may often be pushed or pulled out of the medullary canal and into the adjacent soft tissues percutaneously. Insertion of a percutaneous K-wire, dental pick, or shoulder hook at the site of the fracture may be used to move the fragment out of the medullary canal.
- If the fragment is in the distal fracture fragment, it may be pushed more distally and into the cancellous bone of the metaphysis. This may either be performed with the IM guide rod, a reamer head or an exchange tube.
- If the fragment is small and incarcerated in the bone's isthmus, it may be disrupted and fragmented by the act of reaming. This technique should be used cautiously as it may jam a reamer or cause fracture propagation and iatrogenic comminution.
- If the fragment is obstructing the proximal fracture segment, it may be pushed distally, into the fracture and then into the surrounding soft tissues with a variety of instruments inserted via the entry portal (guide rods, small reamers, exchange tubes).
- Intramedullary cortical fracture fragments may also be retrieved using rigid or flexible intramedullary graspers or similar instruments used by ENT surgeons.

By working through percutaneous incisions, a formal open approach is avoided. Maintaining the surrounding soft tissues minimizes further operative time, surgical dissection, blood loss, and disruption of the local fracture biology. This ultimately reduces the surgical burden to the patients and minimizes the chance of operative and postoperative complications. The technique described and illustrated below is safe, uses preexisting incisions, and allows for extraction or relocation of the incarcerated fragment without excessive surgical trauma to the limb.[1]

Technique

- Once the incarcerated fragment is detected, attempts to ream through the fragment as well as removal by backing up the reamer and ball-tipped guidewire can be made cautiously.
- Before making a formal open approach for fragment retrieval, acquire a long narrow endoscopic grasper (Encision, Boulder, CO) (Fig. 18-34) for fragment extraction.

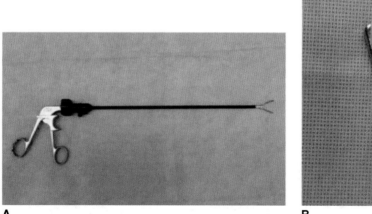
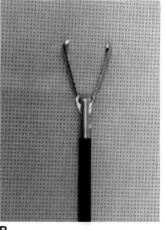

A   **B**

Figure 18-34 I Clinical photographs depicting the endoscopic grasper (Encision, Boulder, CO). The full-length view **(A)** demonstrates the handle and turning mechanism. The close-up view of the distal end **(B)** demonstrates the serrated jaws in detail.

- When a bone fragment is within the medullary canal of the distal femoral bone fragment, the proximal femoral segment should be reamed 1.0 to 1.5 cm larger than intended nail size.
  - This facilitates passage of the intramedullary grasper and may create sufficient medullary space for simultaneous removal of the grasper and the bone fragment.
- Using the same proximal skin incision, the grasper is placed through the existing entry portal and into the canal (Fig. 18-35).
- The grasper is passed down through the proximal segment, across the fracture site and into the distal segment. The fragment is grasped and brought back to just proximal of the fracture site (Fig. 18-36).
- Small bone fragments can be removed entirely from the canal through the proximal entry.

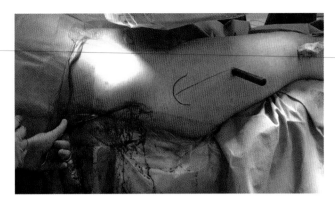

Figure 18-35 | Clinical intraoperative photograph demonstrating the insertion of the grasper through the 3-cm preexisting skin incision in the proximal thigh and femoral entry portal.

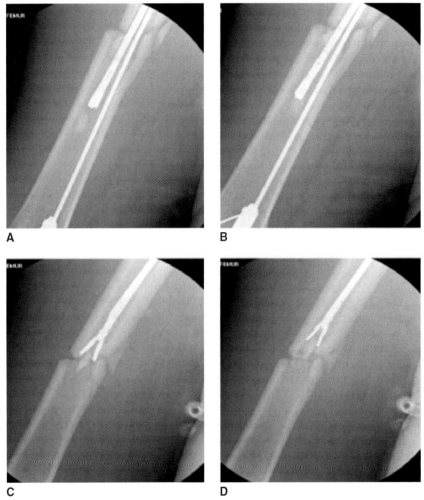

Figure 18-36 | Intraoperative lateral fluoroscopic images demonstrating the endoscopic grasper inside the intramedullary canal **(A)**, grasping one of the incarcerated fragments **(B)**, withdrawal of the fragment back to the fracture site **(C)**, and into the proximal segment **(D)**.

- If, due to size, orientation, or inability to maintain control, the fragment cannot be removed through the proximal fracture, it can be placed in the soft tissues adjacent to the fracture outside of the intramedullary canal.
  - While maintaining control of the fragments, the fracture is manually displaced with a percutaneously inserted instrument (ball-spike pusher), and the fragments were released into the soft tissues adjacent to the fracture site (Fig. 18-37).
- With the fragments out of the way, the guidewire and reamers were passed without incident. Surgical stabilization can continue and routine healing can occur (Fig. 18-38).

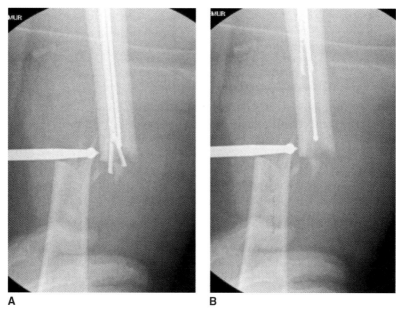

Figure 18-37 I Intraoperative fluoroscopic anteroposterior images demonstrating ball-spike pusher displacing the proximal segment medially. The grasped incarcerated fragment is placed outside the intramedullary canal **(A)** and released into the surrounding soft tissues **(B)**.

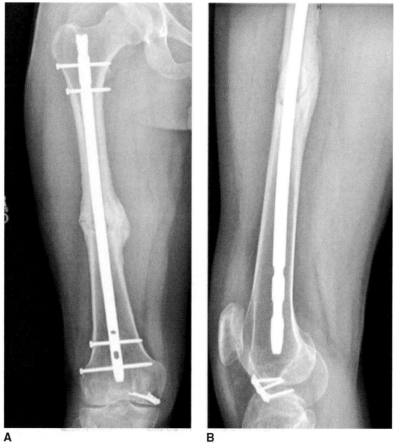

Figure 18-38 I Anteroposterior **(A)** and lateral **(B)** radiographic images at 6-month follow-up visit showing maintained alignment and osseous healing.

Reference

1. Eastman J, Firoozabadi R, Cook L, et al. Incarcerated cortical fragments in intramedullary nailing. *Orthopedics.* 2016;39(3): e582–e586.

Cortical Window for Intramedullary Foreign Body

James Learned

Pathoanatomy

The presence of a ballistic (or other) foreign body within the medullary canal of a long bone can prevent certain common treatments and could potentially make treating future conditions (traumatic or atraumatic/degenerative) more difficult.

Solution

To provide a method of safe extraction of an incarcerated body within the medullary canal whose presence prevents the insertion of intramedullary implants.

Technique

- A 24-year-old male suffered a ballistic femur fracture with incarceration of the major bullet fragment within the medullary canal of the left femur. The fracture was minimally displaced, but extensive comminution was visible on initial radiography (Fig. 18-39).

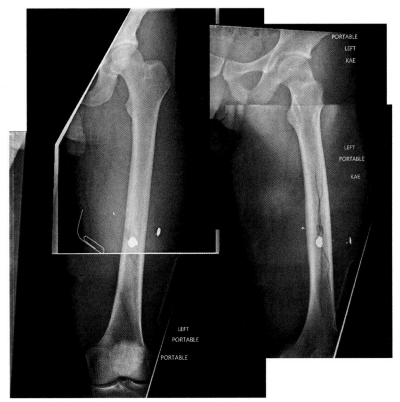

Figure 18-39 I Injury films.

- Aside from the foreign body, the fracture pattern lent itself to intramedullary fixation. However, the position of the bullet fragment made intramedullary nailing difficult and fraught with potential major intraoperative and postoperative complications, such as further incarceration, iatrogenic fracture or displacement, instrument fracture, and potential plumbism.
- Extraction via the antegrade starting point was preferred, but available instrumentation was not of sufficient length, and we doubted there was enough room to grasp the bullet fragment with a pituitary rongeur or other long grasper and for both to pass simultaneous through the femoral isthmus.
- We elected to create a cortical window, using a technique similar to that commonly used for grafting depressed tibial plateau fractures.
- The patient was positioned in the standard semilateral position for intramedullary nailing with the ipsilateral hemipelvis and entire lower extremity prepped in the field.
- A lateral subvastus approach to the femoral shaft was performed after radiographically targeting the position of the fragments, and multiple drill holes were made in a 2- × 3-cm rectangle. Osteotomes were used to connect the drill holes, and an anterior hinge of the periosteum was maintained.

- The ballistic foreign body was easily extracted using a Freer elevator, and copious irrigation was run through the wound. We then proceeded with a standard reamed, antegrade femoral nail with proximal and distal transverse interlocking screws (Fig. 18-40).
- The cortical window fragment was maintained in position with a ball-spike pusher during medullary reaming to avoid eccentric reaming, and the patient was allowed to weight bear as tolerated on the involved limb immediately after surgery.
- The patient returned for a single postoperative visit (Fig. 18-41) but was lost to follow-up after that point.

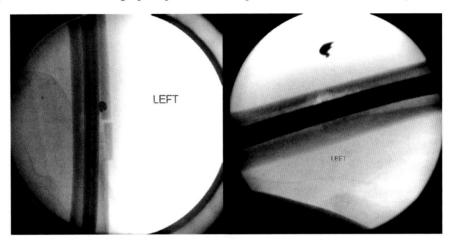

Figure 18-40 ▌ Intraoperative fluoroscopy.

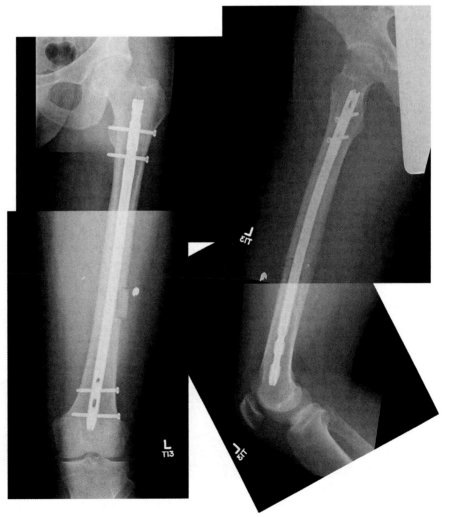

Figure 18-41 ▌ Radiographs at first postoperative visit.

- For segmental fractures, a limited open approach to the proximal fracture allows for accurate reduction and temporary clamp placement.
  - This can remain in place while reaming.
  - This effectively converts the fracture into a simple pattern while addressing the segment most likely to be malreduced.
  - This can simplify treatment and expedite the procedure.
- Blocking screws, wires, or Steinmann pins can be used to effectively narrow the canal near the metaphyseal flares, providing improved ability to obtain and maintain reductions when intramedullary fixation is chosen for fractures in these areas (Figs. 18-42 and 18-43).

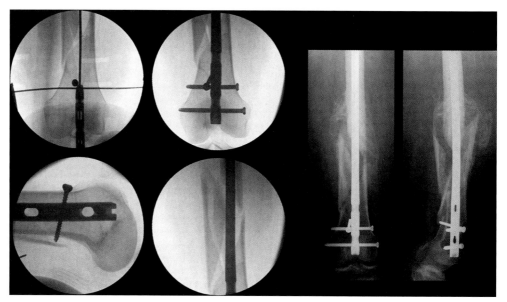

Figure 18-42 I In this distal femoral shaft fracture, a blocking screw was used at the convexity of the deformity to obtain and maintain the reduction.

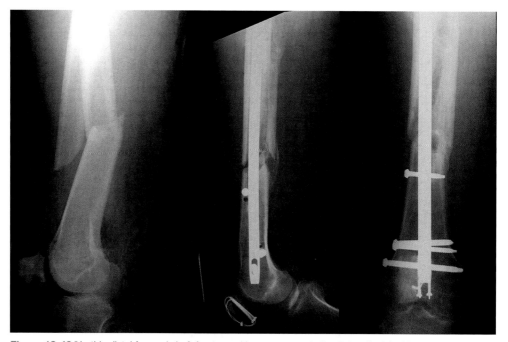

Figure 18-43 I In this distal femoral shaft fracture with an apex posterior deformity, blocking screws were used with an antegrade nail to achieve an anatomic alignment.

- Post nailing, check four things before waking the patient up.
  - The femoral neck for an occult neck fracture.
    - This requires a good AP or internal rotation fluoroscopic view.
  - Symmetry of lower limb lengths and limb segment lengths.
  - Symmetry of lower extremity rotation.
    - Confirm by observing the passive limb rotation with the patient's pelvis level and actively confirm the clinical symmetry of hip rotation.
  - Examine the knee ligaments for the presence or absence of concomitant injury.
  - Palpate the thigh and calf to ensure all compartments are soft.

Troubleshooting: Correcting Length and Rotation Problems

- For objective data regarding rotation, a postoperative CT scan with fine cuts through both knees and hips can provide precise data regarding the fracture rotation and nail rotation by comparing anteversion to the uninjured side.
  - This information is useful in determining which segment to rotate (proximal or distal) and the exact magnitude (Fig. 18-44).

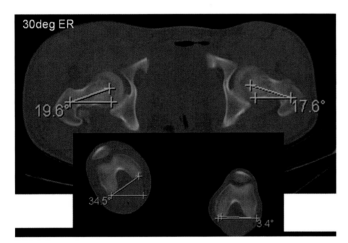

Figure 18-44 CT version studies can identify rotational deformities.

- For correction of rotational malreduction, use Schanz pins in each segment as rotational guides.
  - An external fixator can also be used to maintain length during rotation and may give more precise control.
  - The Schanz pins should be strategically placed around the nail so as not to interfere with subsequent rotation (Fig. 18-45).
- For an overlengthened, yet rotationally correct, limb segment, which needs an axial correction less than the total longitudinal length of the slotted hole, a screw can be placed in the distal portion of the slotted hole, and then the proximal screw removed permitting the fracture to be compressed until the locking screw is seated at the proximal extent of the slot.
  - Similarly, the reverse is also possible for a fracture previously stabilized too short.
  - In this situation, an additional locking screw can be placed in the proximal extent of the slot and the fracture distracted by the length of the slot.

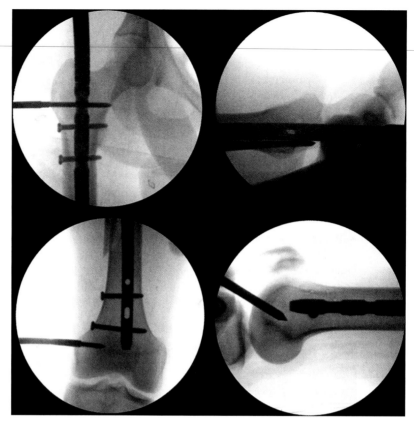

Figure 18-45 To derotate a rotationally malaligned femur, Schanz pins should be placed strategically around the nail prior to removing interlocking screws, to allow for a controlled derotation maneuver.

References

1. McFerran MA, Johnson KD. Intramedullary nailing of acute femoral shaft fractures without a fracture table: technique of using a femoral distractor. *J Orthop Trauma.* 1992;6:271–278.
2. Krettek C, Miclau T, Grun O, et al. Intraoperative control of axes, rotation and length in femoral and tibial fractures. Technical note. *Injury.* 1998;29(Suppl 3):C29–C39.
3. Browner BD. Pitfalls, errors, and complications in the use of locking Kuntscher nails. *Clin Orthop Relat Res.* 1986;(212):192–208.

Chapter 19
Periprosthetic Fractures of the Femur

WILLIAM W. CROSS III
MICHAEL F. GITHENS
M. BRADFORD HENLEY
EDWARD R. WESTRICK
BRANDON J. YUAN

Instruments and Equipment

- Radiolucent flat-top table
- On-table traction device if planning retrograde nail
- Universal distractor or large external fixator
- Tabletop bender
- Large and small standard and modified Weber clamps
- Large and small serrated reduction clamps
- Bone hook/spike pusher
- 2.5-, 4.0-, and 5.0-mm Schanz pins
- K-wires and wire driver/drill
- 18 gauge wire or 1.7-mm cable and wire passer
- Implants
  - Anatomically contoured locking plates
  - Retrograde nail

Patient Positioning

For a Vancouver C femur fracture below a total hip stem, the patient is positioned laterally.

- Allows easy extensile access to the lateral femur and easy limb manipulation.
- Axillary roll.
- Up arm over a universal arm holder.
- Down leg padded and surrounded by folded blankets to create a stable working platform.
- Thin layer of blankets in between the legs.
- Alternatively, prefabricated foam may be used for leg positioning.

For distal femur fractures above a total knee arthroplasty or distal femur interprosthetic fractures, the patient is positioned supine if minimally invasive bridge plating is to be performed with indirect reduction or laterally if direct open reduction of a simple fracture pattern is planned.

- The patient is positioned as high up on the bed as possible if using on-table traction.
- A padded bolster is placed under the ipsilateral torso and hemipelvis and a radiolucent foam ramp under the operative limb.
- Ipsilateral arm is draped over the chest, padded, and secured.

Surgical Approaches

- For a Vancouver C femur fracture below a total hip where an anatomic reduction with interfragmentary compression and neutralization plate placement is planned, an extensile lateral approach is used.
  - An incision following the long axis of the femur is made over the lateral thigh, extending to the level of the distal femoral metaphyseal flare.
  - The IT band is incised sharply, exposing the underlying vastus lateralis.
  - The vastus lateralis is elevated off of the lateral intermuscular septum and femur from distal to proximal.
  - The periosteum should be left intact on the femur.
  - Large perforating arterioles are suture ligated above the intermuscular septum to avoid bleeding.
  - The posterior origin of the vastus lateralis is elevated off the vastus ridge and tagged with heavy suture for later repair.
- Alternatively, if a bridging construct is planned, a limited direct distal lateral approach is used for percutaneous extraperiosteal antegrade or retrograde plate insertion.
- Distal femoral fractures above a total knee arthroplasty or distal femur interprosthetic fractures (between a total hip femoral stem and knee prosthesis) are typically treated with a bridging construct; thus, a limited lateral approach for plate insertion is made.
- If a retrograde nail is planned, the previous total knee incision with a medial parapatellar arthrotomy is used to expose the knee joint.

Reduction and Implant Techniques

Vancouver C Fractures

- Simple patterns including transverse, short and long oblique fractures may be treated with a direct reduction and interfragmentary compression (Fig. 19-1).

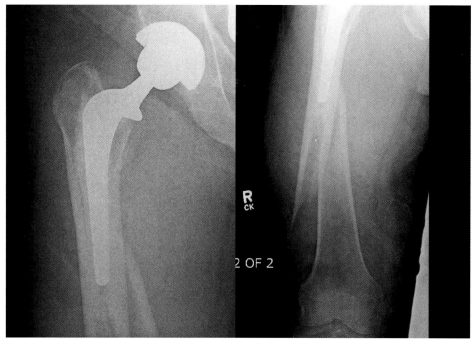

Figure 19-1 ▌ AP radiographs demonstrating a periprosthetic proximal femur fracture with a long oblique pattern. Planned strategy is direct anatomic reduction, lag screw fixation, and long neutralization plate.

- This is achieved with clamp application in appropriate vectors followed by 2.7- or 3.5-mm lag screw fixation (Fig. 19-2).
- Lag screws should be countersunk to distribute compression forces; avoid fracture propagation and interference with plate application.

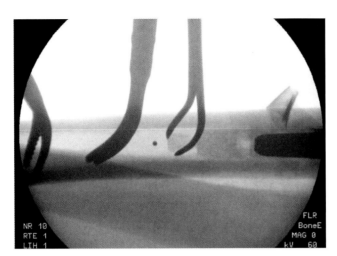

Figure 19-2 | Intraoperative fluoroscopy image demonstrating direct reduction of a long oblique fracture with open clamping. Clamps will be replaced with lag screws in the same vectors.

Biological Application of Cerclage Wire for Anatomic Reduction and Fixation of Periprosthetic Femur Fractures

Brandon J. Yuan
William W. Cross

Pathoanatomy

Periprosthetic femur fractures are often low-energy injuries with spiral or oblique fracture morphologies and minimal comminution. Anatomic reduction of these fractures with rigid interfragmentary compression allows for early weight bearing, which is advantageous in this more elderly patient population. Cerclage wire fixation of periprosthetic femur fractures is often necessary to supplement fixation in the presence of a medullary implant that may prevent more standard lag screw compression across thin, osteoporotic cortices of an oblique fracture.

Solution

Biological application of one or two cerclage wires with minimal soft tissue stripping around a spiral fracture allows for relatively simple reduction of the diaphyseal fracture while simultaneously applying interfragmentary compression without interfering with planned plate application.

Technique

- The fracture is exposed in the standard fashion, using an extensile lateral incision and subvastus approach to the lateral aspect of the femur (Fig. 19-3).
  - Lateral positioning can help to reduce sagittal plane deformity and aids in obtaining length intraoperatively.
- Plan for placement of one or two cerclage wires depending on the obliquity and length of the fracture by sharply releasing (e.g., nicking) the intermuscular septum from the linea aspera at the posterior aspect of the femur for 4 to 5 mm.

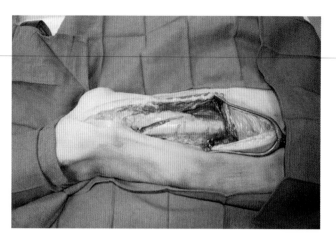

Figure 19-3 | The fracture is exposed through a standard extensile lateral incision and subvastus approach to the femur. Care is taken to expose the fracture without stripping the periosteum.

- Placing a cable passer though this small aperture (Fig. 19-4), a cerclage wire is passed around the femur in a submuscular and extraperiosteal manner with minimal stripping of soft tissue attachments.

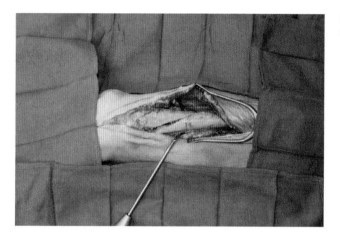

Figure 19-4 | Wire passer is placed around the fracture from posterior to anterior.

- In a similar fashion, a second wire is passed around the fracture (Fig. 19-5).

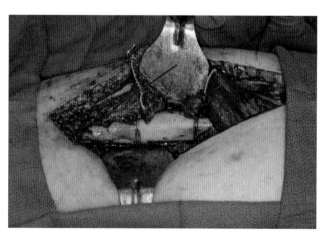

Figure 19-5 | Depending on the length and obliquity of the fracture, two wires can be placed around the fracture.

- The wires are sequentially tightened by the surgeon while an assistant provides traction and rotational control of the distal segment to key in an anatomic reduction of the fracture. If an assistant is not available, a universal distractor is also an effective reduction tool.
- The ends of the wires should be secured toward the anterior side of the femur so the cut ends of the wires will not interfere with later lateral plate application.

- The increasing tension in the wires assists greatly with regaining length along the oblique fracture plane, and often, all that is required is fine-tuning of the rotation of the distal fragment to obtain an anatomic reduction (Fig. 19-6).

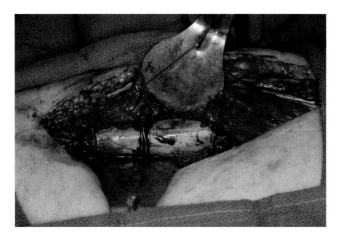

Figure 19-6 ▌ The reduction is fine-tuned as the wires are tightened. The wires should be tightened at the anterior aspect of the femur to allow for lateral plate application.

- Final tightening of the wires secures the reduction and provides interfragmentary compression, even in the presence of a medullary implant (Fig. 19-7).

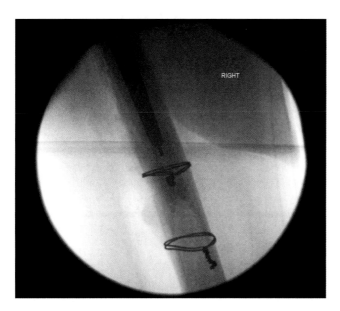

Figure 19-7 ▌ AP radiograph demonstrating anatomic alignment and compression of a periprosthetic fracture in an area of the femur that otherwise would not allow placement of a lag screw.

- Standard lag screws may be added below (or above) the tip of the medullary implant. A lateral neutralization plate can be applied to the femur in the standard fashion on top of the cerclage wires (Fig. 19-8). The wires may remain in situ, or they may be removed after plate application.

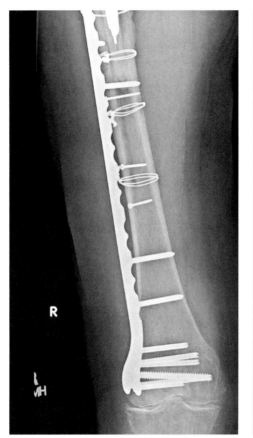 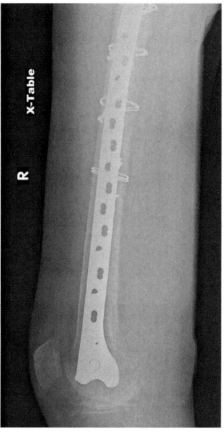

Figure 19-8 ▌ AP and lateral radiographs of a periprosthetic femoral shaft fracture that was reduced and compressed with cerclage wires using the described technique. The fracture was further compressed with lag screws below the cemented implant and neutralized with a lateral locked plate.

- - Transverse patterns may be compressed using a modified straight-straight Weber clamp.
  - Alternatively, a short 3.5-mm LC-DC plate may be placed on the anterior (or anterolateral) femur in compression mode prior to definitive lateral plate placement.
- Comminuted patterns should be treated with an indirect reduction and bridge plating to achieve relative stability.
  - These patterns may be more effectively treated in a supine or sloppy lateral position rather than direct lateral position.
  - Multiple methods may be used for an indirect reduction.
    - Skeletal traction application with a plate-assisted reduction is often successful.
  - Additional manipulative devices include percutaneously applied Schanz pins, bone hooks, and spike pushers.
  - A large external fixator or femoral distractor deployed anteriorly may be helpful in obtaining and maintaining reduction.

- A long lateral plate is applied, spanning the entire femur, obtaining fixation in the proximal and distal metaphyseal femur (Fig. 19-9).

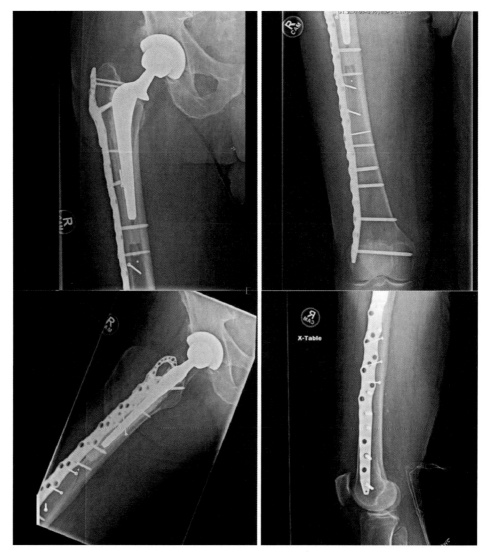

Figure 19-9 I After lag screw placement, the entire femur is spanned with a neutralization plate. Fixation around the stem is achieved with variable angle locking screws.

- A plate spanning the femur from the vastus lateralis ridge to the distal femoral lateral epicondyle will protect from future peri-implant fracture.
- This plate will require contouring with a plate bender to fit appropriately.
- In cases with segmental comminution where overall coronal and sagittal alignment is difficult to judge under fluoroscopy, a flat plate radiograph of the full femur is obtained after a provisional reduction is obtained but before completion of definitive fixation to allow for adjustment before committing to the implant and the reduction.
- Fixation in the proximal femur depends on the size and type of existing hip prosthesis.
  - Current plating systems offer the ability to place smaller (4.0-mm) screws with variable angle technology.
  - This typically allows for several bicortical screws anterior and posterior to the prosthesis stem.
  - Unicortical locking screws may be placed to augment fixation laterally to the femoral component, although they should not be relied upon as the only form of proximal fixation.
  - If no bicortical screw can be placed around the prosthesis, cables should be used in a biologically friendly manner.

Distal Periprosthetic and Distal Interprosthetic Femur Fractures:

- Ensure that the total knee femoral component is well fixed before proceeding with operative reduction and fixation by closely scrutinizing the radiographs, and obtain a CT scan if necessary.
- Most commonly, these injuries involve metaphyseal comminution and should be treated with an indirect reduction and fixation with relative stability (Fig. 19-10).
  - Can be achieved with either a lateral locking plate or retrograde IM nail.
  - Nailing requires a total knee implant with an open box in the femoral component.

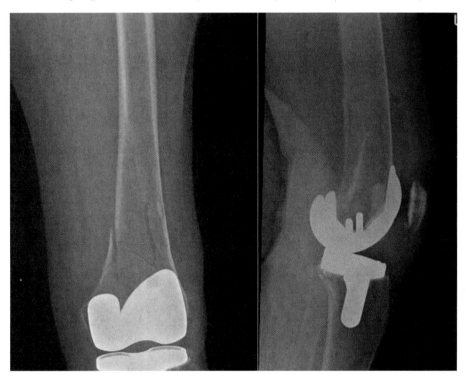

Figure 19-10 | AP and lateral radiographs demonstrating a distal femoral periprosthetic femur fracture above a well-fixed femoral component. While not significantly displaced, this pattern is multifragmentary and should be treated with a relative stability construct.

- Application of distal femoral or proximal tibial skeletal traction may restore length and alignment.
  - The typical deformity in the sagittal plane is an extension deformity.
  - If the distal femoral traction pin is placed in the anterior distal femur, it will aid in reduction of an extension deformity (Fig. 19-11, right).

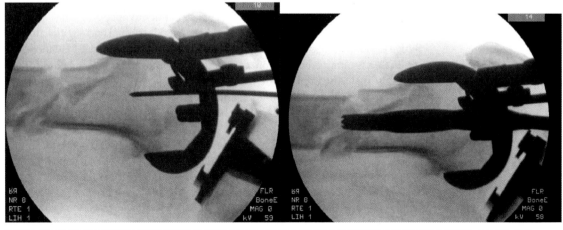

Figure 19-11 | Intraoperative fluoroscopic images demonstrating opening guidewire and reamer position. Length and alignment have been restored with distal femoral skeletal traction placed anteriorly in the distal femur, out of the way of the nailing instruments. Additionally, folded towels placed under the fracture assist in correcting the extension deformity.

- Adding a towel bump under the fracture's apex will also aid in correcting extension.
- If there is overreduction leading to a flexion deformity, the traction pin can be placed in the posterior distal femur or in the proximal tibia.
- Deformity in the coronal plane is less predictable.
- The on-table traction device can be moved from the ipsilateral side to the contralateral side of the table and vice versa to help correct coronal plane malalignment.
- Alternatively, a combination of blocking screws, Schanz pins, bone hooks, and spike pushers may be employed to manipulate the proximal and distal segments directly or indirectly.
- Retrograde IM nailing:
  - The guide pin is placed in the femoral component's open box, and the opening reamer is used to open the medullary canal, taking care not to damage the polyethylene insert or femoral implant (Fig. 19-11).
  - The ball tip guidewire is advanced intramedullary, until proximal to the lesser trochanter.
  - A 10-, 11-, or 12-mm reamer may be advanced through the femoral isthmus as a sounding device to determine nail diameter, but sequential reaming is typically not necessary in this osteopenic patient population.
  - The nail is placed over the guidewire and provisionally held with drilling wires.
  - Full-length flat plate radiographs are obtained to confirm alignment in the sagittal and coronal plane before placing locking bolts.
  - If alignment is suboptimal, there is still opportunity to correct the reduction around the nail in this patient group given their relative osteoporosis.
    - For an extension deformity, the deformity can be corrected by applying a flexion moment to the nail jig, followed by placement of a blocking wire or Poller screw directly behind the nail in either the proximal or distal segment.
    - Alternatively, the nail can be backed out and a blocking screw placed with readvancement of the nail.
    - If correction by manipulation of the nail-mounted targeting jig is insufficient, a 4.0-mm Schanz pin is placed percutaneously from anterior to posterior just above the implant flange and used as a joystick to flex or extend the distal segment.
    - The surgeon may intentionally leave a small extension deformity to ensure the patient achieves full knee extension postoperatively, given that many patients have pre-existing small flexion contractures.
    - For coronal plane angular problems, the same blocking screw and Schanz pin techniques may be used.
    - Once distal interlocking bolts are placed, consider releasing some traction to ensure fracture site bone contact is present and that the fracture is not distracted.
    - Prior to placing proximal interlocking bolts, rotation is confirmed by obtaining a perfect lateral view of the knee, and then, without changing the rotation of the leg or the image intensifier, a lateral hip image is obtained. Version of the femoral neck should match that of the uninjured side's anteversion (±10 to 15 degrees).
    - Proximal interlocking bolts are placed using perfect circle technique in the AP direction.
    - Patients are allowed to weight bear as tolerated as soon as they gain quadriceps control.
- Bridge plating:
  - Indirect, often a plate assisted reduction.
  - If significantly short, consider skeletal traction or a universal distractor.
    - Do not overlengthen. Some surgeons advocate leaving some degree of shortening to encourage union.
  - A lateral locking plate is inserted through a small lateral incision and passed retrograde in an extraperiosteal subvastus lateralis plane.
  - Once length and sagittal plane alignment are obtained, the plate is affixed to the proximal and distal segments with pins or wires.
    - The plate should sit slightly anteriorly on the femoral shaft.
    - The anterior border of the plate should lie directly adjacent to the femoral component's lateral border (Fig. 19-12).
    - Proper plate placement will prevent the introduction of deformity with screw placement.
  - Coronal plane malalignment can be corrected with a whirly-bird device.
    - If unsure of alignment, full-length flat plate radiographs are obtained.
    - Medial metaphyseal comminution is left undisturbed as this serves as a critical healing zone.

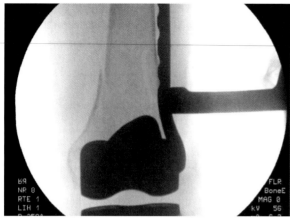
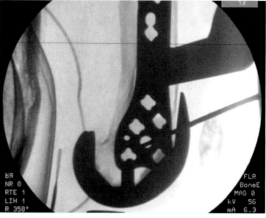

Figure 19-12 | Intraoperative fluoroscopy demonstrating appropriate distal plate placement. The anterior aspect of the distal plate is placed just adjacent to the lateral border of the femoral component. Note the percutaneously applied pin being used to correct sagittal plane alignment on the lateral view.

- The plate is first fixed to the distal segment with a cortical screw to compress the plate to the bone, followed by locking screws.
- If the plate's contour matches the femoral geometry well, it can be affixed to the femoral diaphysis first with a proximal pin and then with a cortical screw.
- If there is a small plate-femur mismatch in the presence of a good reduction, locking screws are used alone to avoid inducing a malreduction with cortical screw placement.
- Construct stiffness is modulated by thoughtful screw spacing and screw density.
  - Too many screws and multiple screws near each other create an overly stiff construct and may induce a nonunion.
- Additionally, unicortical screws can be placed to decrease construct stiffness but should be used sparingly and not in isolation (Fig. 19-13).

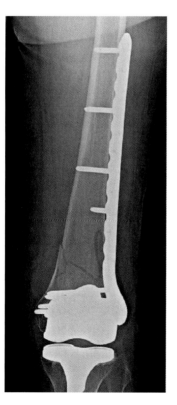
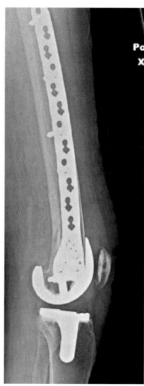

Figure 19-13 | Low screw density, appropriate screw spacing, and a unicortical screw near the fracture have been used to avoid an overly stiff construct.

- In severely osteoporotic patients or in fractures with segmental metaphyseal comminution, additional fixation may be beneficial.
  - Allows early unrestricted full weight bearing.
  - Several options exist to combat this problem.

TIP

Dual Plating for Periprosthetic and Osteoporotic Femur Fractures

Edward R. Westrick

Pathoanatomy

The incidence of periprosthetic femur fractures continues to increase as the number of total hip and knee arthroplasty procedures increases. These fractures are affecting both younger patients and those with worsening bone quality. Salvage of a previously well-functioning prosthesis, rather than conversion to "megaprosthesis," is important, especially in young patients. Similarly, distal femur fractures in patients with advanced osteoporosis present a unique challenge to the surgeon.

Solution

Anatomic reduction and dual plating of periprosthetic femur fractures involving total hip and total knee implants allow salvage of the prosthesis and earlier weight bearing compared to single-plate fixation. Dual plating of osteoporotic intercondylar femur fractures, with vacuous metadiaphyseal bone and anterior cortical comminution, similarly provides stable fixation and allows early weight bearing.

Technique

Sterile Implants/Equipment
- Medium and large pointed reduction clamps
- Femoral distractor or large external fixator
- Shoulder hook/bone hook
- K-wires and wire driver/drill
- Cerclage cables/cerclage wires
- Implants:
  - Periarticular precontoured femur plates, proximal or distal
  - Small fragment nonlocking/locking plate sets
  - Large fragment nonlocking/locking plate sets

Patient Positioning

- For periprosthetic fractures around a total hip arthroplasty, the patient may be placed supine or lateral on a radiolucent table, depending on surgeon preference and the possibility of revision arthroplasty.
- Supine positioning is used for fractures around total knee implants, to allow easier transition, should revision arthroplasty become necessary.
- The C-arm is positioned on the contralateral side of the operating table or on the patient's front if lateral decubitus.

Surgical Approaches

- Determined by the fracture pattern.
- For fractures around a total hip arthroplasty, the previous lateral incision with elevation of the vastus lateralis may be used and is extensile.
  - This would also be the preferred approach for previous anterior total hip arthroplasty.
- For fractures around a total knee arthroplasty, the previous medial or lateral parapatellar arthrotomy may be used, and this allows full visualization of the prosthesis and fracture.
  - This approach also allows easier revision arthroplasty, if necessary.
  - If a medial parapatellar arthrotomy is used, a separate small direct lateral approach may be necessary for placement of the distal screws in the lateral condylar buttress plate.

Reduction and Fixation Techniques

- Spiral femur fractures (Fig. 19-14) around a femoral stem are reduced with multiple pointed reduction clamps.
  - Interfragmentary lag screws and/or cerclage cables are used as necessary.

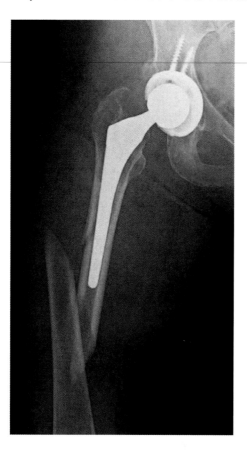

Figure 19-14 ▌ A segmental periprosthetic femur fracture around a well-fixed stem, in an elderly osteoporotic patient.

- The lateral plate is placed in the standard fashion, typically to span the entire femur.
- The orthogonal plate may be placed anteriorly or posteriorly, based on access through the previous incision, and ideally avoiding excessive stripping of fracture fragments.
- Bicortical screws are placed around the femoral stem, in both plates (Figs. 19-15 and 19-16).

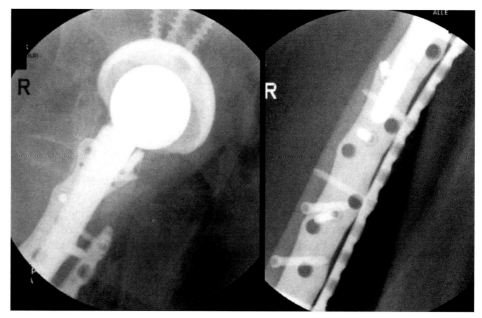

Figure 19-15 ▌ Intraoperative images showing the standard lateral plate, with a separate orthogonal plate, placed posteriorly in this patient. The orthogonal plate can also be placed anteriorly.

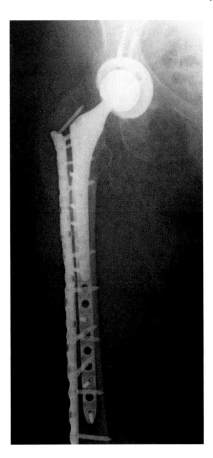

Figure 19-16 | The final fixation construct in the same patient as in Figure 19-15, showing anatomic reduction, independent lag screws, and orthogonal plates. The patient was full weight bearing immediately and healed uneventfully.

- Unicortical locking screws provide insufficient fixation and should be avoided.
- Periprosthetic distal femur fractures typically demonstrate anterior cortical comminution and tension failure of the posterior cortex (Fig. 19-17).

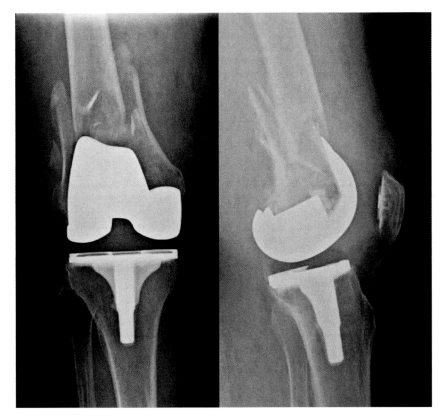

Figure 19-17 | A comminuted periarticular fracture around a previously well-functioning prosthesis, in a young, healthy patient. The prosthesis is well fixed, but there is limited bone stock in the distal segment.

- The fracture reduction is visualized and held with multiple clamps and provisional wires, using techniques outlined previously.
- Though many of these fractures are amenable to retrograde IM nailing, dual plating is another option especially in the presence of canal occluding intramedullary prosthesis stems.
- Either the medial or lateral plate is applied first, depending on location of wires and clamps.
- There are many plate options for the medial aspect of the distal femur, and plate choice depends on surgeon preference and patient anatomy (Fig. 19-18).

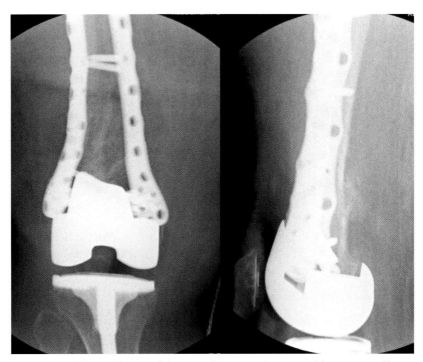

Figure 19-18 | The previous medial parapatellar approach was used for exposure. The reduction was obtained and held with numerous clamps and provisional K-wires, and care was taken to avoid excessive soft tissue stripping. The medial plate is the contralateral side lateral plate (left-sided lateral plate, placed on the medial right distal femur). The lateral plate was placed through the medial parapatellar approach, with a separate lateral incision for distal screw placement, and stab incisions for shaft screws. The patient was full weight bearing immediately, quickly regained full range of motion, and healed uneventfully.

- Care is taken to avoid an overly stiff fixation construct and short working length.
- Large bone defects are filled with bone graft (Figs. 19-19 and 19-20).

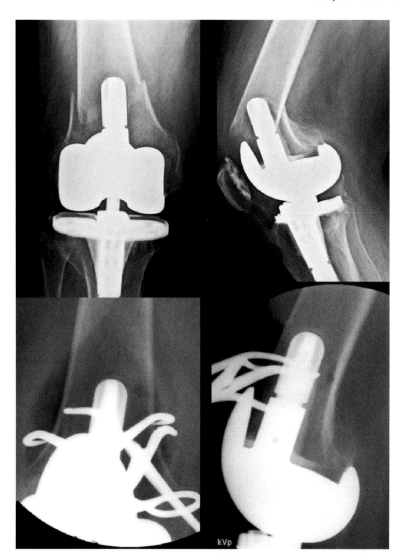

Figure 19-19 ‖ Another example of a periprosthetic femur fracture around a stemmed total knee prosthesis, in a young patient. Anatomic reduction was achieved through a medial parapatellar arthrotomy.

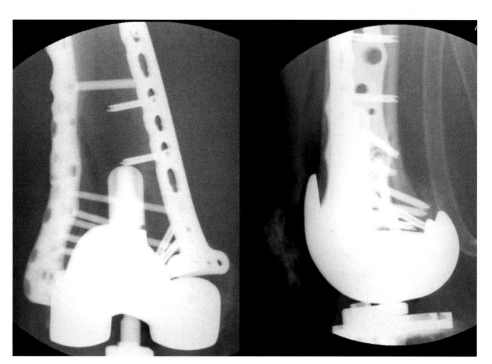

Figure 19-20 ‖ The final fixation construct, showing standard lateral plating, with an additional anteromedial T-buttress plate. The medial plate allowed additional points of fixation in another plane and immediate full weight bearing.

- Osteoporotic patients present a unique challenge, as the typical lateral condylar buttress plate alone is insufficient in those with the poorest quality bone, even with locking screw fixation (Figs. 19-21 and 19-22).

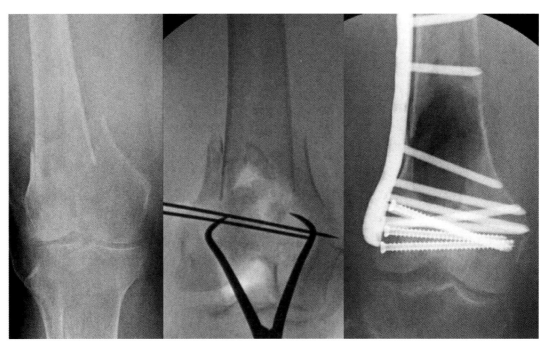

Figure 19-21 ❚ An elderly patient with advanced osteoporosis. The reduction was achieved through an anterior incision and lateral parapatellar approach. Note the large, vacuous metaphyseal bone void.

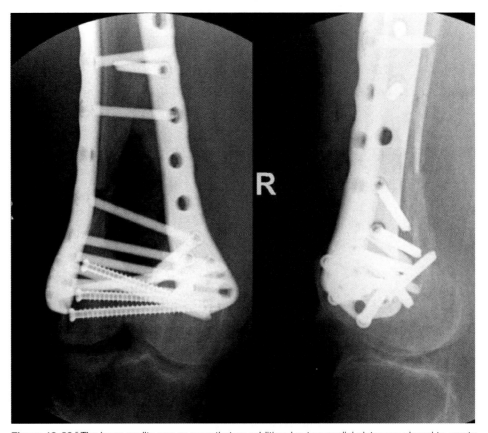

Figure 19-22 ❚ The bone quality was so poor that an additional anteromedial plate was placed to create a stable construct.

- Alternatively, a combined nail + bridge plate construct can be used, which permits immediate postoperative weight bearing.
  - The retrograde nail serves as a centromedial column support while the plate supports the lateral column.
  - When using this technique, unicortical screws or a low density of well-spread bicortical screws is used to prevent an overly stiff construct.
  - Typically, reduction and retrograde IM nailing are performed first as these usually restore sagittal and coronal plane alignment.
  - The distal interlocking bolts are placed from medial to lateral to prevent interference with the lateral plates.
  - The proximal AP interlocking bolts will not interfere with the plate.
  - The plate is placed percutaneously and affixed to the proximal and distal segments with locking screws around the nail.
  - Patients are allowed to weight bear fully as soon as they regain quadriceps control.

Interprosthetic Femur Fractures

- May be either simple patterns or comminuted metaphyseal patterns.
  - Simple patterns are treated with direct reduction and interfragmentary compression followed by lateral plating.
  - Comminuted patterns are treated with indirect reduction and relative stability constructs; either lateral locked bridge plating or IM nailing.
- When plating, the entire femur should be spanned with sufficient implant overlap proximally and distally to avoid inducing an iatrogenic stress riser.
- If the primary implant selected is an IM nail, the stress riser between the femoral component's stem of the hip arthroplasty and retrograde nail is protected with prophylactic plating.
- A combined nail + plate construct can be an excellent construct to treat a highly comminuted metaphyseal fracture in a patient with significant osteoporosis (Fig. 19-23).

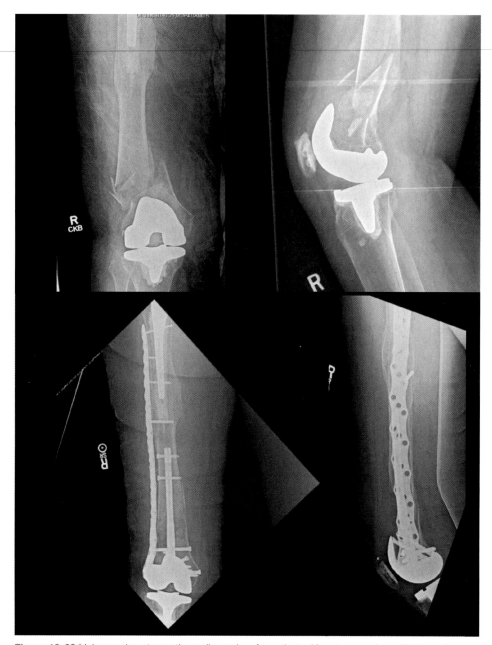

Figure 19-23 I Injury and postoperative radiographs of a patient with osteoporosis and history of multiple fragility fractures who sustained a comminuted interprosthetic femur fracture. A combined nail-plate construct was used to provide sufficient fixation to allow immediate full weight bearing.

Section 7
Knee

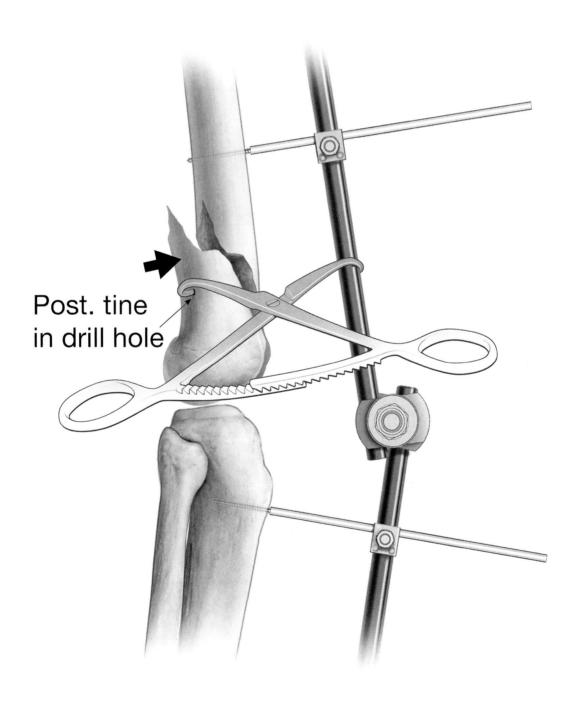

Post. tine
in drill hole

Chapter 20
Distal Femur Fractures

MARK R. ADAMS
MICHAEL J. GARDNER
M. BRADFORD HENLEY
MICHAEL S. SIRKIN
CLAY A. SPITLER
RAYMOND D. WRIGHT JR

Sterile Instruments/Equipment

- Large external fixator
- 2.5-, 4.0-, or 5.0-mm Schanz pins or large K-wires or Steinmann pins for manipulative joysticks
- Large pointed bone reduction clamps (Weber clamps)
- Large quadrangular ball-spike clamp
- Femoral distractor
- Ball-spike pushers
- Shoulder hook/bone hook
- K-wires and wire driver/drill
- Mini-fragment plates or 2.7-mm reconstruction plates
- Smillie knee retractors and "Z retractors"
- Implants
  - Nonlocking condylar buttress plate
  - Locking plate
  - Retrograde nail, if desired
  - Blade plate

Patient Positioning

- The patient is usually placed in a supine position on a radiolucent table.
  - A padded bump is placed under the ipsilateral hip to neutralize hip rotation.
  - The lower extremity is elevated on a soft ramp cushion or other padded bolster to facilitate lateral radiographic imaging.
- Alternatively, lateral positioning can be used for a lateral approach for direct ORIF.
  - This is useful for ORIF of supracondylar distal femur fractures for periprosthetic injuries where the entire femur is to be plated.
  - This is also useful for supracondylar nonunions.
- The C-arm is positioned on the contralateral side of the OR table, opposite the operative extremity.

Surgical Approaches

- Surgical approach is determined by the fracture pattern.

- The *direct lateral approach* may be utilized for the majority of supracondylar and intercondylar femur fractures (Fig. 20-1).

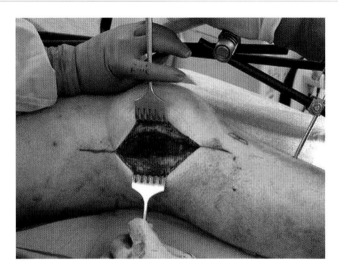

Figure 20-1 I The direct lateral approach can be used effectively for most type C1 and C2 distal femur fractures. The incision is made along the shaft of the femur and often needs to be extended distally to the level of Gerdy's tubercle.

- This approach avoids incision of the quadriceps tendon.
- The distal portion of the vastus lateralis is elevated off of the lateral intermuscular septum.
- It is preferred for its soft tissue sparing benefits.
- If visualization of the distal articular surface is necessary, split and retract the iliotibial band anterior to Gerdy's tubercle and dissect toward the lateral border of the patellar tendon and then curve distally toward its insertion.
  - Avoid an incision crossing the patellar tendon.
  - The distal limb of the incision may be extended distally to the tibial tuberosity lateral to the tendon, to allow for an increased mobilization of the anteromedial soft tissues.
- Allowing temporary limb shortening at the supracondylar level by bayonet apposition of the shaft and metaphyseal portions of the fracture removes the tension from the extensor mechanism, allowing improved medial soft tissue retraction of the extensor mechanism and visualization of the distal articular surface, femoral trochlea, intercondylar notch, and medial femoral condyle, if required (Fig. 20-2).
- Hyperextending the knee with a bump under the heel can also relax the extensor mechanism to improve visualization.

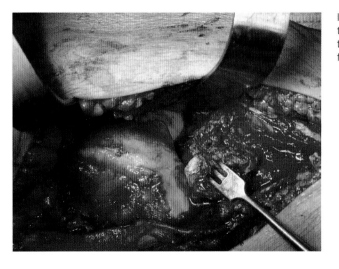

Figure 20-2 I By extending the incision into the lateral part of the fat pad (to the patellar tendon), the distal articular surface of both femoral condyles can be visualized.

■ Placing two "Z" retractors, one superior and one inferior to the patella, facilitates retraction of the extensor mechanism.
- Alternatively, a *lateral parapatellar approach* may be used in cases with significant intercondylar comminution and/or for associated coronal plane fractures (Fig. 20-3).

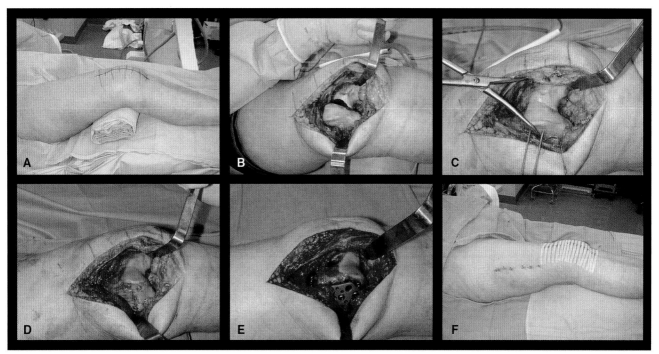

Figure 20-3 I Using a lateral parapatellar approach through a midline or paramedian incision, the articular surface is visualized, and sagittal plane fracture reduction is facilitated **(A, B)**. This approach is anterolateral and thus permits coronal plane fracture fixation (Hoffa fractures) with anterior-to-posterior screws, especially if these involve the medial condyle. The intercondylar articular displacement is then reduced under direct vision, and transcondylar K-wires are placed **(C)**, followed by peripheral screws **(D)**. This allows room for a locking plate to be placed unobstructed **(E)**. The proximal screws may still be inserted percutaneously with this approach **(F)**. (From Nork SE. Supracondylar femur fractures: open reduction and internal fixation. In: Wiss D, ed. *Master Techniques in Orthopaedic Surgery: Fractures*. Philadelphia, PA: Lippincott Williams & Wilkins, 2006, with permission.)

- This approach sacrifices the superolateral geniculate artery to the patella and incises the quadriceps tendon.
- Rarely, a *medial approach* may be used in conjunction with a lateral approach, if necessary, for additional medial condyle access, or for placement of anterior-to-posterior screws for coronal plane Hoffa fractures.
  - The most proximal of the screws should be placed proximally enough so that it is posterior in the femoral condyle, ensuring adequate fixation.
  - This proximal screw can usually be inserted medial (and superior) to the femoral trochlea's articular cartilage.
  - This position is typically proximal to the articular surface (Fig. 20-4).

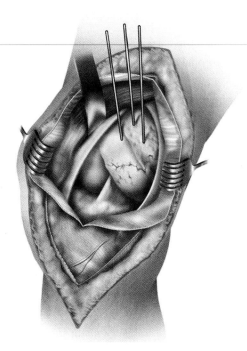

Figure 20-4 ▮ K-wire and screw placement for medial Hoffa fracture. These may be placed percutaneously as cannulated screws or through a small medial parapatellar arthrotomy.

Reduction and Fixation Techniques

- Articular reduction should be performed first.
- Typically, coronal plane (Hoffa) fractures are reduced and provisionally stabilized prior to sagittal plane fractures in the intercondylar region.
  - This sequence may be reversed depending upon the complexity of each fracture.
  - Coronal plane fractures of the lateral and medial condyles can be reduced and compressed with a large pointed reduction clamp.
  - Medial condyle coronal plane fractures may be clamped through the lateral incision.
    - One tine is placed just deep to the extensor mechanism on the anterior aspect of the medial femoral condyle, and the other tine is placed through the intercondylar notch on the posterior medial femoral condyle (Fig. 20-5).

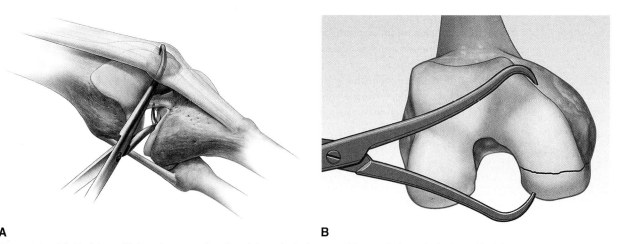

A

B

Figure 20-5 ▮ A, B: A large Weber clamp may be placed through the intercondylar notch through the lateral incision to access some medial femoral condyle coronal plane fracture patterns.

- Multiple anterior-to-posterior K-wires may be necessary to provisionally secure these fractures during screw placement.
- When using nonlocking lateral plates or polyaxial locking plates, Hoffa fractures should ideally be stabilized definitively with interfragmentary lag screws prior to plate placement.
  - However, when using nonpolyaxial locking plate implants, Hoffa fractures may require definitive stabilization after plate placement to avoid interference between the lateral-to-medial plate screws and the anterior-to-posterior Hoffa/condylar screws.
- Fracture location and obliquity in the lateral condyle determines the screw orientation, which should be perpendicular to the fracture plane.
- These are usually 2.7- or 3.5-mm cortical screws (countersunk, if placed through articular cartilage) or headless compression screws placed from anterior to posterior (Fig. 20-6).

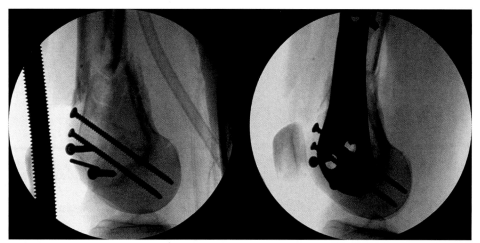

Figure 20-6 | Anterior-to-posterior lag screws for a coronal plane fracture. Note the potential interference with lateral-to-medial locking screws applied through the plate.

- The screws should be angulated approximately 10 degrees from medial to lateral to parallel slope of lateral condyle in sagittal plane and approximately 25 degrees for medial screws (Figs. 20-7 and 20-8).

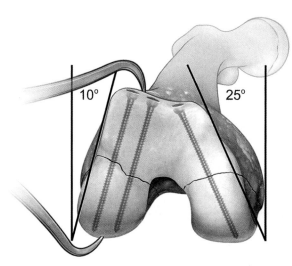

Figure 20-7 | The distal femoral anatomy must be considered with planning and inserting implants for coronal plane fractures. The medial screw starting point may be more medial when inserted through an arthrotomy.

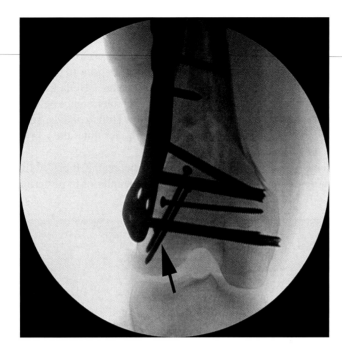

Figure 20-8 I Screws for lateral condyle coronal plane fractures are often placed obliquely for containment within the condyle and parallel to the fracture (*arrow*).

- The screws should be placed in lag fashion and the heads countersunk below the articular surface.
  - These are often inserted through a second small anteromedial incision and medial parapatellar arthrotomy.
- Once the coronal fractures have been stabilized, the intercondylar fracture may be reduced and provisionally stabilized. Loose osseous fragments, soft tissue, and hematoma must be completely removed prior to reduction of the fracture, especially in young patients with dense bone.
- When the fracture configuration allows, a large pointed reduction clamp placed at the level of Blumensaat's line on both the medial and lateral epicondyles will provide balanced compression across intercondylar sagittal plane fractures (Fig. 20-9).

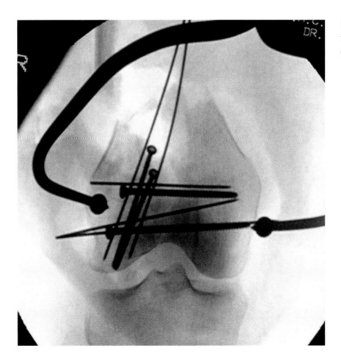

Figure 20-9 I A reduction clamp is placed in the center of each condyle to concentrically compress the intercondylar fracture.

- The clamp tines should be placed near the center of rotation on each condyle, as anterior placement may preferentially compress the intercondylar fracture anteriorly and distract it posteriorly (Fig. 20-10).

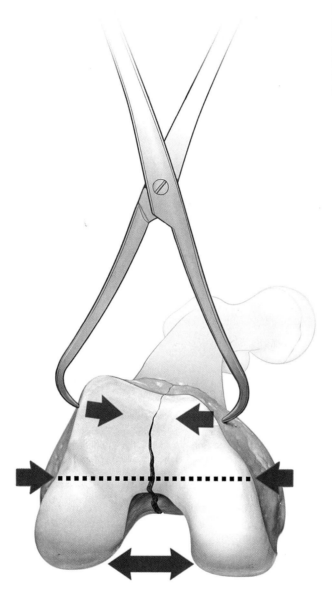

Figure 20-10 | If the intercondylar clamp is placed too anteriorly, the posterior condyles risk becoming distracted (*bottom double arrow*). The ideal clamp placement for balanced fracture compression is relatively posterior on the condyles (*middle arrows and dashed line*) at the level of Blumensaat's line.

- Alternatively, in some fracture patterns, placing one time in the intercondylar notch and the other time on the epicondyle can achieve the appropriate fracture reduction vector (Fig. 20-11).

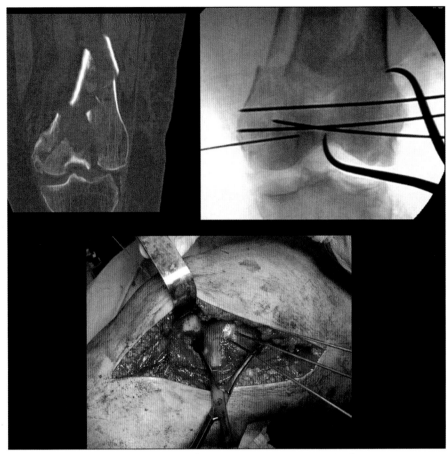

Figure 20-11 When a separate intercondylar or notch fracture fragment has a lateral spike involving the lateral femoral condyle, a reduction clamp placed in the intercondylar notch from the fragment to the lateral epicondyle allows for the appropriate reduction vector.

- ■ This works well if the intercondylar notch is a separate fracture fragment.
- When placed in an epicondyle or condyle, large (2.0- or 2.4-mm) K-wires may be used as joysticks to facilitate reduction of the flexion-extension displacement between the condyles (Figs. 20-12 and 20-13).

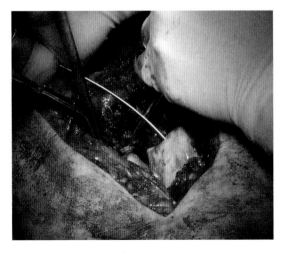

Figure 20-12 The lateral femoral condyle may be angulated/translated/rotated in multiple planes using a K-wire joystick.

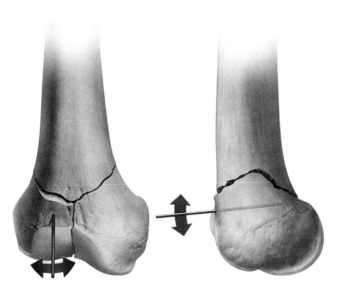

Figure 20-13 I Small Steinmann pins can be inserted anteriorly into the fractured condyle just proximal to the articular surface. These can be particularly effective for internal/ external rotation and flexion/extension reduction maneuvers.

- Multiple K-wires are placed across the fracture as provisional reduction stabilization.
  - Wires should be kept peripherally, just outside the border of the articular cartilage and the epicondyle (vermillion border) to avoid obstructing plate placement (Fig. 20-14).

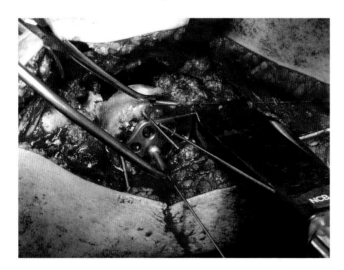

Figure 20-14 I K-wires placed from lateral to medial across the condyles must be kept just below the vermillion border of the distal femur to avoid interference with the plate.

- Wires can also be placed from lateral to medial and then advanced through the medial aspect of the distal femur, out through the medial skin if they may interfere with ideal plate placement, and are critical to fracture reduction.
  - The wires can then be "withdrawn" from the medial side until their blunt ends are flush with the lateral femoral cortex.
  - This removes any K-wire obstruction of the lateral epicondyle for plate application.
- Alternatively, wires can simply be placed percutaneously from medial to lateral to achieve the same effect, but may be a little less accurate than when they are inserted from the lateral side.

- For definitive stabilization, strategically placed screws (usually 3.5 mm) may be placed perpendicular to the fracture anterior or distal to the eventual plate margin. These can be placed so that they are nearly flush with the lateral cortex (Fig. 20-15).

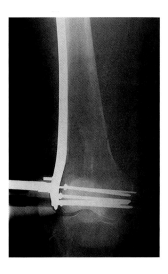

Figure 20-15 ▌ Intercondylar lag screws are placed for articular compression, in a position that will not interfere with the lateral plate placement.

- Intercondylar screws should be placed with the anatomy of the trochlea in mind.
  - Screws placed anteriorly should be placed with a slight (~10 degrees) declination.
  - Additionally, due to the trapezoidal profile of the femoral condyles, bicortical intercondylar screws should not protrude beyond the medial cortex on the "AP" view tangential to the slope of the medial epicondyle.
  - Screw protrusion risks the development of localized synovitis and/or knee pain.
  - To adequately assess the screw tips relative to the medial cortex, internally rotate the femur (or externally rotate the C-arm) 25 degrees (Fig. 20-16).

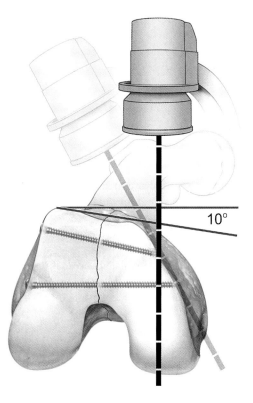

Figure 20-16 ▌ Schematic showing appropriate intercondylar screw angles with respect to the condylar anatomy and fracture plane. Additionally, bicortical screws should not appear to cross the medial epicondyle's cortical border on the AP view due to the trapezoidal shape of the medial condyle. A view tangential to the medial epicondyle may be obtained by rotating the femur internally or the C-arm externally (shadowed C-arm). This allows a more accurate determination of the screw length.

10°

- In cases of more articular comminution, smaller screws (2.0 or 2.4 mm) may be used for stabilization of coronal and intercondylar fracture fragments (Fig. 20-17).

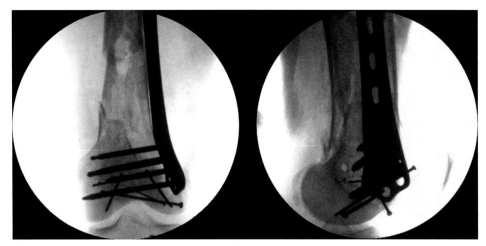

Figure 20-17 In cases of articular comminution, multiple small screws are placed and countersunk for osteochondral fixation.

- Alternatively, a "rim plate" placed along the vermillion border with multiple lag or position screws may be used to stabilize comminution.
- Once the articular segment is reduced anatomically and stabilized, limb length and alignment are restored.
  - Occasionally, there is a cortical interdigitation (i.e., a "direct read") in the supracondylar area immediately proximal to the lateral femoral condyle.
    - Take advantage of this opportunity, provided minimal additional soft tissue dissection is required, by elevating the distal muscle fibers of the vastus lateralis.
  - More often, comminution exists in the metaphysis, and indirect reduction maneuvers are preferable.
- The articular segment is frequently in an extended position relative to the diaphysis due to the attachment of the gastrocnemius and the force of the extensor mechanism (Fig. 20-18).

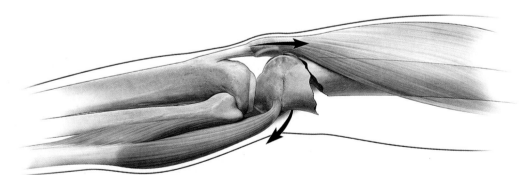

Figure 20-18 Typical deformity of the distal femoral metaphyseal fracture includes shortening and apex posterior. These are due in large part to the pull of the gastrocnemius and the extensor mechanism.

- A femoral distractor can be placed anteriorly to reestablish limb length.
  - Varus and valgus can be manipulated using independent Schanz pins or the plate as a reduction aid (Fig. 20-19).

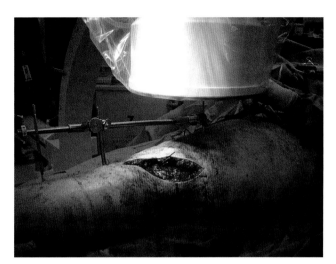

Figure 20-19 I An anterior femoral distractor can facilitate an indirect reduction. Take care to accurately assess the sagittal plane deformity, as this can be accentuated with overdistraction.

- An external fixator placed anteriorly may also be applied to achieve reduction, similar to a provisional spanning frame.
  - Anterior placement in the sagittal plane facilitates locking plate placement as it does not interfere with a lateral operative exposure or application of the plate.
- An anterior Schanz pin may be placed into the distal metaphyseal-articular segment.
  - The pin may be used to manipulate the flexion and extension of the articular segment directly.
  - This pin may be secured to an external fixator, or the previously reduced distal femoral articular fracture segment may be K-wired provisionally after Schanz pin manipulation (Fig. 20-20).

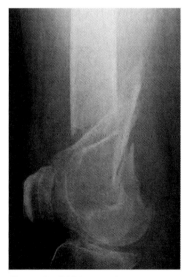 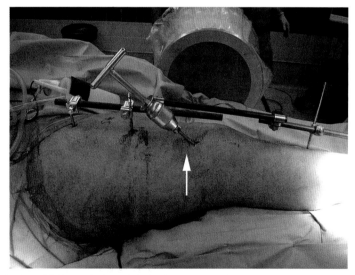

Figure 20-20 I An anterior, percutaneously placed Schanz pin (*arrow*) in the femoral condylar fracture segment can be used to correct a flexion, or more commonly, an extension deformity at the fracture site, as in this case.

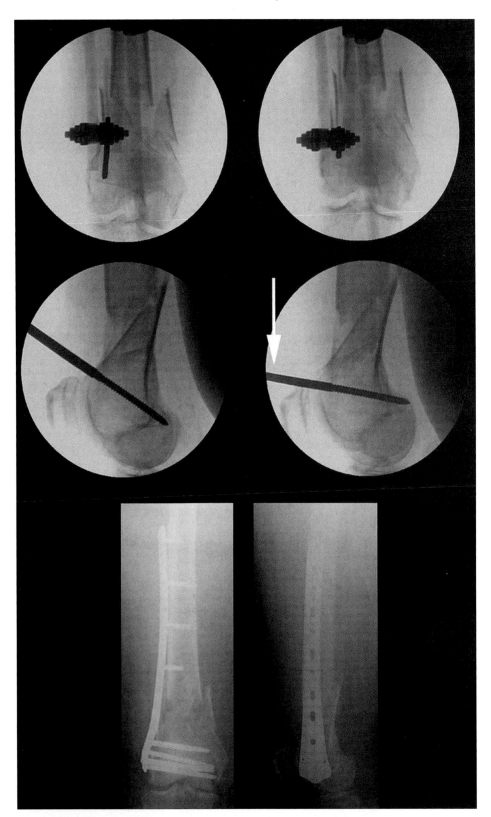

Figure 20-20 (*Continued*)

- A bump placed posteriorly, behind the patient's knee, will also aid in reduction of extension deformity at the fracture site (Fig. 20-21).

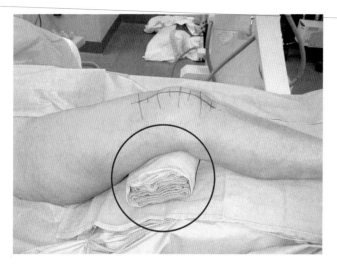

Figure 20-21 I A useful reduction aid is a towel bolster under the apex of the metaphyseal fracture to counteract the forces of the gastrocnemius.

TIP

Sagittal Plane Correction of a Distal Femur Fracture: Posterior to Anterior Clamp

Mark R. Adams
Michael S. Sirkin

Pathoanatomy

The typical sagittal plane deformity of a distal femur fracture is apex posterior due to the pull of the gastrocnemius on the distal segment (Figs. 20-22 and 20-23).

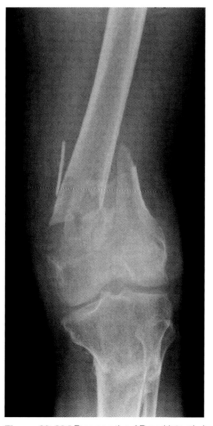 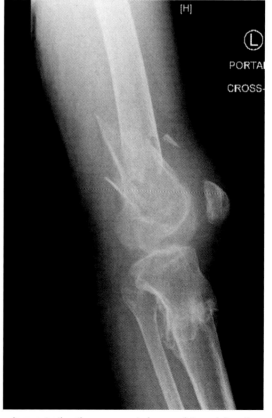

Figure 20-22 I Preoperative AP and lateral views demonstrating the apex posterior angulatory deformity in this distal femoral fracture.

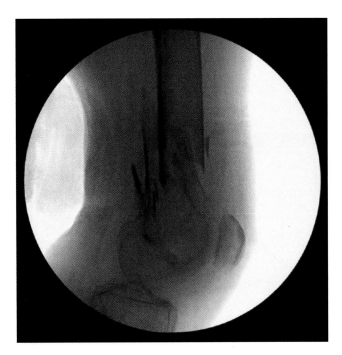

Figure 20-23 I Intraoperative lateral fluoroscopic view demonstrates recurvatum and posterior translation through the knee of distal segment due to pull of gastrocnemius.

Solutions and Techniques

- Correction maneuvers for this deformity include the following:
  - A bump/bolster placed under the distal segment at the apex of the deformity (Fig. 20-23)
  - Schanz pin correction, with pins inserted in the medial and/or lateral epicondyle(s), in the sagittal plane and connected to an anteriorly placed external fixator
  - This technique requires sufficient bone in the distal segment to secure the pin(s).
  - Each pin can be connected to the fixator, either directly to an AP half pin or to a crossbar added to the frame. The connection can be either static using another bar and pin-bar clamps or dynamic, using tensioned elastic Penrose drain(s) or tubing clamped to a neighboring pin or crossbar. Varying the size of the drain (e.g., ½ inches, ¾ inches, 1 inch) and the amount of tension in the elastic can "dial-in" the ideal sagittal plane correction.
- The bar on the anteriorly placed external fixator can also be used to engage the tines of a large clamp placed posterior to anterior.
  - In Figures 20-24–20-26, a large Weber clamp was applied, though other clamps (e.g., quadrangular) will perform similarly.

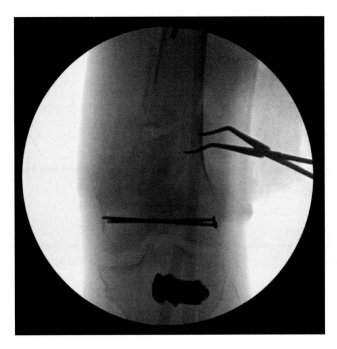

Figure 20-24 I Intraoperative fluoroscopic AP image of a large Weber clamp inserted through lateral approach, tines directed anterior to posterior.

- Pelvic reduction forceps with pointed-ball tips would be another clamp option.
- The posterior tine can be placed through a unicortical drill hole in the posterior or posterolateral aspect of the distal segment, and the anterior tine hooked around the anterior bar of the external fixator.
- This configuration will "flex" the distal femoral segment to counter the apex posterior deformity and will also translate the distal segment anteriorly.

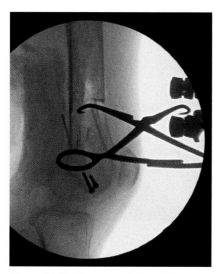
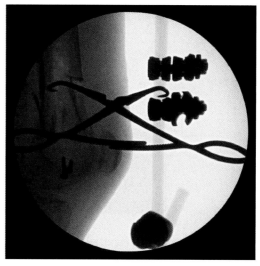

Figure 20-25 I Intraoperative lateral views showing that the large Weber clamp has corrected the extension (apex posterior angulation) and posterior translation of distal segment. The posterior clamp tine is in a drill hole in the posterolateral aspect of the distal segment; the anterior clamp tine is around the anterior external fixator bar.

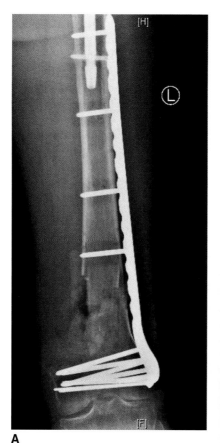
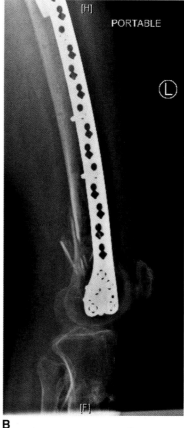

A   B

Figure 20-26 I Postoperative AP and lateral images of final fixation.

- Some reduction of lateral metaphyseal comminution may be necessary to establish length, alignment, and rotation of the distal articular fracture segment relative to the diaphysis.
  - In cases with significant metaphyseal comminution, alignment should be confirmed with an intraoperative radiograph (long cassette) and/or Bovie cord from the center of the femoral head to the center of the ankle joint.
  - In this case, these small fragments may be secured with 2.0-mm straight plates and 2.4-mm screws.
  - The medial metaphyseal comminution should not be manipulated directly, so as to avoid devascularization or soft tissue stripping.
  - If required to gauge reduction, medial comminution should be approximated by pushing or pulling through the fracture's cancellous surfaces via the lateral incision.
- For reduction of the major supracondylar fracture components, multiple simultaneous reduction maneuvers are often necessary (Fig. 20-27).

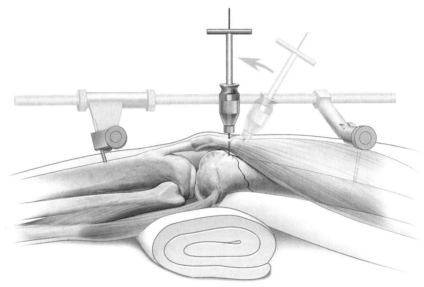

Figure 20-27 | Typical reduction maneuvers for metaphyseal reduction include manual limb traction and manipulation, Schanz pin joysticks, a femoral distractor/external fixator, and strategically placed bumps.

- Once the articular fracture segment has been reduced to the diaphysis, a lateral locked implant is usually used for fixation in fractures with metaphyseal comminution.
  - The plate is inserted submuscularly, deep to the vastus lateralis and extraperiosteally along the lateral cortex of the femur.
  - Once positioned correctly, K-wires are inserted at its proximal and distal ends to secure it provisionally.
  - Its position is confirmed again clinically and radiographically.
  - Next screws are used to secure (or lag) the plate provisionally to the distal articular fracture segment and diaphysis.
  - Length, rotation, flexion, extension, and alignment of the entire femur are then confirmed using intraoperative planar radiographs.
  - Definitive fixation is then inserted sequentially (Fig. 20-28).

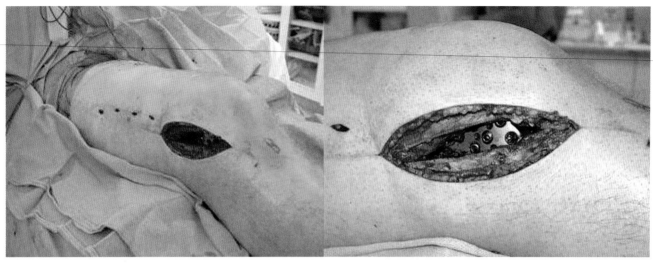

Figure 20-28 I A laterally based locked plate can be slid submuscularly, with percutaneous diaphyseal screws.

- Construct stiffness can be modulated as desired by using unicortical rather than bicortical locking screws, far cortical locking screws, or conventional cortical screws.
- An overly stiff construct may put the patient at risk for metaphyseal nonunion.
- All remaining metaphyseal comminution may be displaced into the medial and/or posterior portion of the metaphysis.
- This theoretically provides a scaffold for bony healing medially and leaves an anterior lateral window for delayed bone grafting, if needed (Fig. 20-29).

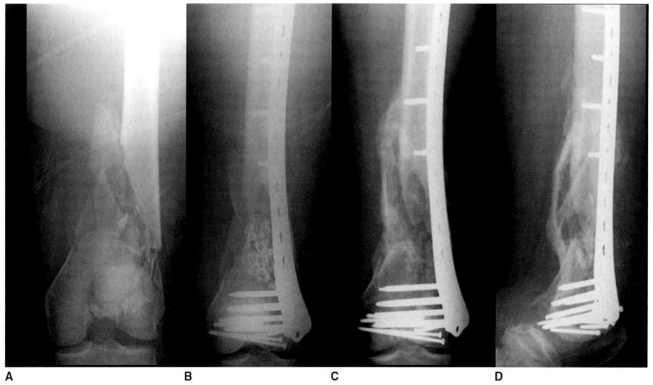

A   B   C   D

Figure 20-29 I An example of a comminuted distal femur fracture **(A)**, with a metaphyseal bone defect remaining after ORIF. The comminution was pushed medially, and antibiotic beads were placed empirically. **(B)**. This facilitated the planned anterolateral bone grafting procedure. The fracture healed uneventfully with posteromedial bridging bone **(C, D)**.

Managing Distal Femur Fractures in the Morbidly Obese Patient

Clay Spitler

Pathophysiology

Morbidly obese patients with supracondylar femur fractures present significant challenges in patient positioning, fracture reduction, and fixation. Many aspects of distal femoral fracture fixation can be challenging in the morbidly obese, including positioning, achieving appropriate coronal and sagittal alignment, and safe postoperative mobilization.

Solution

In positioning, an arm board placed on the side of the uninjured extremity will allow for safe positioning of the patient on a regular or flat-top operating table. Positioning and taping the panniculus away from the operating field will allow for access to the anterior proximal femur. The use of a retrograde nail in conjunction with a lateral locked plate can aid in indirect reduction of the metadiaphyseal fracture and provide increased axial and rotational stability, which decrease the risk of failure with the inevitable weight bearing that occurs during mobilization of the morbidly obese.

Technique

- To use the same flat-top operating table for lower extremity/pelvic fractures in the obese, arm boards placed on the contralateral, uninjured side will provide additional bed width and will not impede fluoroscopic imaging (Figs. 20-30 and 20-31).

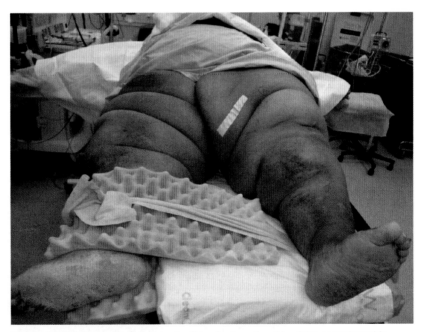

Figure 20-30 | An arm board placed collinearly along the side of the operating table creates additional table width and is used to accommodate an obese patient's increased girth. This is an image of a cantilever-type radiolucent regular operating room table with a weight limit of 1,000 lbs.

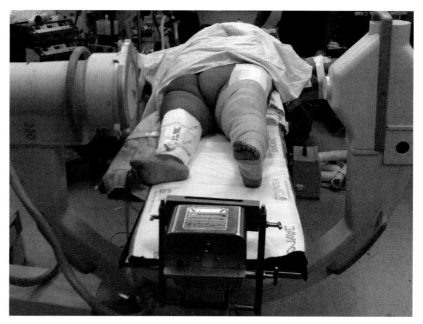

Figure 20-31 I Contralateral arm board does not obstruct fluoroscopic imaging. This patient is on a dual support, radiolucent flat-top operating room table with a weight limit of 500 lbs.

- After standard positioning (e.g., hip bolster) for the planned surgery, if the patient's panniculus is obstructing the surgical field, it may be positioned manually out of the way and held with tape applied to the OR table's rails.
  - Reverse Trendelenburg position assists in positioning the pannus cranially and away from the lower extremities.
  - If securing the panniculus to the chest, one must ensure that the patient can be adequately ventilated prior to beginning the case.
  - In some extreme circumstances, multiple sutures or towel clips have been used to help capture and retract the panniculus out of the surgical field (Figs. 20-32 and 20-33).

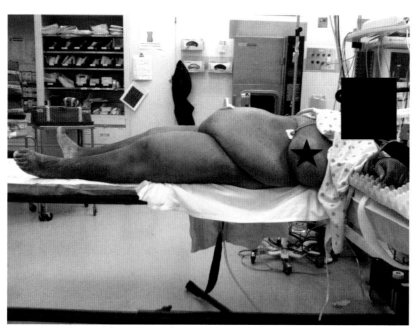

Figure 20-32 I Panniculus overlapping the upper thigh and proximal femur.

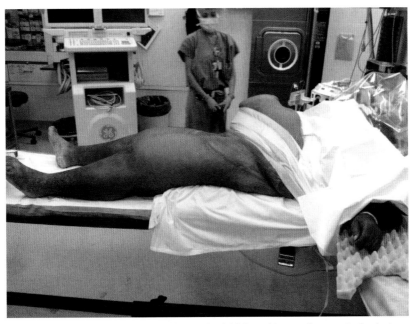

Figure 20-33 ▌Improved access to the proximal thigh and femur after panniculus taping.

- After retracting the panniculus, isopropyl alcohol and chlorhexidine are used to cleanse the newly exposed skin, which is not uncommonly colonized by anaerobic flora and fungus.
- Even when appropriate alignment can be achieved, morbid obesity often prevents their ability to limit weight bearing on the operative extremity and mobilize safely.
- In this select group of patients, the use of an intramedullary nail and a lateral locked plate will provide additional stability, and the implants can aid in indirectly reducing the comminuted metadiaphysis (Fig. 20-34).

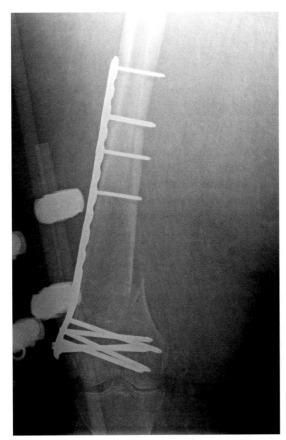

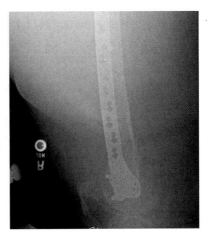

Figure 20-34 ▌AP and lateral images of a malaligned distal femoral fracture after internal fixation. Note the size of the soft tissue shadows.

- A lateral parapatellar approach is used if articular reduction is necessary; otherwise, a tendon-splitting or medial parapatellar approach for a retrograde nail starting point and a direct lateral incision can be used for submuscular plate insertion.
- The reduction should proceed with any necessary articular reduction and fixation with independent lag screws in a manner that will avoid the trajectory of a retrograde intramedullary starting point.
- Provisional reduction can be performed with distal femoral or proximal tibial traction, an external fixator (Fig. 20-35) with pin(s) in the proximal femoral segment, pin(s) in the proximal tibia, and, if needed, a carefully placed pin (outside the path of a nail) in the epiphyseal block to help correct the sagittal and/or coronal plane deformity.

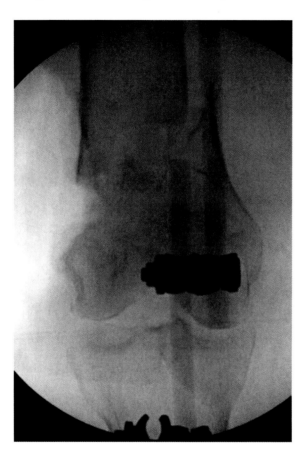

Figure 20-35 I Provisional reduction with external fixator after hardware removal.

- After reducing and fixing the intra-articular fractures, an appropriate length lateral locking plate is selected and fluoroscopically positioned in a submuscular fashion (Fig. 20-36).
- A guidewire for an intramedullary nail is placed using fluoroscopic guidance in the appropriate starting point with the correct entrance angle.
- A medial parapatellar or transpatellar tendon approach is used to create the entry portal through which the ball-tipped guidewire is passed into the proximal femur. Should a long IM nail be desired, the external fixator pins should be placed in the medial proximal femoral metaphysis (Fig. 20-37).
  - Minimal reaming is required in the generally sedentary and osteopenic morbidly obese patients.
  - The referencing guidewire for the lateral locking plate as well as unicortical locking/nonlocking screws in the diaphysis can allow for careful restoration coronal alignment/lateral distal femoral angle.
  - Use of images from the contralateral uninjured side can be a useful for comparison.
- A retrograde nail can then be passed.
  - A short nail will avoid proximal external fixator pins.
  - A long retrograde nail can be used if the external fixator pins were placed strategically outside of the nail path.
  - By virtue of a good starting point and entrance angle in the distal segment and the isthmic-medullary location of the nail in the proximal segment, the nail helps to ensure good sagittal alignment of the comminuted metadiaphysis.

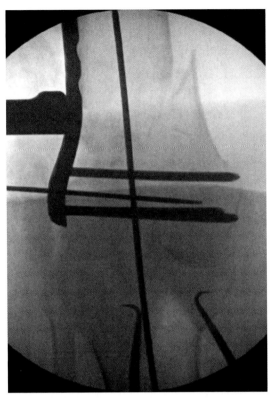 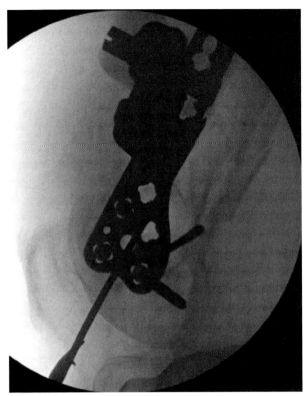

Figure 20-36 ▌ Restoration of appropriate coronal and sagittal alignment of the distal femur using a condylar buttress plate with subsequent placement of a guidewire. Note that the transcondylar screws are directed away from the intended nail path.

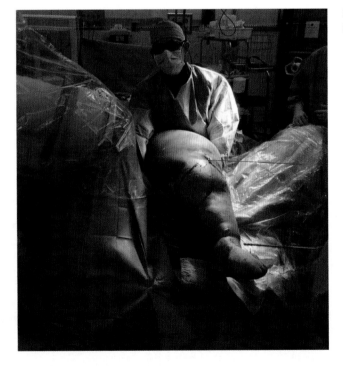

Figure 20-37 ▌ Clinical photograph of retrograde nail guidewire in place.

- In the diaphysis, unicortical locking screws can be placed adjacent to the nail, and nonlocking screws can be aimed around the nail (Fig. 20-38).
- Postoperatively, patients typically require maximal assistance to mobilize with physical therapy and are advised to be partial weight bearing, protected with a walker (Fig. 20-39).

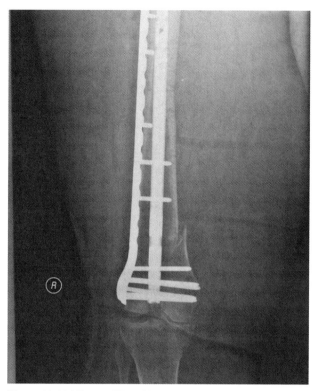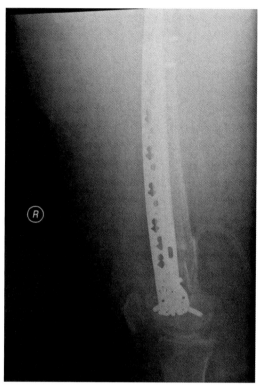

Figure 20-38 I Postop AP and lateral images.

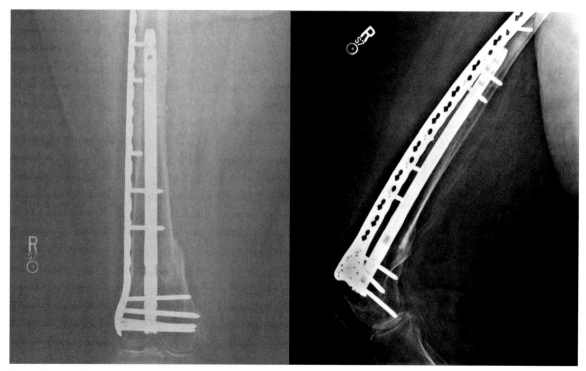

Figure 20-39 I AP and lateral images after fracture healing.

- For isolated medial or lateral femoral condyle fractures with separate trochlear fracture fragment(s), or complex medial Hoffa fractures, a contoured reconstruction plate is a good option and achieves excellent fixation.
  - Plate contour follows articular condylar margin and is placed "extra-cartilagenously" along the rim of the medial (or lateral) femoral condyle in the anterior portion of the medial "gutter."
  - Allows transverse lag screws through plate, if necessary.
  - If proximal extension of a medial plate is necessary, or if this fixation is being used without a lateral plate, it allows anterior-to-posterior plate screws in the shaft to avoid dissection in Hunter's canal and femoral vessel exposure (Figs. 20-40–20-42).

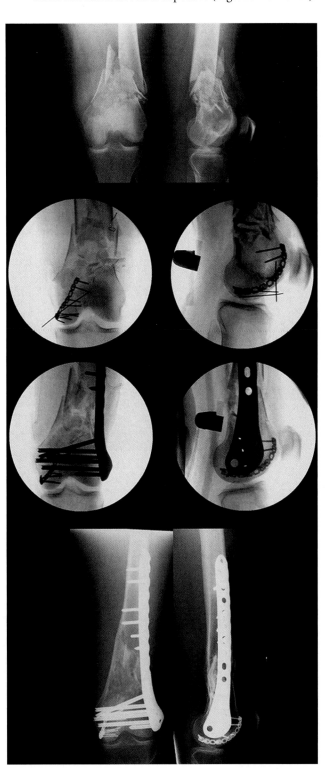

Figure 20-40 I Example using a contoured reconstruction plate along the articular margin for fixation of a medial femoral condyle fracture.

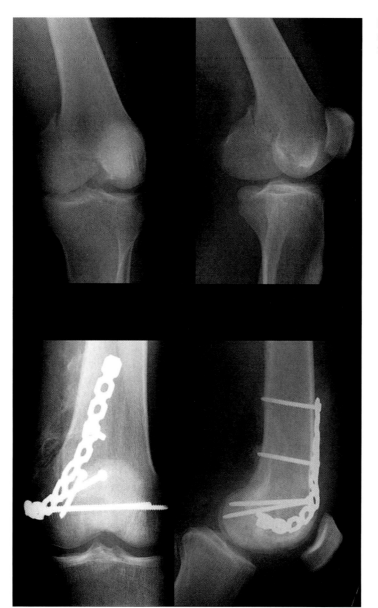

Figure 20-41 I Another plate configuration for an isolated medial femoral condyle fracture.

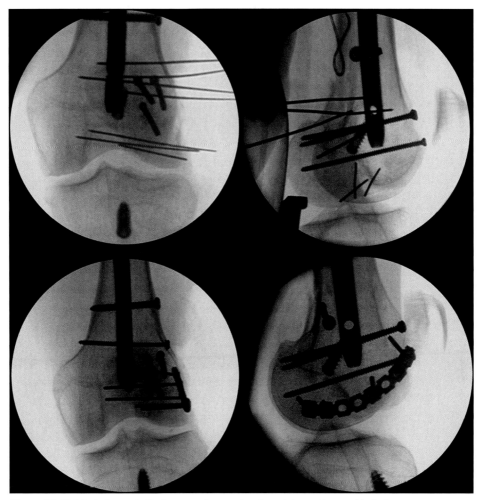

Figure 20-42 I A similar periarticular curved reconstruction plate can be used to buttress multifragmentary lateral condylar and/or trochlear fractures.

Distal Femur Nonunion

- Most commonly occurs in the metaphyseal region, with union of the articular surface.
- May be successfully treated with revision compression plating +/− bone grafting or with IM nailing.
  - If converting to an IM nail, either a retrograde nail or antegrade nail may be placed.
  - The exiting plate may be left in place or the plate may be removed depending on its condition, the desired degree construct stiffness, and whether the articular surface is completely healed or not.
  - If the plate is left in place, selective screws are removed at the articular block for nail placement (Fig. 20-43).

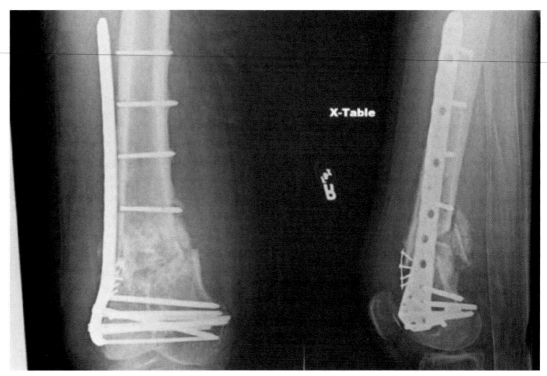

Figure 20-43 I AP and lateral views demonstrate a distal metaphyseal nonunion with failure of all proximal far cortical locking screws.

- Screws in the femoral shaft are exchanged sequentially for unicortical screws during nailing and can either be replaced for bicortical screws around the nail or left as unicortical screws.
- Nailing has the advantage of the reamings acting as bone graft and may negate the need for open autografting.
- Additionally, a nail provides stability along the anatomic axis of the femur, optimizing nonunion loading (Fig. 20-44).

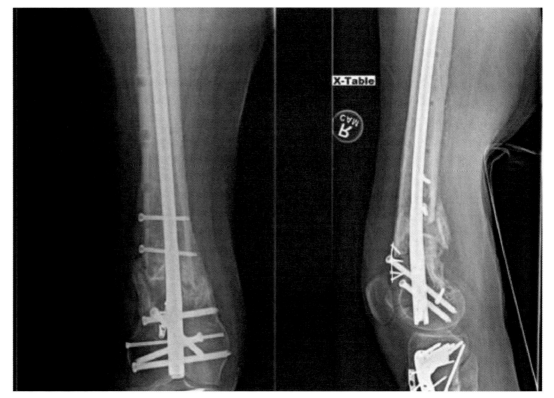

Figure 20-44 I AP and lateral radiographs after nonunion treatment with plate removal and retrograde IM nailing. Note two blocking screws in posterior aspect of metadiaphysis, proximal to the nonunion.

Chapter 21
Patellar Fractures

M. BRADFORD HENLEY

RAYMOND D. WRIGHT JR

Sterile Instruments/Equipment

- Large and small pointed bone reduction clamps (Weber clamps)
- Specialized patellar bone clamps
- Implants
  - Cannulated 3.5- or 4.0-mm screws
  - 1.0-mm cable or 18-gauge wire
  - Minifragment screws for free fragments
  - Minifragment plates (2.0/2.4 mm) for associated coronal plane fracture lines
  - Strong nonabsorbable suture with good handling characteristics, such as no. 5 or no. 2 FiberWire, Ti-Cron, or Tevdek
- K-wires and wire driver/drill
- Beath pins or Hewson wire passer
- Sterile, removable bump for alternate placement behind knee/heel to obtain knee flexion/full knee extension

Patient Positioning

- Supine on a radiolucent cantilever table
- Padded ramp under affected extremity to facilitate lateral imaging
- Bump placed under the ipsilateral hip to limit external rotation of extremity
- Padded tourniquet placed on the thigh if desired

Surgical Approach

- Midline longitudinal incision to deep fascia.
  - A horizontal "smile" incision may be used for improved cosmesis in simple fracture patterns.
    - The medial and lateral ends of the transverse incision should be slightly curved proximally.
    - This approach should not be used if anticipating the patient will need a total knee arthroplasty in the future.
- Fracture is identified and cleansed of clot and fracture debris.
- Flex the knee over the sterile bump to identify and document associated intra-articular pathology, such as chondral injury to the trochlea or femoral condyle.
- Work through lacerations in medial and lateral retinacula to view and/or palpate articular reduction.
  - These can be extended, if needed.

Reduction and Implant Techniques

- Modified tension band
  - Reduction often facilitated with knee in full extension, to relax extensor mechanism especially when there has been retraction of fracture fragments/extensor mechanism.
    - Place a sterile bump behind the heel/distal leg.
  - Grasp major fragments with small pointed reduction forceps for direct manipulation while an assistant clamps major fragments into place with large pointed reduction clamps or a patellar clamp.
  - The large pointed reduction clamp tines should be placed at a depth equal to the midaxis of the patella on the lateral view.
  - A frequently made mistake is to place the clamps too superficially on the patellar poles, overcompressing the dorsal cortex and gapping at the articular surface.
    - Specially designed clamps are available with dual prongs on each tine to grasp the bone though quadriceps and patellar tendons (Fig. 21-1).
  - Fine-tune reduction with dental picks.

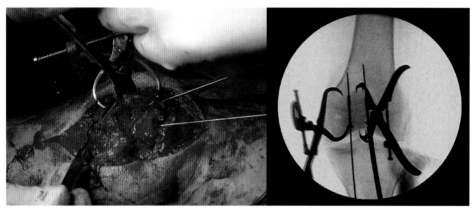

Figure 21-1 Specialized clamps with two prongs on each tine (large Weber clamp is to the left [medial] and patellar clamp is to the right [lateral] on the C-arm view) facilitate grasping the edge of the patella through tendon(s) for manipulation and stabilization.

- Place multiple K-wires in patella for provisional fixation.
- Lag screws may be placed through additional fragments to reconstruct the patella so as to convert a multifragmentary fracture into a simpler two-part fracture with two remaining large fracture fragments and a transverse or short oblique fracture line (Fig. 21-2).
- A surgical tactic should account for the location of screws in the patella (e.g., screws placed horizontally are placed more anteriorly while longitudinally oriented fixation will be placed closer to the articular surface).

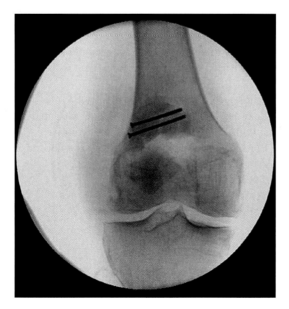

Figure 21-2 Screws placed perpendicular to the fracture lines of additional fragments should be used to sequentially reconstruct the patella into a main proximal and distal fragment.

- ▫ This will avoid the frustration of screw collisions/deflections that compromise fixation and/or quality of reduction.
  - ▫ Horizontally placed screws are best placed from lateral to medial as the lateral patellar facet(s) are narrower than the medial facet(s).
- ● With transverse fracture line reduced and stabilized with clamps and/or additional K-wires, insert smooth guidewires for 3.5- or 4.0-mm cannulated screws from distal (usually the smaller fragment) to proximal (larger fragment), through patella.
  - ▫ Insert to the level of the proximal cortex but not protruding through the cortex (best viewed on the AP image), and measure indirectly (Fig. 21-3).

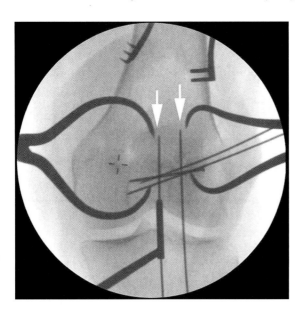

Figure 21-3 ▌The guidewires are inserted to abut the proximal cortex (*arrows*), and indirect measurement is performed.

- ▫ Subtract 2 to 3 mm from measurement, to ensure screw tips do not penetrate the proximal cortex when the head is flush with the near cortex.
- ▫ This ensures that the tension band wire does not develop a stress riser as it is tensioned and bends over the sharp screw edge; additionally, it ensures that the compressive effect of the tensioned wire is transferred to the fracture, rather than to the screw.
- ● After measurement, advance guidewire through proximal patellar cortex, 1 to 3 cm into quadriceps tendon.
  - ▫ Use fluoroscopy or palpation to locate wire.
- ● Separate the tendon's fibers longitudinally to locate the tip of the wire and clamp with a hemostat or Kocher clamp (Fig. 21-4).

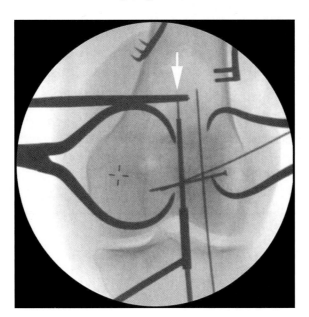

Figure 21-4 ▌After measuring the screw length, the guidewire is inserted through the opposite cortex, and grasped with a clamp (*arrow*) through a split in the quadriceps tendon. The wire is then overdrilled while the wire is held with a clamp.

- Overdrill the wire with cannulated drill while maintaining the grasp on the proximal portion of the wire.
  - This prevents incarceration of the drill on the guidewire and loss of the drill path.
- Overdrill only one wire at a time and then insert a screw.
  - Overdrilling both wires simultaneously risks loss of fracture reduction, if no other K-wires have been used for provisional fixation.
- Screws should be partially threaded or drilled as lag screws if using fully threaded screws.
- Insert 18- or 20-gauge wire, or a 1.0-mm cable, through one of the cannulated screws from distal to proximal.
  - Bring wire limb that exits from proximal screw distally and insert from distal to proximal through the other cannulated screw.
  - Bring the same limb back across patella to meet the other limb, tension the wire (i.e., compress the fracture), and secure.
- Alternatively, a no. 5 braided suture can be used rather than wire for the tension band. This can be passed through the cannulated screws using a Hewson suture passer or stiff angiography catheter.
- In patients in whom fixation of the inferior pole of the patella is tenuous, most often in the setting of osteoporosis, screw fixation may be offloaded to augment osseous fixation.
- A running locking no. 5 braided suture is placed in the patellar tendon with equal length tails for passage through cannulated screws.
- After cannulated screw placement, the suture tails are run through the cannulated screws, and the suture is tied over the bone bridge along the superior pole of the patella.
- Alternatively, the no. 5 suture can be placed through a transverse bone tunnel in the tibial tubercle, run through the cannulated screws, and tied over the superior pole of the patella.
  - To decrease prepatellar symptoms and prepatellar bursitis, place the wire crimp or knot within the quadriceps tendon. If this is not possible, consider drilling a unicortical 2- to 3-mm hole in the anterior patella in which to bury the wire knot or cable crimp (Fig. 21-5).

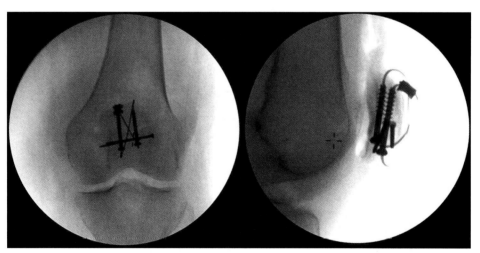

Figure 21-5 Ensuring that the cannulated screw length is short of the proximal cortex prevents crimping the tension band wire at the screw aperture as it exits.

- Dorsal patellar tension plating
  - Clean the fracture, reduce the patella, and stabilize with K-wires.
  - After reduction and provisional fixation, a 2.0-mm straight plate is measured, cut, and contoured to the caudal border of the patella.
  - The most distal hole is then secured to the caudal-anterior patella surface with a 2.4-mm screw.

- The plate is then gradually contoured and tensioned on the anterior surface of the patella by using strategically placed screws (Figs. 21-6–21-8).

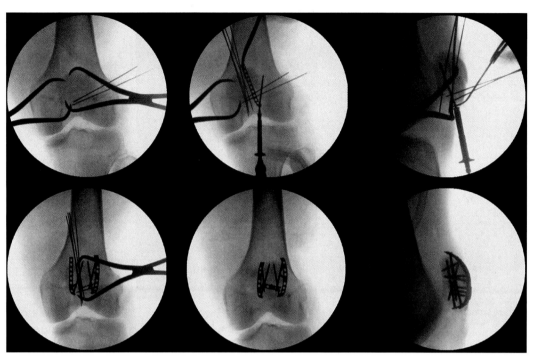

Figure 21-6 | Sequence of reduction and fixation for dorsal patellar tension plating.

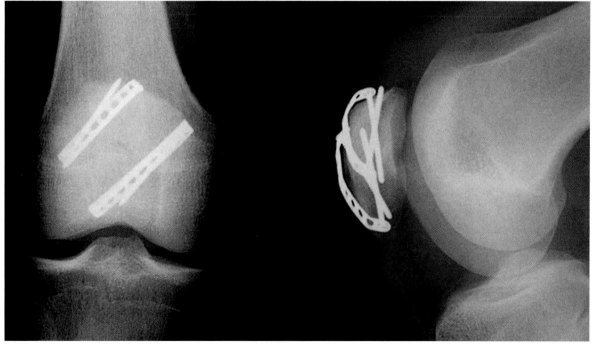

Figure 21-7 | Another case example of patellar tension plating.

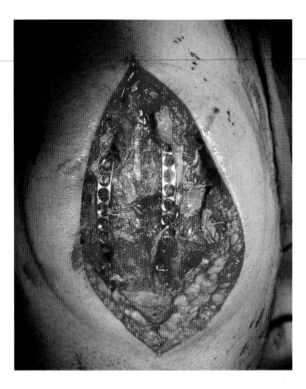

Figure 21-8 | Intraoperative clinical photograph of tension band plates applied to the anterior surface of the patella.

- For complex or revision situations, specialty plates designed for the cuboid and navicular can provide multiple and customizable points of fixation (Fig. 21-9).

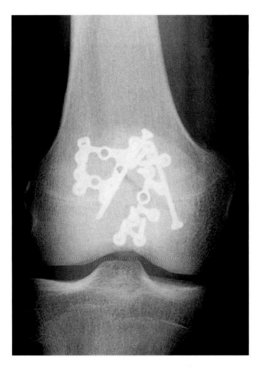

Figure 21-9 | Small fragment specialty foot-specific plates can be used in complex fractures to obtain multiple points of fixation.

- Partial patellectomy
  - Usually necessary for comminuted fractures involving the patella's inferior pole.
    - Leave some bone fragments attached to the patellar tendon to allow for bone apposition and osseous healing following repair (Fig. 21-10).

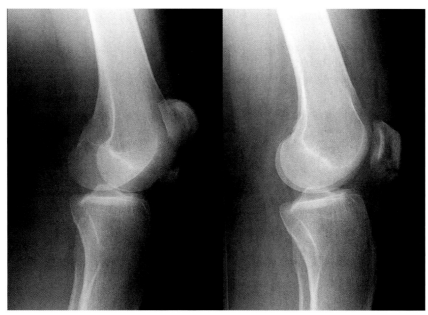

Figure 21-10 | Example of a patient with an inferior pole patellar avulsion fracture, treated with patellar tendon repair. Retention of the comminuted inferior pole allows for bony healing.

- Depending on the patient's size, drill approximately four longitudinal parallel holes at the junction of the anterior and middle thirds of the patella to avoid extension deformity of the residual patella.
  - The most medial and lateral holes should be drilled with a 2.0-mm drill to accommodate one suture strand of nonabsorbable suture.
  - The two inner holes should be drilled with a 2.5-mm drill to accommodate two suture strands (if using no. 5 suture).
- Pass three suture strands (no. 2 FiberWire or no. 5 Ethibond) as locking Krackow stitches in the patellar tendon—medial, central, and lateral.
  - This results in six suture ends at the edge of the patellar tendon.
- Pass the six sutures through the four drill holes from distal to proximal so that the two central holes carry two sutures, and the medial and lateral holes carry only one suture each.
  - Beath pins facilitate suture passage.
    - Oscillate Beath pin partially through the predrilled hole (Fig. 21-11).
    - Place suture strand from patellar tendon through the eyelet in the pin (Fig. 21-12).

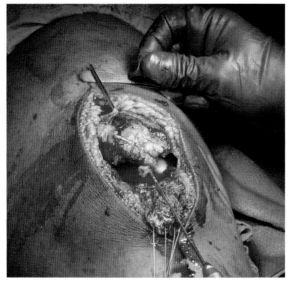

Figure 21-11 | A Beath pin is advanced from distal to proximal through a predrilled longitudinal hole in the patella.

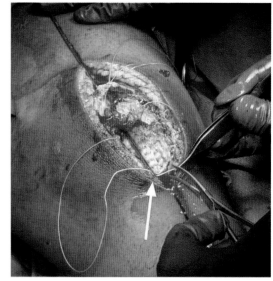

Figure 21-12 | A suture strand from the patellar tendon stitch is placed through the eyelet of the Beath pin (*arrow*).

- The Beath pin is then pulled retrograde from the proximal end, pulling the sutures through (Fig. 21-13).
- Tie each suture strand to its mate strand over the bone bridge between the longitudinal parallel holes.
- Tie the sutures with the knee in extension to achieve apposition (Fig. 21-14).

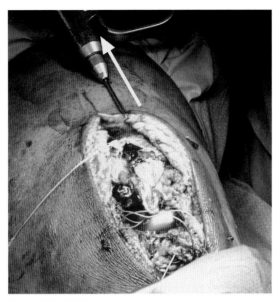
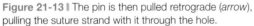
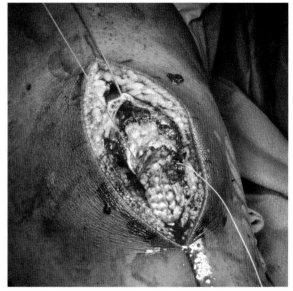

Figure 21-13 | The pin is then pulled retrograde (*arrow*), pulling the suture strand with it through the hole.

Figure 21-14 | Each suture is sequentially tied proximally to its mate strand, completing the repair.

- Once repair is complete, the knee is placed through a range of motion to assure fracture stability and to help guide postoperative rehabilitation.
- The medial and lateral retinacula are closed with robust suture.
- Occasionally, the knots of no. 2 FiberWire may be prominent.
  - This prominence can be minimized by imbricating local soft tissue (usually fibers of quadriceps tendon) over the FiberWire knot with an absorbable 2-0 Dexon suture, thereby burying them.

Chapter 22
Tibial Plateau Fractures

REZA FIROOZABADI
MICHAEL J. GARDNER
MICHAEL F. GITHENS
M. BRADFORD HENLEY
THOMAS M. LARGE

Sterile Instruments/Equipment

- Headlight.
- Tourniquet if desired.
- Femoral distractor.
- Langenbeck and/or Smillie retractors.
- Large and small pointed bone reduction clamps (Weber clamps).
- Large periarticular quadrangular bone clamps.
- Number 2 Ethibond suture for retraction of meniscus after submeniscal arthrotomy and repair of peripheral meniscal detachment (if required); choose a needle with a short radius of curvature (e.g., a GU needle).
- Dental picks and Freer elevators.
- Bone tamps, curved and straight.
- Lambotte osteotomes for metaphyseal cortical window.
  - Alternatively, 2.5- to 4.5-mm drill bits
- Implants: anatomically contoured lateral proximal tibial periarticular plates, standard buttress plate(s), and/or locking plate(s).
  - Long 3.5-mm cortical screws with 2.7-mm low-profile heads
  - Periarticular plate, one-third tubular, or 3.5-mm compression plate for medial or posteromedial buttress (Schatzker type IV)
  - Distal radius 3.5-mm T-plate (old style); also useful for posteromedial side
  - Mini-fragment screws and mini-fragment plates (2.0/2.4 mm) depending on fracture comminution and fracture repair requirements
  - Cancellous allograft, osteobiologic bone void filler (e.g., CaPO$_4$), cancellous allograft, or other product for subchondral support
- K-wires and wire driver/drill.
- Obtain perfect AP and lateral images of the uninjured knee for intraoperative comparison to accurately restore native slope and coronal plane alignment.

Surgical Approaches

- *Anterolateral approach*
  - Positioning
    - Supine on a radiolucent table, foam ramp under the injured extremity
    - Bump under the ipsilateral hip to internally rotate limb for true AP image of knee (so patella is pointing anteriorly)
    - Can place inflatable IV bag bladders under each buttock, which can be inflated and deflated sequentially during the case when switching from one approach to the other

- Distally, skin incision is 1 to 2 cm lateral to the tibial crest, crosses the center of Gerdy's tubercle, and is extended proximally approximately 8 cm proximal to joint line along the midaxial lateral femur at the level of the lateral epicondyle, splitting the IT band in line with its fibers.
- Incise anterior compartment fascia 5 to 10 mm lateral to tibial crest to allow for closure, and elevate anterior tibialis muscle off the periosteum of the proximal tibial metaphysis, starting distally and working proximally, exposing the lateral tibial fracture line.
- Elevate the IT band anteriorly and posteriorly from Gerdy's tubercle, working from distally toward the knee joint.
  - Stop approximately 5 to 10 mm below the knee joint so as to avoid an inadvertent arthrotomy with its bulging lipohemarthrosis.
- Split the fibers of the IT band longitudinally (in line with its fibers), starting proximally (approximately at the level of the lateral femoral epicondyle).
  - Working caudally, elevate the IT band off of the knee capsule both anteriorly and posteriorly.
  - A Smillie retractor placed deep to the IT band can be used to pull its fibers away from the knee capsule as it bulges from hemarthrosis to prevent an unnecessary arthrotomy.
- Work distally toward the knee joint continuing to Gerdy's tubercle.
  - Place the Smillie retractor at the level of the knee joint and retract laterally and posteriorly (protecting the LCL) while releasing the posterior attachment of the IT band to Gerdy's tubercle.
- Continue a posterior release on the proximal tibia, working posterior to the LCL (medial to the LCL and lateral to the tibial plateau and joint capsule), until the anterior capsule of the proximal tibiofibular joint is encountered.
  - The LCL is easily identified if it is placed under tension with a femoral distractor (see below).
- Next, elevate the anterior IT band, again from proximal to distal, off the knee capsule and anterior tibia, continuing toward Gerdy's tubercle.
- Below Gerdy's tubercle, elevate the IT band and anterior compartment fascia toward the lateral border of the patellar tendon until the retropatellar fat pad is accessible.
- Lighten up on the knife just proximal to Gerdy's to avoid entering the joint capsule.
- Placing a femoral distractor at this point facilitates distraction of the knee joint and permits palpation of the lateral collateral ligament, lateral joint space, tibial plateau, and meniscal rim (if present) to allow for an accurate submeniscal arthrotomy incision.
  - Distraction places the knee capsule tension.
  - Additionally, the LCL is placed on tension, clarifying the posterior limit of the submeniscal arthrotomy.
- Submeniscal arthrotomy, multiple sutures for retraction (Fig. 22-1).

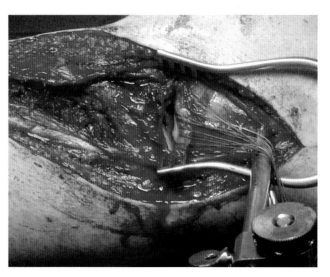

Figure 22-1 I A submeniscal arthrotomy with retraction sutures in peripheral lateral meniscus and a femoral distractor (proximal pin in lateral femoral epicondyle) provide excellent visualization of the lateral tibial plateau.

- Arthrotomy should leave sufficient inferior capsule (tibial coronary ligament) attached to tibia to allow capsular repair.
- Passing capsular and meniscal sutures through plate has the disadvantage of pulling the meniscus inferiorly and away from its anatomic origin.
  - Additionally, capsular disruption and meniscal injury may occur if subsequent hardware removal is necessary.
- Arthrotomy can extend anterior/medial as far as infrapatellar fat pad and patellar tendon.
- Arthrotomy can extend posterior/lateral until LCL and proximal tibiofibular joint are palpable or visible.
  - Typically, the capsulotomy limit is 5 to 10 mm anterior to the popliteal hiatus.
- Occasionally, the joint will be entered and the lateral meniscus cannot be identified.
  - Invariably, this is due to meniscal detachment from the lateral capsule at the meniscal "red zone."
  - The meniscus may be displaced medial to the split in the lateral tibial fracture and usually rests on the cartilage of the depressed articular segment.
  - Often, the meniscus is not so much displaced medially; rather the lateral split fracture component has been displaced laterally.
  - Accurately narrowing the width of the tibial plateau is critical to restoring the lateral meniscal-plateau-femoral condyle relationships.
- A displaced meniscus can often be retrieved with a nerve hook or other curved instrument.
  - A suture is placed into the peripheral margin of the meniscus and is used to continue "delivering" the meniscus laterally to accept additional peripherally placed sutures for repair to its capsular origin.
- *Posteromedial approach*
  - Positioning
    - Supine on a radiolucent table.
    - Elevate the extremity on a radiolucent foam ramp.
    - Bump under the contralateral hip, unless sufficient hip external rotation is possible or simultaneous posteromedial and anterolateral approaches are planned.
    - Can place inflatable IV bag bladders under each buttock, which can bc inflated and deflated sequentially during the case when switching from one approach to the other.
  - Incision is approximately 1 to 2 cm posterior to posteromedial tibial border, but may be more posterior if a posterior plate (rather than posteromedial plate) is needed or more anterior if a medial or anteromedial plate is required (Fig. 22-2).

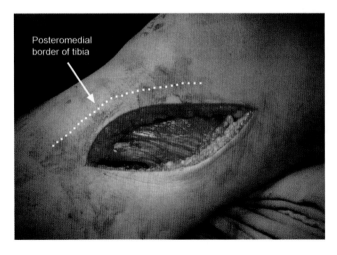

Posteromedial border of tibia

Figure 22-2 I The posteromedial incision is made approximately 2 cm posterior to the tibial border, but may be made more anteriorly or posteriorly according to the fracture pattern and anticipated plate placement.

- Find saphenous vein and nerve.
- Palpate pes tendons through fascia.
- Incise fascia over medial gastrocnemius and follow this fascial incision along the posterior aspect of pes anserinus tendons (Fig. 22-3).

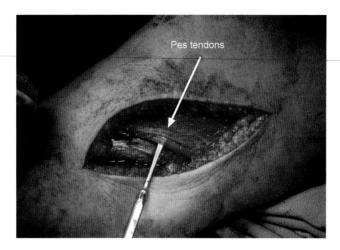

Figure 22-3 I After incision of the deep fascia, the pes tendons are identified and protected and usually retracted anteriorly.

- Work proximal to tendons, if necessary for exposure.
- Elevate the popliteus origin off the posteromedial proximal tibia, and distally elevate a portion of the soleus' origin off the posteromedial tibia.
  - Placing towel bolsters under the knee and ankle lets the gastrocnemius-soleus hang freely for better fracture exposure during the posteromedial approach.
  - Increased mobilization of the pes anserinus is obtained by releasing fascial bands that extend from the semitendinosus and the gracilis to the medial head of the gastrocnemius.
  - Anterior retraction of the pes anserinus tendons away from the proximal medial tibia will reveal the broad tibial insertion of the superficial medial collateral ligament.
  - For more anterior exposure, work in "windows" between tendons of pes anserinus.
- The posteromedial plate is positioned ideally deep to the pes tendons and posterior to the posterior border and insertion of the medial collateral ligament (Fig. 22-4).

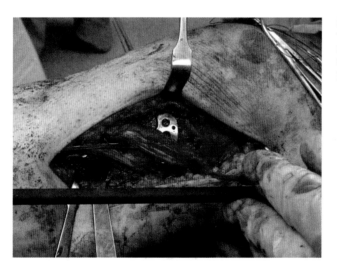

Figure 22-4 I This T-plate is positioned on the posteromedial tibial surface, deep to the soleus and the pes tendons, and posterior to the insertion of the medial collateral ligament.

- The interval between the popliteus and the medial head of the gastrocnemius will lead to the popliteal artery.
- Alternatively, a plate can be placed more posteriorly, rather than posteromedially, depending on the position of the fracture fragment's apex (Fig. 22-5).

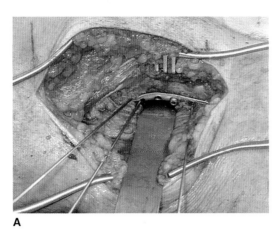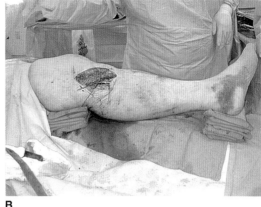

A   **B**

Figure 22-5 In this example, the plate is placed more on the posterior tibial surface, posterior to the hamstring tendons and the medial collateral ligament **(A)**. Bumps under the knee and the ankle allow the gastrocsoleus to hang free to improve fracture site access **(B)**.

- A medial arthrotomy can be performed if required for articular visualization.
- This is typically performed by following the coronal plane fracture proximally to its entry into the chondral surface of the medial plateau.
- Visualization of the articular surface is not as extensive as it is on the lateral side, as the meniscus and medial collateral ligament impede exposure.
- *Direct posterior approach*
  - Excellent approach for fragment-specific posterior fixation; allows access to the posterolateral and posteromedial plateau (Fig. 22-6)

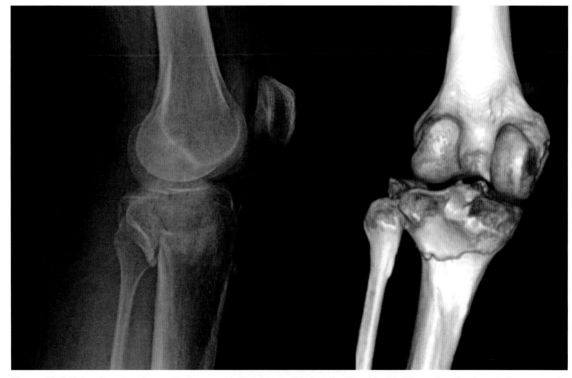

Figure 22-6 Injury imaging demonstrating a posterior shear pattern optimally addressed through a direct posterior approach.

- Typically combined with the anterolateral approach.
- Positioning.
  - Prone on a radiolucent table.
  - Face protected in a prone face mask.
  - Torso rolls on either side of the torso, allowing the abdomen to hang free. Ensure there is not undue pressure on the nipples or ASIS.

- ▪ Nonoperative leg padded with hip and knee slightly flexed.
- ▪ Operative leg with hip neutral to slightly extended and leg on a prone foam ramp to allow unencumbered lateral imaging.
- Incision is an S-shaped incision with a proximal lateral longitudinal limb, the transverse limb crossing the popliteal fossa, and the distal longitudinal limb along the posteromedial tibial border (Fig. 22-7).

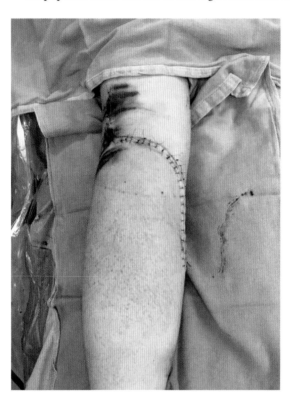

Figure 22-7 | A clinical image demonstrating the skin incision for the direct posterior approach to the left posterior tibial plateau.

- Full-thickness subcutaneous flaps are raised.
- The common peroneal nerve is identified deep to biceps femoris and protected throughout the case (Fig. 22-8).

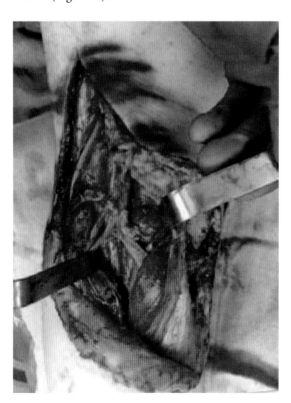

Figure 22-8 | After creating full-thickness skin flaps, the common peroneal nerve (upper left in the image of the left lower extremity) is identified under the biceps femoris and protected. The medial and lateral gastrocnemius heads are retracted exposing the deep saphenous vein.

- Next, the sural nerve is identified distally and traced proximally to the level of the popliteal fossa, between the medial and lateral heads of the gastrocnemius muscle.
- The sural nerve will lead the surgeon to the tibial nerve and the adjacent popliteal artery and veins. Large crossing veins are ligated while exposing the neurovascular bundle (Fig. 22-9).
- The neurovascular bundle is mobilized and can be retracted both medially and laterally for access to specific fragments. The belly of the popliteus is sharply dissected off the posterior tibial plateau to expose the fracture (Fig. 22-10).

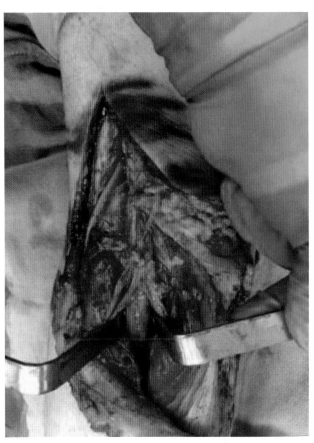

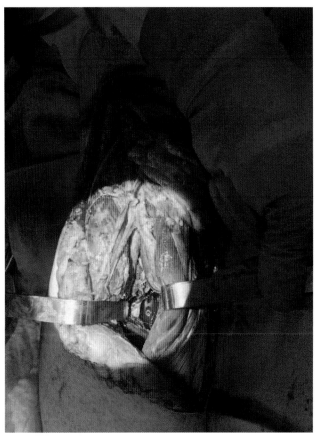

Figure 22-9 ▍ The popliteal artery and tibial nerve are exposed and mobilized to allow medial and lateral retraction.

Figure 22-10 ▍ Retraction of the neurovascular bundle allows access to the posterior tibial plateau.

- Additional exposure to the posteromedial plateau is obtained by using the posteromedial approach described above through the same skin incision (Fig. 22-11).

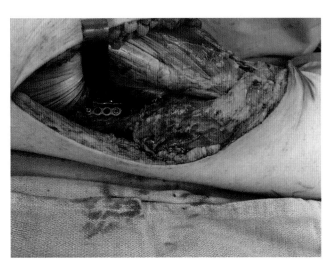

Figure 22-11 ▍ The posteromedial plateau is exposed by retracting the medial head of the gastrocnemius laterally.

- Both windows can be worked simultaneously to achieve reduction and fixation of a large posterior shearing fragment or can be worked individually to address separate posterolateral, posterocentral, and posteromedial fragments.
- Screws are placed carefully as not to interfere with reduction of anterior fragments (Fig. 22-12).

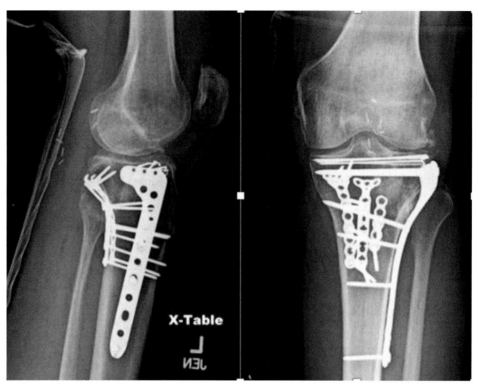

Figure 22-12 ▌ Six months postop radiographs demonstrating a healed bicondylar tibial plateau treated through direct posterior and anterolateral approaches.

Reduction and Implant Techniques

- If a knee-spanning external fixator was placed previously, prep the spanning external fixator into the surgical field to facilitate the sterile limb preparation and draping and to minimize the risk of iatrogenic neurovascular injury.
  - The pin-bar clamps can be removed from the pins and replaced with a femoral distractor if necessary, but the pins should be cleansed with tincture of iodine or similar antiseptic following clamp removal.
  - Ideally, the pins should be left in situ, until the wound is closed and dressed at the end of the case to minimize egress of contaminated fluid and debris on to the surgical field from the pin tracts.
  - After definitive fracture stabilization, it is important to take the knee through a range of motions, but only after the pins are removed, to free any quadriceps adhesions and confirm final ROM and knee joint stability.
    - This is especially important if several weeks have elapsed between injury/fixator application and ORIF.

Use of Femoral Distractor

- Place the proximal distractor pin at the shoulder of the lateral femoral epicondyle.
  - This can be done either percutaneously or at the proximal extent of lateral incision, through the split fibers of the IT band.
  - Distal pin should be placed percutaneously, a bit beyond the anticipated distal end of the plate (Fig. 22-13).

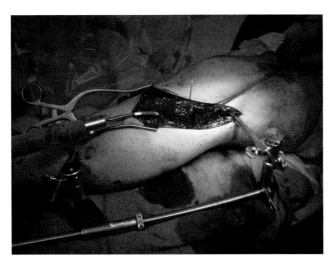

Figure 22-13 | The femoral distractor placed laterally within the lateral incision proximally.

- ▪ Carefully place this incision far enough lateral so that the pin is not crushing the anterior compartment musculature.
  - ● With a lateral distractor, the limb should be placed initially in relative valgus, as distraction creates a varus bending moment when applied.
- ● A distractor placed anteriorly can be used to adjust rotation and sagittal plane alignment.
  - ● With an anteriorly placed distractor, position the limb in extension initially, because the distraction force tends to flex the fracture site.
- ● A second distractor can also be placed medially to restore the medial column length if a preoperative varus deformity exists (Fig. 22-14).

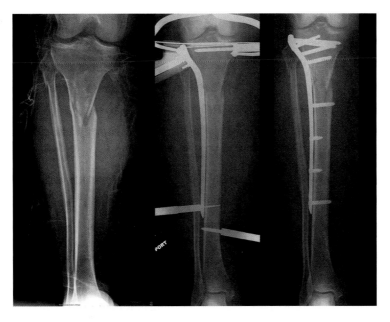

Figure 22-14 | The femoral distractor can be placed medially if a varus deformity exists preoperatively.

- ● This may be placed in conjunction with a clamp and K-wires for articular surface reduction.
- ● After provisional reduction and fixation of the medial plateau, a medial femoral distractor can be left in place to "protect" the medial reduction/fixation from inadvertent or purposeful varus forces applied to the lateral plateau and metaphysis during reduction.
- ● In a metaphyseal fracture, the distractor can be used to manipulate the proximal segment to achieve anatomic alignment and coronal plane rotation.

- Intraoperative planar radiographs after provisional fixation are crucial to determine accurate limb alignment before finalizing fixation (Fig. 22-15).

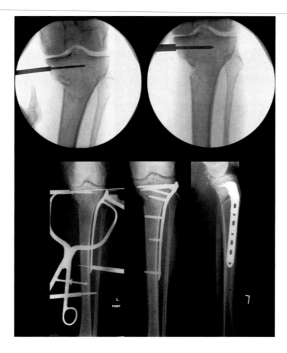

Figure 22-15 | A metaphyseal fracture in varus was reduced indirectly with a medial femoral distractor.

- If femoral distractor sleeves are positioned so that they interfere with visualization of the joint surface or another fracture line on fluoroscopy, changing to the other set of sleeves (e.g., longer to shorter, or vice versa) flips the elbow of the sleeve in the opposite direction to avoid radiographic obstruction.
    - Alternatively, an external fixator may be constructed to be unobtrusive to C-arm visualization and implant placement.

Specific Fracture Patterns

- For *lateral split-depression patterns*, the cortical displacement of the split fragment with an intact rim may be reduced first and provisionally stabilized with clamps and K-wires placed peripherally.
    - If this is chosen, ensure that laterally based K-wires are placed anterior and/or posterior to the articular depression to avoid blocking its subsequent elevation.
- A metaphyseal corticotomy may be created with a large drill bit.
    - Alternatively, 4-mm or more small 2.5-mm drill holes can be created to perforate the metaphyseal cortex in a square of rectangular shape (1 cm × 1.5 cm).
        - These are connected with an osteotome, and the cortical "window" is removed (and saved) for introduction of bone tamps or elevators.
    - Bone tamps are used to elevate the articular surface with the underlying subchondral bone.
    - As it is elevated, the level of the depressed segment is monitored by direct vision through the submeniscal arthrotomy, and after reduction, its relationship to the surrounding articular surface is palpated with a Freer elevator to assess congruity.
    - Avoiding "opening the book" to diminish fragment devitalization, allow the fragments to remain in the correct orientation near their native position(s) and avoid reconstructing free osteochondral fragments outside of the metaphysis (Fig. 22-16).

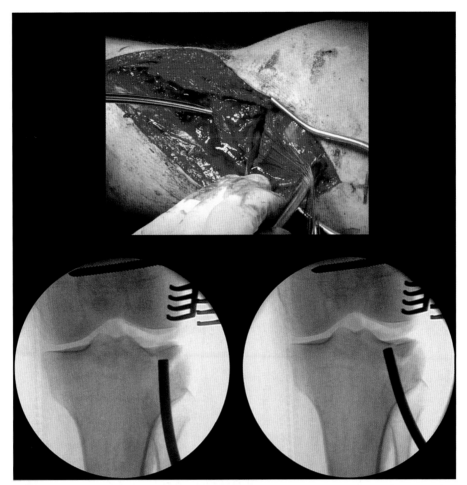

Figure 22-16 I A drill hole or small cortical window, made at the osseous reflection of the lateral plateau, allows access for a bone tamp. Direct articular visualization and palpation with a Freer are used to guide the reduction.

- Multiple areas of articular depression can be elevated en masse with multiple taps of the tamp along multiple points below the depressed fragment(s).
- If the articular fragment to be elevated is not readily accessible due to the location of the corticotomy and the tamp shape, a Steinmann pin can be bent to achieve the desired vector for fragment elevation.
- A K-wire may also be used to drill just below the depressed osteoarticular fragment, its location confirmed with C-arm in orthogonal planes, and subsequently overdrilled with a cannulated drill to create a direct path for an instrument to access the fragment.
- Occasionally, a medial corticotomy allows the best tamp vector for elevation of lateral plateau-depressed articular fragments.
- Multiple prepositioned K-wires are then passed under the elevated fragments. These wires may be bent, cut, and impacted as part of the definitive construct if desired.
- Additionally, allograft bone is impacted into the bone void created by elevation of the depressed fragments for further support.
- Following elevation, a large quadrangular clamp (e.g., with ball spikes) can be used to reduce residual lateral condylar displacement (joint widening) and to compress the articular surface transversely (Fig. 22-17).

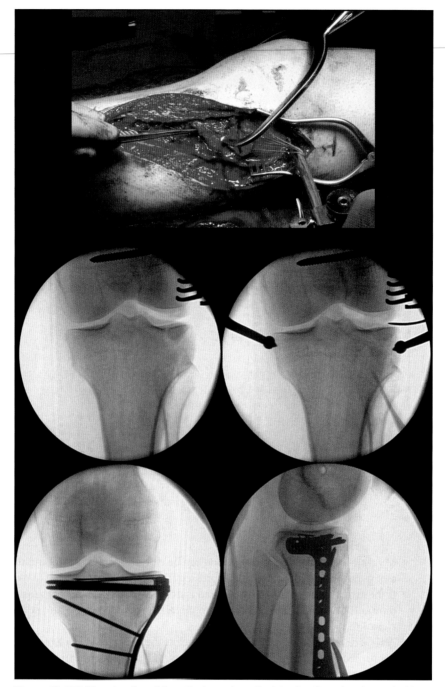

Figure 22-17 I After elevation of the articular surface, the lateral wall can be clamped with the tines placed anterolaterally and posteromedially to compress the articular surface and restore the condylar width.

- When one or both metaphyseal cortices are comminuted or osteoporotic, use a ball-spike clamp over a small plate (e.g., one-fourth tubular plate) or in a hole of the lateral buttress plate.
  - This will distribute the compression forces over a larger surface area and apply more uniform compression of the condyles so as not to penetrate the metaphysis (Figs. 22-18 and 22-19).

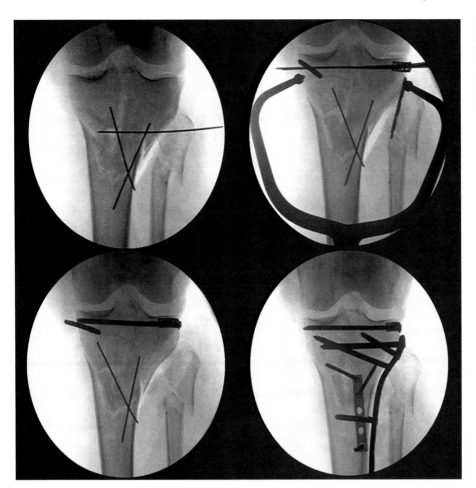

Figure 22-18 | A small malleable plate may be used under the spike of a clamp to distribute the forces in areas of comminution. Note the sagittally placed Schanz pin in the medial tibial condyle, permitting rotational control of this fracture fragment.

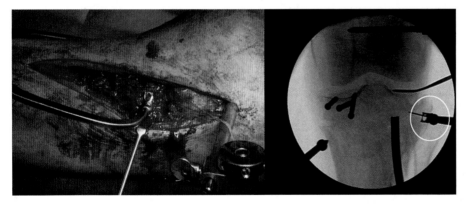

Figure 22-19 | Another example of a quarter tubular plate used as a washer (*circle*) to clamp the lateral plateau to reduce the condylar width in this patient with osteoporosis.

- Intraoperatively, assess the congruity of the radiographic subchondral reduction (line[s]) of both the medial and lateral plateaus with an appropriate C-arm plateau tilt.
  - If one line is clear, while on the same image, the other is not, there is likely a sagittal plane malrotation of one of the tibial plateaus.
  - Sagittal plane malrotations may be corrected with bone clamps and Schanz pin(s) placed anteriorly for fracture segment control prior to compression of the articular surface (Fig. 22-20).

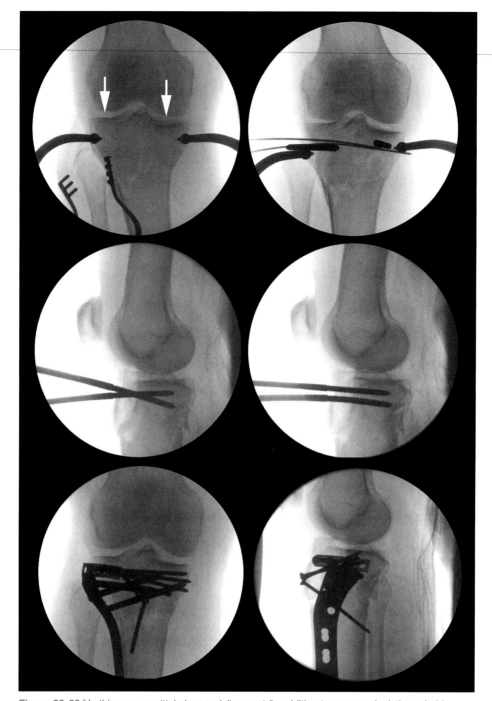

Figure 22-20 I In this case, sagittal plane malalignment (in addition to varus and relative subsidence of the medial plateau) was noted on the AP (*upper left*) and lateral views (*middle left*) (*arrows*). Schanz pins were inserted to derotate both plateaus (*upper right* and *middle right*). This restored the posterior tibial inclination in both plateaus (*middle* and *lower row*).

- *Coronal plane fractures in the lateral plateau* can be compressed and stabilized with 2.4-mm subchondral lag screws placed anterior to posterior just above the rafting screws in the anterolateral plate.
- Reduction and fixation of the posteromedial fragment.
  - Large pointed reduction clamps from anterior to posterior; an old-style pelvic clamp or new-style "goose" neck pelvic clamp helps to avoid excessive pressure on the anteromedial soft tissue.
  - 2.5-mm Schanz pin to joystick.
  - 3.5-mm LC-DC plate contoured with plate-bending press.
    - Stouter plate may be preferable if fracture involves the shaft or is unstable.

      ■ If an antiglide function is needed, a one-third tubular plate, 2.7 LC-DC plate, or 3.5-mm distal radius T-plate is sufficient.
- Femoral distractor or external fixator.
- Proximal screw to lateral fragment, after reduction of lateral plateau.
  - ■ Assistant holds leg up from the lateral side, palpate elbow of lateral plate, and triangulate drill bit (Fig. 22-21).

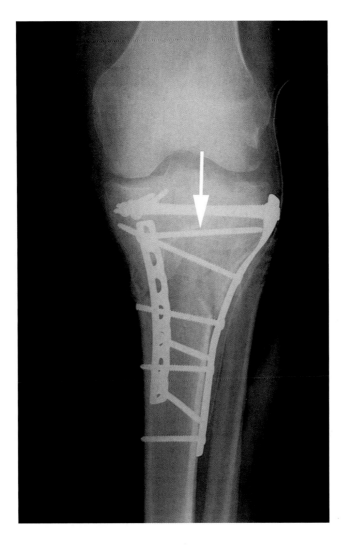

Figure 22-21 I The most proximal of the medial to lateral screws (*arrow*) can be placed bicortically by palpating the anterolateral tibial cortex at the elbow of the plate and triangulating to avoid plate contact.

- In *Schatzker type IV and VI patterns*, the unstable segment is most frequently the distal segment (i.e., the tibial [meta]diaphysis), and the posteromedial fragment is the stable segment.
  - ■ Thus, to reduce the shaft to the intact medial plateau, typically, axial traction, with valgus, extension, and internal rotation forces on the leg, is necessary.
  - ■ Note that this maneuver will tend to place the obstructing structures, such as the gastrocnemius-soleus and hamstrings, under tension.
  - ■ The external fixator may need to be loosened to obtain this reduction.
  - ■ Prior to reduction, multiple long 0.062-inch K-wires are prepositioned along the articular rim of the fragment, aiming toward the intact distal lateral cortex.
  - ■ Along with manipulation of the tibial shaft, the posteromedial fragment may be manipulated with a shoulder hook, spiked pusher or large Weber or goose clamp.
  - ■ Once reduction is obtained, the prepositioned wires are passed. Often, even with multiple wires, the fragment may displace a millimeter or two with clamp removal. This can be corrected with application of a buttress plate, allowing controlled reduction of the fragment.

- If a coronal split exists in a reduced medial articular fragment, anterior-to-posterior subchondral lag screws can be placed below the medial tibial plateau, followed by lateral-to-medial locking screws through a laterally based locking plate.
    - The most proximal locking screws should be placed just distal to the medial subchondral screws to provide them with additional support.
- *Hyperextension varus pattern*
    - Higher rate of vascular and neurologic injury than typical *Schatzker V and VI patterns.*
    - Posterior metaphyseal cortex fails in tension, while the anterior articular surface is crushed (Fig. 22-22).

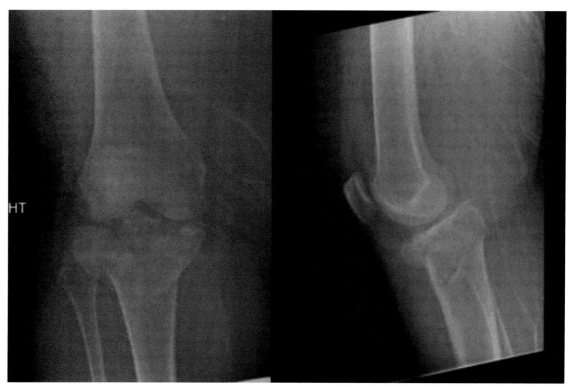

Figure 22-22 I Injury radiographs demonstrating a hyperextension varus bicondylar tibial plateau fracture.

- Often results in comminuted medial and lateral articular surfaces.
- On the lateral injury film, the tibial slope will be negative.
- Critical to restore normal tibial slope and support with anterior implants.
- The medial incision is biased slightly more anterior that the standard posteromedial incision to allow access to the entire medial column.
- Posteromedial fragment typically has a good cortical read because of the tension failure.
    - May be reduced with a large Weber clamp placed in the PCL insertion or posterior rim of the medial plateau and the other tine in the distal segment, docked in a drill hole.
    - Alternatively, a spike pusher placed on the tibial shaft and a shoulder hook on the posteromedial plateau rim may be effective in reversing the negative tibial slope of the posterior fragment.
- The anteromedial fragments are accessed anterior to the anterior border of the superficial MCL through the same medial incision.
- The anterior articular block is elevated using broad osteotomes or a lamina spreader.
- Fixation of the anteromedial fragment(s) is obtained with a T-shaped buttress plate, placed strategically to resist fragment subsidence (Fig. 22-23).

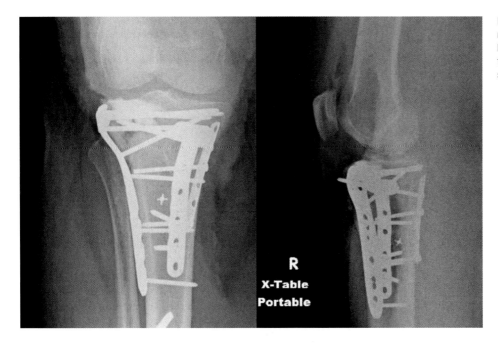

Figure 22-23 | Postoperative radiographs demonstrating anterior buttress plates placed both on the anteromedial and anterolateral surfaces.

- Comminuted articular fragments are reduced radiographically by tamping through a cortical window and held with subchondral wires and allograft bone.
- The lateral plateau is addressed as described above.
- The anterolateral buttress plate is placed more anterior that usual to preferentially buttress the anterior fragments.
  - Often, a large anterior defect persists and requires bone grafting or synthetic bone void filler.
  - Additional structural support may be used for large defects.
  - Cortical allografts (fibula, tricortical iliac crest), tantalum blocks, or spine cage may be used (Figs. 22-24 and 22-25).

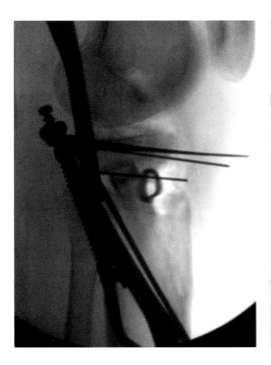
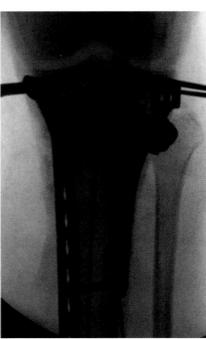

Figure 22-24 | Intraoperative images demonstrating use of allograft fibula for structural support of the articular surface in a hyperextension bicondylar tibial plateau.

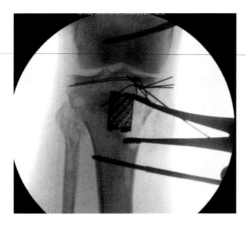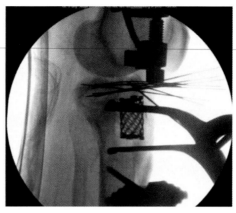

Figure 22-25 | Intraoperative images demonstrating use of a spine cage for structural support of the articular surface in a hyperextension bicondylar tibial plateau.

- If the tibial tubercle is involved as a separate fragment, it should be reduced and stabilized separately.
  - This can be done as the first step if desired and can be accessed through the lateral approach by mobilizing the tissues medial to the incision with or without a distal extension of the incision (Fig. 22-26).

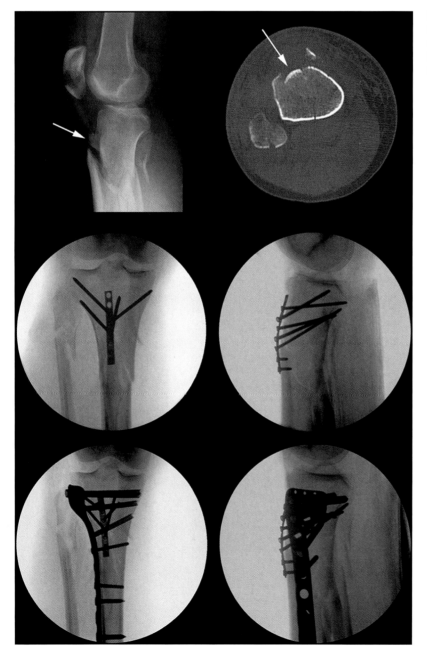

Figure 22-26 | The tibial tubercle is a separate fragment in this case (*arrows*). It was reduced and stabilized using a small fragment plate. This also indirectly reduced a portion of the segmentally comminuted metadiaphyseal fracture.

- If more than a few screws are needed, unicortical screws may be preferable in the anterior plate initially avoiding interference with subsequent reductions and application of screws through other plates (either a lateral plate or a posteromedial plate) (Fig. 22-27).

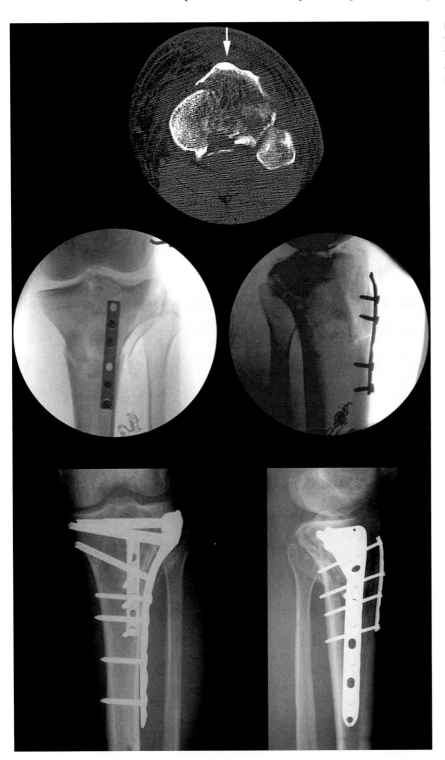

Figure 22-27 When stabilizing a tibial tubercle fracture (*arrow*) associated with a tibial plateau fracture initially, unicortical screws allow unimpeded reduction and implant placement into the other fragments.

- Alternatively, if the tubercle is a large fragment, oblique anterior-to-posterior screws can be used (Fig. 22-28).

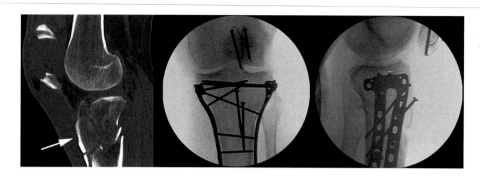

Figure 22-28 ▮ Lag screws may be used for a large separate tibial tubercle fragment (*arrow*).

- Associated fractures of the tibial spines/eminence rarely involve the weight-bearing surface. However, reduction can assist in cortical and articular "reads" and can restore integrity of the cruciate ligaments and meniscal crus.
  - A dental pick or small Freer elevator can be used through a lateral arthrotomy to reduce the central fragment.
  - Stabilization may proceed with K-wires followed by screws (Fig. 22-29).

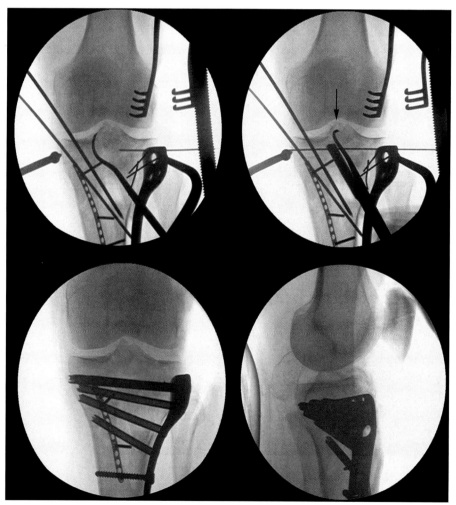

Figure 22-29 ▮ The tibial eminence can be reduced using a small hook through the lateral incision underneath the patellar tendon (*arrow, upper right*).

- K-wires can be placed into the main fragment and advanced through the skin on the contralateral side.
  - These can then be pulled retrograde until they are flush to allow for plate placement (Fig. 22-30).

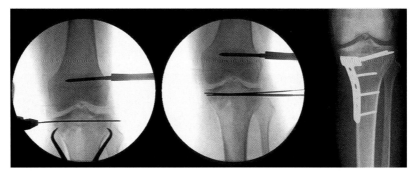

Figure 22-30 I K-wires placed into the main fragment, advanced through the contralateral plateau, and pulled retrograde until flush allows for easier and unencumbered lateral plate placement.

- For an isolated fracture of the posteromedial tibial plateau, the fracture can be reduced under direct vision based on cortical interdigitation.
  - An antiglide plate can be placed on the posterior aspect of the tibia through a posteromedial approach when the patient is supine (Fig. 22-31).

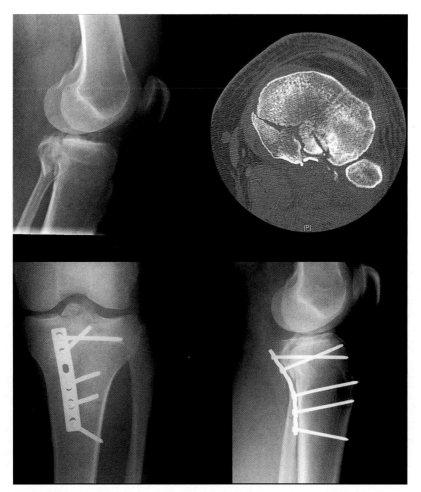

Figure 22-31 I Posterior tibial plateau plating through the posteromedial approach.

- The use of a 2.0-mm buttressing "rim plate" can be effective in applying support or compression to the subchondral and metaphyseal bone as it distributes forces over a larger surface area than screws alone, especially in soft bone. It functions as a large washer.
- Adjunctive techniques to support articular fragments.
  - Using 2.0- or 2.4-mm screws also allows for multiple points of fixation of articular fragments near the subchondral bone.
  - Depending on the anatomic region of comminution, the plate may be placed selectively, anteriorly, anterolaterally, laterally, or medially (Figs. 22-32 and 22-33).

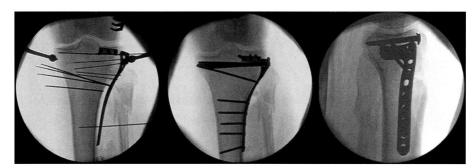

Figure 22-32 | A one-quarter tubular plate with 2.7-mm screws applied as a rim plate placed on the anterior margin of the lateral tibial plateau. This allows compression across a coronal fracture plane and acts as a large washer supporting the screws and elevated articular surface.

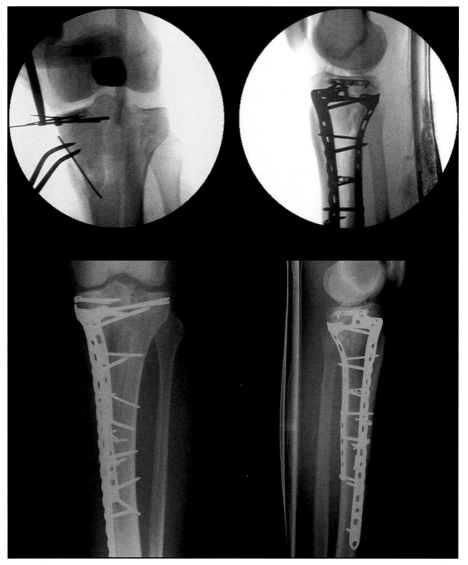

Figure 22-33 | A rim plate can also be placed on the medial plateau to buttress articular segments.

- If comminution of both plateaus is present, a rim plate may be placed along the entire juxta-articular anterior cortical surface.
  - This is helpful in coronal fractures that extend across both tibial plateaus.
  - The plate may be inserted from lateral to medial, under the patellar tendon/infrapatellar fat pad and over the distal insertion of anterior tibial capsule.
  - A small anteromedial incision, placed medial to the patella tendon, facilitates medial screw insertion (Fig. 22-34).

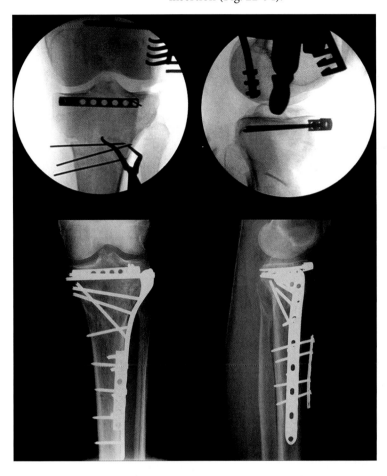

Figure 22-34 ▌ A one-quarter tubular anterior rim plate applied across the entire anterior extra-articular metaphysis of the proximal tibia.

- The anterior-to-posterior screws in these rim plates should be placed proximal to the lateral-to-medial screws inserted through periarticular plates.
- When osteochondral articular fragments are stabilized provisionally with K-wires and are too small for definitive screw fixation, these same K-wires can be used as adjunctive definitive fixation.
  - They can be cut short, bent, and then be impacted flush with the metaphyseal cortex.
  - These function as a subarticular support, buttressing reinforcement (similar to concrete "rebar" or joists).
  - Threaded K-wires likely migrate less often than smooth K-wires, but migration of these periarticular K-wires when associated with stable fixation is rare (Fig. 22-35).

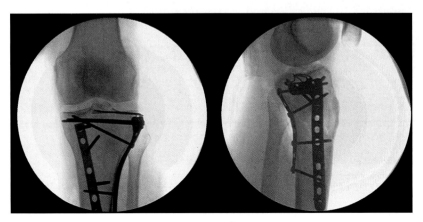

Figure 22-35 ▌ In this case, definitive subarticular K-wires were used for supporting small articular fragments.

- Another technique to capture small fragments is to cut through the two outer holes of a small malleable three- or four-hole plate (e.g., one-third tubular, one-fourth tubular, 2.4 mm, 2.0 mm), leaving one or more intact center hole(s).
  - Each end can be contoured into hooks to create a large linear spiked washer with a larger surface area, similar to a spring plate used for posterior wall acetabular fractures (Fig. 22-36).
  - If the cortical bone is so dense that the hook tips will not penetrate the cortex, two small holes can be drilled with the appropriate spacing to allow the hooks to seat and sit flush with the bone surface.

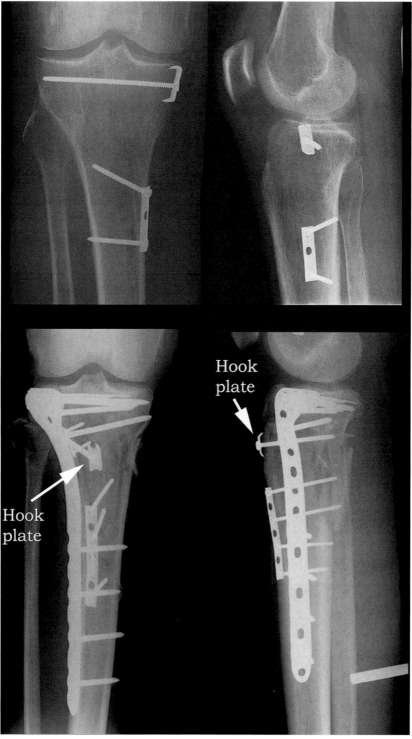

Figure 22-36 I Two examples of hook plates fashioned by cutting a one-third tubular plate to act as a large washer on the tibial plateau.

Foundation Technique for the Profoundly Depressed Tibial Plateau Fracture

Thomas M. Large

Pathoanatomy

Osteoporotic tibial plateau fractures and their associated metaphyseal bone defects are difficult to support and fill with sufficient cancellous allograft given the vacuous tibial metaphysis.

Solution

A foundation of calcium phosphate or calcium sulfate can be used to support the elevated articular surface with a layer of subchondral allograft.

Technique

- Profoundly depressed plateau fractures will have comminuted articular fragments several centimeters below the joint surface. These are usually osteoporotic fractures. They may be unicondylar or part of a bicondylar injury pattern (Fig. 22-37). If unicondylar, the possibility of a concomitant collateral ligament injury should be assessed (e.g., MCL for a lateral plateau fracture).

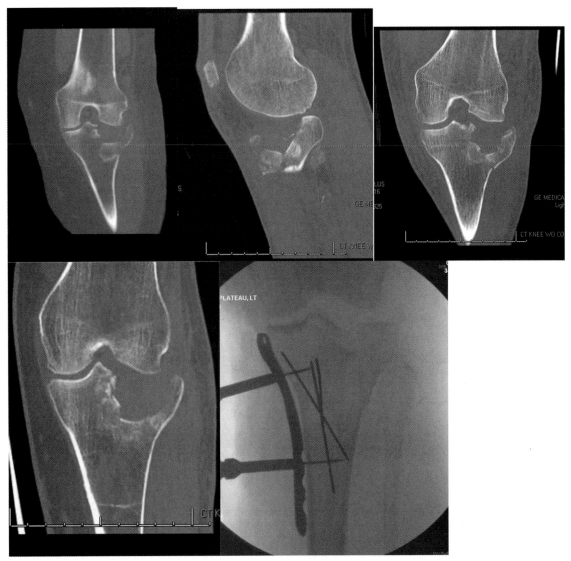

Figure 22-37 ▌ Injury images of a comminuted, osteoporotic, depressed lateral tibial plateau fracture. Note the small, thin, and vertically oriented articular fracture fragments in the central metaphysis.

- The articular fragments are usually thin with little bone attached to the cartilage surface. After elevating these fragments to reduce the joint surface, there remains a large metaphyseal void.
- In osteoporotic individuals, the metaphyseal bone defect below the reduced articular surface and surrounding vacuous metaphysis can be filled with an ever-increasing amount of allograft, which remains unsupported by deficient metadiaphyseal trabeculae.
- If calcium phosphate or calcium sulfate cement is injected directly into the bone void, it may penetrate the joint and disrupt the reduced, interdigitating articular fragments. This may adversely affect healing, and it places a very hard surface directly under these thin joint fragments.
- The "foundation technique" places a layer of physiologically compatible viscoelastic cancellous allograft under the reduced fracture fragments. Below this raft of compacted cancellous bone chips, calcium phosphate, calcium sulfate, or hydroxyapatite is used to fill the remaining large metaphyseal bone void (Fig. 22-38).

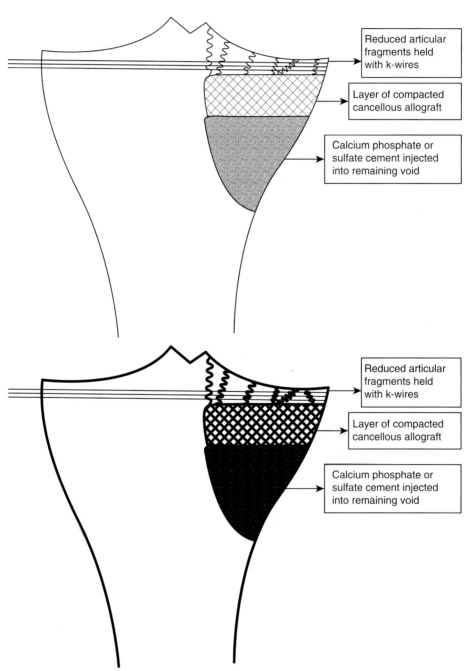

Reduced articular
fragments held
with k-wires

Layer of compacted
cancellous allograft

Calcium phosphate or
sulfate cement injected
into remaining void

Reduced articular
fragments held
with k-wires

Layer of compacted
cancellous allograft

Calcium phosphate or
sulfate cement injected
into remaining void

Figure 22-38 ‖ An illustration demonstrating the layered technique for supporting the articular surface and filling the large residual metaphyseal void after reduction and provisional fixation with subchondral K-wires.

- First, reduce the fracture. Generally, a lateral corticotomy is made in the metaphyseal region, and an impactor is used to elevate the articular fragments into position (Fig. 22-39).

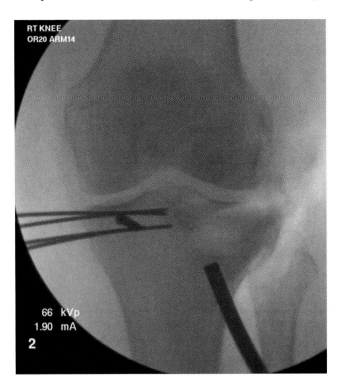

Figure 22-39 | An intra-operative AP image demonstrating pre-positioned K-wires and a tamp in position before reduction of the depressed articular surface.

- Having a raft of K-wires in position medial to the fracture in a juxta-articular location allows these to be easily advanced to hold the articular surface after joint reduction (Figs. 22-39 and 22-40), or alternatively, they can be inserted from the lateral side.
- There are often fragments in the medial aspect of the depression that are oriented perpendicular to the joint line. These may be difficult to reduce from a lateral corticotomy due to their orientation

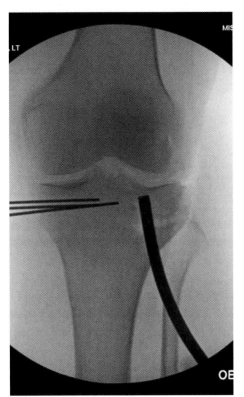

Figure 22-40 | An intra-operative AP image demonstrating tamp assited reduction of the articular surface.

(see Fig. 22-37). A medial corticotomy may be used to elevate these more centrally located, perpendicularly oriented fragments. Once freed from the central metaphysis, a dental pick or Freer elevator can be used to guide them into their reduced positions in the joint surface (Fig. 22-41).

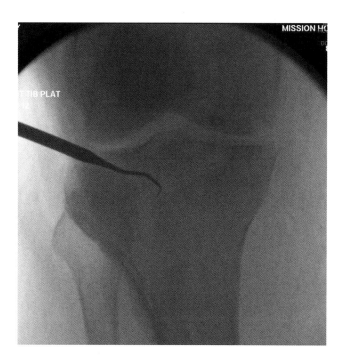

Figure 22-41 I An intra-operative AP image demonstrating use of a dental pick to fine tune the reduction of an independent articular fragment.

- Inspect the reduction using fluoroscopy and direct visualization through the lateral arthrotomy. Headlamp visualization and/or the femoral distractors are useful (Fig. 22-42).

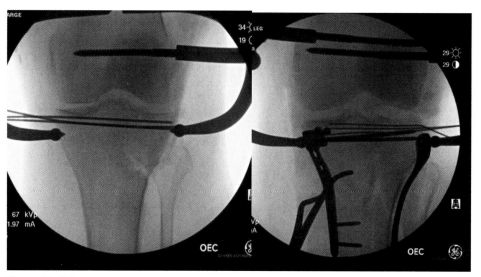

Figure 22-42 I An intra-operative AP images demonstrating use of a quad clamp to reduce the articular width after the joint has been elevated and fixed with K-wires.

- With the joint reduced, consider applying a large periarticular quadrangular-type clamp to maintain the condylar width (Fig. 22-42) and then pack cancellous allograft through the corticotomy under the articular fragments until it is about 1 cm thick (Fig. 22-43).

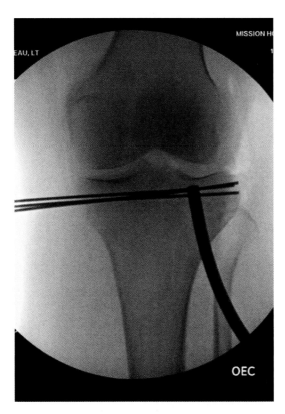

Figure 22-43 ▌ An intra-operative AP image demonstrating use of a tamp to imact crushed cancellous allograft underneath the subchondral bone.

- Inject the calcium phosphate or sulfate cement to fill the remaining void.
- Finally, apply your definitive proximal tibial implant with rafting screws to complete the construct. K-wires are then generally removed although keeping a raft of K-wires or replacing the K-wires with a raft of mini-fragment screws can also be used to augment the construct if needed (Fig. 22-44).

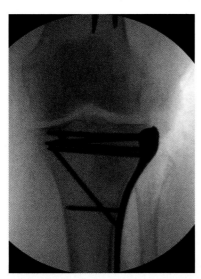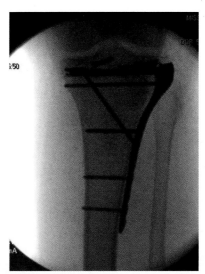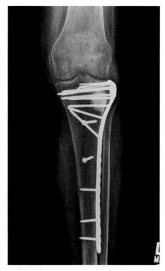

Figure 22-44 ▌ Intra-operative and a post-operative AP images demonstrating injection of the synthetic bone void filler underneath the allograft layer for additional structural support. Subchondral mini-fragment screws can be added so additional articular support.

- This provides a durable result preserving biology at the fracture site while decreasing the risk of subsidence.
- Figure 22-45 shows healed films at follow-up.

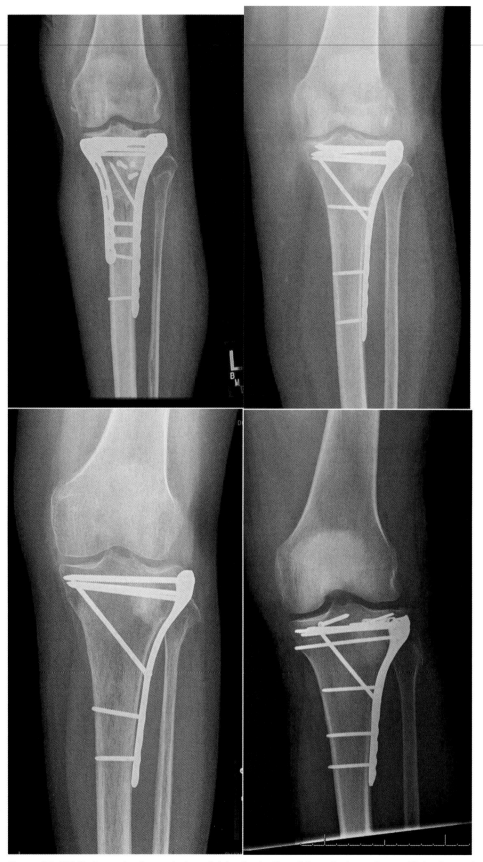

Figure 22-45 I Radiographs demonstrate maintained reduction of the articular surfaces with fracture union.

- *Metadiaphyseal dissociation*
- An effective reduction strategy for severely comminuted fractures includes reassembling the fracture fragments that have the clearest fracture lines.
  - This creates a progressively more stable fracture.
  - The reduction of subsequent fracture fragments is facilitated, much like "doing a jigsaw puzzle."
  - Sequential reductions and fragment stabilization then proceeds (Fig. 22-46).

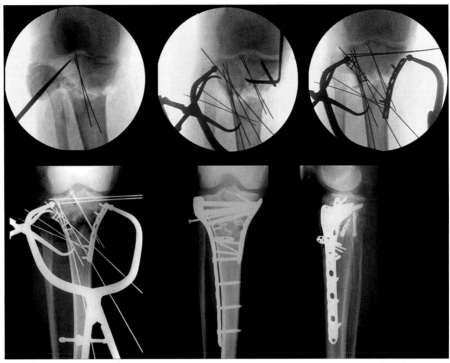

Figure 22-46 ‖ In this severely comminuted tibial plateau fracture, reliable cortical interdigitations (i.e., "cortical reads") are addressed first, and the remainder of the plateau is reduced sequentially to restore alignment.

- When sequentially reconstructing small fragments, small 2.0-mm plates can also be used to stabilize individual cortical fracture lines (Fig. 22-47).

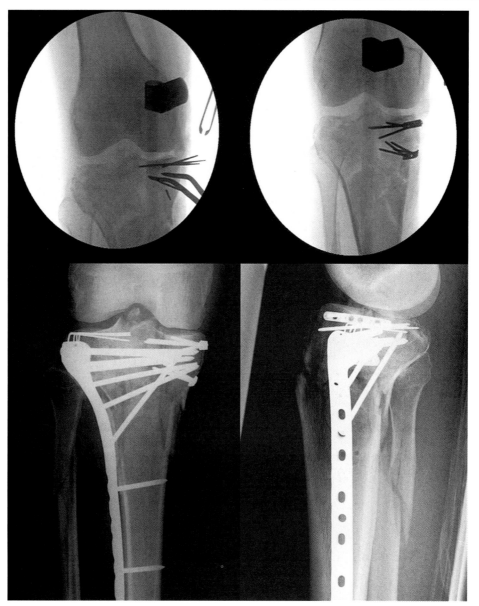

Figure 22-47 I Mini-fragment plates can be used to stabilize individual fracture lines of small periarticular fragments.

- Similarly, small 2.0-mm plates can be used to segmentally stabilize long spiral fracture lines prior to buttress plate placement (Fig. 22-48).

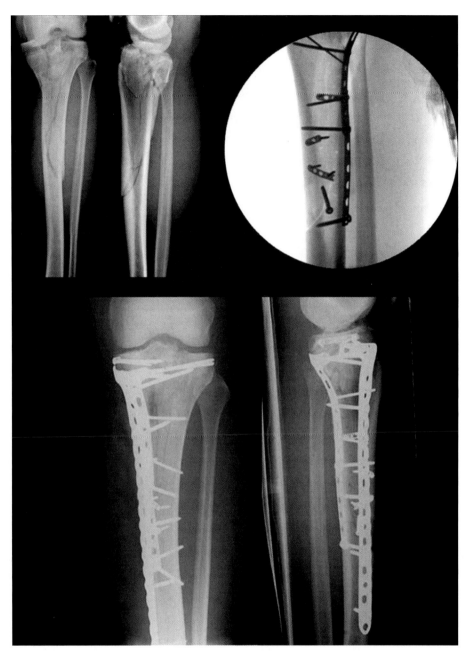

Figure 22-48 ▌ Long fracture lines can be stabilized with 2.0-mm plates and unicortical screws. These provide more stable fixation than do K-wires and do not obstruct subsequent implants. These small plates must be supported by stronger neutralization/buttress plates.

- During the application of a temporizing external fixator, if one of the fracture lines of an articular fragment exits distally in the shaft, it can be reduced and stabilized concomitantly.
  - This converts an AO/OTA type C fracture to a type B pattern, simplifying the definitive reconstructive procedure. The stability of the initial reduction is improved too.
  - The soft tissues must be evaluated carefully to ensure they are amenable to surgical dissection (Fig. 22-49).

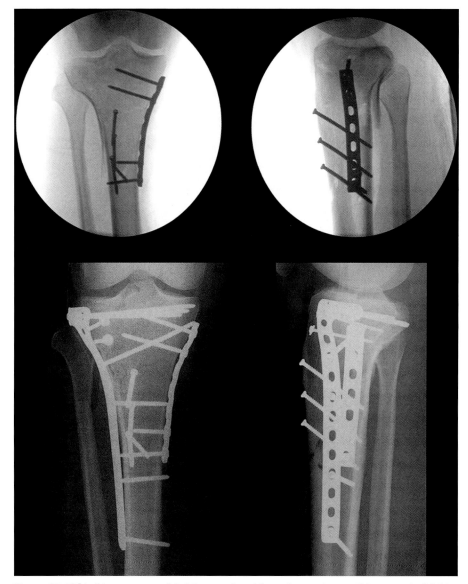

Figure 22-49 I In this case, a medial plate was placed through a posteromedial approach distal to the articular surface at the time of spanning fixator application (external fixator pins are proximal and distal to the C-arm image fields). Several weeks later, when swelling had diminished, final articular repair was simplified.

- If a long medial plate is needed for tibial diaphyseal extension, an anterolateral distal tibial plate from the contralateral side often fits well.
  - This may be applied through a posteromedial approach (Fig. 22-50).

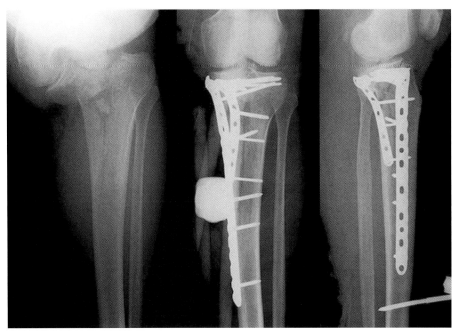

Figure 22-50 | A contralateral anterolateral distal tibial plate may be used on the medial tibial plateau when distal extension is needed.

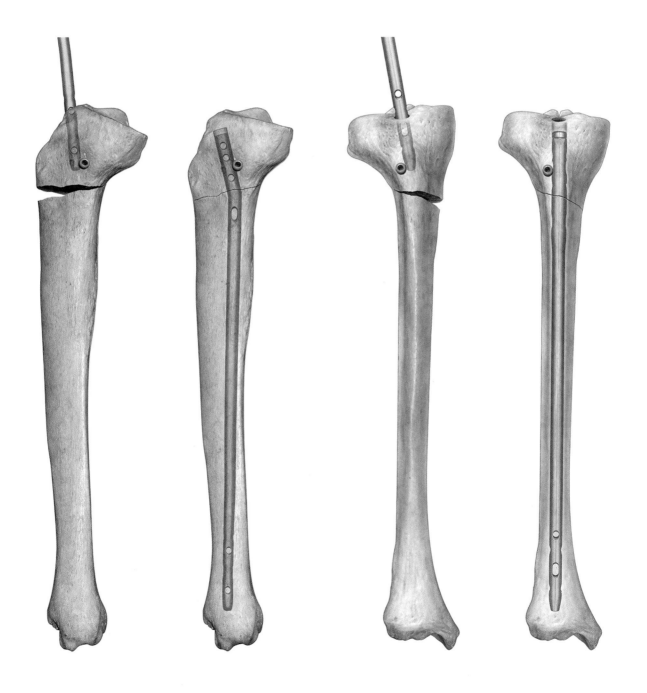

Chapter 23
Tibial Shaft Fractures

ANDREW R. EVANS
MICHAEL F. GITHENS
M. BRADFORD HENLEY
ROBERT A. HYMES
ANNA N. MILLER

Sterile Instruments/Equipment

- Multiple small and large retractors
- Gelpi retractor
- Medium or large radiolucent triangle for limb positioning
- Large and small standard and modified pointed "Weber" bone reduction clamps
- Pigtailed awl or 2.8- to 3.2-mm guide pin and cannulated 8- to 10-mm drill bit
- Implants: small fragment plates and screws (for provisional stabilization of open fractures)
  - Tibial nailing or plating system of choice

Patient Positioning

- Supine.
- Cantilever-type OR table with radiolucent extension (diving board) so that the C-arm is unencumbered for imaging in the AP and lateral planes.
- Place a small bump (rolled towel or blanket) beneath the ipsilateral buttock and flank to neutralize the lower limb external rotation (patella pointed superiorly).
- Consider positioning the ipsilateral upper extremity across the body to avoid shoulder hyperextension and brachioplexopathy.
- If nailing in the semiextended position, elevate the operative leg on a foam ramp to facilitate lateral imaging.
- Exclude the groin and perineum from the operative field with an impervious U-shaped drape.
- Prep and drape the affected lower extremity to the ipsilateral groin.
  - Wrap the toes with an impervious drape (e.g., Ioban, Coban, Viadrape) to minimize toe/toenail-related contamination.
  - For infrapatellar nailing, position the lower extremity over an appropriately sized radiolucent triangular pillow or metal frame.
    - Puts patella tendon on slight stretch, which may facilitate incision placement

Surgical Approaches

Anterior Approach to the Proximal Tibia (for Infrapatellar Tibial Intramedullary Nailing)

- With the knee flexed over the radiolucent triangle, make an incision longitudinally over the midline of the patellar tendon, or medial (or lateral) to the tendon, depending on the fracture pattern and surgeon's preference.
  - This approach portion may also be performed with knee in extension to 30 degrees of flexion.

- Dissect sharply down to the paratenon of patellar tendon.
  - Avoid the occasional infrapatellar branch of the saphenous nerve inferiorly within the subcutaneous tissue.
  - Patellar tendon-splitting approach.
    - Incise the paratenon as a distinct tissue layer, separating its edges from the patellar tendon to facilitate closure.
    - Assess the medial and lateral borders of the patellar tendon through visualization or palpation.
    - Incise the patellar tendon longitudinally in its midline.
      - Use Debakey forceps to retract tendon split, to allow maintenance of single plane in tendon fibers (Fig. 23-1).

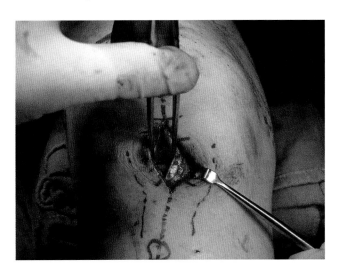

Figure 23-1 I A pair of Debakey forceps placed in the tendon split allows for retraction and extension of the split within the same tendon fiber plane (parallel to and between tendon fibers rather than crossing fibers).

    - Retract the medial and lateral portions of the tendon to visualize the retropatellar fat pad.
    - Atraumatically elevate the fat pad from its distal position, superiorly to visualize proximal tibia.
      - If the insertion point is not approached by elevation of the fat pad and periosteum, beware of injury to menisci or intermeniscal and coronary ligaments.
    - Consider Gelpi or two "L"-shaped retractors (e.g., Langenbeck) to provide visualization and to protect the patellar tendon from reamers.
      - If Gelpi is used, it may be angulated when the knee is placed in flexion by tension on the patellar ligament; this may be avoided by securing the retractor to the leg.
      - A laparotomy sponge placed through finger holes and placed posteriorly around proximal leg will maintain the position of the Gelpi retractor.
  - Paratendinous approach
    - May be performed medially (or rarely laterally) to the tendon.
      - Tibial tubercle is lateral to the intramedullary tibial axis.
      - Skin incision may be chosen to correspond more closely to the planned paratendinous approach.
    - Dissect sharply to the desired edge of the patellar tendon paratenon, and retract it.
- Separate the posterior aspect of the tendon from the retropatellar fat pad bluntly, and sweep the fat pad and anterior periosteum superiorly and posteriorly with a blunt elevator.
- Bovie cautery may be used to assist in elevating the fat pad with the anterior tibial periosteum.
  - Avoid penetration of the joint capsule or injury to the anterior intermeniscal ligament.
- The fat pad should be retracted just far enough to visualize the starting point for the tibial guide pin or awl/nail entry site.[1]
- To facilitate fracture reduction, heel should be elevated slightly off of the table by choosing a triangle of sufficient height.
  - This will permit gravity to assist in restoration of limb length for reduction.
- To correct procurvatum angulation, place bolster or towels posterior to heel or under distal metatarsals, distal to fracture (dorsiflexing foot and increasing apex posterior angulation).
- For recurvatum deformities, place bolster or towels proximal to fracture, allowing distal tibia and foot to sag posteriorly.

Suprapatellar (Retropatellar Approach) for Semiextended Nailing

- Longitudinal skin incision 3 cm long, ending 1 cm proximal to the superior pole of the patella.
- Identify the midline of the quadriceps tendon.
- Make a full-thickness incision through the quadriceps tendon in line with its fibers from the superior pole of the patella to the proximal extent of the incision.
- Manually palpate the patellofemoral joint for plica and ensure adequate space for retropatellar nailing.
- Atraumatically insert the protective cannula to access the standard start site.
- Note, the knee should be flexed between 20 and 30 degrees.
  - Towel bumps are used to flex the knee to the appropriate degree to access the start site.

Lateral Extra-articular Parapatellar Approach for Semiextended Nailing

- Longitudinal incision along the lateral border of the patella, 3 to 5 cm in length, terminating at the level of the proximal tibia.
- Carefully identify the lateral retinaculum distally and incise from distal to proximal without violating the joint capsule.
- Access the starting point by slightly subluxating the patella medially.
  - If the starting point cannot be accessed, a more formal lateral release may be required.
- Nailing proceeds in the semiextended position.

Anterolateral Approach to the Tibial Shaft

- Make skin incision longitudinally 1 to 2 cm lateral to the anterolateral tibial crest.
- Dissect sharply through skin and subcutaneous tissue to the anterior compartment fascia.
- Incise the fascia sharply, approximately 5 mm lateral to the tibial crest, leaving a small fascial flap attached to the tibial crest to facilitate closure of the anterior compartment once fracture fixation has been achieved, if indicated.
- The lateral aspect of the tibial shaft can be exposed by elevating the anterior compartment from the lateral tibial periosteum, leaving the periosteum and periosteal vessels intact.
  - Elevate the muscle from distal to proximal using the natural plane of muscle fiber insertion.
  - This will minimize muscle injury, bleeding, and devascularization.

Posteromedial Approach to the Tibial Shaft

- Most often used for
  - Stabilizing the tibial shaft component of a pilon or tibial plateau fracture
  - Nonunions/malunions
- Make an incision longitudinally 1 to 2 cm posterior to the posteromedial tibial border, being careful not to place incision on the poor and traumatized soft tissues on the medial face of the tibia.
- Dissect sharply through skin and subcutaneous tissue.
  - Dissect to the superficial and deep posterior compartment fascia of the tibia.
- Avoid injury to the saphenous nerve and branch of the saphenous vein.
- Incise the fascia sharply, leaving a 3- to 5-mm flap of fascia attached to the posteromedial tibial border to facilitate later fascial closure if indicated in atraumatic conditions.
- Superficial and deep posterior compartment musculature may be opened or elevated from the posterior aspect of the tibia.
- In the distal third of the tibia, the deep posterior compartment fascia is incised, and the musculature may be elevated off of the posterior tibial periosteum.
  - Posterior soft tissue attachments represent the most robust blood supply to the tibia during fracture healing.
  - Posterior submuscular and periosteal dissection should be limited to prevent further devascularization.

Reduction and Implant Techniques

External Fixation

- Currently, uniplanar external fixation has a limited role in the definitive management of tibial shaft fractures, but can serve as a temporizing technique.
  - May be applied as provisional stabilization to restore limb length, alignment, and rotation in physiologically unstable patients (Fig. 23-2).

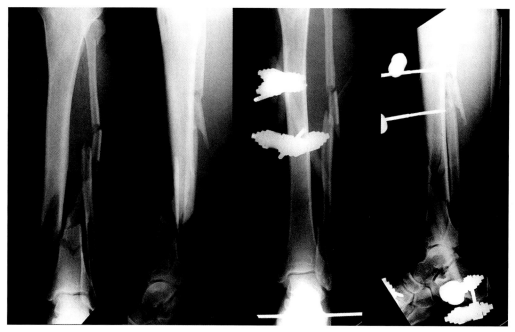

Figure 23-2 ▮ Example of a multiply injured patient with a comminuted open tibial fracture. A damage control approach was used, with tibial external fixation initially. Conversion to intramedullary nailing was performed in 6 days when the patient's hemodynamic profile improved.

- Conversion to internal fixation may be performed without significant increase in infection risk if performed within 5 to 14 days.[2]
- May serve as supplemental fixation to an internal fixation construct, but should avoid contact with the internal fixation devices to prevent contamination via pin tracts.
- Circular tensioned wire (e.g., Ilizarov) external fixation is a particularly useful technique for the management of open tibial fractures with sizeable segmental bone defects (>4 to 6 cm) and is a useful tool in the treatment of deformities and nonunions.
  - Provides the option for management of bone defects with bone transport (controlled mechanical distraction osteogenesis) techniques.

Tibial Nailing

Techniques for obtaining and maintaining reduction while nailing include manual manipulation of the leg, use of a distractor or external fixator, percutaneous manipulation with Schanz pins, percutaneous or open clamping, open reduction and provisional plating, and placement of blocking screws.

Esmarch Bandage for Maintaining Tibia Shaft Reduction during Intramedullary Nailing

Robert A. Hymes

Pathoanatomy

Obtaining and maintaining reduction of the tibia shaft are integral to intramedullary nailing. The majority of closed tibia shaft fractures are manually reduced by the surgeon through traction and gentle manipulation of the fracture fragments into reasonable anatomic alignment. The alignment is then maintained while the guidewire is passed across the reduced fracture site prior to reaming. Maintenance of fracture reduction during reaming and nail insertion simplifies the process. In some fracture patterns, this can be very difficult to achieve with manual manipulation or clamp application.

Solution

An Esmarch bandage can be used during tibial nailing to assist in the maintenance of the reduction.

Technique

After the surgeon aligns the displaced fracture by manipulation, the bandage is wrapped tightly several times around the fractured limb at the fracture site and both proximally and distally (Fig. 23-3A–D).

- The Esmarch should not be so tight as to occlude arterial inflow.

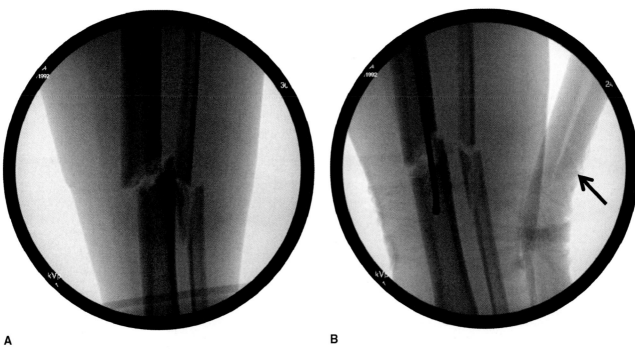

A   **B**

Figure 23-3 ▍ **A:** Intraoperative radiograph of displaced diaphyseal tibia fracture. **B:** Intraoperative radiograph of the reduced fracture stabilized with an Esmarch bandage (*black arrow*).

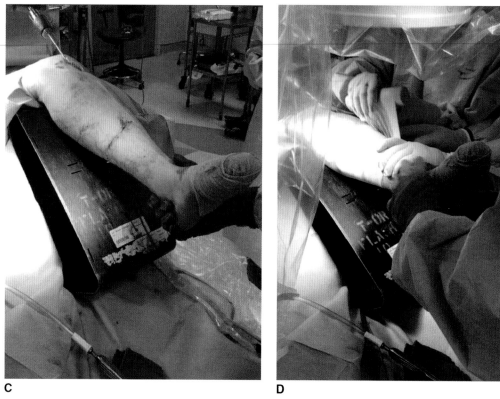

C   **D**

Figure 23-3 ▮ (*Continued*) **C:** Manual reduction of tibia. **D:** Application of Esmarch bandage.

- For the final loop, the bandage is wrapped so as to include the surgeon's hand. This last encircling wrap is then sufficiently loose so as to create a space in which to tuck the residual Esmarch (Fig. 23-4).
- In the majority of cases, this maneuver will maintain the fracture alignment.

Occasionally, after wrapping the Esmarch, additional traction and/or angular corrections are applied to the limb to "fine-tune" the reduction (Fig. 23-5).

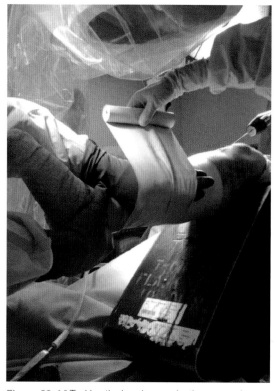

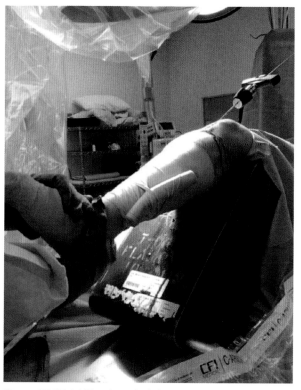

Figure 23-4 ▮ Tucking the bandage under the surgeon's hand to secure the wrap.

Figure 23-5 ▮ Additional manipulation to "fine-tune" the reduction after placement of the wrap.

- It is important to realize that the surgeon must reduce the fracture prior to placement of the Esmarch.
- Application of the bandage is not sufficient to reduce the fracture.

The bandage remains in place during the reaming process as long as the limb remains well vascularized. It may be removed after the nail is seated (Fig. 23-6A–C). Because the reduction of the fracture is maintained and the limb is stabilized by circumferential compression, the process of intramedullary nailing is expedited and usually takes only a few minutes.

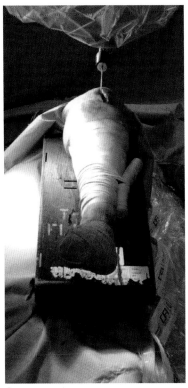

A

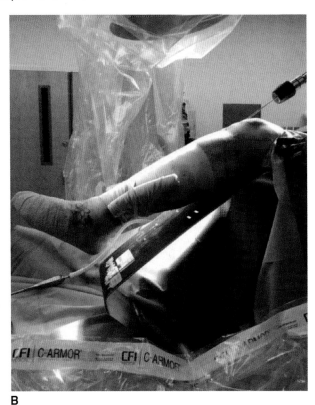

B

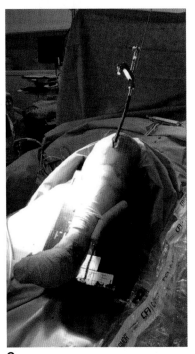

C

Figure 23-6 | A, B: Photograph of Esmarch bandage holding reduced tibia shaft fracture. Note the leg suspended off the radiolucent triangle. **C:** The bandage stays in place until the nail is seated.

- Provisional reduction may be obtained with a medially based femoral distractor.[3]
  - 5.0 × 170 mm Schanz pins.
  - Proximal Schanz pin placement medial to lateral, in proximal tibial metaphysis, posterior to nail insertion point.
    - Pin placed posterior to the midpoint of the anterior-posterior dimension will avoid nail path if at the level distal of the physeal scar.
    - Pin typically placed approximately 1 to 2 cm distal to the articular surface.
  - Distal pin placement medial to lateral in the region of posterior metaphysis/malleolus, near the physeal scar (Fig. 23-7).

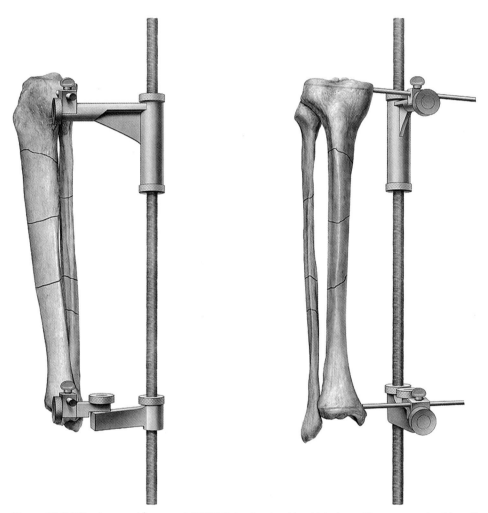

Figure 23-7 I Pin placement for a medial tibial distractor should not interfere with reamer and nail insertion.

- Alternatively, distal distractor pin may be placed into the talar body (in line with tibial axis).
  - Localize starting point medially using fluoroscopy, just distal to anterior colliculus or intercollicular groove of medial malleolus (Figs. 23-8–23-10).

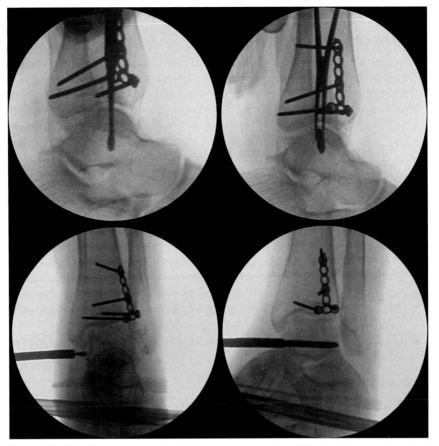

Figure 23-8 In this patient, the distal distractor pin was placed into the talar body, just distal to the intercollicular medial malleolar groove.

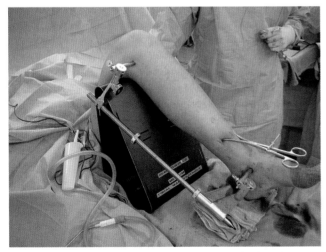

Figure 23-9 Medial femoral distractor used for reduction of a displaced spiral fracture of the distal third tibial fracture. The proximal Schanz pin is placed into the posteromedial tibial metaphysis in the coronal plane. The distal pin is placed into the talar body. A large Weber bone reduction clamp has been placed percutaneously to anatomically reduce and stabilize the spiral fracture.

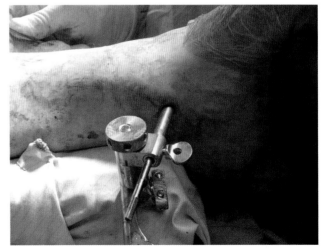

Figure 23-10 Clinical example of Schanz pin placement, medially into the talar body for distractor application. The pin is placed into the central talar body using a small incision at the inferior apex of the anterior colliculus of the medial malleolus.

Cutaneous Landmarks for Medial Talar Body Distractor Pin Placement

M. Bradford Henley
Anna N. Miller

Pathophysiology

For tibial pilon fractures and tibial shaft fractures, restoration of length, alignment, and rotation is critical for fracture reduction. Distraction using a medially based system with a proximal tibial pin and a medial calcaneal pin results in a posteriorly directed force vector. This produced a sagittal plane rotation vector resulting in a recurvatum/extension deformity of the tibial shaft and or distal metaphysis. Furthermore, this distraction vector also results in a torsional moment in the tibiotalar joint and hind foot and places the heel into a "calcaneus"/ankle dorsiflexion position. This reduces intra-articular visualization of the entire tibial plafond when approached either anteromedially or anterolaterally.

Solution

A distractor allows a single surgeon to restore limb length, rotation, and alignment.

- The distal Schanz pin for the distractor may be placed in the posterior tibia, the talus, or the calcaneus, while the proximal pin is usually placed in the proximal tibial metaphysis (for IM nailing) or the metadiaphysis for ORIF of pilon fractures.
- All pins are placed from medial to lateral in the coronal plane. A medial talar body pin is advantageous when used for distraction as the vector is collinear with the long axis of the tibia and results in minimal sagittal plane rotational forces.
- Additionally, a talar pin rarely obscures lateral C-arm images of the distal tibial metaphysis and ankle joint.

Technique

- Cutaneous landmarks alone can be used to place a talar body pin without the need for radiographic imaging. Insertion in the talus avoids possible encroachment of the intramedullary canal and nail path.
- Using a talus pin also avoids pin placement in the distal tibia, which could potentially displace associated posterior malleolar fractures (when IM nailing tibial shaft or distal metaphyseal fractures).
- The talar body's dense bone provides for excellent pin placement and permits distraction colinear with the long axis of the tibia and avoids the talar neck.
- A stab incision is made with a #15 blade (direct the cutting edge of the blade cephalad) directly inferior to the anterior colliculus. This avoids the saphenous vein anterior to the medial malleolus, and the posterior tibial tendon neurovascular bundle distally.
- The anterior and posterior contours of the medial malleolus are visible and palpable. The tip of this palpable subcutaneous landmark is located over the center of the talar body (Fig. 23-11A).
- Using a cannulated guide for a 5-mm Schanz pin, the pin path is first created with a 3.5-mm drill bit (Fig. 23-11B). While drilling, the surgeon holds the foot in neutral, drilling parallel to the dome of the talus, approximating its center of rotation. The Schanz pin is then inserted through the guide (Fig. 23-12A and B).

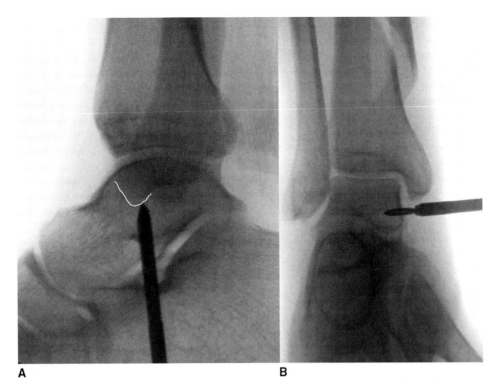

Figure 23-11 | **A:** Lateral radiograph with extracutaneous Schanz pin pointing to tip of anterior colliculus (*white line*). **B:** AP radiograph with tip of 3.5-mm drill bit entering body of talus directly inferior to anterior colliculus.

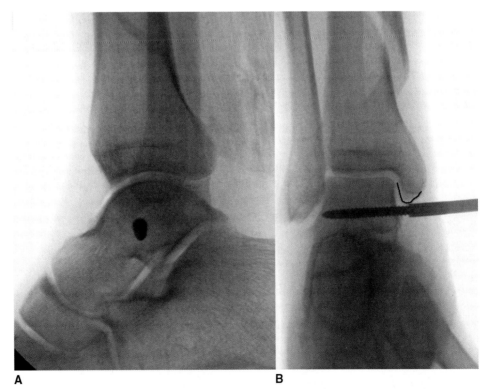

Figure 23-12 | **A:** Lateral radiographic image collinear with shaft of Schanz pin after its insertion into the talar body. **B:** AP image showing Schanz pin inferior to anterior colliculus (*black line*).

● Clinical photos for this technique are presented in Figure 23-13.

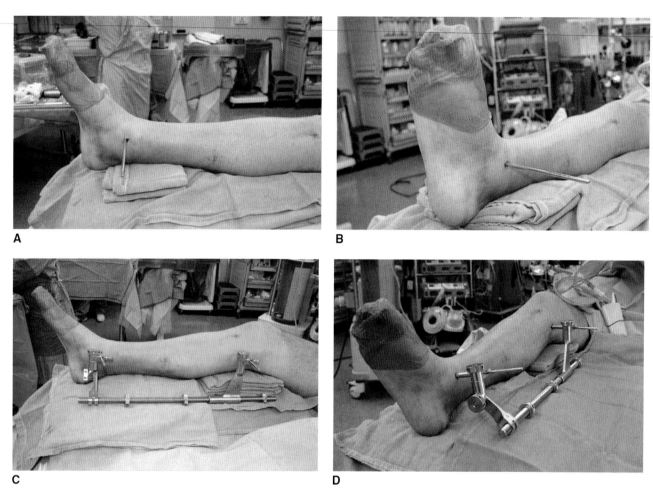

A   B

C   D

Figure 23-13 ❚ Photographs of medial talar pin placement before and after application of the distractor for a tibial shaft fracture. Note distal Schanz pin's position in medial talar body, just distal to anterior colliculus **(A, B)**. Proximal Schanz pin is in posterior tibial metaphysis **(C, D)**. Fixator's hinge/linkage can be used to restore rotation during restoration of limb length.

● Percutaneously placed point-to-point clamp applications are excellent for reduction and compression of closed (e.g., oblique or spiral) tibial shaft fractures (Fig. 23-14).

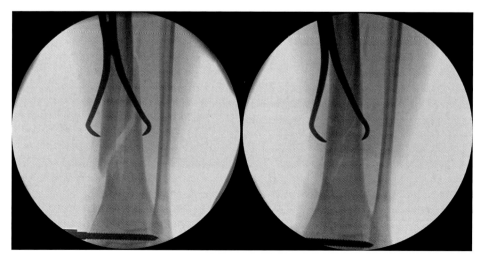

Figure 23-14 ❚ In many fracture patterns, a pointed Weber clamp placed through 0.5- to 1-cm (percutaneous) "stab" incisions can be very effective for fracture reduction.

- Avoid crushing of the skin during clamp application.
- Percutaneous technique minimizes soft tissue injury.
- Incisions for clamp should be based on fluoroscopy, to allow for one tine on each fragment along the ideal vector for interfragmentary compression.
- Large or medium pointed bone reduction clamps (Weber) are ideal for most limbs and fractures.
- Spiral or oblique fractures are most amenable to clamp placement.
- Transverse fractures are easily reduced and compressed with modified Weber clamps.
  - A pilot hole for each tine is placed using a 2.5-mm drill above and below the fracture.
- Retain clamps until interlocking screws are placed.
- Provisional unicortical plating for maintenance of reduction in open fractures is helpful as long as it does not require additional dissection or wound extension beyond that required for adequate debridement (Figs. 23-15–23-18).[4]

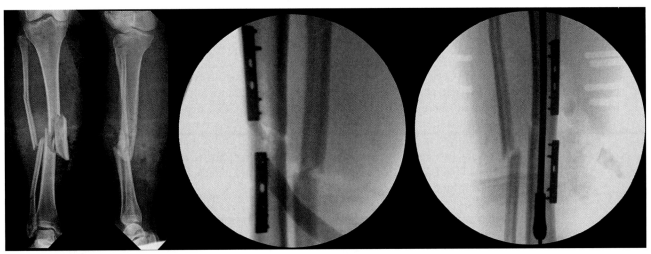

Figure 23-15 | Open segmental tibial shaft fracture. *Left*, initial radiographs; *Center*, provisional unicortical plate fixation; *Right*, preparation of intramedullary canal for nailing.

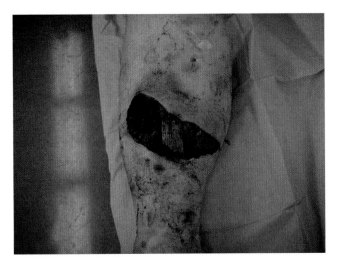

Figure 23-16 | Soft tissue injury of open type 3A segmental tibial shaft fracture at presentation.

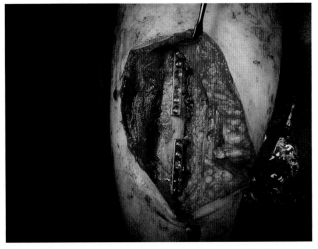

Figure 23-17 | Example of a type 3A segmental open tibial fracture associated with substantial periosteal stripping. After debridement, plates and unicortical screws were used for reduction maintenance during reaming and nail placement.

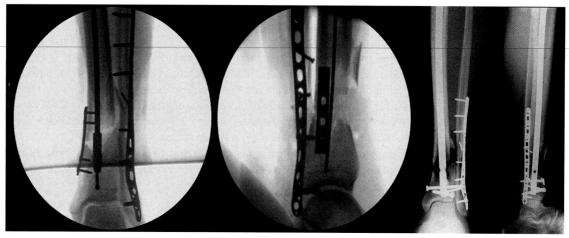

Figure 23-18 I Another example of provisional plating of an open distal tibial fracture, prior to intramedullary nailing. Temporary antibiotic cement beads were placed in this defect prior to closure.

- Thoughtful open reduction of closed fractures for clamping or provisional plating is performed when an accurate reduction cannot be obtained percutaneously.
  - Either an anterolateral or posteromedial approach is used, depending on fracture morphology.
  - Recent literature supports careful open reduction of closed fracture as safe, with no increased rate of infection or nonunion as compared to closed and percutaneous reduction techniques.
  - Blocking (or "Poller") screws or temporary blocking pins/wires can be placed prior to reaming and nail insertion to "recreate" deficient cortices and narrow the effective medullary canal available for the nail (Fig. 23-19).[5]

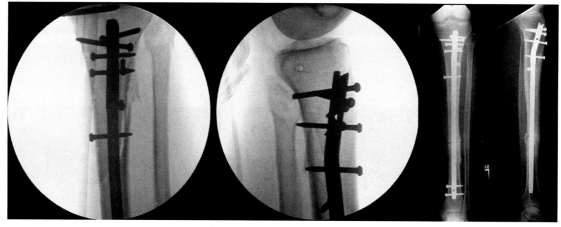

Figure 23-19 I Multiple blocking screws can be used to narrow the effective endosteal pathway, thereby preventing translational and angular deformities. These also add to the construct stability.

- In the setting of oblique or comminuted metaphyseal fractures with a mismatch between the outer nail diameter and the inner diameter of the intramedullary canal (typically, in the metaphyseal or metadiaphyseal region), the nail tends to "seek" the deficient cortex leading to translational/angular deformities.

- These blocking screws are typically placed adjacent to the desired nail path on the concave side of the deformity (Fig. 23-20).

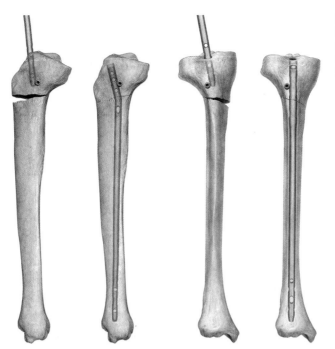

Figure 23-20 | As a general principle, blocking screws are placed adjacent to the nail path, on the concave side of the deformity. This is applicable for both sagittal (**left**) and coronal (**right**) plane deformities.

- Alternatively, Steinmann pins can be used as blocking pins (Fig. 23-21).

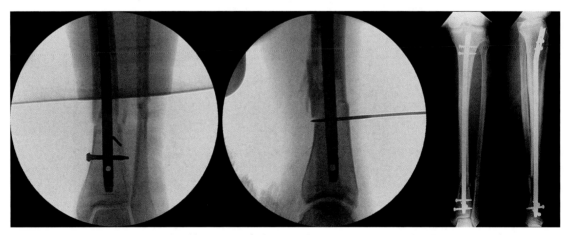

Figure 23-21 | As an alternative to blocking screws, Steinmann pins may be placed to guide the wire and nail along the desired path.

- Pins should be of sufficient diameter so that they are not weakened by adjacent reaming nor deformed by nail insertion.
- Typically, 2.4- to 3.2-mm pins are adequate size depending on the intended application.
- If 3.2-mm pins are used, they may be replaced with 4.5-mm screws.
- If pins are to be removed without replacement by screws, interlocking fixation should be completed prior to pin removal.
- Consider avoiding blocking screws in ballistic fractures as there are often unrecognized fracture lines that may displace or "blow out" when advancing the nail past the blocking screw.

- Nailing of a tibial shaft fracture that involves a concomitant fracture of the tibial plateau or tibial plafond requires provisional and/or definitive articular stabilization prior to reaming and nail insertion (Figs. 23-22–23-24).

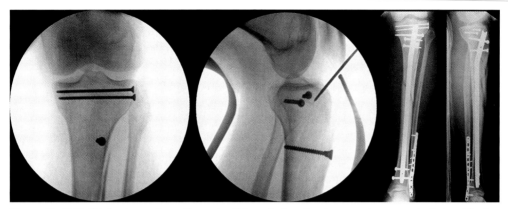

Figure 23-22 | In this fracture pattern with proximal intra-articular extension, percutaneous reduction and fixation of the proximal intra-articular component was placed initially. These implants did not interfere with nail placement.

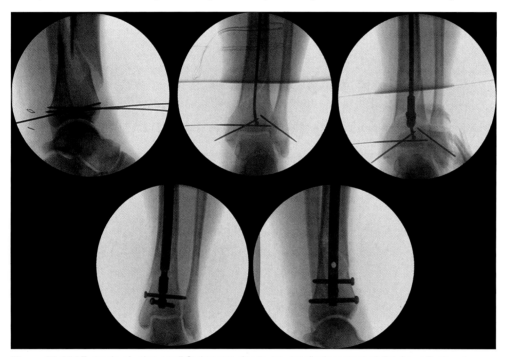

Figure 23-23 | Example of using small Steinmann pins to prevent displacement of distal nondisplaced fractures during nail insertion.

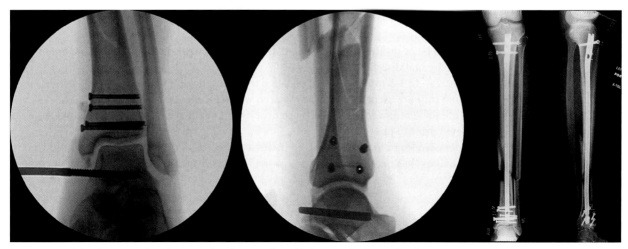

Figure 23-24 | Another example using cannulated screws for ankle fracture fixation while allowing room for distal nail placement.

- CT scanning should be considered for oblique fractures of the distal tibia, as a high incidence of concomitant, often noncontiguous, posterior malleolar and tibial plafond fractures have been described.[6]
- Strategic screw placement allows safe nail insertion around articular fixation.
- Coronal plane articular fractures can be stabilized with a subchondral "rebar" screw configuration (Fig. 23-25).

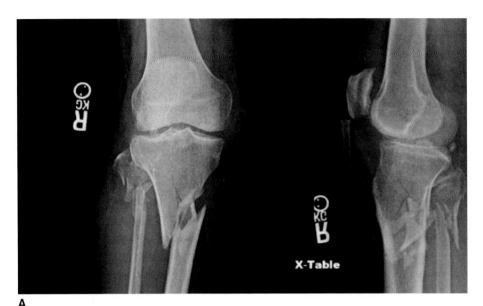

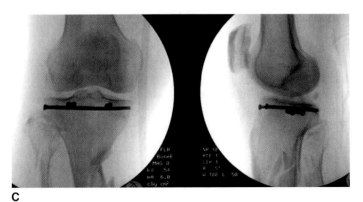

Figure 23-25 I AP and lateral injury images and CT cuts **(A, B)** and intraoperative images demonstrating the rafting rebar technique **(C)** for proximal articular fractures associated with a tibial shaft fracture. The rafter screws are placed carefully to avoid interference with IM nailing **(D, E)**.

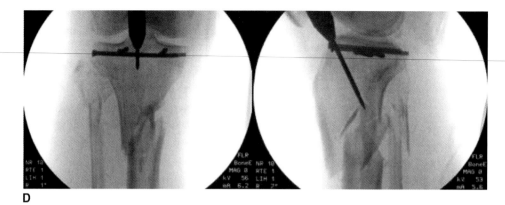

D

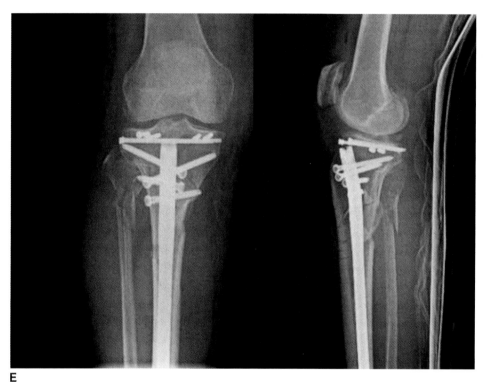

E

Figure 23-25 I (*Continued*)

- For segmental tibial shaft fractures, if the proximal fracture line is in the proximal third of the tibia, even if minimally displaced, stabilization of this prior to guidewire placement may prevent fracture displacement.
  - Adjuncts to reduction and maintenance of reduction include pointed clamp application, strategically placed lag screws, or plate/screws.
  - Nailing in the semiextended position is advantageous as reduction maintenance and imaging are greatly simplified.
- Nail insertion point: locate the starting point for the tibial guidewire.[7]
  - Directly over the medial edge of the lateral tibial spine on an AP fluoroscopic view.
  - Ensure proper rotation by noting patella shadow centrally over femoral condyles and a "normal" relationship of proximal tibiofibular joint.

- At the anterior edge of the tibial plateau on a lateral fluoroscopic radiograph (Fig. 23-26).

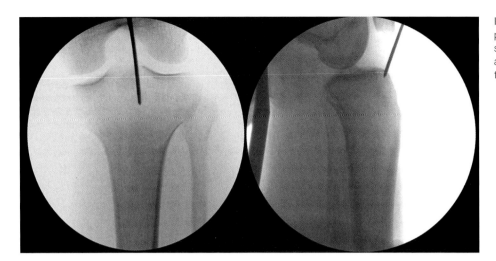

Figure 23-26 | The ideal starting point is just medial to the lateral tibial spine on the AP view and on the anterior edge of the tibial plateau on the lateral view.

- Aim the guidewire centrally in the medullary canal on the lateral view as it passes distally.
  - Generally, the tendency is to be too posterior.
  - Flex knee to minimize impaction on the posterior cortical surface during guidewire passage, reaming, and nail insertion.
- If starting site is acceptable, but wire is trending away from an ideal nail path as it is passed into the proximal tibia, stop passage after only a few centimeters and use starting drill or awl, which is more stiff, to achieve desired path into proximal metaphysis.
- Create a gentle bend approximately 1 cm above the tip of the ball-tipped guidewire to assist in directing the guidewire toward the proper trajectory.
- In revision situations, changing a previous nail path can be difficult.
  - Blocking an off-axis nail entry site may be necessary.
  - Use an intramedullary plate (3.5/4.5 narrow DCP) placed temporarily within the prior nail path to encourage eccentric reaming, thereby moving the entry portal to a preferred location (Fig. 23-27).

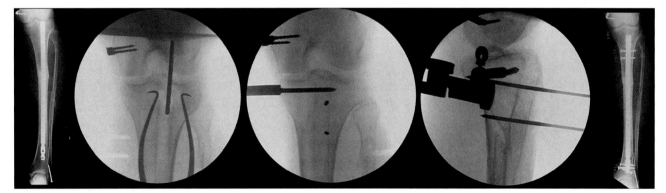

Figure 23-27 | In this patient, a tibial varus malunion developed in part due to an improper starting point. During the revision procedure, an intramedullary plate was used to force the reamer medially thereby creating a new entry portal and nail path within the proximal tibia. Prior to nail insertion, two 3.0-mm Steinmann pins were used to "block" the original nail path, and these were removed only after locking the new nail in its new position. These techniques permitted a much improved reduction and restored limb alignment.

- Consider tying a suture to the plate to avoid losing in canal, or use a graft such as a fibular allograft to fill or partially block an improper starting hole and blocking wires to direct the nail.
- To minimize the posterior translation of the distal fragment in proximal third tibial fractures, sufficient traction must be applied to disengage the posterior tibial cortices so as to permit reduction (e.g., posterior translational displacement) of the distal tibial segment (Fig. 23-28).

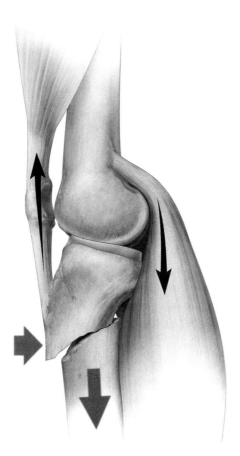

Figure 23-28 ▌ Sagittal plane translational and angular deformity following proximal tibial fracture can be accentuated by the pull of the extensor mechanism and the gastrocnemius muscle (*black arrows*) and shortening of the tibia. It is important to correct this deformity prior to placing internal fixation. Maneuvers include traction on the distal segment to "unlock" the posterior cortex, and posterior translation/"derotation" of the proximal fragment (*gray arrows*).

- Place the tip of the ball-tipped guidewire in the center of the distal metaphysis above the center of the talus on the ankle mortise view and over the center of the talar dome on the lateral ankle view.
  - Use the bent ball tip to pivot the wire path, after the ball is anchored in physeal scar (Fig. 23-29).

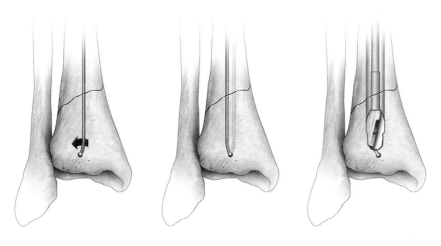

Figure 23-29 ▌ To alter the guidewire position and reamer path, first impact the ball tip firmly into the dense bone of the physeal scar. Rotation around the seated ball tip can rotate the shaft of the guidewire, improving its position prior to reaming.

- Remember that the reamer will only ream to the bend in the wire.
- In dense bone, insertion of the nail beyond the reamed path may result in distraction of the fracture and delay/nonunion.
- Ensure that the wire proximal to the bend is placed in the proper "center-center" position, so as to centralize each reamer within the distal metaphysis.
- Maintain anatomic alignment of the fracture throughout reaming and nail insertion to avoid eccentric reaming and further fracture displacement.
  - Femoral distractor may be useful for this step.
- After nail insertion, avoid fracture distraction.
  - Remove tension on the femoral distractor.
  - Options for compression of the fracture site:
    - Insert distal interlocking screws first.
    - Apply femoral distractor in compression mode.
    - Use the internal compression device built into the nailing system.
    - Retract the nail (backslapping) until compression is achieved (Fig. 23-30).

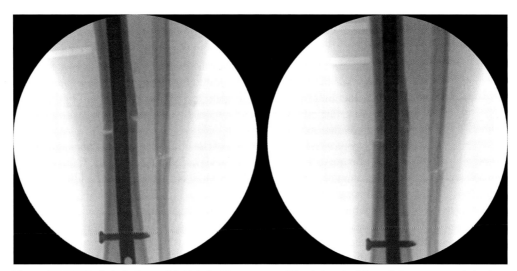

Figure 23-30 | By first placing a distal interlocking screw and "backslapping" the nail, transverse and short oblique fracture gaps can be closed.

- If distal interlocking is to be completed prior to proximal locking (e.g., to compress the fracture through backslapping or compression screw application), the radiolucent triangle may not be removed without removing the nail-mounted proximal targeting guide if the knee is to be placed in extension.
  - However, less knee flexion can be obtained by flipping the radiolucent triangle so that the leg lies on the triangle's hypotenuse and the knee remains sufficiently flexed to protect the prepatellar skin and anterior patella from crush injury from the insertion guide/proximal targeting jig.
- To reduce residual distraction of a tibial fracture after nail insertion and proximal locking, consider the following:
  - Placing the femoral distractor in compression mode.
  - Manually axially impact the limb to eliminate the distraction.
  - Placing distal interlocking screws eccentrically by predrilling the initial pilot hole slightly distally (2 to 3 mm) to the axial equator of the hole in the nail. This can usually eliminate distraction of 2 to 3 mm.
- Supplemental locking bolts in multiple planes should be considered when using nails for fixation of proximal or distal tibial fractures.[8]

- Locking bolts may be placed through a plate to assist as a reduction tool (Fig. 23-31).

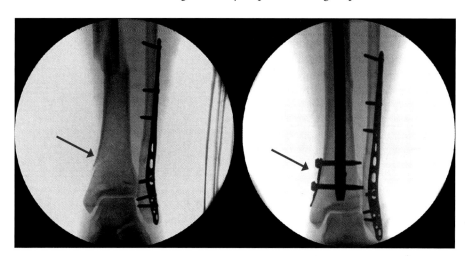

Figure 23-31 I In this case, the distal fracture line remained slightly displaced. A one-third tubular plate was used in conjunction with the interlocking screws as an indirect reduction tool (*arrows*).

Fibular Nailing

- If the fibula can be aligned with little difficulty prior to tibial shaft fracture nailing, consider insertion of an antegrade or retrograde fibular rod to further stabilize the limb's soft tissues and this fracture.
- Fibular reduction can assist the surgeon in realigning the tibia if both the proximal and distal tibiofibular articulations are intact, especially in tibial fractures with segmental bone loss.
- Antegrade fibular nailing.
  - Fluoroscopically, identify the axis of the fibular medullary canal and optimal starting point for nail insertion on the AP and lateral views, collinear with the fibular medullary canal.
  - Make a small longitudinal incision 2 to 5 cm proximal to the fibular head collinear with the fibular canal.
  - Dissect bluntly to the fibular head, avoiding injury to the common peroneal nerve.
    - Nerve is usually located posteriorly and distally to the fibular head, but can be displaced with trauma.
    - If indicated, identify and protect nerve using an open approach.
  - Open the medullary canal with a 2.5-mm drill bit.
  - Introduce a 2.5-mm intramedullary rod (e.g., humeral reaming guide rod or flexible titanium nail).
    - Alternatively, drill entry hole with a 3.5-mm drill to facilitate nail insertion.
  - Once the fibular medullary canal has been accessed and the rod's position confirmed on AP and lateral fluoroscopic views, the rod may be advanced slowly until the tip of the rod has reached the fracture.
  - The fibular fracture should be realigned and the rod advanced into the distal segment(s) for the majority of the fibula's length.
    - Insertion can be aided using an oscillating drill.
  - Prior to seating of the rod at the desired fibular length, the rod should be cut to the appropriate length and bent 180 degrees.
  - The fibular rod may now be seated with the proximal "hook" (cut end) inserted (but not completely sunk) anteriorly (to avoid common peroneal nerve injury) into the fibular head to prevent rotation and loosening of the fixation.
  - Leaving the apex of the proximal rod out of bone facilitates later implant removal if necessary (Fig. 23-32).

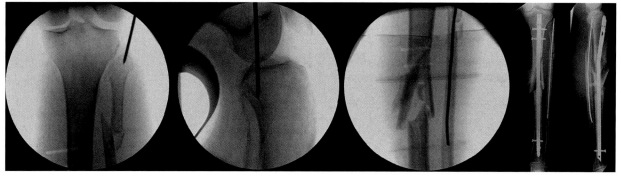

Figure 23-32 I Example of antegrade fibular nailing prior to tibial nailing.

- Retrograde fibular nailing.
  - Fluoroscopically identify the axis of the fibula and optimal starting point for nail insertion on the AP and lateral views.
  - Make a small longitudinal incision 3 to 5 cm distal to the lateral malleolus, in line with the anticipated entry point and collinear with fibular medullary canal on biplanar fluoroscopic views.
  - Dissect bluntly to the tip of the lateral malleolus.
  - Create a starting point using a 2.5- or 3.5-mm drill (Fig. 23-33).

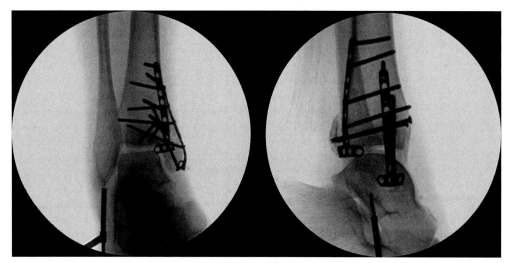

Figure 23-33 I For retrograde fibular nailing, the drill bit is placed on the tip of the fibula, and its position and trajectory are verified on AP and lateral fluoroscopy.

- Open the medullary canal with a 2.5- or 3.5-mm drill.
- Insert a 2.5-mm intramedullary device (e.g., humeral reaming rod) into the distal fibula.
- Once the fibular medullary canal has been accessed and the rod's position confirmed on AP and lateral fluoroscopic views, the rod may be advanced in retrograde fashion.
- The fibular fracture should be realigned, and the rod advanced into the proximal segment(s) for the majority of the fibula's length.
- Prior to seating of the rod at the desired fibular length, the rod should be cut to an appropriate length and bent to prevent migration.

- The fibular rod should now be seated with the distal "hook" (cut end) inserted (but not completely sunk) anteriorly into the lateral malleolus to prevent rotation and loosening of the fixation (Fig. 23-34).
- Leaving the apex of the distal rod out of bone facilitates implant removal, if necessary.

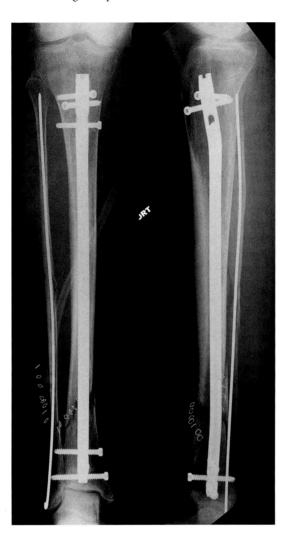

Figure 23-34 | Retrograde fibular rod used to assist in reduction and augment limb stability of an open tibial and fibular fracture.

Plating of Tibial Shaft Fractures

- Percutaneous or minimally invasive plate fixation of tibial shaft fractures is an option in certain situations.
  - Internal fixation of tibial shaft fractures in skeletally immature patients
  - Compression plating of simple midshaft tibial fracture patterns; though intramedullary nailing remains preferred in most cases
    - Medial plates are often best avoided in open fractures and in closed fractures with injured anteromedial soft tissues.
  - High-level athletes to minimize risk of anterior knee pain
  - Burn, infection, or other soft tissue trauma at nail insertion site
  - Obliterated canal
  - Canal too small
  - Long-term external fixator
  - Medullary osteomyelitis (prior nailing)
  - Selected nonunions or malunions
- Selected nonunions or malunions.
- Bridge plating of comminuted segmental tibial shaft fractures.
  - Management of fractures located at the proximal or distal metadiaphyseal junctions[9]
  - Management of fractures involving the tibial shaft and tibial plateau or pilon (Fig. 23-35)
- Minimize soft tissue stripping and further devascularization of the fracture zone.

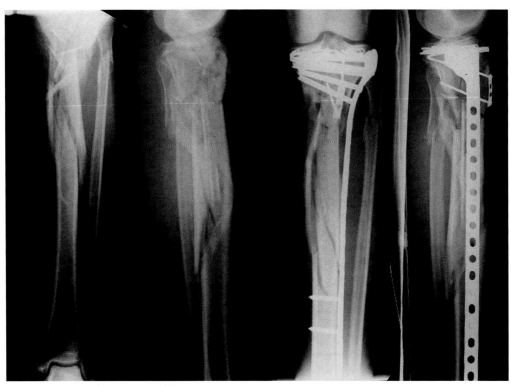

Figure 23-35 | Bridge plating can be an effective option for high-energy proximal tibial fractures.

Proximal Tibiofibular Joint Disruption

- More common in high-energy injuries.
  - Associated with high-energy tibia fractures
  - Knee dislocations
  - Rarely an isolated injury
- May have concominant peroneal nerve injury.
  - More common after posterior dislocation
- If persistent dislocation after tibial shaft fixation, consider reduction and fixation.
- Compare proximal tib-fib joint with radiographs of the uninjured knee.
- An externally rotated lateral view shows this joint well.
- Typically can be reduced using percutaneously placed quad clamp, large Weber clamp, or shoulder hook (Fig. 23-36).

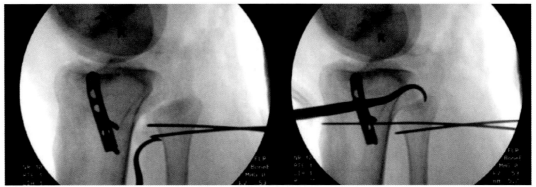

Figure 23-36 | Intraoperative lateral view demonstrating reduction of a dislocated proximal tibiofibular joint with a shoulder hook.

- Place a guidewire for a 3.5- or 4.0-mm screw from the fibular head into the proximal tibia and confirm location and reduction on all three views (AP, lateral, externally rotated lateral) (Fig. 23-37).

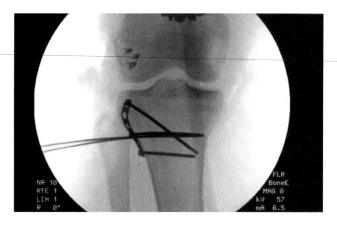

Figure 23-37 I The reduction is maintained with a K-wire and a guidewire for a cannulated screw is placed.

- Once the reduction and wire placement is confirmed accurate and safe, a screw (with or without a washer) is placed over the wire (Fig. 23-38).
- If the fibular head is not easily palpable and open approach is required to avoid injury to the peroneal nerve.

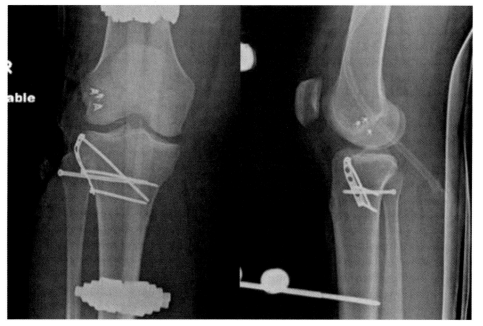

Figure 23-38 I Postoperative images demonstrate reduction and fixation of a dislocated proximal tibiofibular joint.

References

1. Tornetta P III, Riina J, Geller J, et al. Intraarticular anatomic risks of tibial nailing. *J Orthop Trauma.* 1999;13:247–251.
2. Nowotarski PJ, Turen CH, Brumback RJ, et al. Conversion of external fixation to intramedullary nailing for fractures of the shaft of the femur in multiply injured patients. *J Bone Joint Surg Am.* 2000;82(6):781–788.
3. Rubinstein RA Jr, Green JM, Duwelius PJ. Intramedullary interlocked tibia nailing: a new technique (preliminary report). *J Orthop Trauma.* 1992;6:90–95.
4. Dunbar RP, Nork SE, Barei DP, et al. Provisional plating of Type III open tibia fractures prior to intramedullary nailing. *J Orthop Trauma.* 2005;19:412–414.
5. Krettek C, Miclau T, Schandelmaier P, et al. The mechanical effect of blocking screws ("Poller screws") in stabilizing tibia fractures with short proximal or distal fragments after insertion of small-diameter intramedullary nails. *J Orthop Trauma.* 1999;13:550–553.
6. Boraiah S, Gardner MJ, Helfet DL, et al. High association of posterior malleolus fractures with spiral distal tibial fractures. *Clin Orthop Relat Res.* 2008;466:1692–1698.
7. Schmidt AH, Templeman DC, Tornetta P, et al. Anatomic assessment of the proper insertion site for a tibial intramedullary nail. *J Orthop Trauma.* 2003;17:75–76.
8. Nork SE, Barei DP, Schildhauer TA, et al. Intramedullary nailing of proximal quarter tibial fractures. *J Orthop Trauma.* 2006;20:523–528.
9. Vallier HA, Le TT, Bedi A. Radiographic and clinical comparisons of distal tibia shaft fractures (4 to 11 cm proximal to the plafond): plating versus intramedullary nailing. *J Orthop Trauma.* 2008;22:307–311.

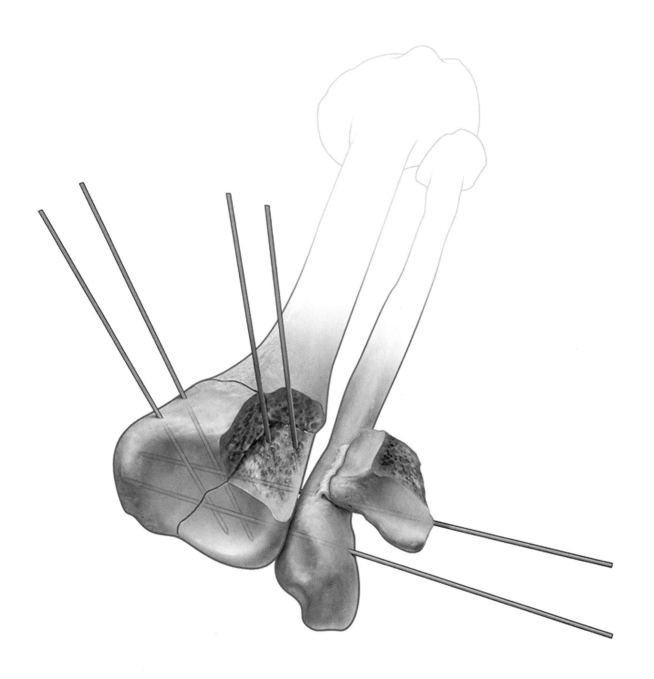

Chapter 24
Pilon Fractures

JOSEPH COHEN
CHRISTOPHER DOMES
MICHAEL J. GARDNER
MICHAEL F. GITHENS
CLAY A. SPITLER
LISA A. TAITSMAN

Sterile Instruments/Equipment

- Headlight
- Tourniquet if desired
- Femoral distractor
- Large and small pointed bone reduction clamps (Weber clamps)
- Dental picks and Freer elevators
- Osteotomes for articular disimpaction
- Implants: anatomically contoured distal tibial periarticular plates, locked and/or nonlocked; medial and lateral
  - Small fragment plates and screws
  - Periarticular plates
  - Mini-fragment screws and mini-fragment plates (2.0/2.4 mm) depending on fracture requirements
  - Long solid or cannulated 3.5-mm screws for medial column fixation
  - Cancellous allograft chips
- K-wires and wire driver/drill

Surgical Approaches (Fig. 24-1)

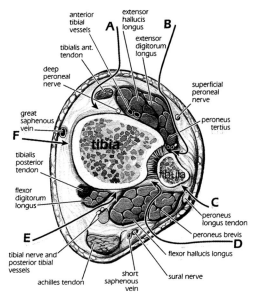

Figure 24-1 I Cross-sectional schematic showing the intervals for common approaches to pilon fractures. *A*, anteromedial; *B*, anterolateral; *C*, posterolateral (fibula); *D*, posterolateral (tibia); *E*, posteromedial. *F*, medial. (From Howard JL, Agel J, Barei DP, et al. A prospective study evaluating incision placement and wound healing for tibial plafond fractures. *J Orthop Trauma.* 2008;22:299–305, with permission.)

Anteromedial Approach

- Positioning
  - Supine on a radiolucent table.
  - Bring the patient to the foot end of the table.
  - Place a small bump under the ipsilateral hip and torso.
  - Place a pneumatic tourniquet on the ipsilateral thigh if desired.
  - Elevate the leg on a soft ramp cushion to facilitate lateral radiographs and apply exclusionary drape lower limb (Fig. 24-2).

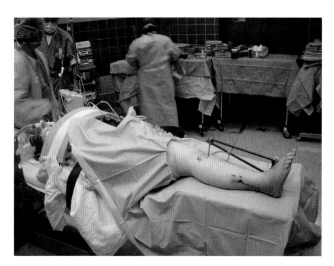

Figure 24-2 | Supine patient positioning for anteromedial or anterolateral approach to a pilon fracture.

- Incision starts proximally, 1 cm lateral to tibial crest.
- Curves medially, approximately 60 to 80 degrees at joint line.
- Continues to a point 1 cm distal to medial malleolus (Fig. 24-3).

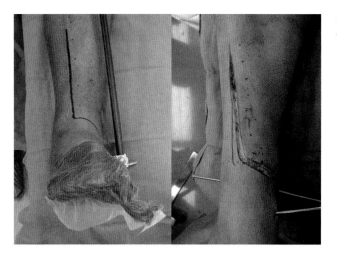

Figure 24-3 | Incision for an extensile anteromedial approach for pilon fractures.

- Superficial dissection to fascia, sweep subcutaneous tissue off fascia, working medially, just to margin of the tibial crest (Fig. 24-4).

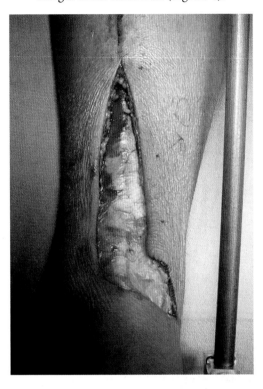

Figure 24-4 I Superficial dissection of an anteromedial approach to the level of the fascia.

- Make full-thickness incision in fascia and periosteum just medial to anterior tibialis tendon and elevate with soft tissue flap.
  - Take care not to violate the tendon sheath, which is elevated extraperiosteally or with periosteum at fracture site (Fig. 24-5).

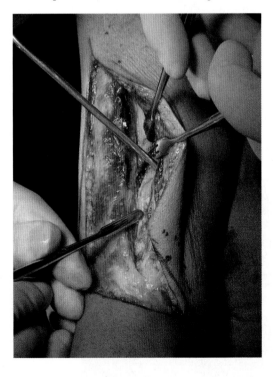

Figure 24-5 I A full-thickness flap is elevated just medial to the anterior tibialis tendon that allows for anatomic closure.

  - Alternatively, elevate the subcutaneous layer off the periosteum medially, and make a separate "window" incision in periosteum, as needed.
    - This results in less periosteal stripping but leaves a thinner subcutaneous flap and perhaps should be avoided in poor hosts (smokers, elderly, those with compromised vascularity, etc.).

- Avoid the greater saphenous nerve and vein medially in the distal limb of the incision. Retract vein medially, if necessary.
- Make arthrotomy over dominant anterior (sagittal) fracture line.
- Use a laminar spreader in the metaphyseal fracture line, if necessary, to expose the metaphyseal and articular surface.
  - Take care not to injure or comminute cortical interdigitations, especially in patients with brittle bone or osteopenia (Fig. 24-6).

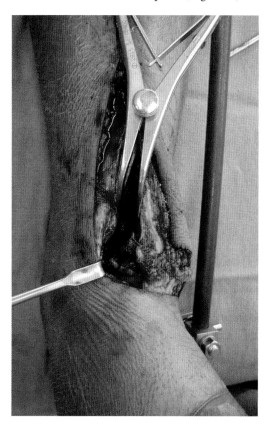

Figure 24-6 ‖ Depending on the fracture pattern, the fracture gap may be distracted for access to the articular fragments.

- Deep closure is critical.
  - Reapproximate soft tissue edges of full-thickness flaps using absorbable braided suture.
  - Place all sutures and clamps provisionally.
  - After all are in place, use sutures to mobilize retracted soft tissues "en mass." Then tie each suture sequentially.
  - Skin is closed with Allgöwer-Donati stitches using 3-0 nylon sutures (Fig. 24-7).

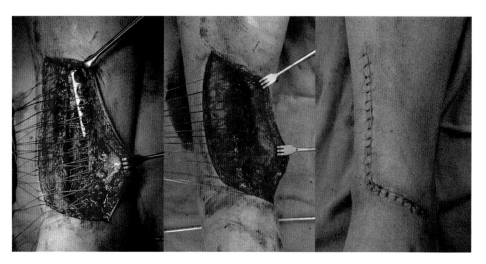

Figure 24-7 ‖ The full-thickness deep layer is closed with interrupted absorbable suture, and clamped prior to tissue mobilization and knot tying. This allows distribution of tissue tension, ensuring a watertight closure and minimizing tissue tearing. Interrupted Allgöwer-Donati sutures are placed to minimize the skin edge hypoxia.

Anterolateral Approach

- Positioning
  - Supine on a radiolucent table.
  - Bring the patient to the end of the table.
  - Place a small bump under the ipsilateral hip and torso.
  - Place a pneumatic tourniquet on the ipsilateral thigh if desired.
  - Elevate the leg on a soft ramp cushion to facilitate lateral radiographs.
- Incision is longitudinal, 2 to 4 cm lateral to tibial crest proximally approximately halfway between the tibia and fibula; distally, it is in line with the fourth ray of the foot.
- The proximal extension of the incision is usually limited to approximately 7 cm above the joint line due to the orientation and origin of the crossing anterior compartment muscles.
  - The proximal screws in the plate can be inserted percutaneously after assessing the location of the superficial peroneal nerve. With percutaneous placement of proximal screws in the plate, the deep peroneal nerve and vascular structures are at risk and should be avoided during drill and screw insertions.
- At the level of the ankle joint, the incision is centered over the mortise.
- Extends distally in line with the fourth metatarsal over the talar dome and proximal neck, if necessary (Fig. 24-8).

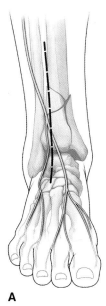
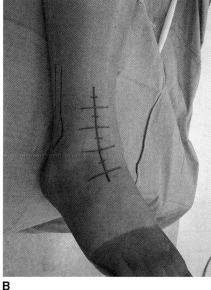

A   **B**

Figure 24-8 I **A:** This schematic demonstrates the location of the anterolateral surgical incision. The incision is typically placed in line with the fourth metatarsal and centered at the ankle joint. The proximal extension is usually limited by the origin of the anterior compartment musculature. **B:** A typical incision location and length. This allows for the exposure of the articular surface for reduction and placement of plates at the distal tibial metaphysis. Proximal plate placement and fixation typically requires an additional approach more proximally or, more frequently, multiple small incisions for lateral to medial screw placement. Distally, the talar neck may be exposed to allow for the placement of a pin in the talus and for distraction across the ankle joint. (From Nork SE, Barei DP, Gardner MJ, et al. Anterolateral approach for pilon fractures. *Tech Foot Ankle Surg.* 2009;8(2):53–59, with permission.)

- Identify superficial peroneal nerve in superficial dissection (Fig. 24-9).

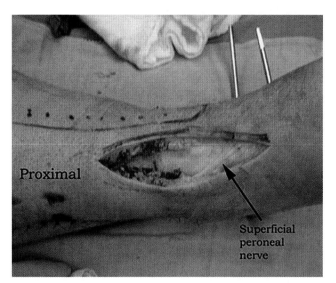

Proximal

Superficial peroneal nerve

Figure 24-9 I With an anterolateral approach, the superficial peroneal nerve must be identified superficial to the fascia. (From Nork SE, Barei DP, Gardner MJ, et al. Anterolateral approach for pilon fractures. *Tech Foot Ankle Surg.* 2009;8(2):53–59, with permission.)

- Retract the anterior compartment medially with its deep peritenon and tenosynovium, to expose the joint capsule.
  - It is easiest to start laterally at the tubercle of Chaput (Fig. 24-10).

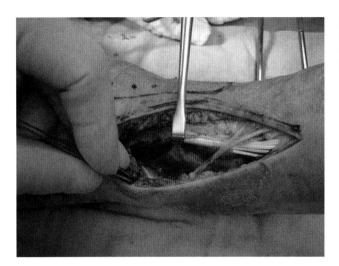

Figure 24-10 ▌ The anterior compartment is retracted medially. Try to keep the anterior compartment tendons surrounded with their peritenon.

- Cautious subperiosteal elevation of the anterior compartment from the distal metaphyseal tibia should be done with a Freer rather than a knife to avoid injury to the deep peroneal nerve and accompanying anterior tibial artery.
- These structures may be entrapped in the metaphyseal fracture zone with anterior crush–type patterns.
- Find the sagittal fracture plane and incise the periosteum vertically from the metaphysis to the joint, if not already disrupted by the injury.
- "T" the joint capsule tangentially to the distal tibia, leaving a rim of capsular tissue ("coronary ligament") (Fig. 24-11).
  - If possible, protect the lateral anterior malleolar artery (a branch of the perforating artery, which in turn is a branch of the peroneal artery), which lies transversely on the ankle capsule and anastamoses with the anterior tibial artery.

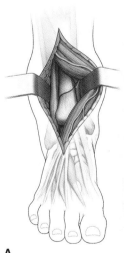
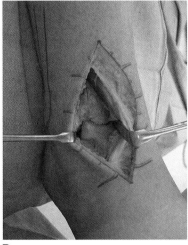

Figure 24-11 ▌ A: The deep dissection allows for the exposure of the distal tibial metaphysis after medial retraction of the entire anterior compartment. B: After an arthrotomy of the ankle joint, the distal tibia and the talar neck are exposed. The anterior tibiofibular ligaments are left attached to the anterolateral articular segment. (From Nork SE, Barei DP, Gardner MJ, et al. Anterolateral approach for pilon fractures. *Tech Foot Ankle Surg.* 2009;8(2):53–59, with permission.)

A   B

Posteromedial Approach

- Positioning
  - Supine or prone on a radiolucent table.
    - If prone, allow sufficient space between the dorsum of foot and table for ankle dorsiflexion.
  - Bring the patient to the foot end of the table.
    - If prone, consider moving the patient a bit distal to the foot end of the table, so as to facilitate ankle dorsiflexion.
  - Place a pneumatic tourniquet on the ipsilateral thigh if desired.
  - Elevate the leg on soft ramp cushion to facilitate lateral radiographs.
  - Consider a bump under the contralateral hip to externally rotate the affected leg, improving access for reduction and hardware placement.
- Difficult to visualize the joint (unless a distractor is used); most helpful for extra-articular cortical reductions.
- May be a necessary approach if one or more posterior compartment structures are entrapped within a posteromedial fracture line (e.g., tendon of the posterior tibialis).
  - Carefully evaluate the CT scan for posterior structure entrapment, particularly when a displaced posteromedial fracture line is present.
- Incision is centered between the Achilles tendon and the posteromedial tibial border, over PT/FDL/FHL tendons of posterior compartments.
- Several intervals or "windows" can be chosen to approach the fracture for reduction and fixation: between the tibia, the posterior tibialis, the flexor digitorum longus, the posterior tibial neurovascular bundle, and the flexor hallucis longus.
  - One or more windows may be used depending on the location of the fracture line(s) and desired implant placement and screw orientation (Fig. 24-12).

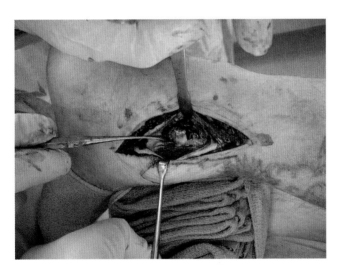

Figure 24-12 ▌ Posteromedial approach to a left ankle in the prone position. The posterior tibialis tendon is retracted anteriorly and the flexor digitorum longus and neurovascular bundle are retracted posteriorly for access to the posteromedial distal tibia.

Posterolateral Approach

- Positioning
  - Semilateral or prone
    - Lateral allows for simultaneous anterior exposure with adequate hip rotation.
    - If prone, see above for positioning tips (see also Fig. 24-12).
  - Bring the patient to the foot end of the table.
  - Place a pneumatic tourniquet on the ipsilateral thigh if desired.
  - Elevate the leg on a soft ramp cushion to facilitate lateral radiographs.
- Difficult to visualize joint (unless a distractor is used); most helpful for cortical reductions.
- Incision is centered between the Achilles tendon and the posterior fibular border, if no prior fibular incision.
- Protect sural nerve crossing from middle of leg to lateral retromalleolar region distally.
- Interval is between FHL and peroneal tendons.

- Dissect lateral to medial to expose posterior tibia.
- Femoral distractor within incision to the calcaneus can help restore length.

Reduction and Implant Techniques

- To obtain intraoperative distraction of the articular surface, a small Schanz pin (4.0-mm pin, predrill with 2.5-mm bit) can be placed in the talar body/neck for a distractor.
  - The threaded distractor rod should be placed posteriorly, and the talar pin should be placed just distal to the articular surface in the talar body/neck.
  - This configuration allows for slight plantar flexion of the talus as well as axial distraction across the tibiotalar joint.
  - This improves visualization of the articular surface and does not distract through the subtalar joint.
  - If an anterolateral approach is used, the pin can be placed within the surgical wound.
  - The entry point in the talar body/neck is exposed by incising the fascia of the extensor digitorum brevis and elevating the muscle belly (Figs. 24-13 and 24-14).

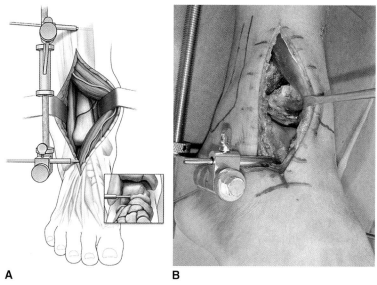

A   **B**

Figure 24-13 ▮ **A:** After the placement of a small femoral distractor from the tibia to the talar neck/body junction, the joint is distracted. This allows for complete visualization of the entire articular surface of the distal tibia. **B:** A clinical example of left tibial pilon fracture after the placement of a small femoral distractor. Visualization of the joint can be improved with head lamp illumination. (From Nork SE, Barei DP, Gardner MJ, et al. Anterolateral approach for pilon fractures. *Tech Foot Ankle Surg.* 2009;8(2):53–59, with permission.)

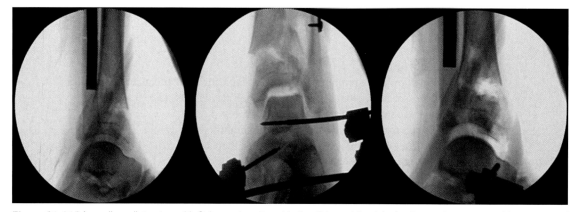

Figure 24-14 ▮ A medium distractor, with Schanz pins placed in the tibia and the talar body, creates more working space at both the metaphyseal defect behind the articular surface and the articular surface itself (*left*, predistraction; *center* and *right*, postdistraction).

- An alternative to a lateral distractor is a medial distractor.
    - Both the tibial and talar body/neck pins can be placed percutaneously.
    - This allows unencumbered access to the anterolateral incision.
- For additional distraction, the spanning frame can be tensioned through the calcaneus to distract the posterior aspect of the joint.
    - Talar neck pin distraction then allows for anterior joint distraction and slight plantar flexion (Fig. 24-15).

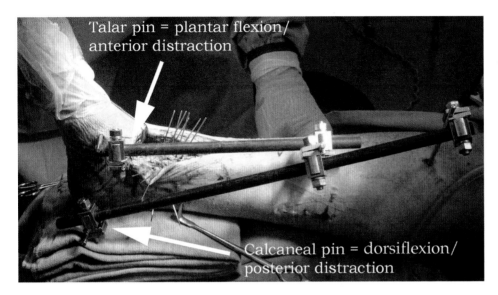

Figure 24-15 | External fixation used for articular distraction, posteriorly through a calcaneal pin and anteriorly through a talar neck pin.

- Medial talar body pin placed just distal to tip of the anterior colliculus of medial malleolus results in straight axial distraction across the ankle joint.
    - Distraction is usually without ankle dorsi- or plantar flexion as long as distraction moment is collinear with longitudinal axis of leg-ankle (from a proximal medial tibial pin).
- It may be difficult to distract across the ankle joint with significant metaphyseal comminution, especially if the medial malleolus or medial metaphyseal column is a free fragment.
    - In this case, it may be beneficial to apply a mini-fragment plate across metaphysis to allow articular distraction (Fig. 24-16).

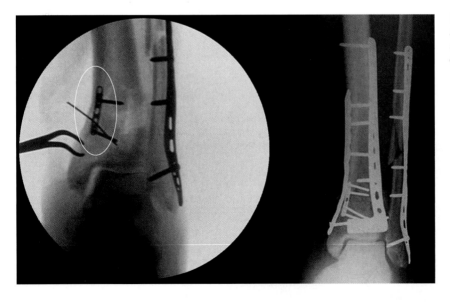

Figure 24-16 | A mini-fragment plate across the metaphysis will allow provisional stabilization to allow articular distraction (*left, circle*).

- A "skid zone" (marginal impaction of the anterior aspect of posterolateral fragment) is frequently present denoting the path of the talus associated with the initial trauma and its impaction/dislocation/subluxation (Fig. 24-17).

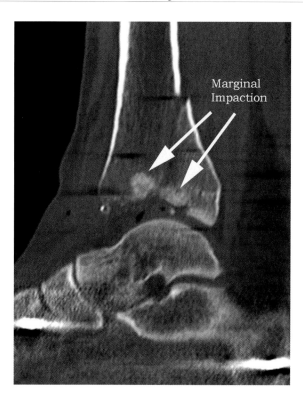

Marginal
Impaction

Figure 24-17 | Sagittal CT image reformations should be analyzed for anterior marginal impaction of the Volkmann fragment.

- Use a curved osteotome followed by a straight osteotome to disimpact the impacted metaphyseal and subchondral bone with the attached articular surface.
- Alternatively, stacked osteotomes can be used in succession to reduce the articular surface (Figs. 24-18 and 24-19).

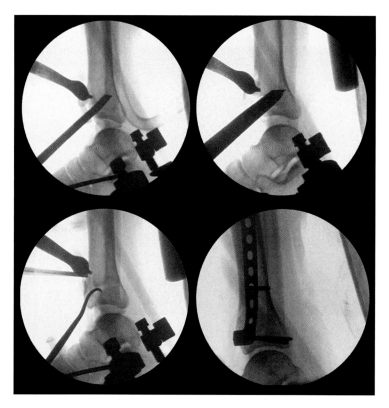

Figure 24-18 | Stacked osteotomes can be used in succession to disimpact the articular surface.

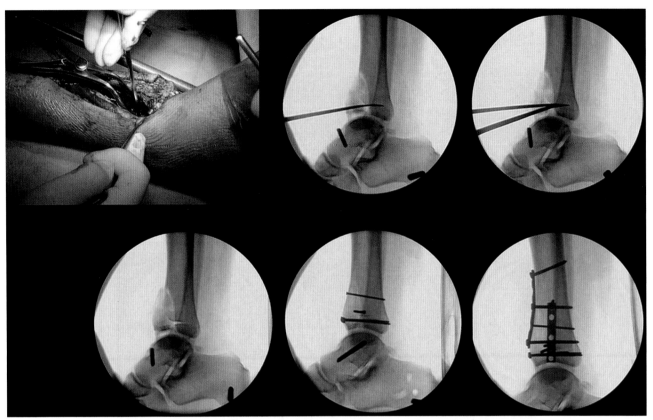

Figure 24-19 | Another example of using osteotomes to disimpact and reduce the "skid zone" of anterior articular surface of posterior fragment. A rim plate is then placed to secure the disimpacted Volkmann fragment, and final fixation is applied.

- Support disimpacted articular fragments with K-wires and fill the bone void with cancellous allograft chips.
- If the posterior Volkmann fragment is not impacted, but is displaced, the typical deformity assumed by this fragment is sagittal plane malrotation in dorsiflexion.
  - Reduction of this fragment is critical.
  - There are several options to achieve this.
    - The anterior cancellous surface of the posterolateral fragment can be accessed either after the Chaput fragment is rotated externally on the AITFL or through metaphyseal comminution.
      - This permits exposure to central articular comminution, hematoma and debris, and the posterior Volkmann fragment.
      - The posterior fragment can then be derotated and pinned into place using K-wires from the tibial shaft angling distally (Fig. 24-20).

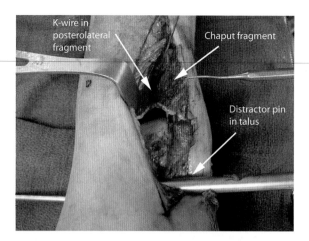

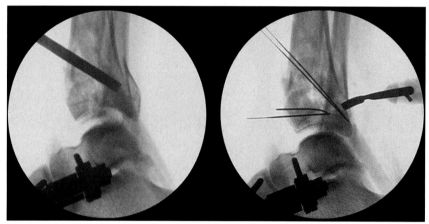

Figure 24-20 I The Volkmann posterolateral fragment can be accessed through the fracture site anteriorly.

- Alternatively, after reduction, the Volkmann fragment can be provisionally stabilized with two or three K-wires inserted percutaneously, from lateral to medial through the fibula (transfibular K-wires).
    - The wires' bicortical points of fixation in the fibula serve to increase their cantilever bending stiffness.
    - Since they are placed outside of the immediate operating field, subsequent pilon fracture repair proceeds unimpeded.
- A clamp tine can be passed through a posterolateral approach, through either a small stab incision or the previous fibular incision.
    - Depending on the fracture pattern, available clamp configuration, and the size of the Volkmann fragment, the clamp tine may be placed either anterior to the peroneal tendons and posterior to the fibula or posterior to the peroneal tendons.
    - The tine will cross the posterior syndesmotic ligaments and will then be placed onto the posterior malleolus fragment (Fig. 24-21).

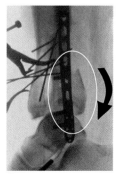
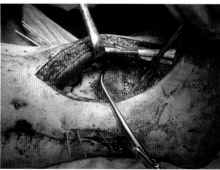
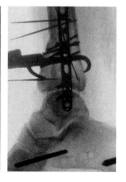

Figure 24-21 I The posterolateral Volkmann fragment is typically displaced in dorsiflexion (**A**, *circle, rotational arrow*). A critical step in the overall reduction strategy is addressing this reduction. This can be reduced by using a pointed Weber clamp through a small posterolateral approach **(B)**. On a lateral fluoroscopic view, the position of the fragment is improved and is stabilized provisionally using an antegrade K-wire from the tibial shaft.

A   B

- Alternatively, a shoulder hook or small elevator can be inserted percutaneously to manipulate and compress the Volkmann fragment.
    - Anterior-to-posterior K-wires can then be placed across the fragment to stabilize it provisionally (Fig. 24-22).

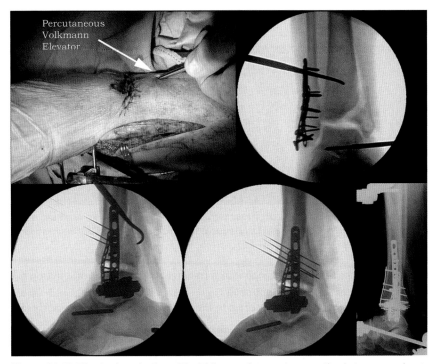

Figure 24-22 ‖ To obtain reduction of the Volkmann fragment, one option is to use an elevator or hook through a percutaneous approach.

- Place one tine of a large pointed reduction clamp through the interosseous membrane, taking care to avoid the posterior tibial neurovascular bundle (Fig. 24-23).

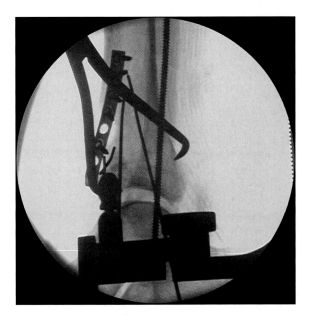

Figure 24-23 ‖ A clamp may be placed through the syndesmosis to reduce the posterior Volkmann fragment.

■ Alternatively, a 2.5-mm threaded Schanz pin can be placed into the fragment through the anterior window and can be used to rotate the fragment.

■ A separate posterolateral approach may be used to anatomically reduce the proximal spike of the posterior malleolus fragment.

● An antiglide plate should be placed at the apex of the fracture's spike.

● Screws placed should be short enough not to interfere with unreduced anterior fragments (Fig. 24-24).

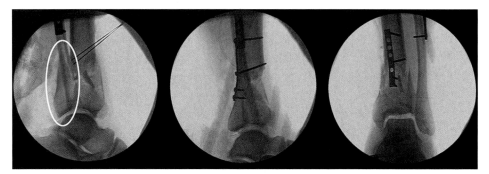

Figure 24-24 I Provisional plate placement with short screws can be used. Anatomic reduction of the spike of the proximal cortex indirectly reduces the articular surface of this fragment (*left*, Volkmann fragment in *circle*).

■ If a large displaced osteochondral fragment is present, its orientation can be marked and the fragment removed temporarily.

● This facilitates direct access to the Volkmann fragment anteriorly (Fig. 24-25).

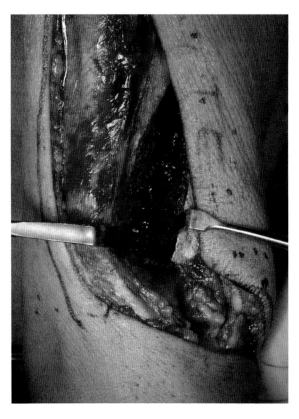

Figure 24-25 I Temporary removal of a large osteochondral fragment facilitates access to the posterior Volkmann fragment through the fracture for manipulation and reduction.

■ Another option for reducing the Volkmann fragment is through the metaphyseal fracture, via the anterolateral or anteromedial approach.

● A small hole (2.0 to 2.5 mm) is placed in the central portion of the fragment by drilling from anterior to posterior.

● Use a dental pick, shoulder hook, or threaded pin to manipulate the fragment and correct the sagittal plane rotation.

● Secure its position with K-wires.

- If Volkmann fragment reduction is performed as a first step, this can provide a stable segment to which the remainder of the articular surface may be reduced (Fig. 24-26).

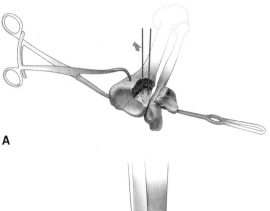

Figure 24-26 | Multiple effective options exist for Volkmann fragment reduction, including anteriorly placed K-wires (**A,B**), clamp placement (**A**), posterolateral shoulder hook placement (**A,B**), or an antiglide plate (**B**).

A

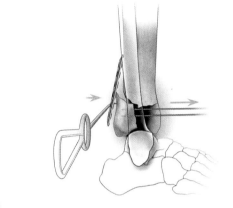

B

- The remainder of the articular segment can be reduced to this stable and reduced fragment (Figs. 24-27 and 24-28).

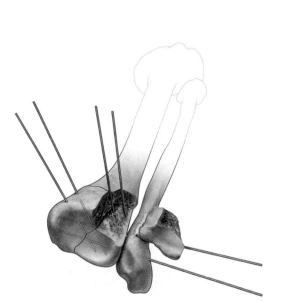

Figure 24-27 | Following reduction of the posterolateral fragment, a typical reduction sequence proceeds with central comminution (not shown) and the medial fragment.

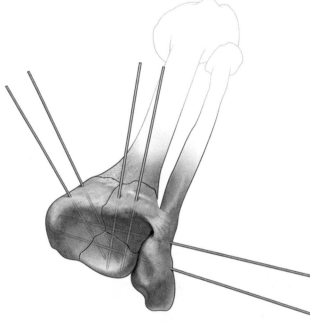

Figure 24-28 | As a final step, the anterolateral Chaput fragment is reduced and K-wires are inserted.

- Anterior rim plate
  - Useful for sagittal plane compression of articular surface.
  - To span the entire surface of the anterior cortex of the distal tibia, a 2.0-mm ten-hole plate can be contoured.

- Hooks may be created at one (or both) end(s) by cutting through a hole and bending the remaining hole edges for additional fixation (Fig. 24-29).

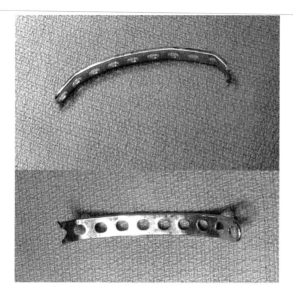

Figure 24-29 I A 2.0-mm rim plate can be used as a buttress for articular compression. A plate length of 10 holes allows for fixation across the entire cortical surface of the distal tibia, though shorter plates may also suffice.

- The articular surface is first reconstructed and stabilized provisionally with K-wires (Fig. 24-30).

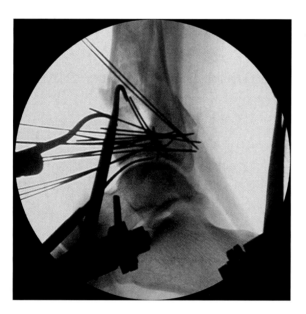

Figure 24-30 I Reduction of the articular surface is first performed, which can be visualized directly and palpated with a blunt elevator.

- The rim plate is then applied to the distal aspect of the anterior tibial cortex (Fig. 24-31).

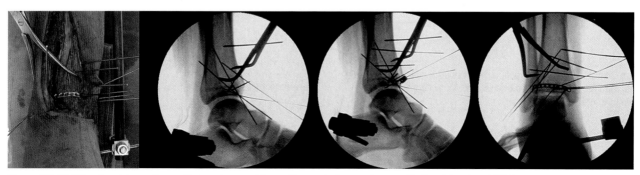

Figure 24-31 I The rim plate on the cortical surface and its position and alignment are verified on lateral and AP fluoroscopy.

- Using lateral fluoroscopic guidance, anterior-to-posterior screws are placed (Fig. 24-32).

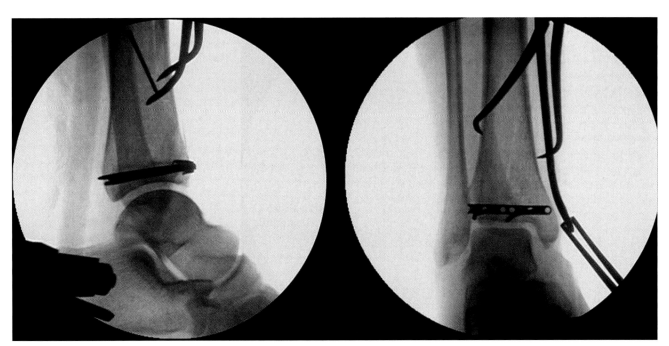

Figure 24-32 ‖ 2.4-mm lag screws are placed from anterior to posterior under fluoroscopic guidance.

- Alternatively, a five-hole 2.0-mm straight plate can be used to span a single fracture line and capture several larger articular fragments.
- Again, 2.4-mm screws are placed in a lag fashion (Fig. 24-33).

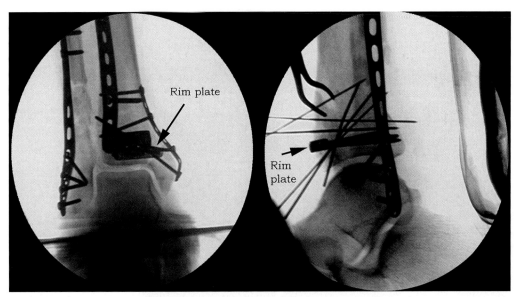

Figure 24-33 ‖ A smaller rim plate can be used selectively for individual fracture lines.

- A six-hole plate should be selected if fixation into a medial malleolar fragment is needed (Fig. 24-34).

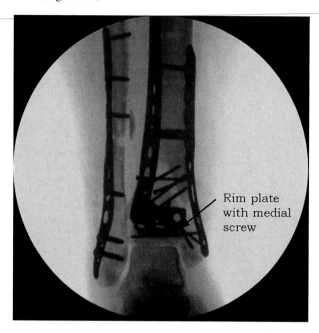

Figure 24-34 I A six-hole plate should be used for screw placement into a medial malleolus fragment.

Rim plate with medial screw

- A more laterally placed rim plate can be used for a separate Chaput fragment (Fig. 24-35).

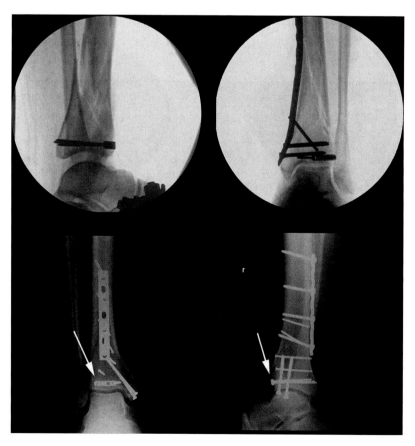

Figure 24-35 I Two examples of small rim plates (*arrows*) with selective fixation into the anterolateral Chaput fragment.

- One side of two adjacent holes can be cut to form a "side" hook plate.
  - This allows the tab to be bent along the axis of the plate and to bend the plate in the plane of its flat surface, similar to a reconstruction plate (Fig. 24-36).

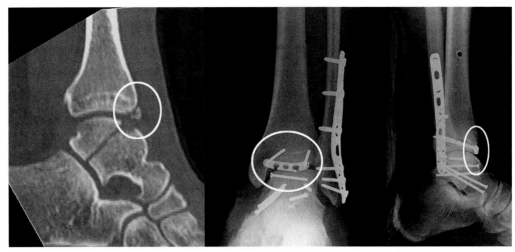

Figure 24-36 | A mini-fragment plate can be used to create a side hook to capture small periarticular fragments (*circles*).

- If multiple small osteochondral fragments are present anteriorly, a malleable maxillofacial 2.0-mm plate can be contoured and placed along the anterior rim of the distal tibia as a buttress (Fig. 24-37).

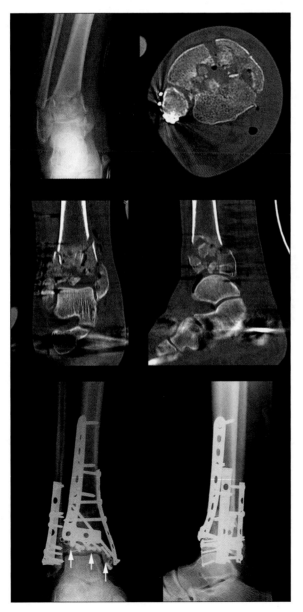

Figure 24-37 | A malleable 2.0-mm plate (*arrows*) can be contoured to the distal tibial rim to buttress small osteochondral fragments.

- After reduction of the distal segment and its articular surface, if the articular block is displaced from the shaft, it can be reduced with a Schanz pin or other instruments to the distal diaphysis.
- Long oblique fractures are amenable to clamping, although ideal clamp location may crush skin and soft tissues.
  - To obtain an accurate clamp vector and avoid crushing soft tissues, the clamp may be "extended" by placing a percutaneous unicortical screw, with the head at the level of the skin.
  - Docking the clamp tine into the screw allows effective clamping without crushing soft tissues (Figs. 24-38 and 24-39).

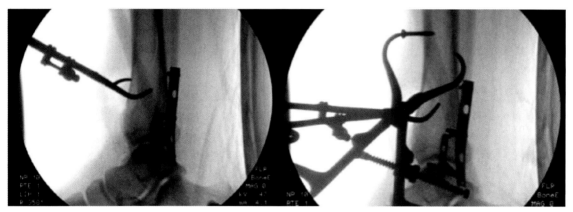

Figure 24-38 I Fluoroscopic images demonstrating placement of a unicortical screw as a "clamp extender" to allow accurate clamp vector while avoiding undue pressure on the soft tissues.

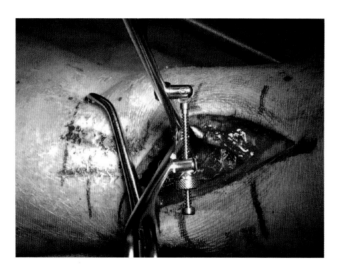

Figure 24-39 I An intraoperative image demonstrating clamp application in the head of a 3.5-mm screw placed percutaneously as a "clamp extender."

- If the articular block is translated relative to the tibial shaft, the external fixator or a spiked pusher can be used to manipulate the tibial shaft to align it with the joint segment (Fig. 24-40).

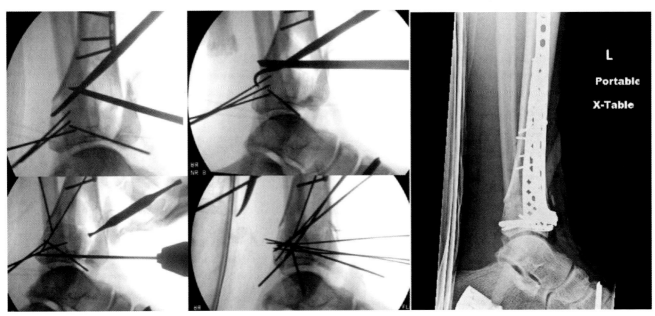

Figure 24-40 I Multiple methods are available for reduction of a displaced Volkmann fragment. These intraoperative images demonstrate use of an osteotome and shoulder hook for fragment disimpaction and mobilization. A threaded Schanz pin may be used for additional fragment manipulation. Lastly, the entire articular block may be indirectly reduced to the shaft using the external fixator.

- Repair can then proceed with K-wire provisional fixation followed by definitive plate and screw stabilization (Fig. 24-41).

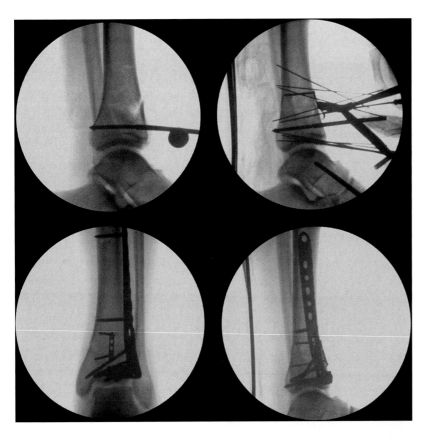

Figure 24-41 I A Schanz pin can be used to derotate the entire articular block. Reduction and provisional fixation can then continue with K-wires and plates.

Lag Screw "Macro Reduction"

Clay Spitler, MD

Pathoanatomy

Some comminuted fractures have large, widely displaced fragments for which improved alignment would be helpful in spite of a plan for bridging internal fixation. Clamp application in this situation often makes application of a bridge plate difficult.

Solution

The use of a well-placed lag screw can act as a clamp with minimal soft tissue trauma, both improving alignment and allowing for easier application of a bridge plate without clamp interference.

- Simple fractures are best treated with direct reduction and rigid fixation, and comminuted fractures are best treated with relative stability.
- Articular fractures require anatomic reduction with rigid fixation, whereas comminuted metaphyseal segments are best treated with bridge plating and relative stability.
- The soft tissues around periarticular fractures of the lower extremity often dictate the available surgical approaches that are possible and can prohibit the ideal approach for fracture fixation.
- When bridging a comminuted metaphyseal segment, there are times when the length, alignment, and rotation of the limb have been restored, for example by a universal distractor, an external fixator, or an intact fibula. Fracture gaps with unacceptable displacement may persist between large fragments in the comminuted zone. In some cases, it is advantageous to bring these fracture fragments into closer apposition prior to bridge plating. Clamp application can improve this alignment, but clamps frequently hinder or obstruct plate application. Understanding the orientation of fracture planes from a preoperative CT scan can allow for application of a percutaneous lag screw. These screws can act as a reduction clamp, performing a "macro" reduction, improving the alignment of the fragments, and allowing for the application of a bridging plate.

Technique

- Example of a closed type 43C tibial pilon fracture associated with an intact fibula (Fig. 24-42).

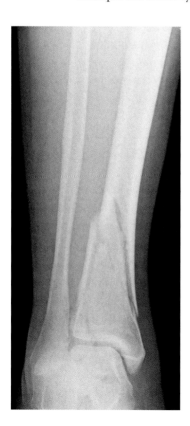
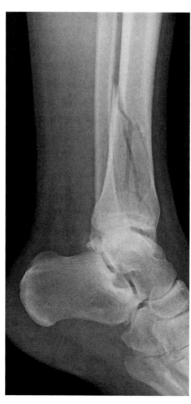

Figure 24-42 | AP and lateral images of a closed type 43C tibial pilon fracture.

- A 3.5-mm lag screw is placed into the large displaced comminuted metaphyseal bone fragment (Fig. 24-43).

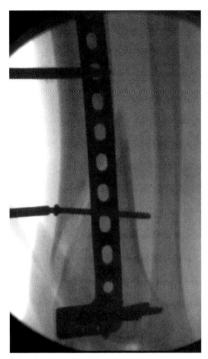 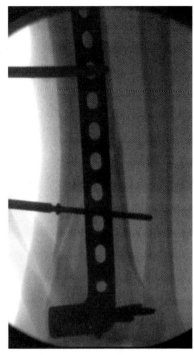 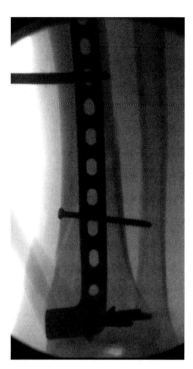

Figure 24-43 I Sequential tightening of a lag screw results in an indirect reduction.

- Bridge plating then proceeds, typically with indirect reduction techniques to achieve near-anatomic alignment. After plate placement, the "macroreduction" lag screw is then removed in order to allow for appropriate interfragmentary motion to promote secondary bone healing (Figs.24-44 and 24-45).

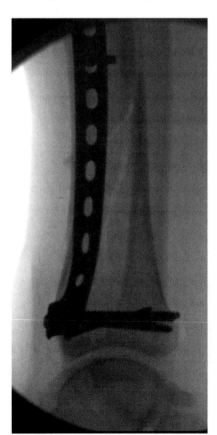

Figure 24-44 I Removal of "macro reduction" lag screw after bridge plating.

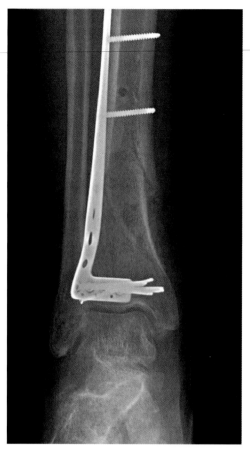
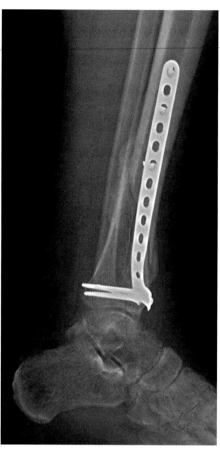

Figure 24-45 | AP and lateral radiographs of the healed fracture.

- Another example: open 43C pilon, talar dome osteochondral fracture and tongue-type calcaneal fracture (Fig.24-46).

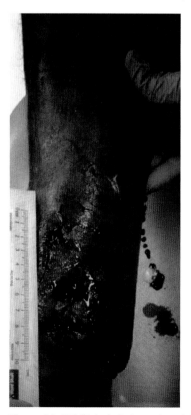
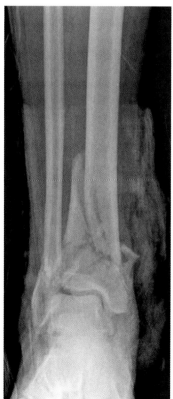
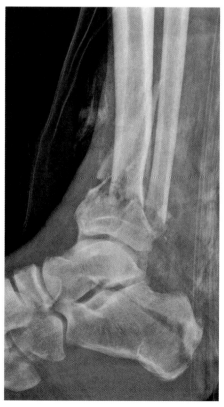

Figure 24-46 | Clinical photograph and AP, lateral radiographs of an open type 43C pilon fracture with an associated fracture of the fibula, talar dome osteochondral fracture, and tongue-type calcaneal fracture.

- First, the fibular is reduced and plated, and then the intra-articular portion of the fracture is stabilized through a limited periarticular incision (Fig. 24-47).
- Next, the pathway for a percutaneous 3.5-mm lag screw is prepared. Its position and placement are determined based on a preoperative CT scan (Fig. 24-48).

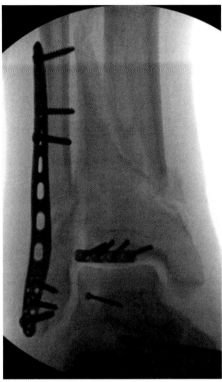

Figure 24-47 ▍Fluoroscopic image after tibial articular reduction and fibular fixation.

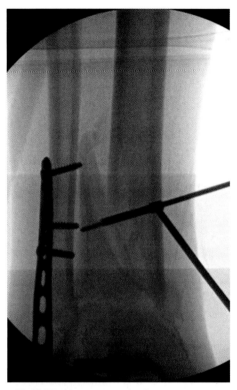

Figure 24-48 ▍Pathway preparation for a percutaneous "macro reduction" lag screw.

- The lag screw is inserted and tightened sufficiently to allow an anterolateral plate to be inserted through the limited periarticular incision (Figs. 24-49 and 24-50).

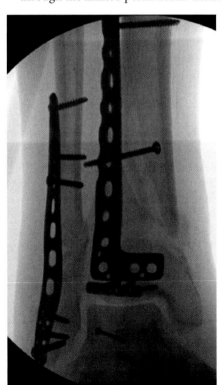

Figure 24-49 ▍Application of a bridge plate after "macro reduction" screw is tightened sufficiently.

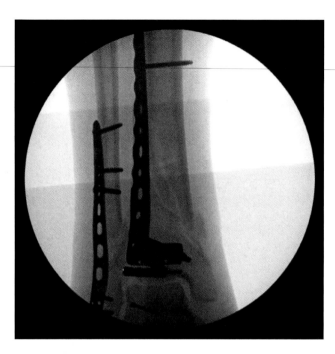

Figure 24-50 I Mortise image after further stabilization and removal of the lag screw.

- Final fixation radiographs show restoration of limb length and alignment (Fig. 24-51).

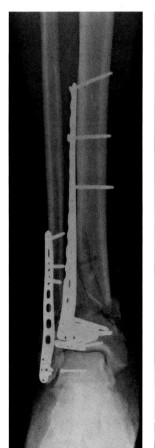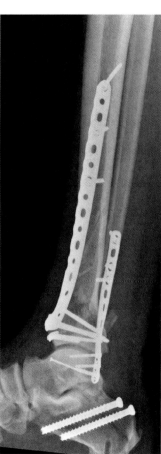

Figure 24-51 I AP and lateral radiographs after fixation is complete.

- To stabilize the reduced articular segment to the metaphysis through an anterolateral approach, an anterolateral plate may be placed (Figs. 24-52 and 24-53).

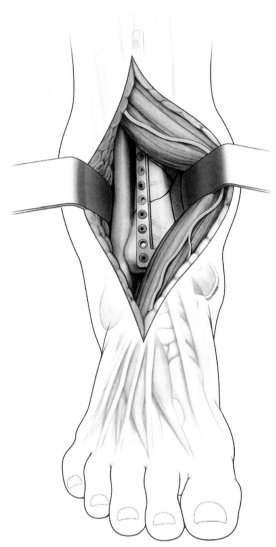

Figure 24-52 ▌ After the reduction of the articular surface, an anterolateral plate can be slid in a submuscular fashion through the anterolateral approach. The plate is fixed to the distal articular block followed by fixation proximally to the tibial diaphysis. (From Nork SE, Barei DP, Gardner MJ, et al. Anterolateral approach for pilon fractures. *Tech Foot Ankle Surg*. 2009;8(2):53–59, with permission.)

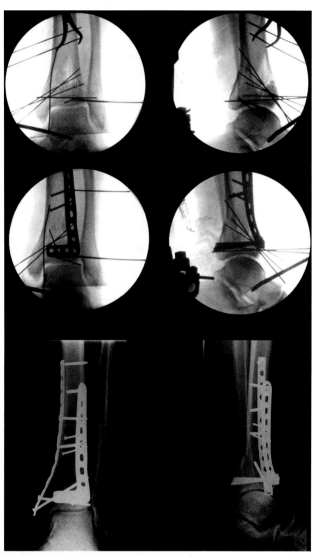

Figure 24-53 ▌ Radiographic example of an anterolateral plate placed through an anterolateral approach.

Suture-Assisted Plate Guidance for Pilon Fractures
Lisa Taitsman
Christopher Domes
Joseph Cohen

Pathoanatomy

An anterolateral approach is often used in the operative management of pilon fractures. The neuro-vascular bundle can be injured when inserting a plate from distal to proximal using the anterolateral approach during stabilizing of pilon fractures. This is a concern when a skin and soft tissue bridge remains between the anterolateral approach at the ankle and the proximal incision used for diaphyseal screw placement. Screws placed without direct visualization increase the risk of nerve or vessel injury.

Solution

A suture can be placed in the most proximal hole in the plate to facilitate its safe passage under the neurovascular bundle. The suture also helps guide the end of the plate as it is advanced proximally minimizing additional soft tissue stripping and allowing for a more accurate plate placement.

Technique

- The anterolateral approach to the pilon and ankle joint is performed by making a skin incision in line with the fourth ray.
- The retinacular layer is incised, and the tendons are retracted from lateral to medial to provide access to the ankle joint. The neurovascular bundle contained within the soft tissue (Fig. 24-54) is retracted with the tendons.

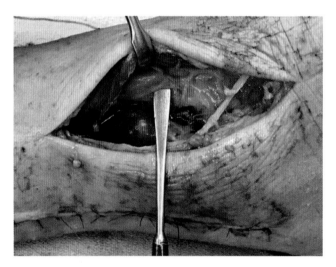

Figure 24-54 In a right lower extremity, the superficial peroneal nerve is seen coursing superficial to the retinaculum and the structures of the anterior compartment. A small Langenbeck retractor has elevated the muscle-tendon units of the anterior compartment, and a Freer elevator demonstrates the anterior tibial artery and veins and the accompanying deep peroneal nerve.

- A separate incision is made proximally, adjacent to the lateral aspect of the tibial crest at the proximal end of the desired plate. The fascia of the anterior compartment is incised, and the muscle is elevated extraperiosteally from the tibia.
  - Care is taken to not injure the neurovascular bundle.
- A soft tissue bridge remains intact between the two incisions.
- The pilon fracture is reduced and provisionally stabilized with Kirschner wires. The plate is selected and a suture is tied to the proximal hole in plate (Fig. 24-55).

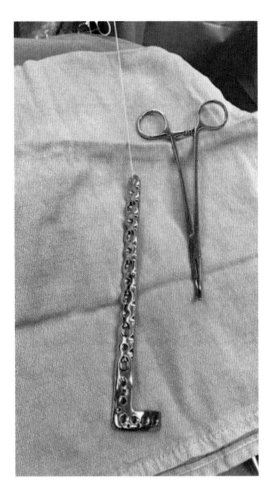

Figure 24-55 I A suture is tied to the proximal hole in the plate.

- Once the surgeon is ready to place the plate, a retractor is placed in the distal incision to elevate soft tissues including the neurovascular bundle. It is important to confirm by direct visualization that the neurovascular bundle is protected by the retractor. A long clamp is passed from the proximal incision to the distal incision (Fig. 24-56).
- The tip of the clamp is visualized in the distal incision and confirmed to be under the retractor, thus between the soft tissue (neurovascular bundle) and the bone. The end of the suture is placed into the clamp (Fig. 24-57).

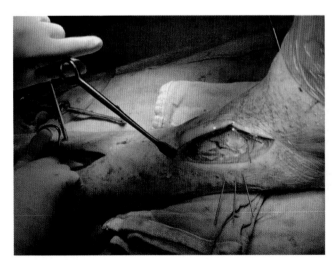

Figure 24-56 I A long clamp has been passed underneath the structures of the anterior compartment, from proximal to distal and visualized in the distal incision.

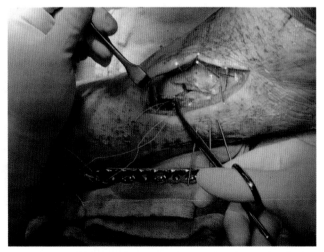

Figure 24-57 I The end of the suture (attached to the proximal hole in the plate) is grasped by the clamp.

- The clamp with the suture is pulled up and out through the proximal incision (Fig. 24-58).
- The plate can then be guided proximally along the tibia, safely under the neurovascular bundle and positioned in the appropriate location (Fig. 24-59). The plate is fixed in place and the suture is cut and removed.

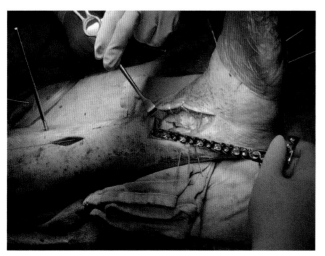

Figure 24-58 ▌ After the clamp has been withdrawn from the proximal incision, tension is applied to the suture and the plate is guided proximally to its extraperiosteal location.

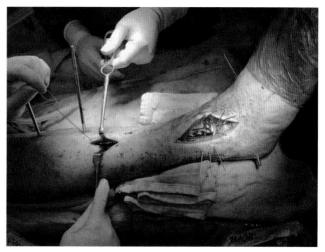

Figure 24-59 ▌ Once the plate is confirmed to be in its final position, it is stabilized with K-wires, the proximal suture is removed, and definitive fixation ensues.

- If an anteromedial approach is performed, a medial plate may be advanced subcutaneously from distal to proximal through the medial extent of the incision.
  - Avoid injury to the greater saphenous vein and nerve when extending the transverse limb of the incision medially.
  - Proximal screws may be placed percutaneously (Fig. 24-60).

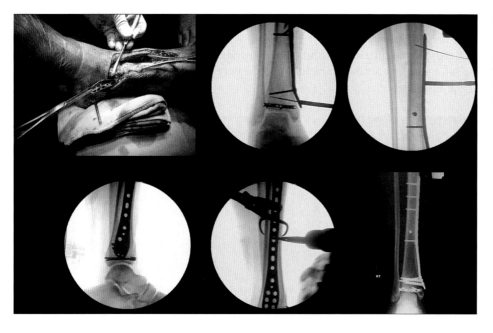

Figure 24-60 ▌ Depending on the need for medial stabilization, a plate can be slid through the medial extent of an anteromedial approach. The plate can then be stabilized distally, and the proximal screws can be placed percutaneously.

- An anterolateral plate may also be placed through an anteromedial approach, depending on the fracture pattern.

- If the pilon fracture resulted in a valgus deformity, and the medial malleolus failed in tension, a small tensioned plate can be used to stabilize this fragment.
  - In this pattern, a large buttress plate is not necessary for medial column fixation (Fig. 24-61).

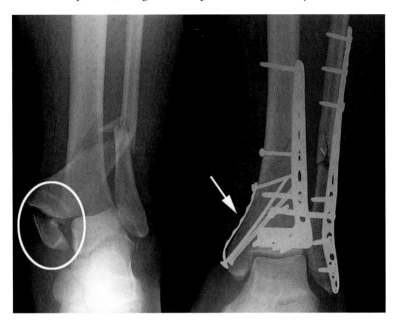

Figure 24-61 ‖ When the medial malleolus fails in tension (*circle*), a small fragment tension plate (*arrow*) adequately stabilizes this fragment.

- A dorsal distal radius plate designed for the contralateral side fits well on a large medial malleolus fragment (Fig. 24-62).
- New advances in plate technology allow fragment-specific fixation through a single plate. This may be advantageous in highly comminuted patterns.

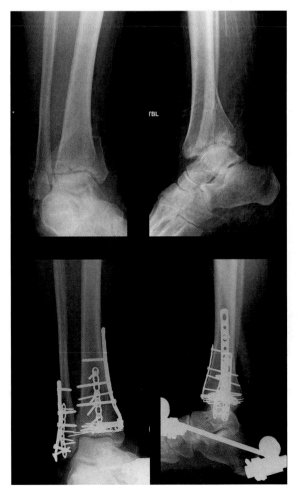

Figure 24-62 ‖ Example of a left dorsal distal radius plate applied to the large medial malleolus fragment in the right pilon fracture.

Special Situations and Techniques

- Analyze the axial CT for presence of posteromedial tendon(s) (posterior tibialis/flexor digitorum longus) in fracture site.
  - This will significantly impede indirect reduction of fracture planes, such as reducing a posteromedial fracture line from an anterior approach (Fig. 24-63).

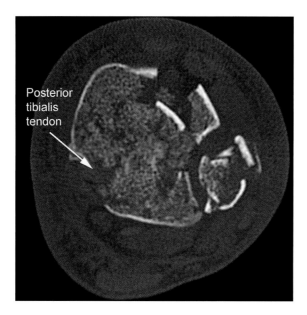

Figure 24-63 I On the axial CT scan, the posterior tibialis tendon can be seen in the fracture site. This requires attention prior to reduction of this fracture line. Use of a femoral distractor, which aids significantly with articular reductions, may be an impediment when a tendon is interposed in a fracture plane. As the limb segment is lengthened and the tendon is placed under tension, tendon mobility is reduced and reduction is impeded. Loosening the distractor will usually facilitate the maneuver to extract the tendon.

- In cases where the Chaput and Volkmann fragments are small and unable to be captured by implants, the syndesmosis will likely remain unstable, and a transsyndesmotic "positioning" screw should be considered (Fig. 24-64).

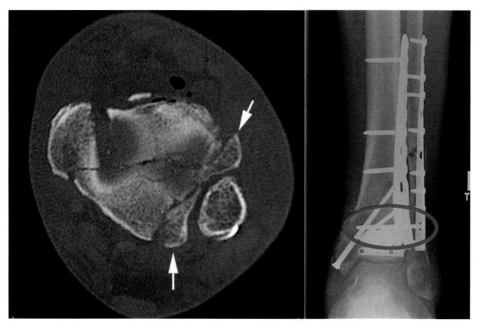

Figure 24-64 I When the Chaput and Volkmann fragments are small (*arrows*), transsyndesmotic fixation should be anticipated (*circle*).

- An alternative approach to temporizing fixation is to convert a type C to a type B pilon fracture if the soft tissues and fracture type allow.
  - This is best performed through a posteromedial (sometimes posterolateral) approach using small fragment plates and screws.
    - While more malleable plates are preferred for distal metaphyseal fractures, a 3.5-mm LC-DC plate should be considered for fractures involving the tibial diaphysis.

- This step can be performed initially through a clean open wound or as an intermediate stage while the anterior soft tissue edema resolves.
- Definitive articular reduction is greatly facilitated after this is performed by creating a stable column as a base for the staged reconstruction (Fig. 24-65).

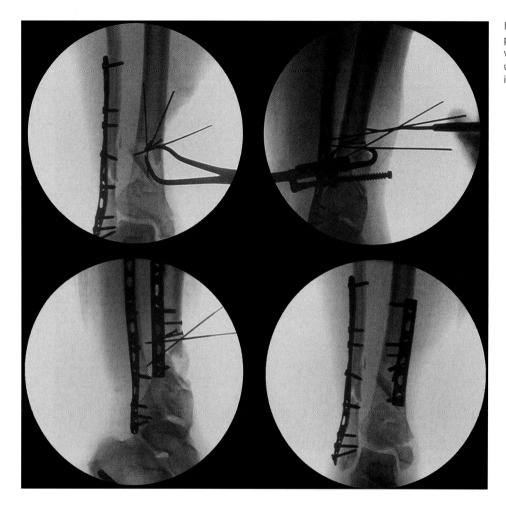

Figure 24-65 ∎ In this case, a large posteromedial articular fragment was stabilized to the tibial diaphysis using a small fragment plate and independent lag screws.

- To reduce posterior fragments from an anterior approach, lag screws in multiple directions can be used to pull in multiple sequential vectors (Fig. 24-66).

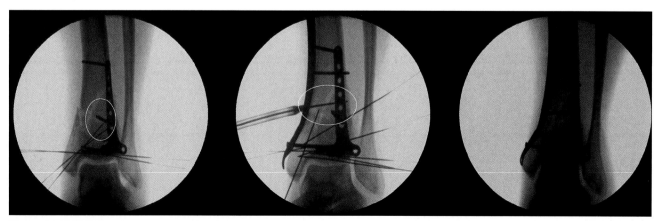

Figure 24-66 ∎ Initially, a lag screw was placed from anterior to posterior to reduce a displaced posterior fragment (*left, circle*). To reduce the coronal plane displacement, the first screw was loosened and a second screw was placed from medial to lateral (*center, circle*).

- If the fracture pattern is predominantly posterior, a posterior plate may be preferable and is best applied through a posteromedial or posterolateral approach.
  - A periarticular plate designed specifically for this location or a plate designed for the contralateral proximal tibia fit well after some contouring (Fig. 24-67).

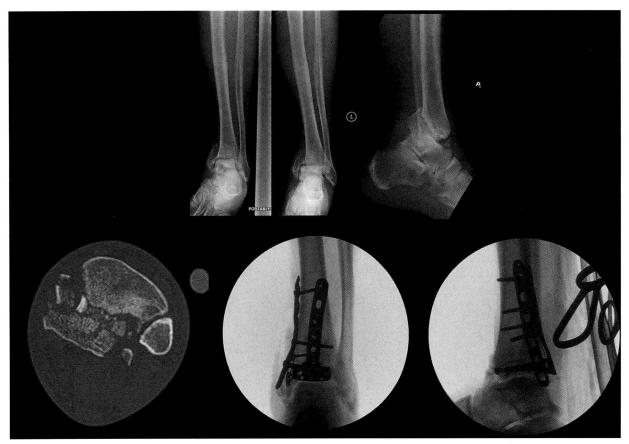

Figure 24-67 I When the fracture fragments are posterior, a periarticular buttress plate may be placed posteriorly through a posterior approach.

- A liability of a posterior approach is the difficulty visualizing the articular surface.
  - An anterior approach allows direct reduction of the medial extent of the fracture line as well as the articular surface, and the posterior fragment can be stabilized with anteroposterior lag screws (Fig. 24-68).

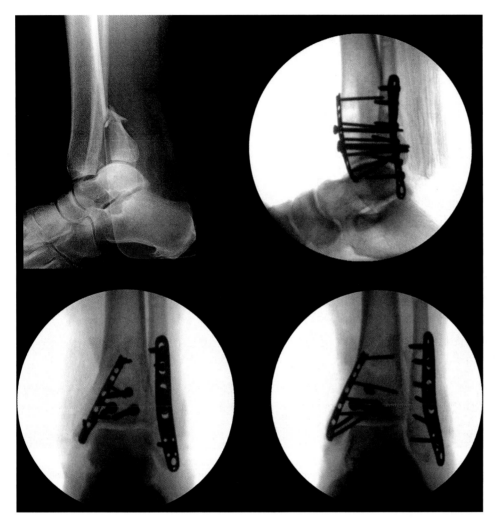

Figure 24-68 | To address a posterior type B pilon from an anterior approach, medial dissection allows visualization of the cortical fracture line and removal or repositioning of intercalary articular comminution. Joint distraction allows direct inspection of the intra-articular reduction. Anterior-to-posterior or posterior-to-anterior lag screws can be placed to stabilize the fragment.

- Depending on the fracture pattern, another valuable reduction strategy is to first obtain a reduction of the medial malleolar fragment by interdigitating its cortical fracture lines.
  - This then becomes a stable foundation on which to reduce the remaining fracture fragments.
  - Initially, the medial plate should be placed provisionally with unicortical screws.
  - After reduction of the entire fracture, these unicortical screws can be replaced with bicortical screws.

- The plate can be inserted subcutaneously, in either direction, so a formal extensile medial approach for reduction and plate application is not needed routinely.
  - This avoids making an incision through injured medial soft tissues as is common in these injuries (Fig. 24-69).

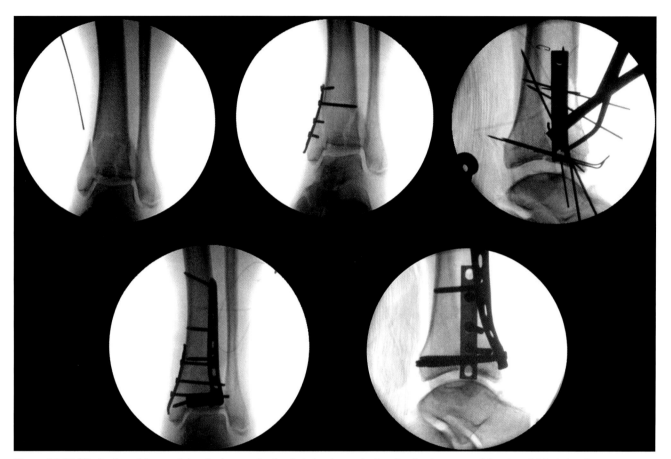

Figure 24-69 I Reduction of the medial malleolus may be the first step in repair of a pilon fracture, especially when it fails in tension. Anatomical reduction using cortical interdigitations followed by provisional fixation creates a stable fragment to which the remaining tibial plafond components may be reduced. The small medial incision is marked with a K-wire. After the medial malleolar fracture is reduced, a small fragment plate is placed extraperiosteally, followed by insertion of unicortical screws. The remainder of the fracture is then reduced to the stable fragments.

- If the fibular fracture is transverse, not comminuted, and minimally displaced, an intramedullary fibular screw or wire can be used for stabilization.
  - Cortical interdigitations should provide rotational stability.
  - If rotationally unstable, a second screw can be used to neutralize forces.
  - Be aware that open reduction is the surest method of achieving an anatomical fibular reduction.
  - A 2.5-mm drill should be used first, and a 3.5-mm drill can be used in the distal fragment to achieve compression.
    - A triple-fluted 2.5-mm drill bit is preferred to a double-fluted drill bit as it is easier to control and less likely to "wander" at its entry point.
    - The drill should be oscillated to minimize the risk of cortical perforation as it contacts the endosteal surface obliquely.
  - The starting point on the lateral view is critical and is similar to any intramedullary nail, in that it will affect reduction of the fracture.

- It can be offset to achieve tension or compression in the desired direction in the sagittal plane (Fig. 24-70).

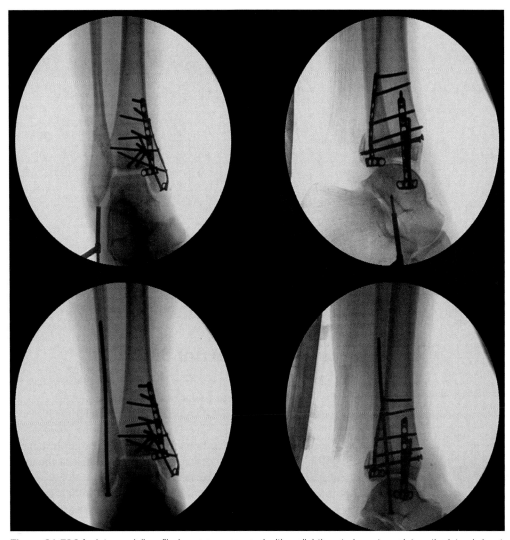

Figure 24-70 | An intramedullary fibular screw was used with a slightly anterior entry point on the lateral view to correct the apex posterior fracture deformity.

- To fill the metaphyseal voids with cylindrical small cancellous dowels, use a 4.5-, 5.5-, or 6.5-mm drill guide to harvest cancellous bone "plugs."
  - The proximal tibial metaphysis is a useful donor site.
  - Alternatively, autograft may be obtained by making one of more stab incisions in lateral calcaneus.

- It is possible to make several passes at different angles to obtain several cylinders of bone graft (Fig. 24-71).

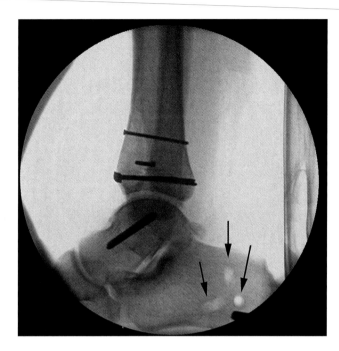

Figure 24-71 I To obtain local cancellous bone graft that is more compact and has some structural integrity, a 4.5-, 5.5-, or 6.5-mm drill guide can be used to harvest from the calcaneus through stab incisions (*arrows*).

Maintaining the External Fixator

- Consider maintaining the external fixator for B- and C-type pilons where there is significant anterior crush associated with anterior talar escape.
  - May be necessary to maintain the reduction of the talus under the plafond, even after definitive fixation
  - More commonly used to protect fixation and prevent early anterior talar escape
- Obtain sterile flat plate x-ray (lateral view) of the full length tibia at the end of the case to ensure the talus remains directly under the plafond.
- If the talus is anterior or anterior fixation is tenuous, maintain the external fixator with a posterior vector to keep the talus under the plafond and offload the anterior fixation (Fig. 24-72).
- External fixator is removed at 6 to 8 weeks (Fig. 24-73).

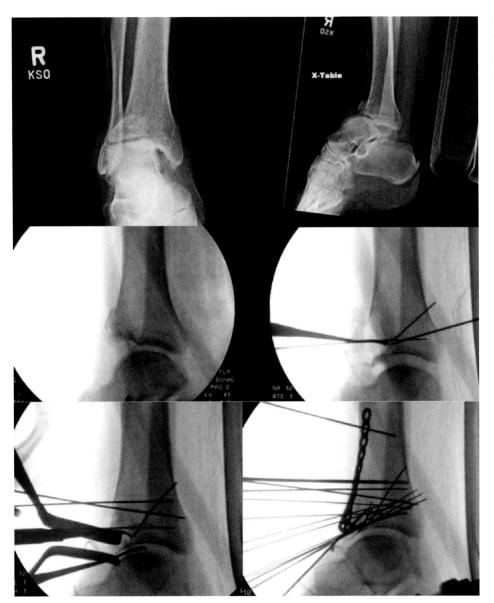

Figure 24-72 I Injury and intraoperative images of an OTA B-type pilon with anterior talar escape and significant anterior comminution.

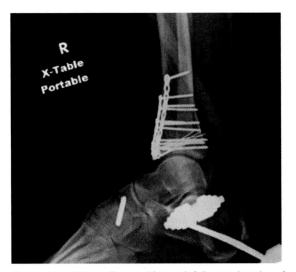

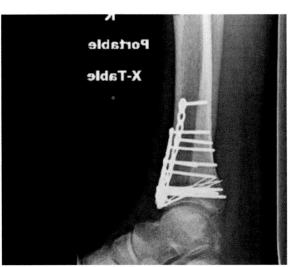

Figure 24-73 I Immediate and 3-month follow-up imaging of a pilon fracture for which the external fixator was maintained for 6 weeks. The external fixator was maintained to protect the delicate reduction and fixation and maintain the talus in a reduced position underneath the tibial plafond.

Chapter 25
Ankle Fractures

DAVID P. BAREI

DAPHNE M. BEINGESSNER

M. BRADFORD HENLEY

ERIC D. FARRELL

MICHAEL J. GARDNER

JESSICA HOOPER

ZACHARY V. ROBERTS

MATTHEW P. SULLIVAN

NIRMAL C. TEJWANI

Sterile Instruments/Equipment

- Tourniquet if desired
- Small pointed bone reduction clamps (Weber clamps)
- Small serrated bone reduction clamps
- Dental picks and Freer elevators
- Laminar spreader for fibular "push screw"
- Large quadrangular ball-spike clamp for syndesmosis reduction
- Implants: Anatomically contoured periarticular fibular plates (lateral or posterolateral), one-third tubular plates; 2.0 and 2.4 plates/screws
  - Long 3.5-mm (or 4.0-mm) cortical screws for syndesmosis
  - Long 3.0-, 3.5-, or 4.0-mm cortical, cancellous, or cannulated screws for medial malleolus/anterior colliculus
  - Minifragment screws and minifragment plates (2.0/2.4 mm) for independent fibular lag screws and for posterior or medial malleolar comminution, depending on the fracture pattern
- K-wires and wire driver/drill

Surgical Approaches/Positioning

- Variable and depends on the injury pattern
- Supine with a bolster under the ipsilateral hip for most lateral malleolar, bimalleolar, and trimalleolar injuries
  - Consider no bolster for isolated medial malleolar fractures (or posteromedial approaches to posterior malleolus), providing adequate internal/external hip rotation for imaging ankle and mortise.
- Lateral or prone position facilitates access to the posterior malleolus.
  - Prone position makes ORIF of lateral and medial malleoli accessible but provides a less familiar perspective.
  - Lateral position may allow for reduction and fixation of the medial malleolus following fixation of the posterior and/or lateral malleolus, assuming the patient's hip anatomy allows adequate external rotation.

- Posterolateral approach
  - Plane between posterior border of fibula and peroneal tendons
  - May be preferable
    - For concomitant access to the posterior malleolus (interval between flexor hallucis longus [FHL] and peroneal tendons), if necessary.
    - Allows a separate anterolateral approach for pilon fractures.
    - There is less risk of injury to the superficial peroneal nerve.
    - The implant is not directly under the skin incision.
- Posteromedial approach
  - Several "windows" may be used to access the posterior portion of the medial malleolus and posterior malleolus: anterior to the PT tendon or posterior to the PT/FDL tendons.
  - Generally, FHL is retracted posteriorly and laterally with the posterior tibial neurovascular bundle.

Reduction and Fixation Tips

Fibula Fractures: Rotational Mechanism

- Most spiral fibular fractures (SER-type fracture patterns) are amenable to 2.4- or 2.7-mm lag screws (in addition to plate fixation of the fracture).
  - May be placed independently, prior to lateral plate placement, or through a posterolateral plate.
  - Posterior-to-anterior placement avoids soft tissue stripping anteriorly.
- K-wires for provisional fixation
  - Transcutaneous K-wire placement from anterior to posterior avoids interference with posterolateral plate (Fig. 25-1). Wires are removed after plate application.

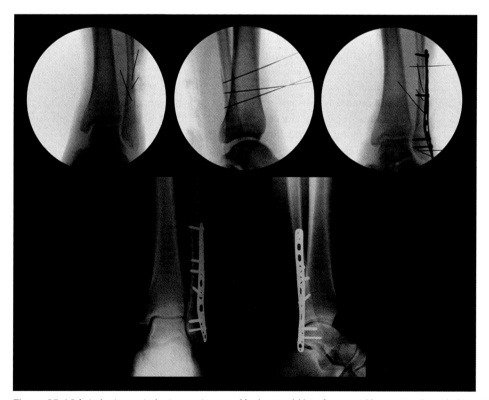

Figure 25-1 I Anterior-to-posterior transcutaneous K-wires avoid interference with a posterolateral plate and posterior-to-anterior lag screw.

- Consider use of small lag screws for more proximal (Weber C) fractures.
  - 2.0-, 2.4-, or 2.7-mm screws provide excellent fixation and have a small head that will not interfere with plate application (Fig. 25-2).

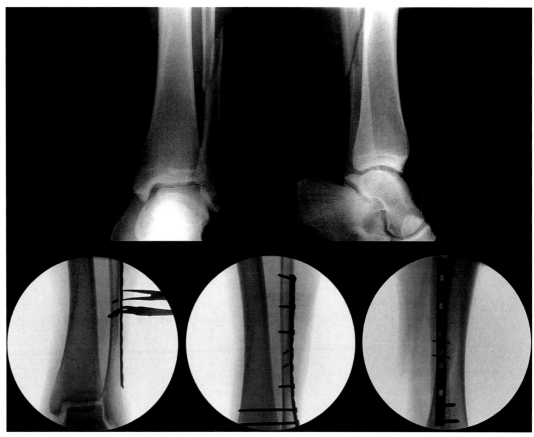

Figure 25-2 ▮ Two minifragment lag screws achieve excellent interfragmentary compression and do not impede neutralization of plate placement.

- Keep the plate posterolateral distally (Fig. 25-3).
  - Longer, posterior-to-anterior distal screws in the lateral malleolus may provide better distal fixation as they are frequently 24 to 30 mm in length.
  - Often allows bicortical screw placement with screw tips exiting anteriorly, away from the articular cartilage of ankle joint.

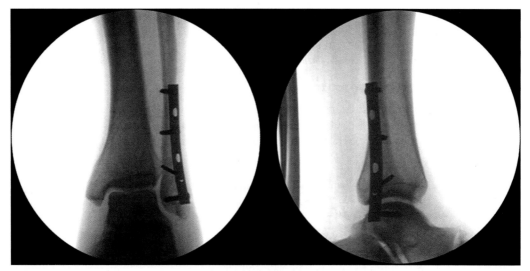

Figure 25-3 ▮ Posterolateral plating of the distal fibula is attractive for several reasons. Applied posterolaterally, the plate is mechanically suited to prevent the shortening and posterolateral translation that occur in most SER-type fractures. Additionally, the lag screw can be placed through the plate and anchored proximally in the thicker anterior cortical bone. The posterior-to-anterior screw(s) in the distal fragment also tend to be longer (24 to 30 mm), thus improving the distal fixation. This case demonstrates the use of a one-third tubular plate, a 2.7-mm lag screw, and 3.5-mm proximal and distal screws.

- Antiglide plate position on fracture apex is biomechanically favorable.
- Reduced implant prominence and low frequency of hardware removal with posterior placement.
- Lag screws may be placed through the plate after antiglide and distal/proximal fixation to augment compressive fixation force at fracture.
  - Use of a 2.7-mm lag screw leads to less screw head prominence and less potential for irritation of the peroneal tendons (see Fig. 25-3).
  - An additional benefit of placing a 2.7-mm lag screw through the plate is the ability to replace it with a slightly larger screw if insufficient fixation is suspected.
    - Permits "rescuing" the interfragmentary lag screw fixation with a slightly larger 3.5-mm lag screw (usually with a 2.7-mm head) when 2.7-mm lag fixation is inadequate
- To augment distal fixation, consider converging the tips of the distal screws.
  - "Interlocking" the screws with each other can improve the fixation by allowing interference fit between the threads of the two screws (Fig. 25-4).

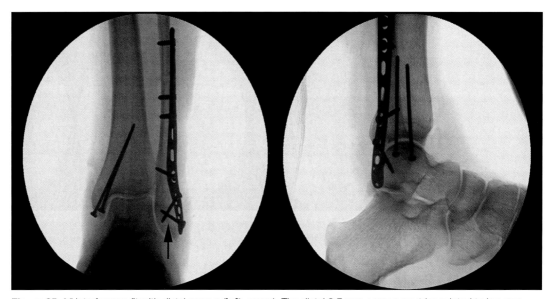

Figure 25-4 ▌ Interference fit with distal screws (**left**, *arrow*). The distal 2.7-mm screws are triangulated to improve fixation with interference between the threads of the two screws.

TIP

ORIF Fibula with 2.7- and 2.4-mm Reconstruction Plates
Eric D. Farrell

Pathoanatomy

Open reduction internal fixation of fibula fractures can be accomplished with many types of implants. Despite newer "anatomic" locking plates, obtaining fixation of all significant fragments such as Wagstaffe's tubercle can be difficult in certain fracture patterns.

Solution

A technique for fibular fixation using a 2.7-mm reconstruction plate placed posterolateral with the addition of a 2.4- or 2.0-mm plate can help secure comminuted distal fractures.

Technique

Equipment
- 2.7-mm reconstruction plate and screws
- 2.4-mm or 2.0-mm locking plate and screws
- 3.5-mm drill bit

Case Example: A 27-year-old male sustained a left trimalleolar ankle fracture while playing soccer. The patient was splinted by the emergency department and followed up in clinic (Fig. 25-5A–C).

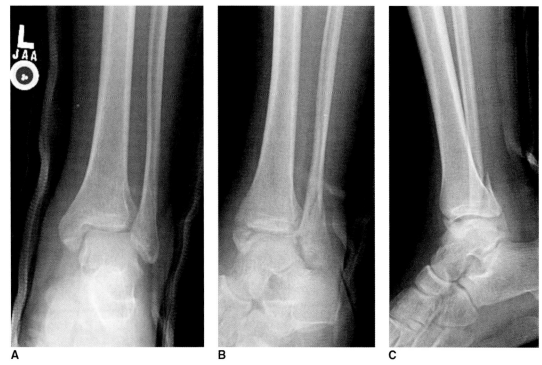

A   **B**   **C**

Figure 25-5 ▮ **A–C:** AP, mortise, and lateral radiographs of a trimalleolar ankle fracture. The images fail to show the comminution of the anterior aspect of the distal fibula.

- He was taken to the OR 10 days postinjury, after the soft tissue envelope had improved.
- A posterolateral approach to the fibula was used; the peroneal tendons retracted posteriorly.
  - The position of the superficial peroneal nerve is noted for protection.
- The fracture is reduced, clamped (Fig. 25-6), and secured with K-wire(s); the length of the 2.7 recon plate is determined and then cut to length.

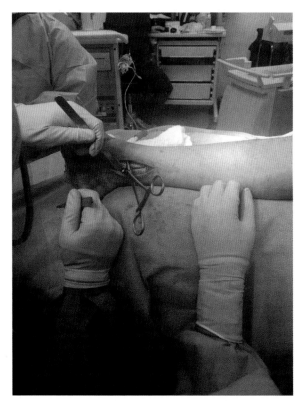

Figure 25-6 ▮ Exposure of the lateral and posterolateral fibula with reduction clamp stabilizing the main fracture fragments.

- Tip: The rough portion of the drill's chuck can be used to smooth the cut edges of the plate.
- Other plates may be used alternatively.
- If a syndesmotic screw is needed, the corresponding hole in the plate can be enlarged to accommodate a 3.5 screw without any risk of "catching" or binding to the plate.
  - In addition, the syndesmotic screw may need to be angled in the plate, also necessitating a larger plate hole. In this particular case, the syndesmosis was exposed, visualized, and noted to be unstable when stressed.
- To accomplish this, a 3.5-mm drill is used to enlarge the syndesmotic hole once it is determined in which hole the screw will reside.
  - The plate is clamped tightly with one or two large pliers or vice grips. The 3.5-mm drill is then started at full speed and placed completely coaxial with the hole. The drill bit is then slowly advanced into the hole. Note: Do not start the drill with the bit already in the hole (Fig. 25-7).

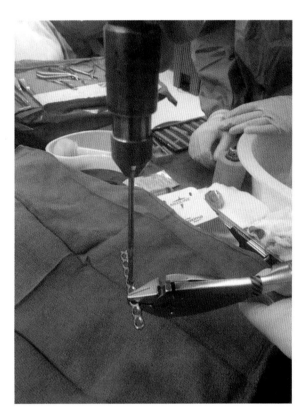

Figure 25-7 | Drill has been started on full-speed and then advanced into the hole.

- While the drill is on full speed, the bit is moved in and out of the hole as the drill angle is changed slowly so as to enlarge the hole (Fig. 25-8A and B).

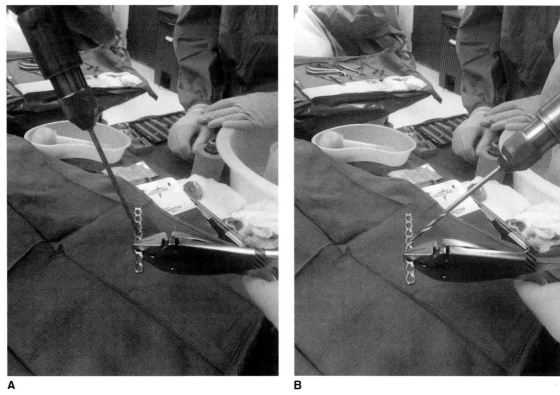

A   **B**

Figure 25-8 I **A and B:** Angle of drill bit is slowly changed as the drill is maintained on full speed.

- Once the hole is enlarged sufficiently, the plate is flipped and the process repeated from the plate's other side (Fig. 25-9A and B).

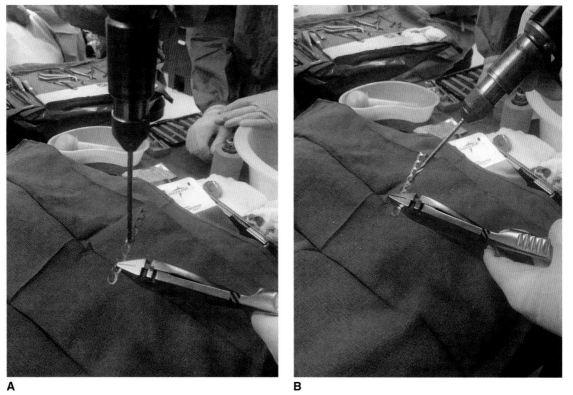

A   **B**

Figure 25-9 I **A and B:** Plate has been flipped revealing the "unbeveled" texture and the enlarging process repeated.

- The plate is then rinsed with sterile saline and fixation of the fracture continued (Fig. 25-10).
- The cut end of the plate should be placed proximally to decrease the risk of peroneal tendon irritation.
- In this case, there was an anteromedial fragment that was not visualized on the initial x-rays. The location of the fragment precluded fixation using the posterolateral plate. The decision was made to secure this fragment with a 2.4 recon plate.
  - TIP: A 2.4 or 2.0 plate can be placed anteriorly to secure Wagstaffe's tubercle. Once the plate is contoured, it is secured distally with one or two screws. One of these may be a locking screw. If the plate is undercontoured, when the proximal nonlocking screws are engaged, the underlying tubercle will be stabilized in compression (Fig. 25-11).

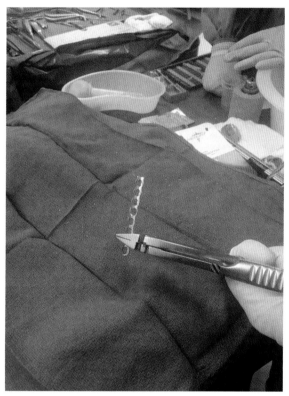

Figure 25-10 | Completed hole enlarging. Note the size of the #4 hole.

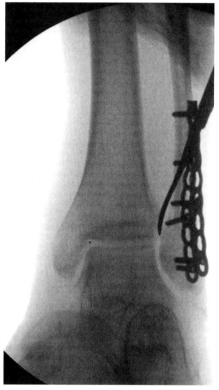

Figure 25-11 | Posterolateral 2.7 recon and anterior 2.4 recon plates have been placed and syndesmosis assessed.

- Following fibular fixation, the medial malleolus is reduced and fixed with one or two lag screws (Fig. 25-12).
- In this case, a single bicortical 3.5 screw was used for fixation. Two smaller screws could have been used instead (Fig. 25-13).

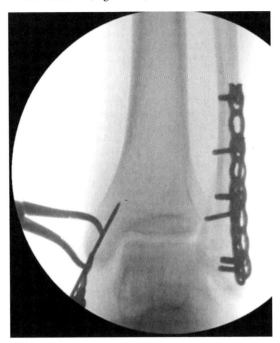

Figure 25-12 | Medial malleolus has been exposed through a small incision and reduction held with point-point tenaculum and K-wire. The fragment was noted to be small with an oblique fracture line.

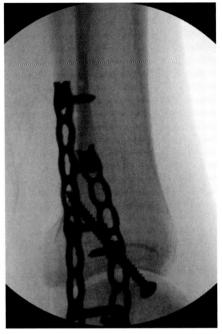

Figure 25-13 | Medial malleolus screw has been place in bicortical fashion, perpendicular to the fracture line with good compression and stability.

- The final fixation needed is the syndesmotic screw.
  - A clamp may be collinear to the syndesmosis to maintain the reduction. A 1.6 or 2.0 K-wire can then be added for additional stability to prevent anterior or posterior translation.
  - Under fluoroscopic guidance, the syndesmotic screw is drilled with a 2.5-mm drill and drill sleeve, and then, the proximal three cortices are tapped (Fig. 25-14A and B).
  - When placing self-tapping syndesmotic screw in young patients/good bone, it is beneficial to tap the near tibial cortex or insert the screw into the near cortex of the tibia and then remove the screw followed by readvancing the screw to the far cortex. This may help prevent subtle widening of the syndesmosis due to the "cork-screw effect," which allows the screw to spin without advancing as the tibial hole is advanced into the tibia. If there is good fibular/tibial bone quality and/or if the screw threads contact with the edge of the plate screw hole, the fibula can displace laterally along the screw's axis.

Figure 25-14 | **A and B:** Syndesmotic screw being drilled, then measured for four-cortices fixation.

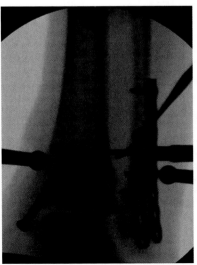

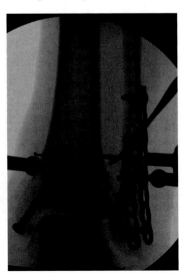

A   B

- Once all fixation has been placed, fracture reduction and implant placement is scrutinized with multiple views of fluoroscopy (Fig. 25-15A–D).
- Final films are shown in Figure 25-16A to C.
- Five-month postop x-rays are shown in Figure 25-17.

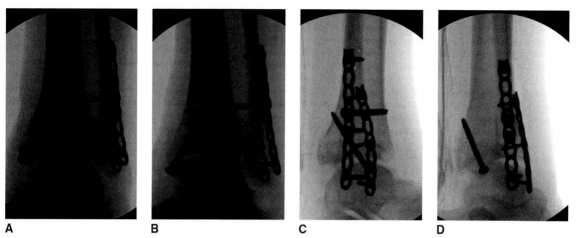

Figure 25-15 | A–D: AP, lateral, and mortise fluoroscopy views. Note bicortical fixation of the medial malleolus screw in Figure 25-15C. Anterior position/screw length of the 2.4 plate and confirmation of syndesmotic screw placement are reflected in Figure 25-15C and D.

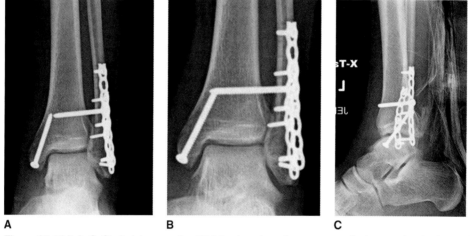

Figure 25-16 | A–C: Sterile intraoperative AP, lateral, and mortise x-rays confirming good reduction and safe placement of implants.

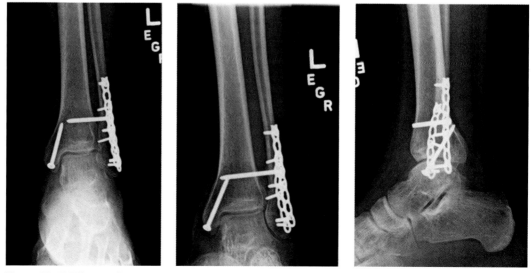

Figure 25-17 | Five month postoperative x-rays.

Fibula Fractures: Abduction Mechanism

- Transverse or short oblique fibular fractures with variable comminution are usually the hallmarks of these injuries.
- Use fragments to help determine length, alignment, and rotation of the fibula.
  - Use x-rays of the contralateral ankle for comparison.
  - Recreate the "dime sign."
  - Compare fibular lengths.
  - Compare the fibulotalar articulation (lateral talar facet/gutter) for symmetry.
  - Reconstitute "Shenton's line" of the ankle mortise at the distal lateral tibiofibular articular (Fig. 25-18).

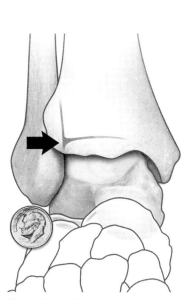 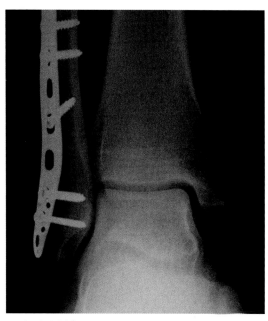

Figure 25-18 I Several radiographic markers can be helpful for reconstructing the anatomic fibular length in comminuted fractures. These include the "dime sign" (seen as the dime at the distal end of the fibula) and the fibular Shenton's line (*arrow*).

- Minifragment screws are useful to reconstruct the comminuted fragments.
- Stacked one-third tubular plates, or a thicker periarticular plate, can increase the stiffness of the fixation construct across comminuted segments.
  - When applying a stacked plate construct, tie the two plates together at each end with a 2-0 resorbable suture to make them easier to handle (Fig. 25-19).

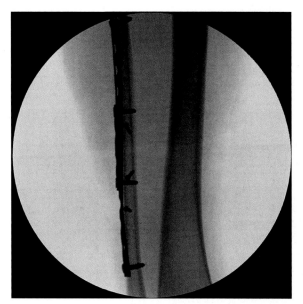

Figure 25-19 I Stacking one-third tubular plates can stiffen the lateral construct and help support areas of comminution. Tying the plates together with 2-0 suture(s) makes them easier to manipulate.

- Use indirect reduction technique for restoration of the fibular length.
  - Stabilize the plate distally with multiple K-wires and/or screws.
  - Insert a bicortical fibular screw proximal to the plate.
  - Apply a laminar spreader to distract and restore length (Fig. 25-20).

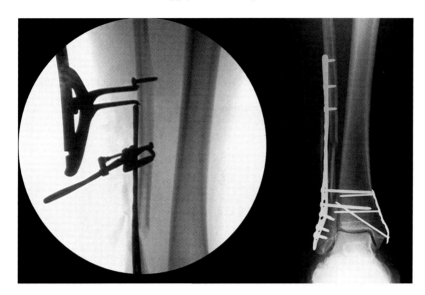

Figure 25-20 I Use of a push screw with a laminar spreader to restore fibular length indirectly.

- Control the plate with a Verbrugge or serrated clamp to maintain proximal plate-bone apposition.
  - These clamps permit translation of the plate along the fibular shaft, thereby permitting restoration of the fibular length.
- When using indirect reduction techniques, initially support the distal fixation with wires through the plate and/or one screw.
  - The use of multiple wires placed distally helps prevent loss of fixation during indirection reduction techniques.
  - When screws are used alone in soft bone, distraction forces may result in cavitation of metaphyseal bone, potentially compromising definitive distal screw fixation.
  - Place the wires bicortically and orthogonally to the plate or at a slightly more acute angle (i.e., 60 to 90 degrees) so as to maintain contact of the plate and bone during distraction.
  - Remove these wires with a pliers and not a drill to decrease the likelihood of breakage of any bent wires during removal.
  - This minimizes stressing the screw-bone interface without distracting against definitive screws (Fig. 25-21).

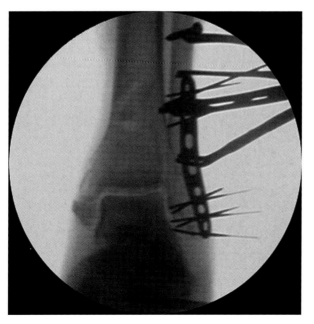

Figure 25-21 I A laminar spreader between a push screw and the proximal edge of the plate is a good tool to help restore the fibular length. This figure shows the plate fixed to the distal fragment with K-wires alone, a useful technique to keep from stressing distal fixation during the reduction process.

- Use a small anterior fibular plate to augment fixation if significant comminution of either medial or lateral malleolus (Fig. 25-22).

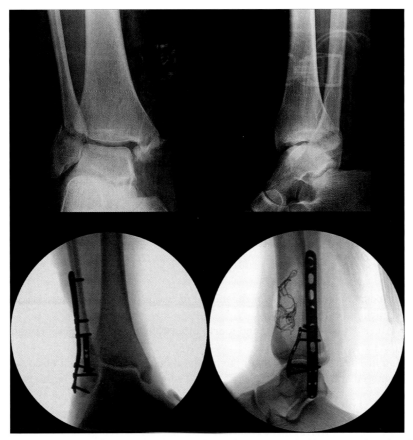

Figure 25-22 ▍ In this bimalleolar fracture, the fibula was treated with a posterolateral periarticular plate and an anterior minifragment plate for stabilization of comminuted intercalary fragments.

Fibular Fractures: Adduction Mechanism

- The fibular fracture is typically a perisyndesmotic or an infrasyndesmotic transverse (or short oblique) fracture.
  - May be suitable for medullary screw fixation.
  - Requires a rotationally stable fracture pattern (i.e., fragment interdigitation and compression).
  - Overdrill the starting hole with a 3.2- or 3.5-mm drill to make the screw insertion easier.
  - Use long 2.5-mm calibrated drill bit to prepare the medullary canal of the fibula and estimate the screw length.
  - Starting point is critical. Make sure that it is center/center on the AP and lateral views and collinear with fibular canal, if not collinear. Then, angulation at the fracture site may occur if the screw is stiffer than the reduction afforded by fracture interdigitation.

- Alternatively, a small tensioned plate can provide sufficient rotational stability of small fibular avulsion fragments (Fig. 25-23).

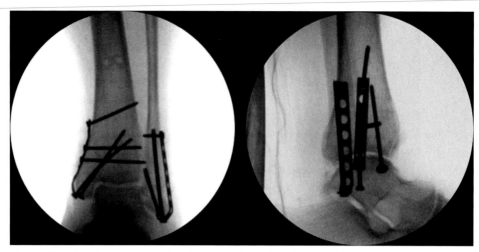

Figure 25-23 | A minifragment tension plate for fibular avulsion fracture stabilization.

- Consider smaller implants for the medial malleolus when the fracture is comminuted and/or the fragments are small.
  - Anterior and/or posterior one-fourth tubular plates with 2.7-mm screws or 2.4/2.0 plates and screws.
- Marginal articular impaction of the medial shoulder of the plafond often exists. Ensure this is diagnosed and treated with "elevation" and supportive grafting (Fig. 25-24).

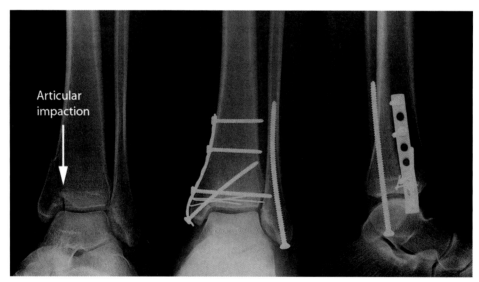

Figure 25-24 | Fixation of the supination adduction injury: the medial plafond impaction has been reduced and stabilized with wires and bone graft. An antiglide plate buttresses the medial malleolus, and a medullary screw stabilizes the fibula.

Medial Malleolar Fractures

- Approaches should provide surgical exposure and visualization from the anterior ankle joint to the posterior tibialis tendon, as well as the cortical surface.
- For large fracture fragments, two 3.5- or 4.0-mm cancellous lag screws or two 3.5-mm cortical screws inserted using a lag technique are usually sufficient, depending on the size of the fracture fragment (Fig. 25-25).

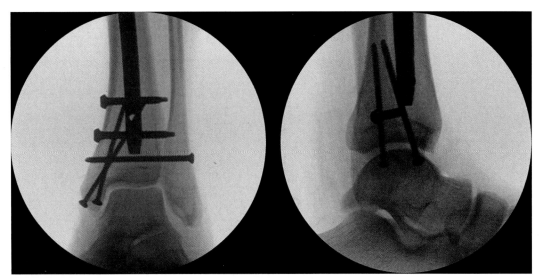

Figure 25-25 ▌ Two 3.5 cortical screws, inserted using lag technique, are used to fix this medial malleolar fracture.

- Consider smaller screws (3.0/2.7/2.4 mm) for anterior or posterior collicular fractures.
- Placing bicortical medial malleolar lag screws can increase the strength of the medial fixation and are useful in osteoporotic bone.
  - For easier insertion, place provisional K-wires away from, but roughly parallel to, the anticipated screw trajectory.
  - These can be used as an external visual guide during screw insertion.
  - Overdrilling the near cortex will make it easier to find the hole with the screw tip.
  - Tapping both cortices will assist in screw insertion as the screw may skid along the endosteal surface due to the obtuse angle of intersection (Fig. 25-26).

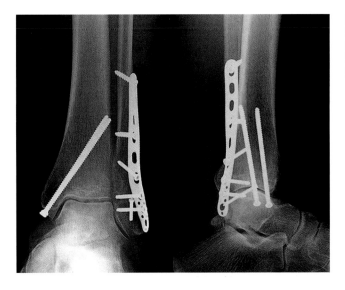

Figure 25-26 ▌ Improve medial fixation by placing bicortical 3.5-mm screws (with 2.7-mm heads). This may be especially important in patients with osteoporotic bone.

- When drilling the far cortex, advance the drill bit slowly to avoid bending or breaking the drill bit.
  - If the drill bit bends, remove the bit and create a distal cortical hole by drilling the lateral tibial cortex with a stiffer instrument, such as a 2.4-mm smooth Steinmann pin.
- Another method of obtaining bicortical fixation is to use a K-wire, a cannulated drill bit, and a cannulated tap to create both the gliding and threaded holes for lag screw fixation.
  - After creating the screw path, fix the fracture with noncannulated screws.
- In osteoporotic bone, be careful not to overcompress the fracture.
  - The denser metadiaphyseal bone permits good screw purchase and may result in fracture angulation and a malreduction.

- 2.0-mm plates are useful for comminuted or multifragmentary avulsion medial malleolus fractures (Fig. 25-27).

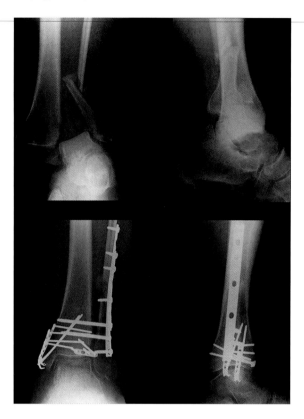

Figure 25-27 | 2.0-mm straight plates with 2.4-mm screws are useful implants for comminuted medial malleolus fractures. Note the stacked one-third tubular plates to increase the rigidity of the lateral fixation across the intercalary comminution. The avulsed Chaput fragment has been repaired with a four-hole 2.0-mm straight plate.

The Chaput (or Tillaux-Chaput) Fracture Fragment and/or the Wagstaffe-Le Forte Avulsion Fracture Fragment

- May be approached through a separate anterolateral approach, if fibular approach is sufficiently posterior to provide for an adequate skin bridge.
- A 2.0-mm straight plate placed anteriorly is used both as a tension band and as a washer or spiked washer for fixation.

The Posterior Malleolus

- Fracture morphology—the lateral view underestimates the size of the posterior malleolar fracture fragment and the articular involvement.
  - Consider using a lateral view with approximately 30 degrees of external limb rotation for a view tangential to the fracture line.
  - This view, in addition to a mortise view, guides the direction of lag screw fixation.

- May be addressed by exploiting the lateral or medial malleolus fracture.
- Direct reduction and ORIF through posterolateral or posteromedial approach (Fig. 25-28).

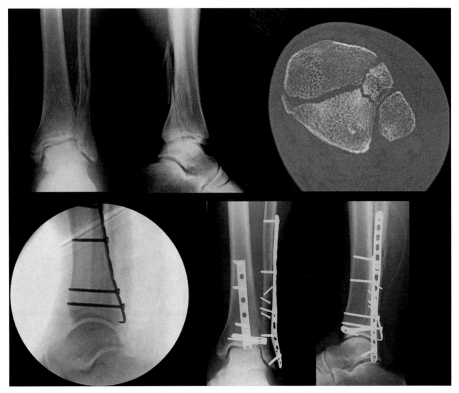

Figure 25-28 ▌ Posterior antiglide plate. This large posterior malleolus fracture was reduced using a posterolateral approach with the patient in the lateral position. A one-third tubular plate (fashioned as a hook plate) was used with 3.5-mm screws. The fibular fracture was reduced and fixed subsequently through the same skin incision. Alternatively, a posteromedial approach anterior to the posterior tibial tendon would allow direct access to the fracture (figure) but would not be ideal for orthogonal screw placement. The Chaput fracture was repaired through a separate, smaller anterolateral approach with a quarter tubular plate and 2.7-mm screws.

- Posterolateral approach
  - The posterolateral approach allows access to the cortical surface of the posterior tibia, but limited access to the ankle joint.
    - The fracture is accessible superiorly and laterally above the posterior tibiofibular ligament and along its posteromedial border.
    - The posterior tibiofibular ligament prevents access to the lateral fracture border, except above the ligament near the fracture's apex.
  - It is helpful to obtain a CT scan preoperatively to identify the interfragmentary fragments or articular impaction that will block the reduction of the posterior malleolus.
  - The fracture plane is usually best imaged with some external rotation (variable), tangentially to the fracture plane, which can be determined more accurately using the CT scan's axial images to identify the orientation.
  - Lateral or prone positioning can be used.
  - The skin incision is along the posterior border of the peroneal tendons.
  - Dissect posterior and medial to the peroneal tendons to access the posterior malleolus distally.
    - Develop the plane anteromedial to the peroneal tendons to access the medial border of the fibula.
      - Do not injure the posterior tibiofibular ligament running transversely.
      - Reflect the FHL but preserve the peroneal artery, which courses along the interosseous membrane deep to this muscle.
    - Alternatively, access the posterior surface of the fibula through the FHL/peroneal interval.
      - This is much easier with patient prone.
  - To minimize dissection, a portion of the posterior malleolar fragment can sometimes be accessed for cleaning and reduction through the medial malleolar fracture, if present, or through the fibular fracture (prior to its reduction).

- A one-third tubular or smaller plate placed in an antiglide position with supplementary lag screws is usually a sufficient fixation for this fracture.
  - Alternatively, smaller plates can effectively buttress a small posterior malleolar fragment; 2.4- and 2.0-mm straight or T-plates should also be considered.
- Clamp application can be necessary for anatomic articular reduction (Fig. 25-29).

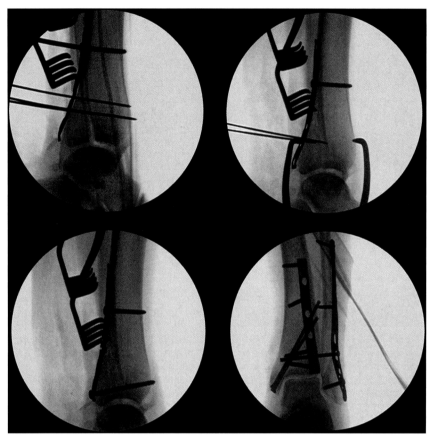

Figure 25-29 | If indirect reduction with a plate does not obtain an anatomical articular reduction, place a clamp tine through a small anterior incision and the other tine directly on the Volkmann fragment (**upper right**).

- Posteromedial approach
  - Patient may be positioned prone or supine, assuming that there is adequate hip external rotation to allow access and reduction. Alternatively, a "figure of four" position of the limb with the patient positioned supine can be used.
  - Allows direct access to the fracture plane.
  - Fibula is not "in the way" with this approach compared to the posterolateral approach.
  - Several "windows" may be used to access the posterior malleolus: posterior to the PT tendon and anterior to the FDL tendon, posterior to the PT and FDL tendons, and anterior to posterior tibial neurovascular bundle or posterolateral to PT/FDL and NV bundle, retracting FHL laterally.
    - Generally, the interval is posterior to the PT/FDL, while the FHL is retracted posteriorly and laterally with posterior tibial neurovascular bundle.
  - Occasionally will require both posterolateral and posteromedial approach (Figs. 25-30 and 25-31).

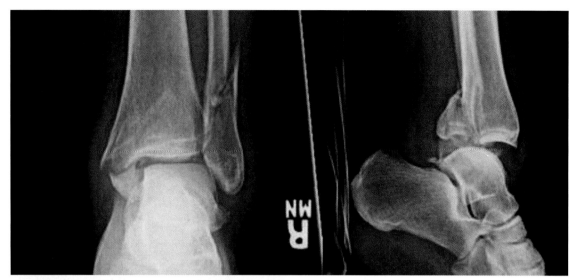

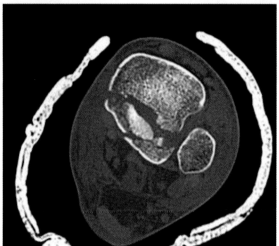

Figure 25-30 | Injury x-rays and CT scan demonstrate a complex trimalleolar ankle fracture with a segmental posterior malleolus. Simultaneous posteromedial and posterolateral approaches will allow for fragment-specific reduction and fixation.

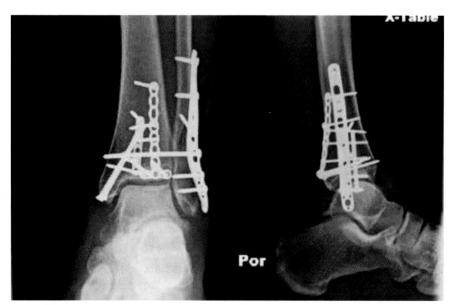

Figure 25-31 | Postoperative radiographs demonstrate accurate reduction and fragment-specific fixation achieved through simultaneous posteromedial and posterolateral approaches. A separate small anteromedial approach was used for reduction of the medial malleolus.

- Indirect reduction
  - Indirect reduction with screw fixation of the posterior malleolus is an attractive option in trimalleolar ankle fracture patterns as it allows the patient to be positioned supine for the entire procedure.
  - Disadvantages are reliance on indirect or percutaneous methods to manipulate the posterior malleolus, radiographic assessment of the reduction, and a less secure fixation construct.
    - A shoulder hook or large pointed bone reduction clamp (Weber) is a useful tool to manipulate and reduce the posterior malleolus percutaneously (Fig. 25-32).

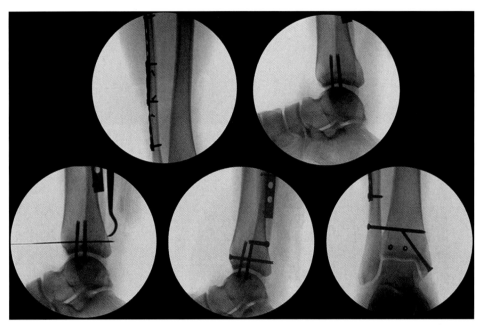

Figure 25-32 I Initial anatomical reduction of the diaphyseal fibula fracture in this trimalleolar ankle injury provides near anatomic reduction of the posterior malleolus. Note that if the fibular plate continued distally, it would obscure the radiographic assessment of the posterior malleolar reduction. A shoulder hook is used to manipulate the Volkmann fragment into a more distal position using fluoroscopic guidance (**lower left**). The posterior malleolus is stabilized using anterior-to-posterior cannulated lag screws and the syndesmotic reduction is secured with a transsyndesmotic 4.0-mm cortical screw.

- Anatomical reduction of the fibula will often reduce the posterior malleolus indirectly.
  - However, plate fixation of the fibula can obscure the radiographic assessment of the articular surface and the posterior malleolar fracture plane.
  - Use K-wires or lag screws to provisionally stabilize the fibular reduction prior to reduction of the posterior malleolus.
  - Apply definitive fibular fixation after articular reduction is confirmed radiographically.

- Scrutinize the AP and lateral views for a medial (and posterior) double density, potentially indicating a posteromedial fracture fragment.
  - Consider obtaining a CT scan to further assess (Fig. 25-33).

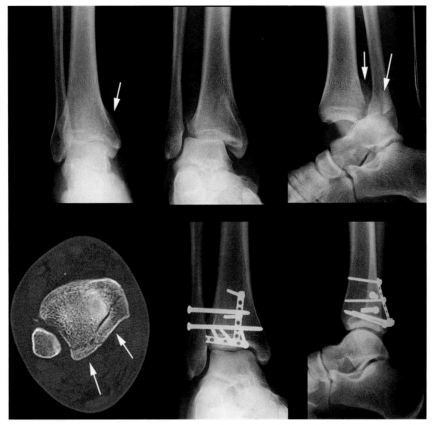

Figure 25-33 | A double density was seen medially on the AP view (*arrow*, **upper left**) and posteriorly (*arrows*, **upper right**). A CT scan was obtained to further evaluate the morphology of the posterior distal tibia (*arrows*, **lower left**). This injury was treated with a posteromedial approach and a transverse minifragment plate to stabilize both the posterolateral and posteromedial fragments.

Syndesmosis

- When comminution of the incisura exists, or for patients with an old or chronic syndesmotic injury, consider an open syndesmotic reduction (Fig. 25-34).

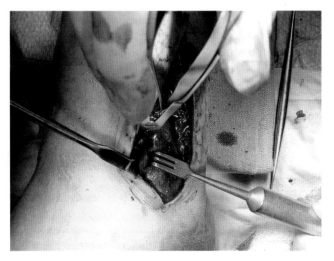

Figure 25-34 | The distal tibiofibular syndesmosis can be approached by extending the posterolateral incision sufficiently to permit soft tissue retraction (shown) or through a separate anterolateral incision in line with the fourth metatarsal. A laminar spreader is used to distract the disrupted joint so that interposed hematoma, callus, ligaments, or fracture fragments can be cleared from the tibiofibular articulation.

- Sagittal plane instability.
  - Check for fibular and talar subluxation in the sagittal plane using the lateral view.

- After reduction maneuvers, use a percutaneously placed periarticular or linear bone clamp and place one or two 0.062-inch K-wires to provisionally stabilize the ankle mortise and syndesmosis.
  - This is followed by definitive fixation (Fig. 25-35).

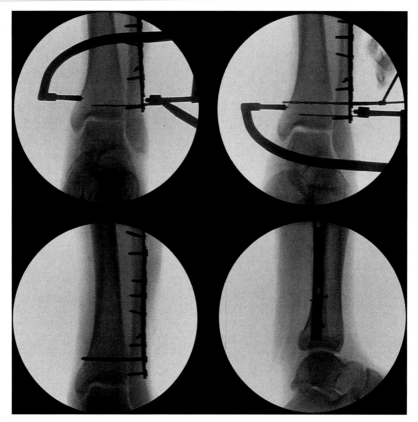

Figure 25-35 I The syndesmosis is first reduced and stabilized using a linear bone clamp. The reduction is assessed on both the AP and lateral views, and a 0.062-inch K-wire is used to maintain reduction and as additional temporary stabilization. Definitive fixation is then applied.

- Syndesmosis screws may be inserted through a lateral fibula plate as the location of this plate facilitates screw insertion, which is orthogonal to the incisura (see Fig. 25-35).
  - Ideally, these screws should be inserted perpendicular to the incisura and orthogonal to the fibula (same figure below).
  - However, syndesmotic screws placed through a posterior or posterolateral fibular plate may cause the fibular to translate anteriorly along the screw's trajectory if the fibula is not stabilized in a reduced position prior to creating the path for the interosseous screw.
  - Thus, it is important to provisionally stabilize the syndesmotic reduction with one or two trans-syndesmotic K-wires prior to drilling the syndesmosis screw path, especially if placed through a posterolateral fibula plate.

Anatomic Closed Reduction and Internal Fixation of Syndesmosis Injuries

Matthew P. Sullivan
David P. Barei
Daphne M. Beingessner

Pathoanatomy

An accurate and anatomic syndesmosis reduction is difficult to achieve reproducibly.

Solution

Understanding the patient's contralateral anatomy and radiographic images

Technique

- The first step to getting the reduction of syndesmosis "correct" is to identify what "correct" is. Contralateral fluoroscopic images are essential. Both lateral and mortise views of the uninjured side should be obtained before prepping the injured leg and may reveal subtle anatomic variations (imperfect "dime sign" in this particular patient) (Fig. 25-36).

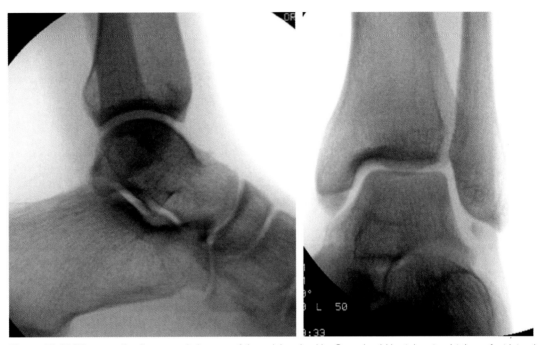

Figure 25-36 ▌ Preoperative fluoroscopic images of the uninjured ankle. Care should be taken to obtain perfect lateral and mortise views, as they will be essential for comparison during surgery.

- If the surgeon forgets to acquire these images prior to positioning and prepping the injured leg, a perfect lateral of the uninjured ankle can be obtained without too much difficulty by externally rotating the uninjured ankle through the drapes.
- A limited anterolateral approach to the syndesmosis may aid in reduction and stabilization.
  - This approach is classically made in line with the fourth ray between the tendons of extensor digitorum and peroneus tertius. Given the limited nature of this approach, it is helpful to localize the incision under fluoroscopy.
  - The superficial peroneal nerve is usually found in the subcutaneous tissues deep to this skin incision.
- The anterior inferior tibiofibular ligament is usually torn in midsubstance. Alternatively, an avulsion of the tubercle of Chaput or Wagstaffe tubercle may be encountered.
- The distal tibiofibular articulation is directly posterior and slightly superior to the ligament.
  - The joint may be entered by gentle lateral displacement of the lateral malleolus. A smooth laminar spreader may be of assistance.
  - Cleanse the joint by removing any interposed soft tissue or ligament.
- Gently reduce the joint by squeezing the ankle between your thumb and fingers.
  - Thumb pressure over the lateral malleolus with gentle anteroposterior translation and internal/external rotation of the fibula should allow it to centralize within the incisura.
  - This should be confirmed by direct observation.
- While maintaining the reduction, insert a 0.062-inch Kirschner wire across the tibiofibular syndesmosis for provisional stabilization.

- This allows the surgeon to confirm the reduction on fluoroscopy and compare it to the uninjured side (Fig. 25-37).

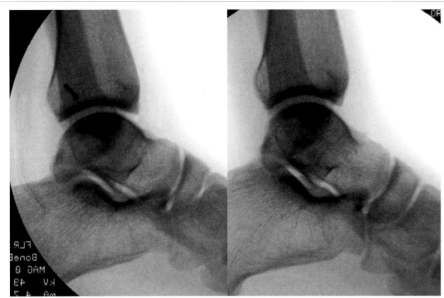

Operative Ankle   Contralateral Ankle

Figure 25-37 | Following syndesmosis reduction and insertion of a 0.062-inch Kirschner wire, a perfect lateral of the operative ankle is compared to the uninjured side. Particular attention is paid to the relationship between the anterior and posterior cortices of the tibia to those of the fibula. A symmetric reduction can be seen in operative extremity as compared to the uninjured side.

- The critical point of comparison here is the anterior-posterior relationship of the fibula to the tibia (to assess AP translation) and the relative size of the fibula to the tibia (to assess fibular rotation).
- As long as the K-wire bisects the incisura, gentle mediolateral compression across the syndesmosis may be performed if the mortise appears wide on the mortise fluoroscopic image and this is confirmed by direct observation.
- Our preference is to use a large spin-down Weber clamp, which we feel is more precise than a quad periarticular clamp.
  - Avoid aggressively compressing with this clamp (Fig. 25-38).

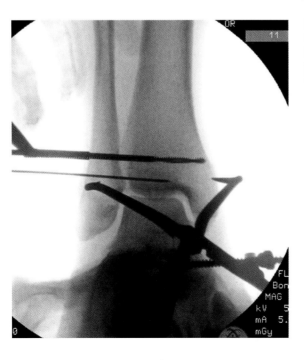

Figure 25-38 | A large spin-down Weber clamp is used to provide precise yet gentle compression during fixation while the transsyndesmotic K-wire prevents anterior translation of the fibula within the incisura.

- At this point, the surgeon may choose any number of fixation constructs; and again, final fluoroscopic images should be compared to the uninjured side prior to the conclusion of the procedure (Fig. 25-39).

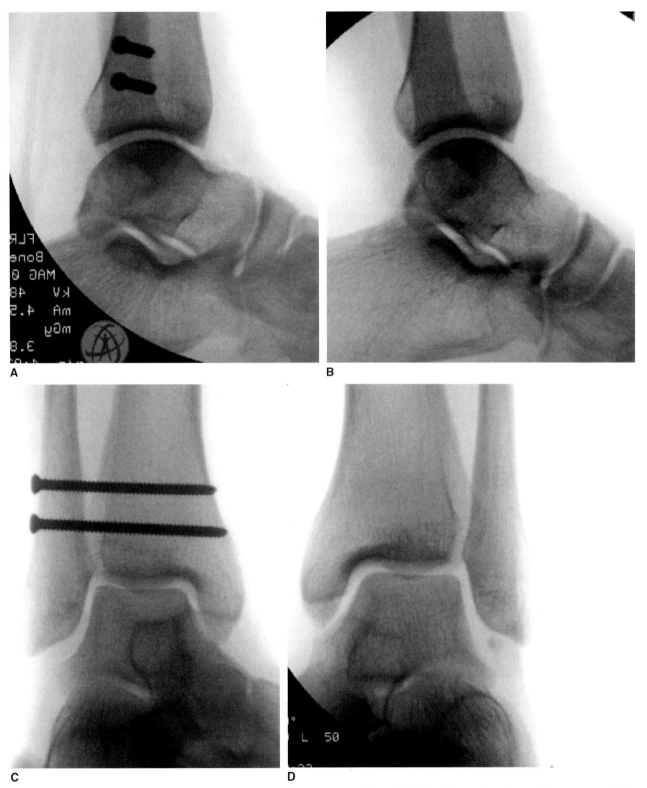

A

B

C

D

Figure 25-39 | Final comparison views (lateral and mortise) of the injured to uninjured side should be performed to confirm an anatomically reduced syndesmosis.

- The protruding tips of screws in a lateral or posterolateral fibular plate may cause a syndesmotic malreduction as a long screw may encroach upon the tibial incisura, thus preventing a concentric reduction of the fibula (Fig. 25-40).

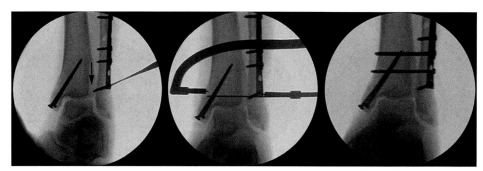

Figure 25-40 ▌The long screw in the distal end of the one-third tubular plate on the fibula prevents anatomic reduction of the syndesmosis (*arrow*, **left**). Note the apparent widening of the syndesmosis despite the symmetric appearance of the tibiotalar joint space. The distal screw has been shortened and an open reduction of the syndesmosis has been preformed (**center**). Syndesmotic fixation is complete and the clamp has been removed (**right**).

- If the syndesmotic injury involves an avulsion of the tibial insertion of the anterior syndesmotic ligament (Chaput or Tillaux-Chaput tubercle), an open reduction and fixation with a small hook plate ensures anatomic repair of this ligament (Fig. 25-41).

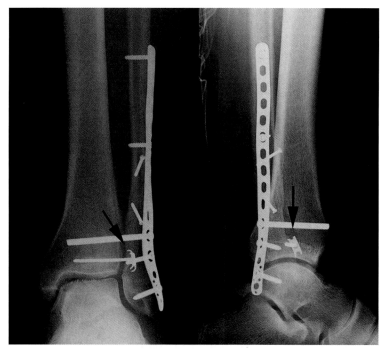

Figure 25-41 ▌Open reduction of an avulsion-type syndesmotic injury with a small hook plate, made by modifying a three-hole 2.0 straight plate (*arrows*). This was supported with a quadricortical syndesmotic screw.

- The syndesmosis may be overtightened if comminution is present on the fibular or tibial side of the syndesmotic joint (Fig. 25-42).

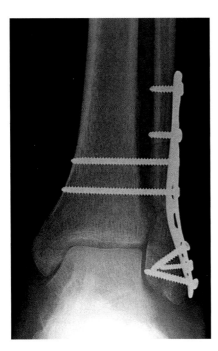

Figure 25-42 I Be cautious if there is significant comminution involving the syndesmotic area. If the fracture disrupts the articular areas on either side of the distal tibiofibular articulation, the syndesmosis can be overtightened.

TIP | Use of a Neutralization Plate for Syndesmotic Fixation of the Ankle

Jessica Hooper
Nirmal C. Tejwani

Pathoanatomy

Injury at the ankle syndesmosis most commonly occurs as a result of excessive external rotation of the dorsiflexed ankle, causing disruption of the interosseous ligamentous complex (Figs. 25-43 and 25-44).

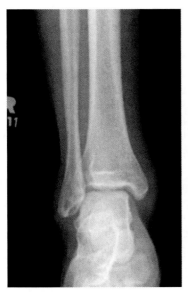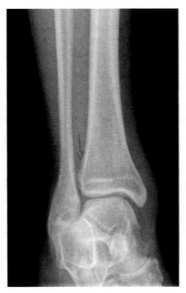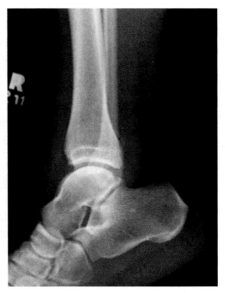

Figure 25-43 I Injury films, from left to right, AP, mortise, and lateral views of the right ankle demonstrating no fracture on these ankle images. Loss of tibiofibular overlap best seen on the mortise view is suggestive of syndesmotic injury.

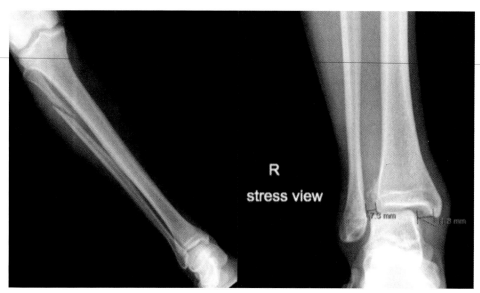

Figure 25-44 I Injury leg films, at left, AP of the right tibia and fibula demonstrating an oblique Weber C high-fibula fracture. At right, stress view of the right ankle demonstrating clear disruption of the distal tibiofibular articulation and medial clear space widening.

Anatomic reduction of the fibula into the incisura and secure fixation to limit fibular rotation are both important to successful treatment of this injury.

Solution

- The ideal method of syndesmotic fixation should provide fixation without limiting normal ankle motion, and this is contingent on an anatomical reduction of the distal tibiofibular joint.
  - When screws are used, they should be centered in the fibula so as to avoid eccentric placement with risk of fracture of the cortex and loss of fixation.
- We present a reproducible method for reduction and fixation of isolated syndesmotic injuries using a short (two- or three-hole) one-third tubular plate applied to the posterolateral surface of the fibula that allows secure anatomic reduction and optimal screw placement.

Technique

- The patient is positioned supine on a standard table. Following induction of anesthesia, a bolster is placed under the ipsilateral hip to eliminate external rotation of the extremity. A radiolucent ramp is placed under the operative leg to facilitate intraoperative fluoroscopy. Bring in fluoroscopy to obtain a true mortise (~15 degree internal rotation) view of the ankle. Holding the ankle in neutral dorsiflexion, use a large bone reduction clamp to center and maintain the fibula into the incisura of the tibia. Check the appearance of reduction with a fluoroscopic view.
- Next, place a radio-opaque straight instrument or drill bit on the anterior aspect of the distal tibia at the expected screw location approximately 2 cm proximal to the ankle. Tip: Using fluoroscopic guidance, make the instrument parallel to the ankle mortise, and draw a line on the skin. No further fluoroscopic imaging is needed until all screws have been placed.
  - The line drawn on the skin now represents the desired transverse trajectory of the syndesmotic screws. It provides a visual check for the operating surgeon, thereby reducing operative time and radiation exposure.
  - Directly lateral to this line, make a lateral longitudinal incision approximately 3 to 4 cm long over the posterolateral aspect of the fibula. Protect the superficial peroneal nerve if it is encountered. Then, expose the fibula in an extraperiosteal fashion.
  - Tip: Apply a short (two-/ three-hole) small-fragment one-third tubular plate to the posterolateral aspect of the fibula, centered over the line drawn parallel to the ankle mortise.

Use of a short plate provides several advantages over syndesmotic screws or suture button fixation:

- The plate acts as a washer to apply uniform pressure on the fibular cortex for one or more screws.
- A three-hole plate may be preferred over a two-hole plate because it allows the central hole to be used for clamp placement, which keeps the screws centered on the bone.

- Screw centralization prevents fracture of the cortex of the fibula by a screw placed too anterior or posterior and associated loss of syndesmotic fixation.
- Slightly posterolateral placement of plate on fibula reduces hardware prominence and may help orient screws perpendicular to the syndesmosis.
- If using a three-hole plate, place a small pointed reduction clamp in the center hole to keep the plate centered over the bone. If using a two-hole plate, use a small serrated reduction clamp to affix the plate to the fibula, taking care to keep the plate centered on the bone.
- In healthy bone, place two 3.5-mm cortical screws through the proximal and distal holes in the plate in a tricortical fashion (Figs. 25-45 and 25-46).

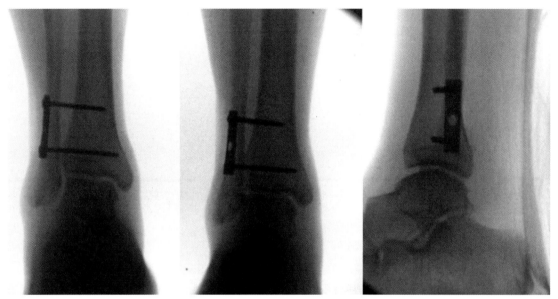

Figure 25-45 | Final fluoroscopic images after syndesmotic fixation with a three-hole plate and two tricortical 3.5-mm screws. From left to right, AP, mortise, and lateral views of the ankle demonstrate anatomic reduction of the syndesmosis, restoration of the ankle mortise, and screws parallel to the mortise.

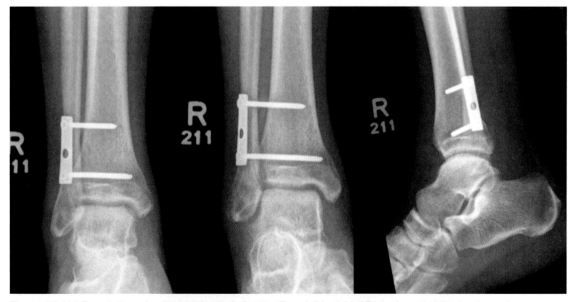

Figure 25-46 | Case 1, 6 weeks after syndesmotic fixation. From left to right, AP, mortise, and lateral radiographs demonstrate the hardware in appropriate position without loss of syndesmotic reduction.

- The trajectory of the screws should be parallel to the drawn line representing the ankle mortise and directed from posterolateral to anteromedial on an AP radiograph such that the incisura is crossed perpendicularly. Obtain complete fluoroscopic views of the ankle (anterior-posterior [AP], mortise, and lateral views) to ensure that the syndesmosis is anatomically reduced and the hardware is appropriately positioned.
  - Consider quadricortical fixation in patients with poor bone quality (osteoporosis, osteomalacia) and in those with altered sensation (diabetics with peripheral neuropathy).
- If fixation of the medial malleolus is required, as in the case of a true Maisonneuve fracture, it may be easily combined with this technique of syndesmotic fixation without modifying either fixation technique (Figs. 25-47 and 25-48).

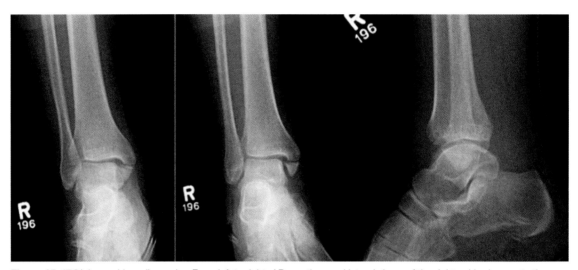

Figure 25-47 ▌ Injury ankle radiographs. From left to right, AP, mortise, and lateral views of the right ankle demonstrating a transverse fracture of the medial malleolus.

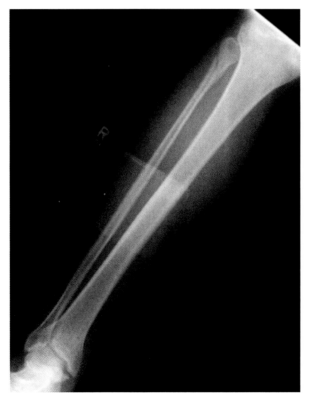

Figure 25-48 ▌ Injury leg radiograph. AP view of the right tibia and fibula demonstrating an oblique fracture of the fibular neck and a transverse fracture of the medial malleolus. No stress view was needed in this case; the presence of fractures in both bones indicates that the syndesmosis was disrupted as the energy imparted by the injury traveled from the medial malleolus to the proximal fibula.

- We recommend initial fixation of the medial malleolus to allow for more accurate assessment of syndesmotic reduction on the mortise view of the ankle.
- The medial malleolar screws provide a "goalpost" for the distal syndesmotic screw, another visual cue to judge its trajectory (Figs. 25-49 and 25-50).
- Once the incisions are closed, place the patient in a short leg splint. The splint should be kept in place for 2 weeks, at which time the sutures are removed and the patient is placed in a CAM boot to allow ankle range of motion.
- The patient should be kept nonweightbearing for a total of 6 weeks following surgery and then may be advanced to weightbearing as tolerated.

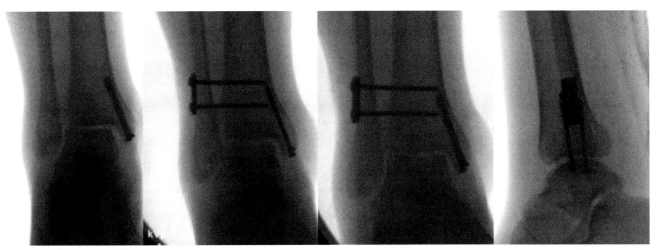

Figure 25-49 ▌ Fluoroscopic views of the right ankle. At left, mortise view of the ankle following fixation of the medial malleolus with two cannulated screws. AP, mortise, and lateral views of the ankle following fixation of the medial malleolus and syndesmotic fixation with a two-hole plate.

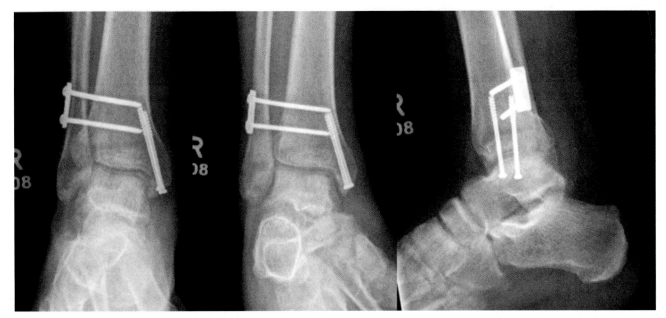

Figure 25-50 ▌ Case 2, 6 weeks after operative fixation. From left to right, AP, mortise, and lateral radiographs demonstrating hardware in appropriate position without loss of reduction.

Fixation Considerations in Osteoporotic Bone (Figs. 25-51 and 25-52)

- Augment fibular fixation with syndesmotic screws.
- Double plate the fibula.
- Consider locking implants.
- Use multiple syndesmotic screws through a plate.
- Use bicortical medial malleolar screws.
- Be gentle during clamp application. Do not comminute fragments.

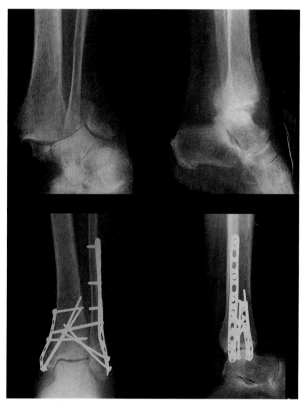

Figure 25-51 I In this osteoporotic ankle fracture-dislocation, both a medial plate and multiple transsyndesmotic screws were used to augment fixation.

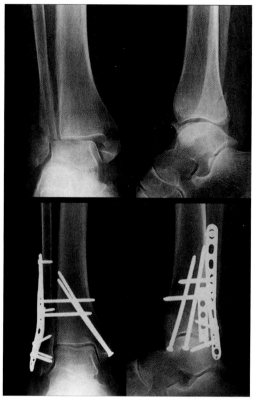

Figure 25-52 I Another osteoporotic ankle fracture stabilized using similar principles.

Chapter 26
Talus Fractures

DAVID P. BAREI
DAPHNE M. BEINGESSNER
MICHAEL L. BRENNAN
MATTHEW GARNER
MICHAEL F. GITHENS
SEAN E. NORK

Sterile Instruments/Equipment

- Tourniquet if desired
- Headlight
- Small pointed bone reduction clamps (Weber clamps)
- Dental picks and Freer elevators
- Schanz pins (2.5 to 4.0 mm)
- Universal distractor or external fixator (small)
- Micro-oscillating saw if medial malleolar osteotomy needed
  - 3.5- to 4.0-mm cancellous and cortical screws for osteotomy fixation
- Implants
  - Mini- and small-fragment screws and mini-fragment plates and screws (2.0/2.4/2.7/3.5 mm)
  - Autograft, cancellous allograft, or other bone substitute for structural defects
- K-wires and wire driver/drill

Positioning and Imaging

- Supine at the foot end of the radiolucent cantilever table.
- Small bump underneath the ipsilateral hip.
- Three views are used to assess talar fracture reductions: lateral of the talus/ankle, Canale view, and ankle mortise.
- Prone position for posterior talar body fractures when a posteromedial or posterolateral approach is planned.

Surgical Approaches

- Simultaneous medial and lateral approaches for talar neck fractures.[1]
  - Two approaches are needed invariably, as it is difficult to assess reduction on opposite side of the talus, if inferred from side approached by single incision.
- Anterolateral incision is in line with the fourth ray of the foot (Figs. 26-1 and 26-2).
  - Sharp dissection, full-thickness flaps.
  - Avoid superficial peroneal nerve in proximal incision.
  - Develop interval between long toe extensors and extensor brevis musculature.
    - Brevis musculature typically retracted plantar/lateral.
    - Avoid branches of dorsalis pedis artery, muscular branches to EHB and EDB, and lateral tarsal artery.

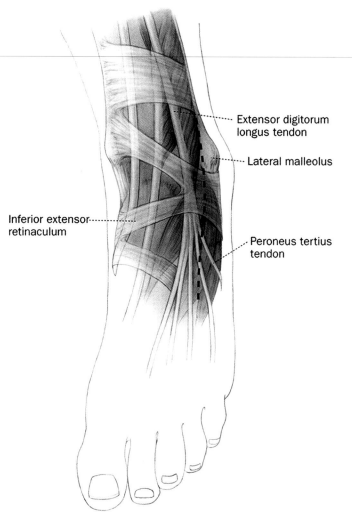

Figure 26-1 ▌ Incision for an anterolateral approach for a talus fracture. (From Vallier HA, Nork SE, Benirschke SK, et al. Surgical treatment of talar body fractures. *J Bone Joint Surg Am.* 2004;86(1_suppl_2): 180–192. Reprinted with permission.)

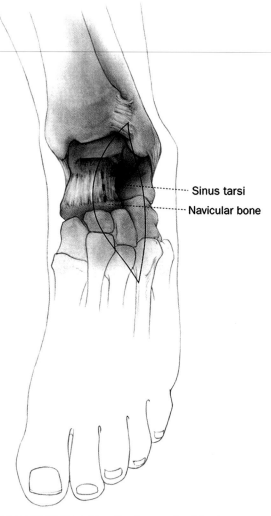

Figure 26-2 ▌ Deep dissection for an anterolateral approach to the talus. (From Vallier HA, Nork SE, Benirschke SK, et al. Surgical treatment of talar body fractures. *J Bone Joint Surg Am.* 2004;86(1_suppl_2): 180–192. Reprinted with permission.)

- Retract anterior compartment tendons medially.
- Reflect or excise sinus tarsi fat.
- Visualization should include the lateral dome of the talus, lateral process of the talus, lateral talar neck, lateral talar head, and the talofibular articulation.
- Dissection plantar to the lateral process of the talus allows access to the posterior facet of the subtalar joint, facilitating reduction and/or debridement of osseous and chondral debris.
  - Anteromedial approach is between anterior and posterior tibialis tendons (Figs. 26-3 and 26-4).
  - From anterior medial malleolus to navicular.
  - Deltoid protected.
  - Plantar dissection avoided.
  - Incise the talonavicular joint capsule, proximal to medial tarsal artery.
  - Expose the dorsomedial talar neck and medial body.
  - Visualization includes medial talar dome, medial talar neck, and talar head.
    - Retraction of capsule and dorsal soft tissues allows visualization of the anterior aspect of the talar dome to the lateral side.
    - Plan incision to allow medial malleolar osteotomy depending on the fracture pattern.

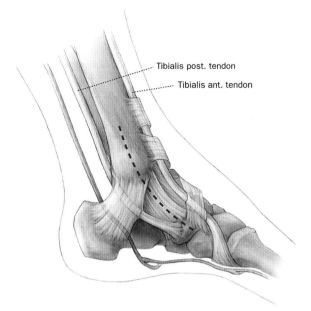

Figure 26-3 I Plane of an anteromedial incision. (From Vallier HA, Nork SE, Benirschke SK, et al. Surgical treatment of talar body fractures. *J Bone Joint Surg Am.* 2004;86(1_suppl_2):180–192. Reprinted with permission.)

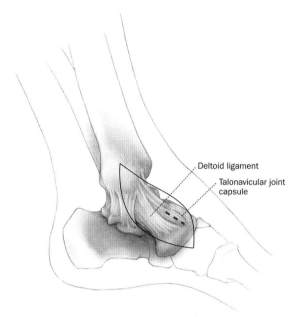

Figure 26-4 I Deep dissection for an anteromedial approach. (From Vallier HA, Nork SE, Benirschke SK, et al. Surgical treatment of talar body fractures. *J Bone Joint Surg Am.* 2004;86(1_suppl_2): 180–192. Reprinted with permission.)

Anterolateral and Anteromedial Approaches

Matthew Garner
Daphne Beingessner

Pathoanatomy

- **Vascular supply of the talus:**
  - Talar neck and body fractures often result in disruption of their arterial blood supply.
  - Care should be taken to minimize iatrogenic injury at the time of surgical intervention to limit the risk of nonunion and avascular necrosis.
  - The talar body and neck are supplied by three arterial branches:
    - Posterior tibial artery
      - Artery of the tarsal canal (dominant supply)
        - Supplies the majority of the talar body
      - Deltoid branch of posterior tibial artery
        - Often the only intact arterial blood supply in displaced fractures of the talar neck or body
        - Supplies medial talar body
    - Anterior tibial artery (dorsalis pedis)
      - Direct branches supply the talar head and neck.
    - Perforating peroneal artery
      - Artery of the tarsal sinus supplies talar head and neck.

Solution

Use vascular sparing surgical approaches and small universal distractors or external fixators to restore length and alignment prior to fixation of talar neck fractures.

Techniques

- Simultaneous medial and lateral approaches (Vallier HA, et al. *J Bone Joint Surg.* 2003;85A: 1716–1724).
  - Two approaches are invariably needed, as it is difficult to assess reduction on opposite side of the talus if inferred from side approached by single incision.

- Begin with anterolateral approach.
- Anterolateral approach
  - Incision is in line with the fourth ray of the foot (Fig. 26-1).
  - Sharp dissection, full-thickness flaps.
  - Avoid superficial peroneal nerve in proximal incision.
  - Develop interval between long toe extensors and extensor brevis musculature.
    - Brevis musculature typically retracted plantar/lateral.
    - Avoid branches of dorsalis pedis, muscular branches to EHB and EDB, and lateral tarsal artery.
  - Retract anterior compartment tendons medially.
  - Reflect or excise sinus tarsi fat.
  - Visualization should include the lateral dome of the talus, lateral process of the talus, lateral talar neck, lateral talar head, and the talofibular articulation.
  - Dissection plantar to the lateral process of the talus allows access to the posterior facet of the subtalar joint, facilitating debridement of osseous and chondral debris.
- Localizing medial incision:
  - Place Freer elevator through the anterolateral incision and across the fractured talar neck to the medial soft tissues (Fig. 26-5).
  - Mark medial incision just inferior to Freer elevator.

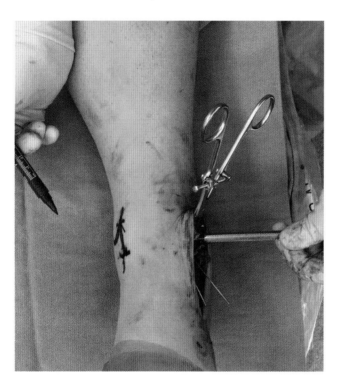

Figure 26-5 I Use of Freer elevator over anterior talar neck through anterolateral incision to localize the level of the medial incision.

- Anteromedial approach (Figs. 26-3 and 26-4):
  - Interval is between the anterior and posterior tibialis tendons.
  - Incision from anterior medial malleolus to navicular.
  - Deltoid is protected to preserve ligament and blood supply.
  - Plantar dissection is avoided.
  - Incise talonavicular joint capsule, proximal to medial tarsal artery.
  - Expose dorsomedial talar neck and medial body.
  - Visualization includes medial talar dome, medial talar neck, and talar head.
    - Retraction of capsule and dorsal soft tissues allows visualization of the anterior aspect of the talar dome to the lateral side.
  - Plan incision to allow medial malleolar osteotomy depending on fracture pattern.

- Posteromedial approach
  - Used to access posterior talar body fractures and posteromedial process fractures.
  - With application of a distractor, one can visualize the posterior one-half of the talar body.
    - This exposure can be improved further by performing a gastrocnemius recession.
  - Position prone, with the patient's feet at the end of a radiolucent cantilever table.
  - Elevate the operative extremity on a prone foam ramp or blanket ramp to facilitate lateral imaging.
  - Incision just medial to the Achilles tendon, without entering the paratenon (Fig. 26-6).
  - Achilles tendon is retracted laterally to expose the underlying FHL muscle belly (Fig. 26-7).
  - Elevate and retract the FHL along with all deep posterior compartment contents medially.
  - Incise capsule of ankle joint to expose posterior talus (Fig. 26-8).

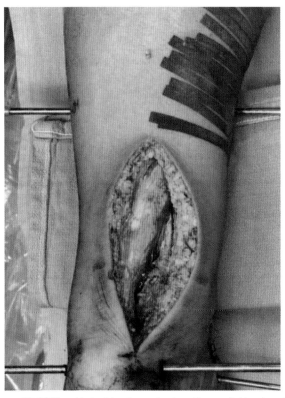

Figure 26-6 I The skin incision is made along the medial border of the Achilles tendon. The paratenon is not violated.

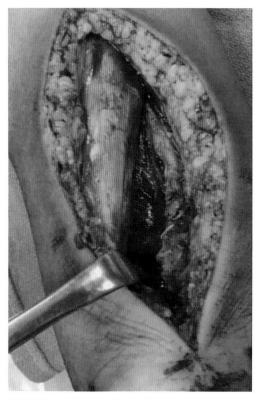

Figure 26-7 I The Achilles is retracted laterally to expose the underlying FHL muscle belly.

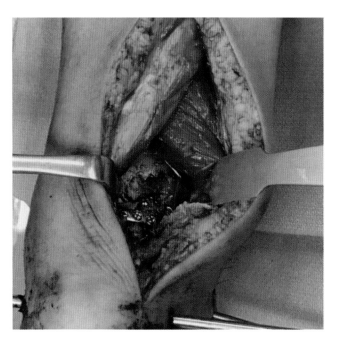

Figure 26-8 I The Achilles is retracted laterally, while the FHL and underlying deep posterior compartment structures are retracted medially to expose the tibiotalar and subtalar joint capsules.

- Use a K-wire through the incision in the posterior malleolus of the tibia to maintain retraction of FHL.
- Ankle dorsiflexion with distraction exposes a large portion of the talar body.
- The surgeon can view both the tibiotalar and subtalar joint from this approach.

Reduction and Fixation Tips

Extruded Talar Body Reduction

- Talar body is typically extruded posteromedially, adjacent to the neurovascular and tendinous structures contained within the tarsal tunnel.
- Very difficult to reduce in an awake patient, but an attempt is worthwhile in the ED with conscious sedation.
- Basic principles include the following:
  - Knee flexion to relax gastrocnemius musculature
  - Longitudinal traction applied to the calcaneus
  - Countertraction applied to the posterior aspect of the distal femur
  - Valgus angulation of the calcaneus
  - Direct pressure over the talar body toward the mortise

- When this does not work
  - A symmetrical external fixator can be created in an attempt to create adequate space to reduce the dislocated talar body.
  - Insert transcalcaneal Schanz pin.
  - Insert two bicortical tibial shaft Schanz pins (medial and lateral).
  - Construct biplanar frame connecting the lateral tibial pin to the lateral aspect of the transcalcaneal pin and medial tibial pin to the medial aspect of the transcalcaneal pin.
  - Medial and lateral open-ended compressor-distractor devices will create symmetric, controlled distraction between the calcaneus and the tibial plafond to accept the talar body.

- When this does not work
  - Ensure that the distraction provided by an external fixator is adequate.
  - Proceed with two exposures described (anterolateral and anteromedial).
  - Remove entrapped soft tissue, if present, that may impede relocation.
  - Perform direct manipulation of the body with a bone hook or placement of a Schanz pin into a nonarticular surface of the talar body.

- When this does not work
  - Medial malleolar osteotomy (rarely required)

Talar Neck

- Use cortical interdigitations for reduction; more commonly, this is on the lateral side or inferomedially, as impaction/comminution is typically dorsomedially.
- Some vertical neck fractures traverse the anterior chondral surface of the talar body.
  - Often the chondral interdigitations along this portion of the fracture provide an excellent assessment of reduction accuracy.
- Visually assess the quality of reduction, medially and laterally using both incisions.
  - Subtle rotational and angulatory malreductions can be appreciated from one side or the other.
- Radiographic correlation requires understanding of the normal talar relationships with the rest of the foot.
  - Talar axis on the AP view.
    - Common malreduction deformity is varus.
  - Talar axis on the lateral view.
    - Common malreduction deformity is extension, especially in high-energy fractures.
    - These high-energy injuries often require tricortical or cancellous bone graft to "strut" the area of impaction and comminution (dorsally) so as to restore the talar-first metatarsal angle.
    - The talar-first metatarsal angle should be nearly parallel on the AP and lateral radiographs.

- The anterior and middle facets are on the talar head fragment; the posterior facet is on the body fragment.
  - Check to ensure that these are congruent radiographically.
- A contiguous or noncontiguous lateral process fracture is often associated with a talar neck fracture.
  - Lateral process fractures should be reduced and fixed whenever possible.
  - Consider biasing the proximal portion of the anterolateral incision slightly more plantar if a neck fracture involves the lateral process. This will allow improved access to the lateral process without compromising access to the neck.
  - Reduce dental picks and provisionally hold with multiple small K-wires.
  - Definitive fixation with a 2.0-mm T-plate.
  - If the lateral process is multifragmentary, K-wires are cut, bent, and impacted as part of the definitive fixation.

- Managing circumferential comminution
  - Difficult problem.
  - Small external fixator from the distal medial tibia to the medial aspect of the navicular and from the fibula to the lateral aspect of the navicular will allow controlled restoration of talar neck length and angulation.
  - Radiographically reduce the anterior and middle facet (i.e., head fragment) and the posterior facet (i.e., body fragment) to the calcaneus.
  - If these joints are congruent, then the talar neck length is correct.

Provisional Fixation

- Multiple retrograde K-wires from both the anteromedial and anterolateral exposures.
  - Avoid placing wires in the fibula or across the tibiotalar/subtalar articulations.
- A femoral distractor with Schanz pins in the medial distal tibia and the cuneiforms can be used to aid in fracture visualization and reduction (Fig. 26-9).

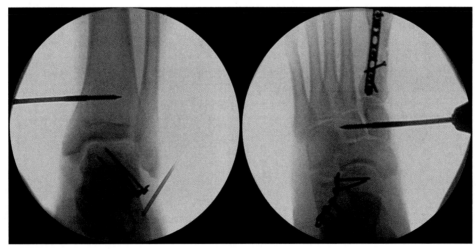

Figure 26-9 | A universal distractor placed from the tibia to the midfoot can restore talar neck length.

- A Weber clamp can be used to compress across the talar neck fracture.
  - The posterior tine of the clamp is placed posterior to the medial malleolus, avoiding neurological, vascular, and tendinous structures (Fig. 26-10).

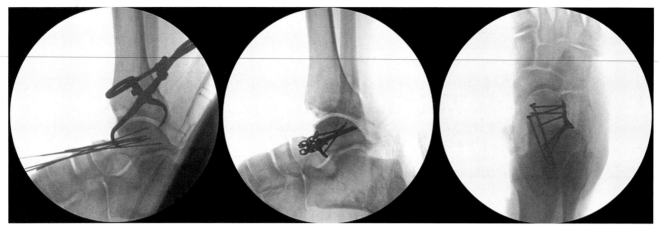

Figure 26-10 I A clamp may be placed across the talar neck to compress noncomminuted fracture lines.

- When access to the talar body is limited due to a proximal neck fracture (or one that extends into the anterior portion of the talotibial articulation), fracture reduction can be facilitated by stabilizing the talar body prior to addressing the fracture.
  - This can be performed by plantar flexing the foot so as to bring the fracture into view (avoid being obscured by anterior lip of the tibia).
  - The talus is held in this plantar-flexed position by placing one or two small Steinmann pins from the tibia or fibula into the talar body (avoid the weight-bearing articular surface).
  - Reduction of the midfoot onto the stabilized hindfoot is thereby facilitated as only one fracture fragment is freely mobile.
- A K-wire can be placed transversely across the talar head segment through both incisions to manipulate the distal talar neck fragment.
  - Avoid dorsal dissection over the talar neck to minimize vascular disruption (Fig. 26-11).

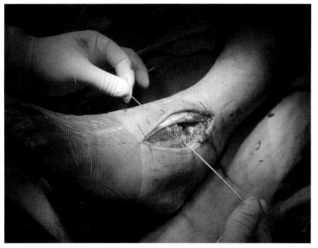
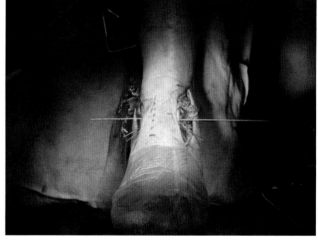

Figure 26-11 I A K-wire placed through the distal fragment is useful for multiplanar manipulation.

- Alternatively, use dental picks and elevators to reduce the fracture.

Definitive Implant Placement

- K-wires are mechanically weak, so screws are favored for definitive fixation.
- Despite posterior-to-anterior screws identified as more mechanically sound than anterior-to-posterior screws, small- and mini-fragment implants placed anteriorly are favored for comminuted fractures and are preferred currently.
  - 1.5-, 2.0-, 2.4-, 2.7-, and 3.5-mm screws.
  - Plates are 2.0- or 2.4-mm mini-fragment implants.
  - Many of these can be found on modular hand or modular foot sets.
  - Both straight plates and T-plates are useful.
  - Make sure to verify the maximum screw lengths in implant sets.

- After fracture reduction and provisional stabilization, definitive fixation usually begins on the lateral side, unless there is no medial comminution.
  - In fractures without comminution, an anatomic reduction, and good bone quality, screw fixation alone is satisfactory.
- Plating a talus is not intuitive, but is an excellent technique for fixation.
  - The lateral aspect of the talus is more amenable to plate application than the medial side.
  - Typically, a four- or five-hole 2.0-mm straight plate is contoured with approximately 50 to 70 degrees of bend (extension) to follow the extra-articular surface along the lateral talar neck, between the talar head and lateral process (Figs. 26-12–26-16).
  - Ensure this plate does not impinge on the fibular facet of the talus with foot eversion and abduction.

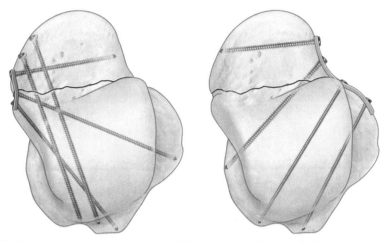

Figure 26-12 ▌ Typical implant placements for the medial talar column include longitudinal screws, countersunk in the talar head, and small plates (*left*). A small portion of the overhanging navicular tuberosity can be removed to facilitate implant placement without functional consequence. For the lateral column of the talus, plate fixation is used across the typically tension failure fracture line. The methods shown are used in multiple combinations depending on the fracture requirements.

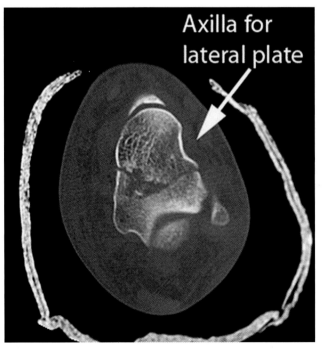

Figure 26-13 ▌ CT scan demonstrating the lateral talar plating surface. Note the lateral tension failure and the medial talar neck comminution.

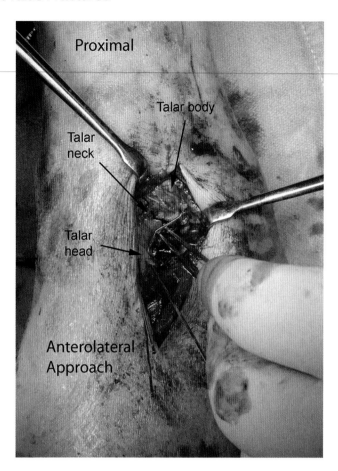

Proximal

Talar body

Talar
neck

Talar
head

Anterolateral
Approach

Figure 26-14 | Clinical example of a lateral plate application for a talar neck fracture.

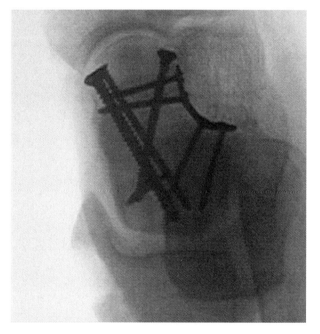

Figure 26-15 | Fluoroscopic example of typical implant position for a talar neck fracture.

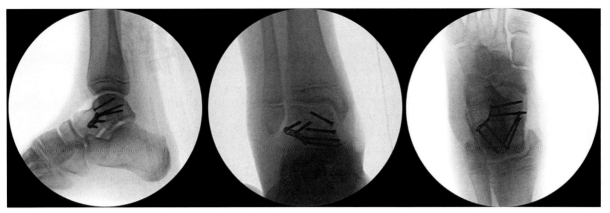

Figure 26-16 | Another example of a talar neck fracture stabilized with a lateral plate and medial column screws.

- When additional fixation through a plate is desired, a 2.0-mm T-plate can be used, with the horizontal portion of the "T" placed vertically along the anterior portion of the talar neck, just proximal to the talar head articular margin.
  - This allows additional fixation into the talar head through the plate (Fig. 26-17).

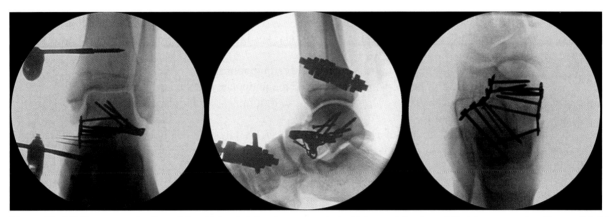

Figure 26-17 | Case example of medial and lateral plating for a comminuted talar neck fracture. A T-plate was used on the medial side for additional distal fixation.

- Medial-sided plating is more difficult, as there is very little space available between the chondral surfaces of the talar head and the anteromedial talar body.
  - Flatter surface.
  - Fully invert foot to determine proximal extent of plate placement without impinging on medial malleolus.
- Screws placed independently of the plate are typically 2.7 or 3.5 mm.
  - Commonly, these screws are used to neutralize the medial column of the talus and act as a fully threaded strut across the medial portion of talar neck, so as not to shorten the medial column (varus).
  - The foot is abducted at the talonavicular articulation uncovering the medial chondral surface of the talar head.
  - Screws are placed through the chondral surface with the screw heads countersunk.
    - For improved access to the medial talar head, a small portion of the overhanging navicular tuberosity may be removed.
  - Similar principles are applied when placing lateral longitudinal screws.
- Bone defects of the neck are managed with morselized bone graft or structural bone graft depending on the size of the defect and stability of the fracture reduction.

TIP Reduction and Fixation Tips

Daphne Beingessner
Matthew Garner

- Use cortical interdigitations for reduction; more commonly, this is on lateral side or inferomedially as dorsomedial impaction/comminution is common.
- Some vertical neck fractures traverse the anterior chondral surface of the talar body.
  - Often, the chondral interdigitations along this portion of the fracture provide an excellent assessment of reduction accuracy.
- Visually assess the quality of reduction, medially and laterally using both incisions.
  - Subtle rotational and angulatory malreductions can be appreciated from the one side or the other.
- Radiographic correlation requires understanding of the normal talar relationships with the rest of the foot.
  - Talar axis on the AP view
    - Common malreduction deformity is varus.
  - Talar axis on the lateral view
    - Common malreduction deformity is extension, especially in high-energy fractures.
    - These high-energy injuries often require tricortical or cancellous bone graft to "strut" the area of impaction and comminution (dorsally) so as to restore the talar-first metatarsal angle.
    - The talar-first metatarsal angle should be nearly parallel on the AP and lateral radiographs.
  - The anterior and middle facets are on the talar head fragment; the posterior facet is on the body fragment.
    - Check to ensure that these are congruent radiographically.
- A through and through K-wire can be placed to manipulate distal talar neck fragment.
  - Avoid dorsal dissection over the talar neck to minimize vascular disruption (see Fig. 26-11).
- Provisional fixation:
  - Length and alignment of comminuted talar neck fractures can be difficult to assess, and fracture reduction may be difficult to maintain while definitive fixation is placed.
  - Preoperative imaging of the contralateral, uninjured extremity, including three views of the foot and a talar neck view (Canale view), can be helpful in assessing restoration of neck length, alignment, and fixation.
  - Multiple retrograde K-wires from both the anteromedial and anterolateral exposures (Fig. 26-18).
    - Avoid placing wires in the fibula or across the tibiotalar/subtalar articulations.

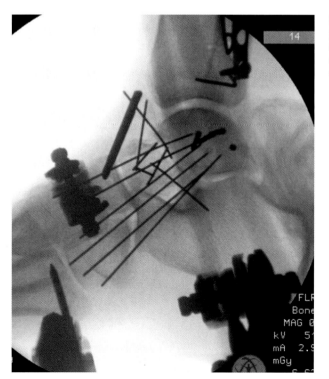

Figure 26-18 | Radiograph demonstrating provisional fixation with retrograde K-wires across the fracture. Image also demonstrates 4.0-mm Schanz pins placed into the cuneiforms laterally and the navicular medially.

- Managing comminution:
  - Distraction of a comminuted, impacted talus fracture using a small external fixator or small universal distractor can help restore length and alignment and can also hold reduction while provisional and/or definitive fixation is placed.
    - Schanz pins are placed in the medial distal tibia and fibular shaft. Midfoot pins can then be placed medially into the navicular or cuneiforms and laterally into the navicular or cuneiforms.
    - If an external fixator is already in place, bars can be connected to the existing medial and lateral external fixator pins or bars instead of placing new pins into the distal tibia or fibula.
    - External fixator bars or a universal distractor should be placed inferiorly to permit visualization through the surgical incisions (Fig. 26-19).

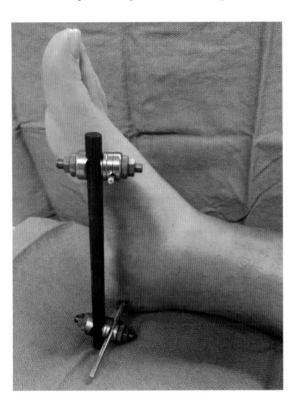

Figure 26-19 | Clamps and bars (or a small universal distractor) are placed inferior to permit distraction of the medial and lateral columns while permitting access to the planned surgical incisions. Distraction can be performed using a universal distractor or distraction clamps found in standard external fixator sets.

  - Distraction in line with the talar neck both medially and laterally can be adjusted to restore length and varus/valgus alignment (Fig. 26-20).

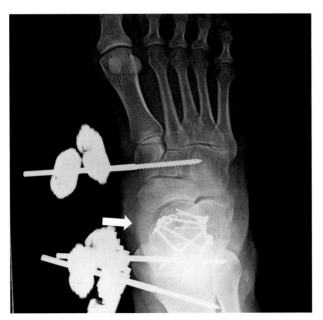

Figure 26-20 | Intraoperative alignment radiograph demonstrating medial distraction through an external fixator pins and a 2.0-mm T-plate bent into a fixed-angle device and placed medially (arrow). The bent portion of the T-plate functions as a strut preventing varus collapse of the talar head in the setting of severe, circumferential comminution.

- Radiographically reduce the anterior and middle facet (i.e., head fragment) to the calcaneus and the posterior facet (i.e., body fragment) to the calcaneus.
- If these joints are congruent, then the talar neck length is correct.
- Definitive implant placement:
  - K-wires are mechanically weak, so screws are favored.
  - Despite posterior-to-anterior screws identified as more mechanically sound than anterior-to-posterior screws, small and mini-fragment implants placed from anteriorly are favored for comminuted fractures and are currently preferred:
    - 1.5, 2.0, 2.4, 2.7, and 3.5 mm screws.
    - Plates are 2.0- or 2.4-mm mini-fragment implants.
    - Many of these can be found on modular hand or modular foot sets.
    - Both straight plates and T-plates are useful.
    - Make sure to verify the maximum screw lengths in implant sets.
    - Locking plates are useful in cases of comminution where fixed-angle constructs are preferable.
  - After fracture reduction and provisional stabilization, definitive fixation usually begins on the lateral side, unless there is no medial comminution.
    - In fractures without comminution, an anatomic reduction, and good bone quality, screw fixation alone is satisfactory.
- Preventing varus collapse:
  - Severe comminution of the medial and lateral talar neck can make fixation difficult.
  - Plating of the medial or lateral talar neck can often prevent varus collapse:
    - The lateral side of the talus is more amenable to plate application with more surface area available.
      - A 3- to 5-hole 2.0- or 2.4-mm plate can be used with a 50- to 70-degree bend permitting placement along the extra-articular surface of the talar neck between the talar head and lateral process.
    - Medial-sided plating is more difficult, as there is very little space available between the chondral surfaces of the talar head and the anteromedial talar body.
      - Medial plating can be accomplished with a 2.0-mm straight plate.
      - When additional fixation through a plate is desired, a 2.0-mm T-plate can be used, with the horizontal portion of the "T" placed vertically along the anterior portion of the talar neck, just proximal to the talar head articular margin.
      - In cases of severe comminution and loss of length, a 2.0-mm T-plate or straight plate can be contoured into a fixed-angle "blade plate" to provide medial support and prevent varus collapse of that talar head (Figs. 26-20 and 26-21).

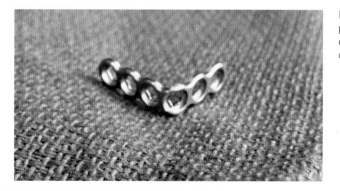

Figure 26-21 | A 2.0-mm locking straight plate bent into fixed-angle device and contoured for medial talus to prevent varus collapse.

Talar Head Fractures

- Most commonly, an articular shear pattern resulting from a talonavicular subluxation or dislocation (Fig. 26-22).

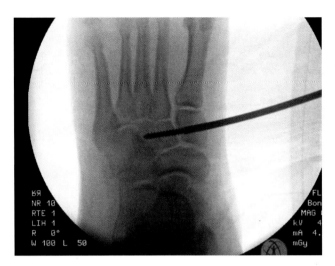

Figure 26-22 | A fluoroscopic image demonstrating a medial talar head fracture resulting from a shearing mechanism. A medial distractor is used to aid in visualization of the injury and facilitate reduction.

- More commonly seen in combination with a talar neck or body fracture than in isolation.
- Medial talar head shear fracture is more common than lateral.
- May be addressed through the anteromedial incision described above.
  - A medial distractor aids in fracture visualization (Fig. 26-22).
  - Additionally, a portion of the medial corner of the navicular may be removed with a rongeur for fracture reduction and implant placement.
- Reduction is preformed with dental picks and joystick K-wires (Fig. 26-23).

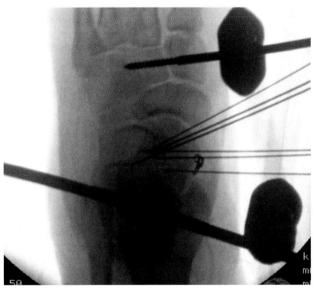

Figure 26-23 | The reduction is achieved with K-wires functioning as joysticks as well as dental picks and held with multiple small K-wires.

- Definitive fixation is achieved with buried 2.0-mm lag screws.
- If fracture morphology allows, a small buttress plate may be placed on the medial talus, just off the cartilaginous border of the medial talar head (Fig. 26-24).

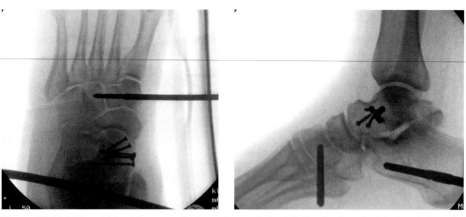

Figure 26-24 I AP and lateral fluoroscopic views demonstrate definitive fixation of a talar head shear fracture with buried lag screws and a small buttress plate.

Talar Body Fractures

- Goal: Restoration of articular surface of both the talar dome (tibiotalar articulation) and the posterior facet (subtalar articulation).
- CT scans are useful.
  - Use the CT scan to determine the best approach.
  - Study the location of the major fracture lines relative to the medial and lateral malleoli.
  - Determine if osteotomy of the medial or lateral malleolus would aid in visualization, reduction, and/or fixation.
- Three major approaches
  - Anteromedial—may be extended with medial malleolar osteotomy if needed.
  - Anterolateral—may be extended with lateral malleolar osteotomy if needed (rare).
  - Posteromedial—may be extended with medial malleolar osteotomy if needed.
- Visualization is improved with the use of a small femoral distractor or external fixator and headlamp illumination.
- Talar body fractures affect the talar portion of the subtalar articulation (posterior facet).
  - Posterior facet fragments are typically impacted into the cancellous surface of the talar body and impede reduction of larger peripheral fragments.
    - Identifying and reducing displaced and impacted posterior facet fragments is typically the initial focus, followed by reduction of the talar dome and peripheral fragments.
- Provisional fixation is performed with multiple K-wires.
- Definitive fixation is with multiple mini-fragment screws (1.5, 2.0, 2.4, 2.7 mm).
- Osteonecrosis and delayed union are increased.
  - With major joint fracture lines or crush injury
  - With associated dislocation

Posteromedial Talus Fractures

- Fracture reduction and posteromedial plate is placed through posteromedial approach for posterior talus fractures (Figs. 26-25 and 26-26).
  - Position prone.
  - Headlamp is very helpful; distractor is usually necessary.
    - Pin in medial distal tibia and medial posterior tuberosity of the calcaneus.

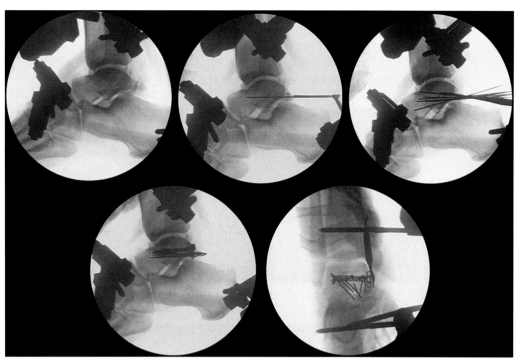

Figure 26-25 ❚ Case example of posteromedial talar fracture plate placement.

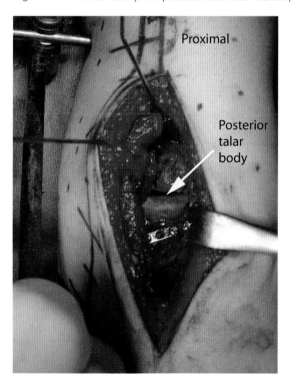

Proximal

Posterior
talar
body

Figure 26-26 ❚ Clinical view of posterior talar body following operative fixation. The K-wires retract the FHL.

- The primary working interval is between the Achilles (retracted laterally) and the entire deep posterior compartment (retracted medially).
  - Occasionally, additional intervals will need to be exploited to access more medial fracture fragments. Most commonly, this involves working between FHL and the neurovascular bundle.
- The subtalar joint is first assessed for articular impaction.
  - This is disimpacted with a Freer elevator or narrow osteotome and provisionally held with K-wires.
- Next, comminuted intercalary fragments are reassembled and held with wires. This may require creating a "working window" between major fracture fragments.
- Lastly, large fracture fragments are reduced and held with wires.
- Definitive fixation of individual fragments may be achieved by independent buried 2.0- or 2.4-mm lag screws, depending on fracture morphology.

- Summative fixation is achieved with a 2.0-mm straight or T-plate placed horizontally along the posterior talar body, along the vermillion border below the talar dome cartilage (Figs. 26-27 and 26-28).
    - Multiple 2.0- or 2.4-mm lag or position screws are placed through the plate and into the talar body, taking care not to place them in the subtalar joint.

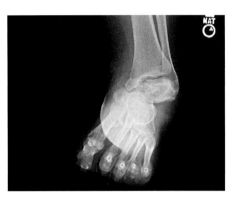
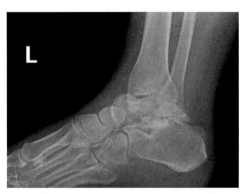

Figure 26-27 I Injury films demonstrating a medial subtalar dislocation with associated posterior talar body fracture.

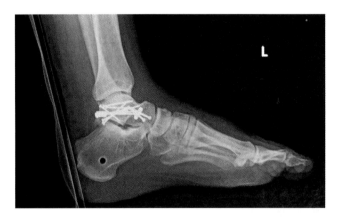

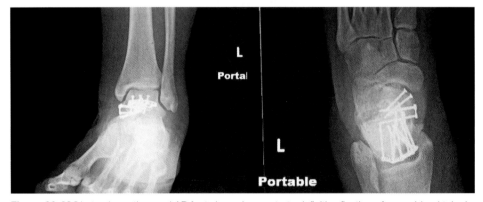

Figure 26-28 I Lateral, mortise, and AP foot views demonstrate definitive fixation of a combined talar head shear and posterior body talus fracture.

Lateral Process Fracture

- Transverse incision beginning at the distal tip of the fibula and extending anteriorly 2 to 3 cm, parallel to plantar border of the foot (Fig. 26-29).

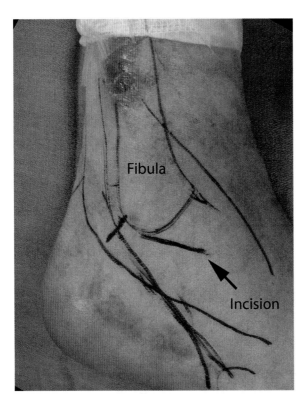

Figure 26-29 | Incision marked for exposure of the lateral talar process.

- Direct reduction.
- Often a contoured 4-hole 2.0-mm plate is of appropriate size.
  - Cut outer two holes to form each end into a hook, leaving central two holes for 2.4-mm screws (Fig. 26-30).

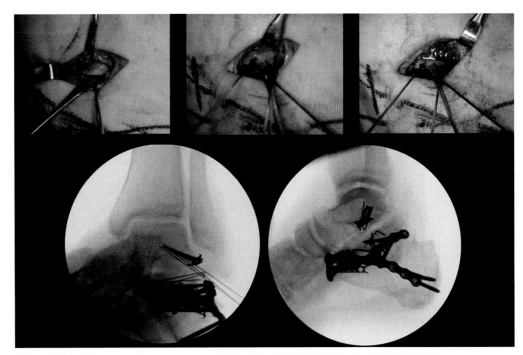

Figure 26-30 | Clinical and fluoroscopic examples of lateral talar process reduction and fixation.

Posterolateral Talus Fracture

- Distractor from the fibula to calcaneus
  - Drill the fibula with a 2.5-mm drill.
  - Place a 4-mm short-threaded Schanz half pin into the fibula.
  - Place a similar Schanz pin in the calcaneal tuberosity from lateral to medial.
  - Dorsiflex the ankle.
  - An 8-mm bar with two clamps provides distraction.
  - A distractor is then applied to provide distraction of the lateral column of the ankle (Fig. 26-31).

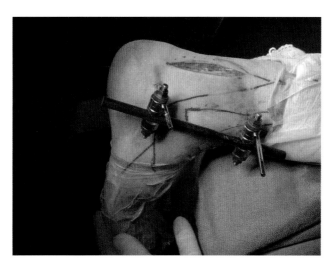

Figure 26-31 | An external fixator used as a distractor between the fibula and calcaneus.

- Posterolateral approach
  - A posterolateral approach is made to the ankle directly lateral to the Achilles tendon, with care being taken to stay outside the Achilles tendon sheath.
  - Dissection is medial to the sural nerve.
  - Use a Doppler probe to ensure incision is medial to the peroneal artery (Fig. 26-32).

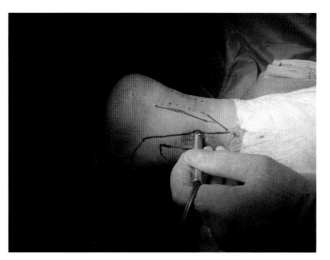

Figure 26-32 | A vascular probe ensures that the posterolateral incision does not endanger the peroneal artery.

- Dissect to the level of the capsule.
- The capsule is incised, providing direct access to the subtalar joint as well as to the tibiotalar joint (Fig. 26-33).

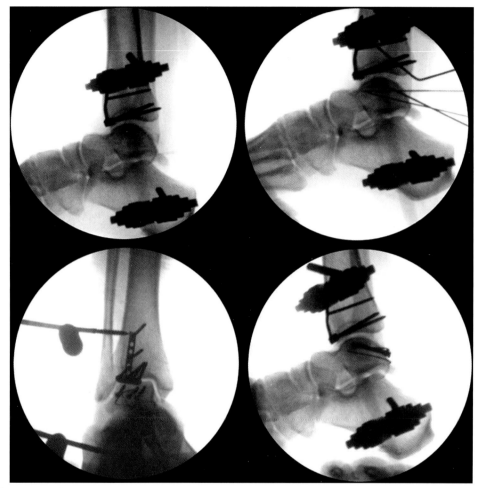

Figure 26-33 | Case example of posterolateral talar fixation for a talar body fracture.

Reference

1. Vallier HA, Nork SE, Benirschke SK, et al. Surgical treatment of talar body fractures. *J Bone Joint Surg Am.* 2003;85-A:1716–1724.

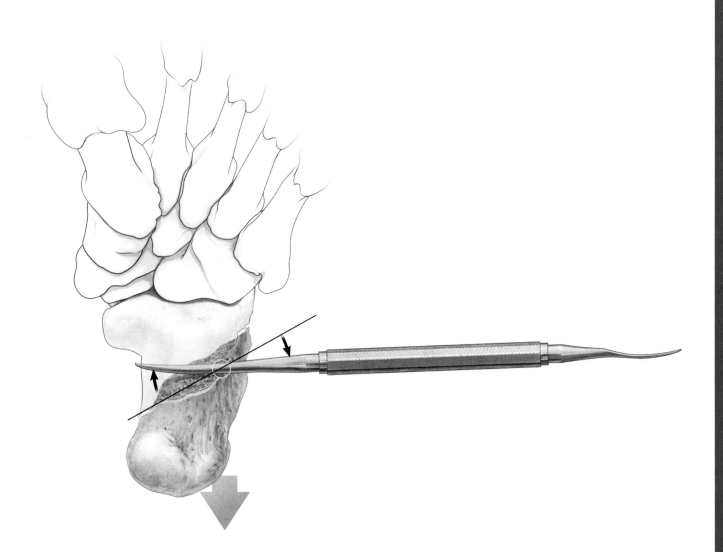

Chapter 27
Calcaneus Fractures

MICHAEL L. BRENNAN

PETER A. COLE

ANTHONY J. DUGARTE

DANIEL N. SEGINA

BRAD YOO

Sterile Instruments/Equipment

- Tourniquet
- Headlight
- Large pointed bone reduction clamps (Weber clamps)
- Laminar spreader
- Dental picks and Freer elevators
- Shoulder hook
- Schanz pins (2.5 to 4.0 mm)
- Femoral distractor (small)
- Implants
  - Mini- and small-fragment screws and minifragment plates (2.0/2.4/2.7/3.5 mm)
  - Calcaneal plates, locking or nonlocking
  - Autograft, cancellous allograft, or other bone substitute for structural defects
- K-wires and wire driver/drill

Positioning

- The patient is positioned in the lateral decubitus position.
  - Take care to pad all bony prominences, including down greater trochanter, fibular head (peroneal nerve), and elbow (radial nerve).
- See Chapter 1 for full description.

Surgical Approach

- Extensile lateral approach, as described by Benirschke and Sangeorzan.[1]
- Vertical limb should be approximately 1 cm anterior to the Achilles tendon.
  - The vessel that supplies the flap can be located with a Doppler.
  - Proximal extension of the vertical limb should be performed without injuring this vessel.

■ Take caution not to injure the lateral calcaneal artery, which is directly across the vertical limb and supplies the majority of the flap (Fig. 27-1).

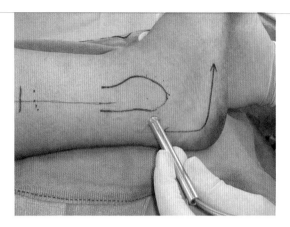

Figure 27-1 I Doppler showing the position of the arterial inflow to the lateral heel flap.

● To determine the course of the sural nerve, mark a point one thumb breadth posterior to the distal tip of the fibula, and connect it to the base of the fifth metatarsal (Fig. 27-2).

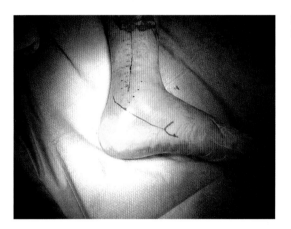

Figure 27-2 I The approximate course of the sural nerve based on the fibula and the fifth metatarsal.

● Gently curve incision, and make horizontal limb along the glabrous border of the heel (Fig. 27-3).

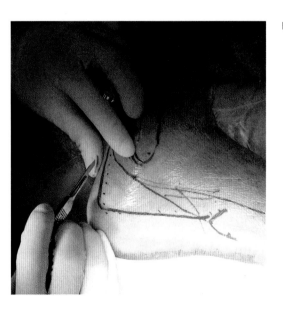

Figure 27-3 I The lateral extensile incision.

- Meticulous subperiosteal elevation of soft tissues off of the lateral wall.
  - Place small rakes under periosteum, and avoid separating soft tissue layers.
  - Elevate the calcaneofibular ligament.
  - Dissect beneath the osseous reflection of the peroneal sheath, and elevate the peroneal tendons anterosuperiorly.
  - 0.062-inch K-wires can be inserted into the fibula and talus, and bent for soft tissue retraction.
    - Be mindful of point pressure on soft tissues.
- Alternatively, and depending on fracture pattern and acuity, a percutaneous approach or sinus tarsi approach may be used.

Reduction and Fixation Techniques

- Spanning calcaneus external fixation (Figs. 27-4 and 27-5).
- Used to restore calcaneal morphology early, particularly for joint depression and broken tongue–type patterns with significant shortening, height loss, varus, and lateral translation.
  - Place the frame medially to preserve lateral soft tissues for lateral exposure after soft tissues heal.
  - A medial incision is made over the medial cuneiform.
  - A 170- × 5.0-mm Schanz half pin is placed from the medial to the middle of the lateral cuneiform.
  - A second 170- × 5.0-mm Schanz half pin is placed via the percutaneous incision through the medial tibia to provide a point of fixation on the tibia.
  - External fixation clamps are then applied, and a bar is placed from the cuneiform pin to the tibial pin.
  - A third 5.0-mm Schanz pin is placed in the calcaneal tuberosity via a medial incision.
    - This pin is placed bicortically but NOT transcutaneous on the lateral side.
  - Distraction is then applied via a pin-bar clamp to the already established bar apparatus from the medial cuneiform to the tibia, forming a "T."
  - A distraction vector of height, length, and translation is facilitated to disimpact the fracture.
    - This facilitates the restoration of anatomic height and length at the time of definitive reconstruction.
  - Additional distraction vectors can be applied as needed through additional bars.
  - A laminar spreader between two pin-bar clamps or a pin-bar clamp and a universal chuck can be used to medialize the tuberosity fragment.
  - After the distraction has been achieved, lateral, axial, and AP views of the foot document the position of the pins and distraction that is achieved.

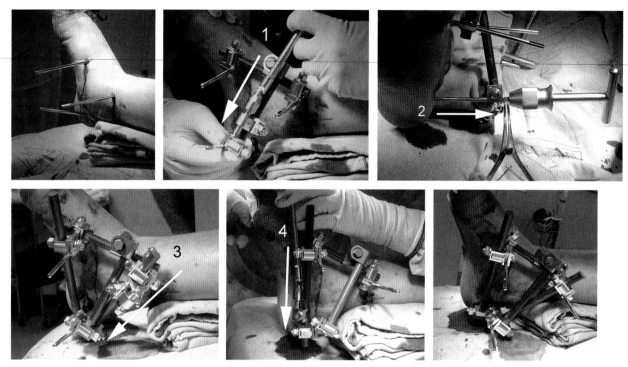

Figure 27-4 ❚ Calcaneal external fixation placement. Half pins are placed medially in the cuneiforms, the calcaneal tuberosity, and the distal tibia. Length is reestablished initially (*1*), followed by reduction of the tuberosity varus and translation (*2*). Height and length are once again fine-tuned (*3*, *4*).

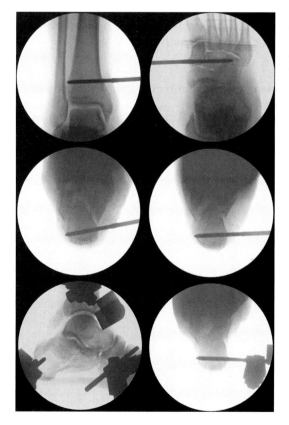

Figure 27-5 ❚ After placement of Schanz pins in the distal tibia, cuneiforms, and calcaneal tuberosity (**top row**), the calcaneal height, length, varus, and translation are progressively reduced (**second and third rows**).

Calcaneal External Fixation

Peter A. Cole
Anthony J. Dugarte

Pathoanatomy

Fractures involving the calcaneus occur in the context of a vulnerable soft tissue envelope. Soft tissue complications with ORIF of calcaneus fractures are frequent historically.

Solution

Similar to other lower extremity fractures in which treatment is often staged (e.g., unstable tibial plateau and tibial pilon fractures), calcaneus fractures may be also managed with a temporizing external fixator.

Technique

A medially based, 3-pin ExFix for calcaneus fractures can be used to improve calcaneal position with regard to length, height, and alignment in order to maintain optimal tension on the soft tissue envelope, to promote edema resolution, and to facilitate future surgery with the intention to mitigate soft tissue complications.

Rationale for temporizing calcaneal external fixation (ExFix)

- Placement of an ExFix is low risk.
  - Theoretically, there should be no more risk for pin site wounds in the context of calcaneus fractures as there would be for pilon fractures where the practice is acceptable and often the standard of care.
- Provisional external fixation and staged management of lower extremity articular fracture are principled surgeries.
- Restoration of skin tension and heel cord length obviates future problems.
  - If left untreated, even in a delayed fashion, morbidity in the treatment of calcaneal fractures is compounded.
- Improving the position of the tuberosity with an ExFix provides for a definitive care management plan if the patient is deemed a poor surgical candidate.
  - For example, if the patient has comorbidities or is noncompliant, placing the tuberosity in a proper position for healing restores heel dimension and contour, allowing for future fitting of footwear.
- Tongue-type and joint depression–type calcaneus fractures may require different configurations, which need to be implemented into the pin montage.
- Geriatric patients with osteoporosis may warrant hydroxyapatite-coated pins to improve durability of fixation.

Indications

- Displaced calcaneus fractures, open or closed

Contraindications

- Incompletely ossified calcaneus in skeletally immature patients
- Patients with chronic foot ulcers and peripheral vascular disease
  - May predispose patients to deep pin tract infection and osteomyelitis
- Nondisplaced fractures

Preoperative Planning

- Imaging.
  - Lateral calcaneus and Harris axial views obtained for injured and noninjured side (Fig. 27-6)

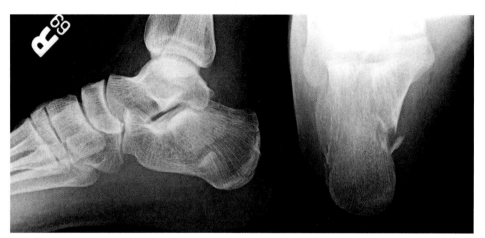

Figure 27-6 ‖ Lateral (**left**) and Harris axial (**right**) views demonstrating two comminuted, minimally displaced fractures involving the middle and posterior thirds of the calcaneus. Both fractures likely enter the posterior facet of the talocalcaneal joint and the middle facet of the talocalcaneal joint.

- The length of the calcaneus by virtue of the anterior process or cuboid involvement should be assessed in addition to the height as determined by the Böhler angle (Fig. 27-7).

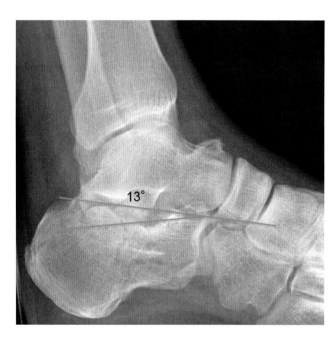

Figure 27-7 ‖ Lateral x-ray demonstrating a Böhler angle of 13 degrees.

- Additionally, on the axial view, varus alignment should be appreciated.

- This step may be done by x-ray analysis, though a computed tomography (CT) scan evaluation of two-dimensional reconstructions, in particular semicoronal and sagittal views, is also useful (Fig. 27-8).

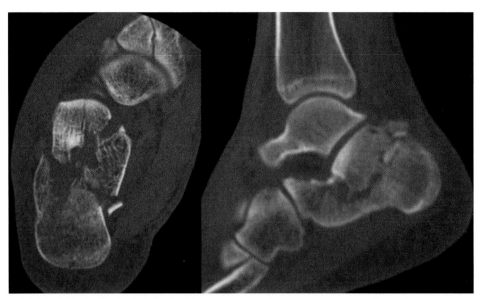

Figure 27-8 | Semicoronal (**left**) and sagittal (**right**) computed tomography displaying a comminuted, mildly displaced intra-articular four-part right calcaneal fracture that involves the posterior and anterior facets of the talocalcaneal and calcaneocuboidal joints.

Patient Positioning

- Because the pin frame is a medial ExFix, the patient should be supine.
- C-arm should be positioned ipsilateral to the injured limb.
  - In this fashion, Harris axial and lateral views can be obtained intraoperatively to assess reduction.

Approach

- First pin should be used in the distal tibia, in the supramalleolar region.
  - This position should avoid impaling the saphenous neurovasculature.
- Second pin should be placed through a 1-cm incision through medial calcaneus, approximately 1 cm from posterior edge of heel and 1 cm proximal to subglabrous skin.
  - The calcaneal pin should be oriented perpendicular to the mechanical axis of the tuber, which is frequently in varus.
- The third pin should be at the base of the first metatarsal (Fig. 27-9).

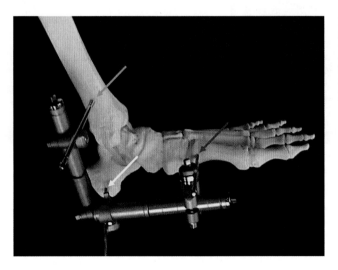

Figure 27-9 | The medial profile view of a model of a medial multiplanar external fixator for a calcaneus fracture demonstrating pin placement in the distal tibia (*blue arrow*), posteromedial calcaneus (*yellow arrow*), and base of the first metatarsal (*red arrow*) or in the medial and middle cuneiform

- Generally, 5-mm Schanz pins are used in the calcaneus and tibia, and a 4-mm pin is used in the base of the first metatarsal.
- All three pins should be bicortical, but should not penetrate the opposite lateral skin.
- Hydroxyapatite-coated pins are used in osteoporotic patients.

Pearls

- First, achieve restoration of length by distracting between the first metatarsal and calcaneus pin.
  - This reorients the calcaneal tuberosity from initial varus to neutral.
- After length is restored, tuberosity height and Achilles length are restored by distracting between the tibia and calcaneus pins.
- Beware of overdistraction.
  - Avoid distraction across foot compartments or neurovascular structures as this may result in tibial nerve dysfunction.
  - Some small ExFix frames are designed to employ distraction once they are placed on the patients and can be useful in patients presenting late.
- Every attempt should be made to perform calcaneus ExFix within 3 days of injury.
  - If presentation is delayed 5 to 7 days after injury, provisional external fixation should be reconsidered.
- The joint depression injury drives the posterior facet into the tuberosity and prevents the Böhler angle from being completely restored.
  - Therefore, this angle is unlikely to normalize prior to ORIF.
- If the patient has tongue-type fracture, place a 5-mm Schanz into the tongue fragment and drive just distal to the subchondral bone so a reduction maneuver may be employed before the pin is attached to the frame
  - Understanding the pathoanatomy of tongue-type lesions is critical. The tongue fragment must be incorporated into the frame to avoid soft tissue complications at the posterior heel/Achilles insertion.
  - The frame can be left in place temporarily until soft tissue swelling resolves sufficiently to permit ORIF or can be left as definitive treatment for no <6 to 8 weeks (Fig. 27-10).

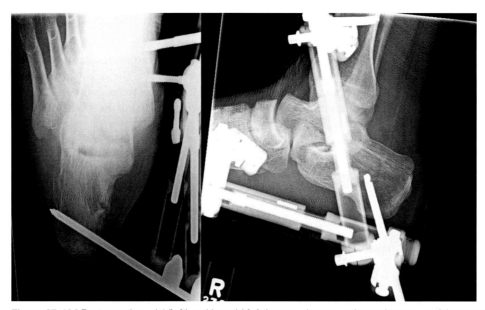

Figure 27-10 ▌ Postoperative axial (**left**) and lateral (**right**) x-rays demonstrating maintenance of the anatomical position of the calcaneus, in terms of height, length, and neutral alignment.

- A "kickstand" may be added to the frame based on patient desire in order to assist in limb elevation and to keep pressure off of the heel and foot (Fig. 27-11).

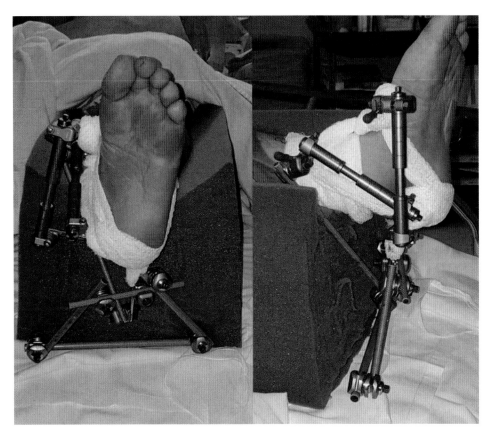

Figure 27-11 | Example of the optional kickstand configuration, which elevates the foot and ensures pressure is kept off of the calcaneus.

Postoperative Management

- Wound care
  - Pin tract care should proceed aggressively to avoid pin tract infections.
  - Skin tenting should be relieved at the pin-skin interface.
  - Showering is permitted with soap and water with ExFix in place.
  - Elevation should be mandated in the preoperative setting, prior to ORIF.

- Rehabilitation
  - Active and passive ROM with toe stretching in extension should be instituted as soon as the patient can tolerate and is mandatory to prevent claw toe formation.
  - Continue skin and soft tissue management until swelling resolution to allow for ORIF or minimally invasive fixation measures.
  - 6 to 8 weeks for closed ExFix management, followed by a period of progressive weight bearing as tolerated (WBAT).

Tongue-Type Fractures

- High vigilance must be maintained for threatened posterior soft tissues.[2]
- Tongue variant with impaction.
  - Via a small incision posteriorly, a Schanz pin is placed into the tuberosity to provide a manipulative reduction of the tuberosity and to disimpact the articular segment from the critical angle of Gissane (Fig. 27-12).

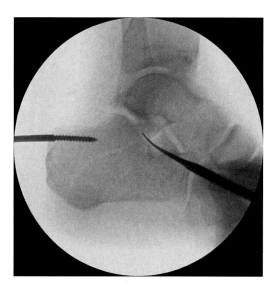

Figure 27-12 I For reduction of tongue-type fractures, a Schanz pin can be placed in the displaced tuberosity fragment and used as a joystick. When the fracture involves the posterior facet, a small incision allows for direct palpation with an elevator to ensure articular congruity.

- A sinus tarsi approach is made just distal to the tip of the fibula to assess the articular reduction.
  - The reduction is then provisionally stabilized with a series of percutaneously placed 0.062-inch wires (Fig. 27-13).

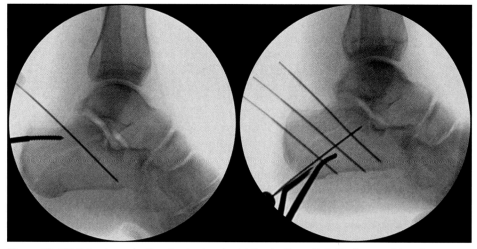

Figure 27-13 I Following reduction, the fracture is stabilized with multiple K-wires provisionally.

- The most anterior K-wire is just anterior to the Achilles insertion, and the remaining K-wires are placed posterior to the first one.
  - If necessary, a small incision is made medially, and additional manipulation of the tuberosity can be performed using a large pointed clamp or a shoulder hook.

- Axial K-wires are then placed from posterolateral to anteromedial into the sustentaculum (Fig. 27-14).

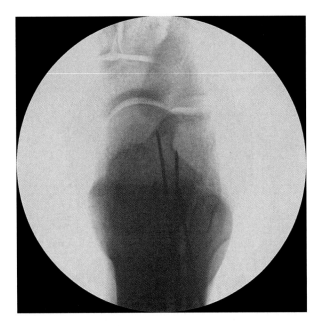

Figure 27-14 ∥ An AP view of the foot demonstrates wire and subsequent screw placement into the sustentaculum, which provides good bone for implant anchorage.

- After all K-wires are placed, using lateral and Harris axial views to confirm reduction and K-wire position, a 3.5-mm cannulated screw is placed over the middle wire in a lag fashion.
    - This provides compression and is tightened down to anchor through the plantar cortex.
    - The remaining superior to inferior screws are then placed over the K-wires.
    - Axial cannulated screws are then placed through a small incision over the two axial K-wires (Fig. 27-15).

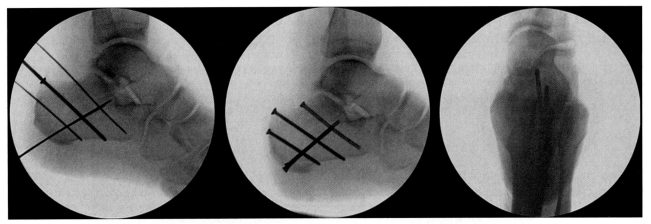

Figure 27-15 ∥ Multiple cannulated or noncannulated screws are then placed for definitive fixation.

- A small plate may be utilized as a washer to prevent perforating the cortex with the screwhead.
- Tongue-type fracture (alternative technique No. 1)
    - Use an elevator through a segment of the extensile incision to disimpact the posterior facet.
    - Use 2.5-mm Schanz pin posteriorly in tuberosity to assist in reduction.
    - When reduced, place lateral to medial lag screws across the posterior facet and longitudinal screws to stabilize the tongue fragment (Fig. 27-16).

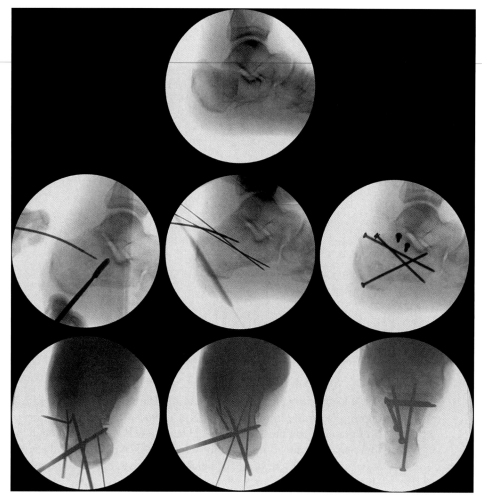

Figure 27-16 ▌ Depending on the fracture pattern, an elevator can be used to elevate the posterior facet fragment.

- Tongue-type fracture (alternative technique No. 2)
  - Percutaneous clamp across the fracture line.
  - Make incision at the edge of the glabrous skin laterally in line with the extensile incision.
  - Slide clamp deep to the heel pad and clamp inferior cortex of tuberosity (Fig. 27-17).

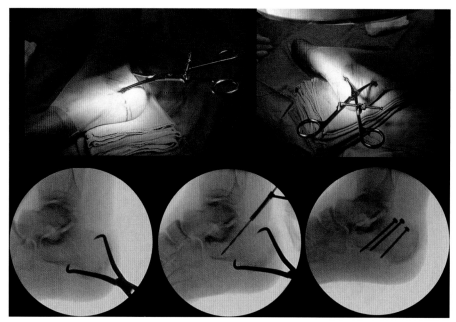

Figure 27-17 ▌ A large pointed reduction clamp can also be very effective for fracture reduction.

- Tuberosity avulsion fracture
  - Skin is particularly at risk with this injury.
  - Reduce emergently, and closely monitor the skin.
  - Directly clamp through stab incisions, followed by K-wires and lag screws (Fig. 27-18).

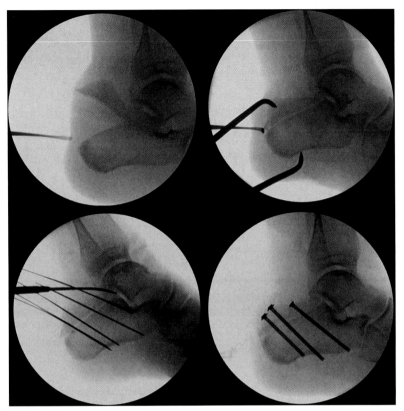

Figure 27-18 I Widely displaced tuberosity fractures can place the posterior soft tissues at risk of necrosis, and emergent treatment should be considered.

- Medial process fracture
  - Anchors a large portion of the plantar fascia and facilitates a competent windlass mechanism.
  - Displaced medial process fracture (> approximately 1 cm) can result in a painful heel and altered gait mechanics, if not reduced and stabilized.
    - Heel pad is displaced medially.
  - Following reduction using an oblique incision, taking care to protect the medial plantar nerve, a cervical H-plate is ideally suited for stabilization (Fig. 27-19).

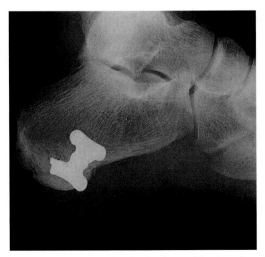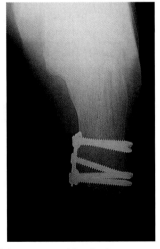

Figure 27-19 I Example of reduction and fixation of medial process avulsion fracture.

- Joint depression fractures
  - Many fractures have very predictable and consistent fracture line configurations.
    - It is important to learn the three-dimensional fracture pattern and fragment positions and to preoperatively plan reduction sequence and techniques and implant placements (Fig. 27-20A).

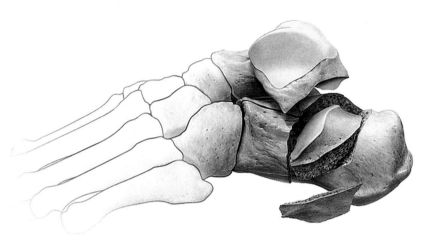

A

Figure 27-20A I Lateral view of a typical joint depression calcaneal fracture pattern. The primary fracture line runs from the angle of Gissane posteromedially and separates the sustentaculum from the remainder of the calcaneus. The posterior facet fragment is depressed, and the lateral wall displaces laterally. In this example, there is a sagittal plane secondary fracture line in the anterior process.

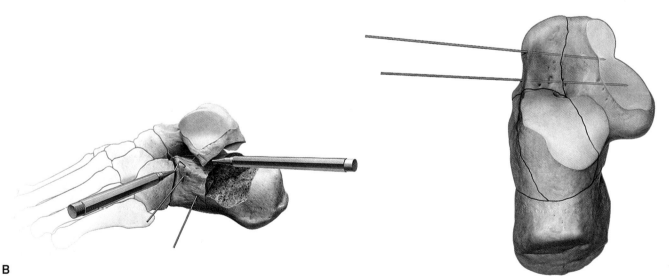

B

Figure 27-20B I Reductions typically proceed from anteromedial in a posterior and lateral direction. Dental picks and other reduction instruments are used to reduce the anterior process fracture lines under direct vision, and K-wires are placed provisionally from lateral to medial. The position of these wires is also demonstrated from a superior vantage point.

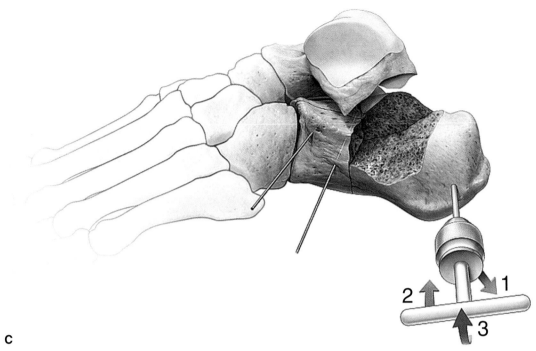

C

Figure 27-20C | Next, the posterior facet is disimpacted or can be completely removed and placed on the sterile back table. A Schanz pin is inserted in the posteroinferior corner of the incision from lateral to medial. This is used to manipulate the tuberosity out of its typical deformity. The usual tuberosity reduction maneuvers include (1) posteroinferior translation (to restore height and length); (2) medial translation (to reduce lateral displacement); and (3) valgus rotation (to reduce varus deformity).

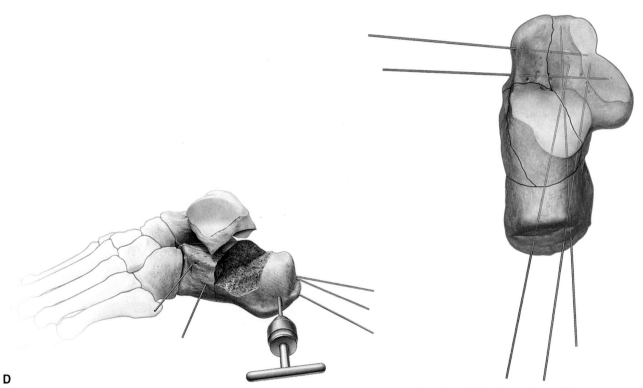

D

Figure 27-20D | With the tuberosity reduced, axial K-wires are placed percutaneously from the tuberosity into the anteromedial sustentaculum fragment.

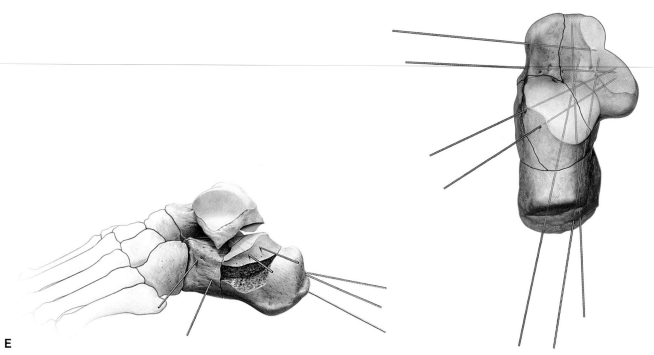

E

Figure 27-20E I With the anterior process and the tuberosity reduced, a defect should remain that allows for anatomic reduction of the posterior facet fragment. The anterior aspect of the posterior facet at the angle of Gissane often provides a critical reduction assessment. Additionally, the posterior aspect of the articular fragment should be assessed at the junction with the tuberosity fragment. K-wires are then placed from the posterior facet into the sustentaculum.

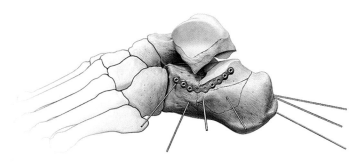

F

Figure 27-20F I The lateral wall is then replaced. A small curved plate positioned along the angle of Gissane allows for lag screws in the posterior facet and the anterior process fractures.

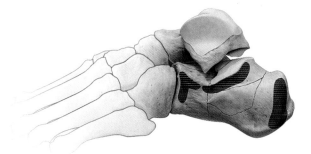

G

Figure 27-20G I Several anatomic regions of the calcaneus offer strong bone for optimal implant anchorage. These include the anterior process, the angle of Gissane, the subchondral bone of the posterior facet, and the posterior aspect of the tuberosity.

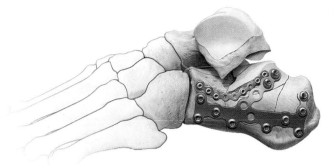

Figure 27-20H ▮ Finally, a calcaneal plate of appropriate size is placed with strategic screw placement to complete fixation.

H

- Reduction of the tuberosity is critical in restoring the overall morphology of the calcaneus and the spatial relationship of the facets to each other.
  - It is particularly important to focus on reduction in the region of the critical angle of Gissane and the anterior process.
  - When addressing this, ensure visualization is possible medially at the level of the middle facet.
  - It is possible to work anterior to the interosseous talocalcaneal ligament without destabilizing it.
- Because the posterior facet is relatively long in its anterior to posterior dimension, make sure the posterior surface is evaluated from a posterior-superior vantage point through the vertical limb of the incision.
- Place a 4.0-mm Schanz pin laterally, and use a 4.5-mm drill guide for manipulation (Fig. 27-21).
  - This avoids the hand getting in the way of visualization.

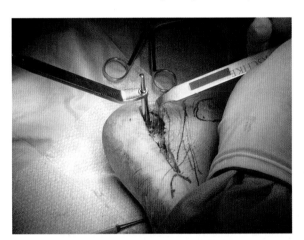

Figure 27-21 ▮ Use a drill guide or Schanz pin holder for efficient manipulation of the Schanz pin in the tuberosity.

- A laminar spreader can be helpful to reestablish the tuberosity length and height (Fig. 27-22).

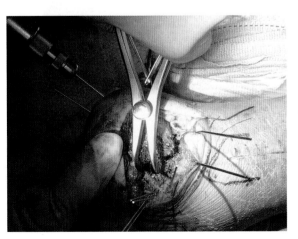

Figure 27-22 ▮ A laminar spreader can be used to disimpact the posterior facet from the tuberosity.

- Aim K-wires and nonlocking screws from the lateral wall with a slight anterior vector to obtain purchase in the strong sustentacular bone medially (Fig. 27-23).

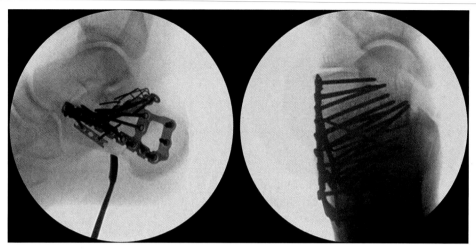

Figure 27-23 ▌K-wires and screws are preferentially anchored in the strong bone of the sustentaculum.

- Screw positions and lengths can be verified on the AP view of the foot.
- Fracture comminution and impaction between the posterior facet and posterior tuberosity often leave a large cancellous void between these anatomic landmarks.
  - A tricortical iliac crest auto-/allograft can be used to occupy this void area and aid in structural support of the posterior facet (Fig. 27-24).

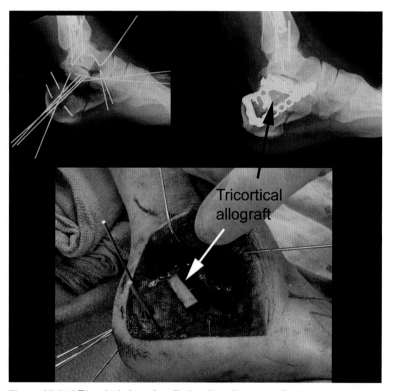

Figure 27-24 ▌Tricortical allograft or fibular allograft can be effective in providing mechanical support for the elevated articular segment.

Technique to Assist in Calcaneal Tuberosity Reduction

Brad Yoo

Pathoanatomy

- The primary fracture line creates discontinuity between the calcaneal tuberosity and the distal anterior process segment (Fig. 27-25A–C).
- The asymmetric tension from the posterior tibialis and gastrocsoleus complex, along with the axial injury mechanism, results in a displaced tuberosity. The displacement is one of varus alignment, cranial displacement, and axial length shortening.

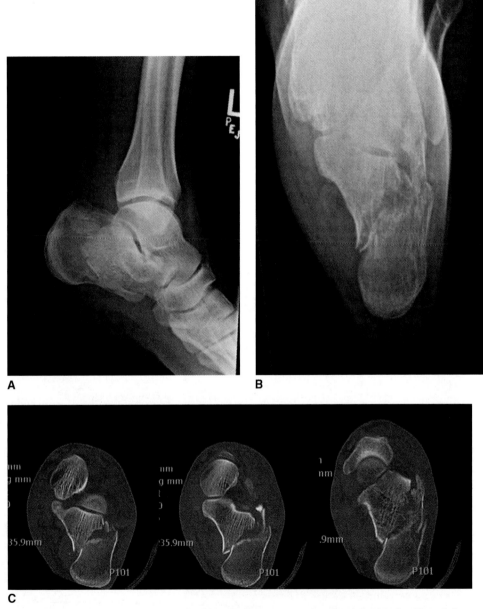

A   **B**

C

Figure 27-25 ‖ **A:** Harris axial radiograph with typical appearance of a primary fracture line through the os calcis. **B:** Lateral radiograph of the same fracture. **C:** Axial computed tomography images of the same fracture.

Imaging

- Radiographic imaging of the medial fracture line is essential to an accurate reduction. The patient is placed in a lateral decubitus position, with the feet positioned to allow obstruction-free imaging (Fig. 27-26A and B).

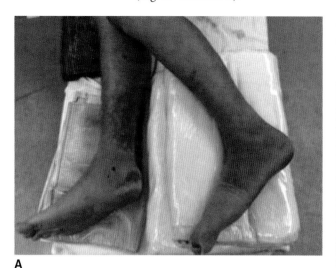
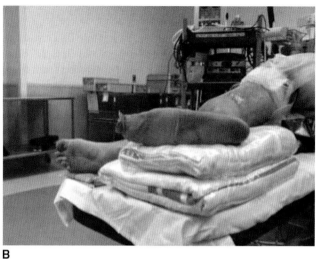

A   **B**

Figure 27-26 I **A and B:** Feet positioning during the lateral extensile calcaneal approach.

- The fluoroscopy unit is oriented around the patient to obtain lateral, AP foot, and Harris axial views (Fig. 27-27A–C). The Harris axial and lateral views provide the most useful perspective in assessing the reduction of the tuberosity.

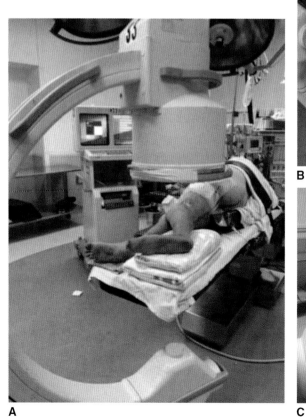
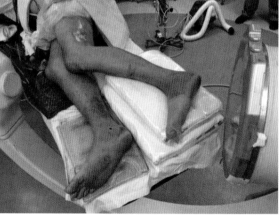

B

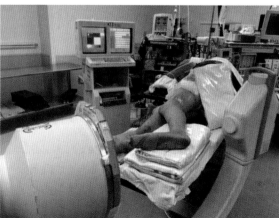

A   **C**

Figure 27-27 I **A:** Fluoroscopy unit orientation for a lateral heel view. **B:** Fluoroscopy unit orientation for an AP foot view. **C:** Fluoroscopy unit orientation for a Harris axial view.

Technique

- An external fixator pin placed from lateral to medial in the tuberosity or from posterior to anterior in the axial plane will help manipulate the fragment. These types of joysticks are frequently under-powered as the sole reduction device and become loose quickly.
- As an adjunct to the tuberosity joysticks, a lever may be employed through the primary fracture line, using the fracture edge of the medial calcar as a fulcrum. A joker elevator or stout Freer is useful (Fig. 27-28A–C).

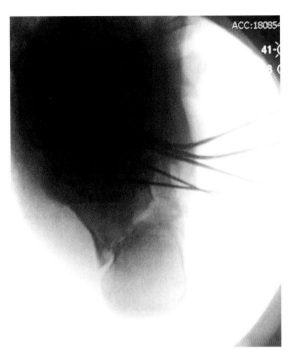

A

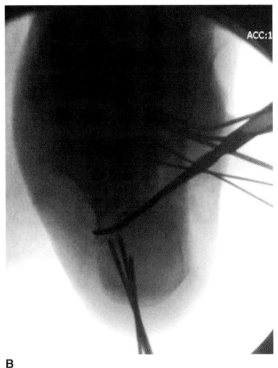

B

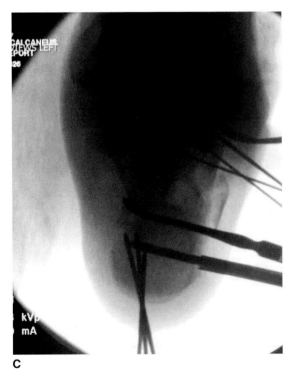

C

Figure 27-28 | **A:** Fluoroscopic Harris axial image demonstrating the tuberosity displacement and the primary fracture line. **B:** Introduction of a lever through the primary fracture line, with medial edge of the fractured calcar as a fulcrum. **C:** The tuberosity is levered into position and the reduction held with the advancement of axially placed Kirschner wires. The tuberosity is no longer in varus, and its height has been reestablished.

- Axially placed Kirschner wires may be preliminarily placed into the tuberosity.
- A lateral to medial directed Schanz pin in the tuberosity can assist in reducing the varus during the levering maneuver.

- A large fragment drill sleeve may be placed over the Schanz pin to stabilize the pin, prevent excessive penetration, and assist in manipulation of the tuberosity fragment.
- Once the reduction has been executed, the tuberosity reduction can be temporarily held as the Kirschner wires are advanced (Fig. 27-29).

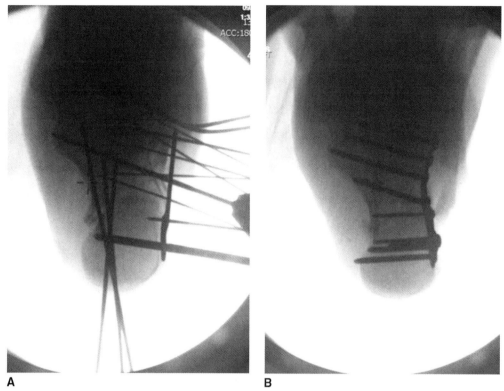

A   **B**

Figure 27-29 ▮ A and B: The sustentaculum is being prepared for screw insertion. Compression of the plate against the tuberosity will further improve reduction of the tuberosity.

- Compression of the fracture to the plate will help reduce residual tuberosity translation (Fig. 27-30).

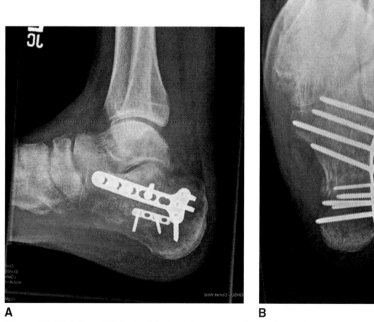

A   **B**

Figure 27-30 ▮ A and B: Lateral and axial postoperative radiographs.

TIP

The Utility of the Distractor in Calcaneal Fracture Reduction

Daniel N. Segina

Pathoanatomy

Traditional fixation strategies for displaced intra-articular calcaneal fractures (DIACF) involve anatomic restoration of the articular injury. Additional reconstructive goals include restoration of calcaneal morphology, especially calcaneal height, width, and coronal alignment. Because formal open approaches often require a waiting period to allow for soft tissue swelling to resolve, fracture fragments are often difficult to mobilize using traditional techniques.

Solution

The use of a strategically placed Schanz pin into the posterior tuberosity is a well-established technique to aid in morphologic restoration (Figs. 27-31–27-33).

Another helpful strategy to assist in calcaneal morphology restoration involves the use of a medially placed distractor.

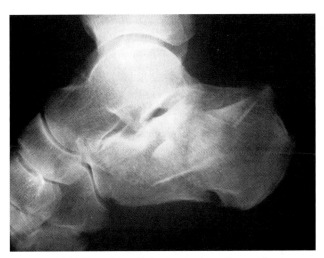
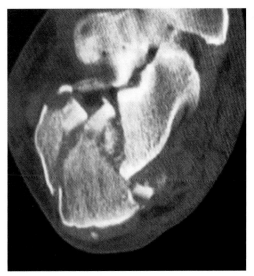

Figure 27-31 I Comminuted joint depression calcaneal fracture.

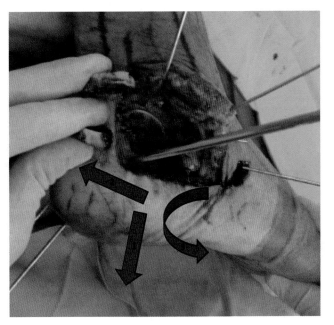

Figure 27-32 I Lateral extensile approach using Schanz pin to effect reduction translational and angular forces. First (*arrow-1*) axial length is restored; second (*arrow-2*) the tuberosity is derotated out of varus; and third (*arrow-3*) the tuberosity is translated medially so that the medial border of the is aligned on the Harris axial image.

Technique

- The patient is placed at the foot of a radiolucent "cantilever-type" OR table in the lateral position and prepped and draped.
- The injured extremity is externally rotated to allow for access to the medial tibia and the medial posterior tuberosity (Fig. 27-33).

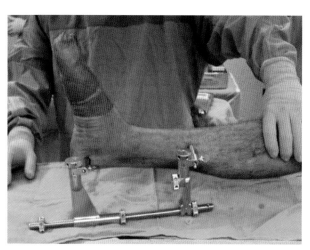
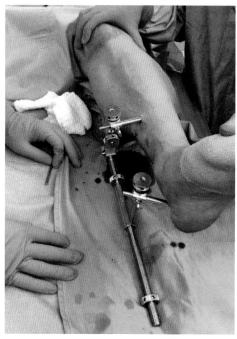

Figure 27-33 ▍ Intraoperative views of the externally rotated extremity after application of a universal distractor. Note that the position of the pins and the distractor (posterior and medial) will allow for unencumbered C-arm imaging.

- A 5.0-mm terminally threaded Schanz pin is placed in the tibial diaphysis with a second 4.0-, 5.0, or 6.0-mm terminally threaded Schanz pin applied to the medial posterior tuberosity. Careful placement is necessary to allow for unobstructed calcaneal fluoroscopic imaging.
  - Another aid is to invert the C-arm and improve calcaneal imaging including lateral and Harris views (Figs. 27-34 and 27-35).

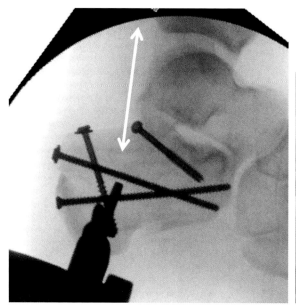
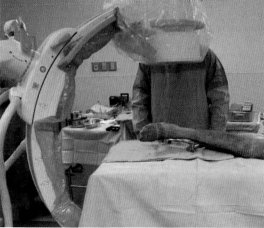

Figure 27-34 ▍ Lateral image obtained with the distractor in place and the corresponding position of the C-arm in the clinical setting. The distraction vector is shown by the *white arrow*.

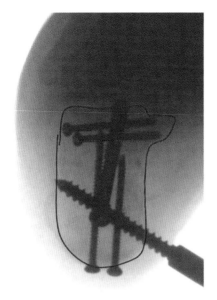
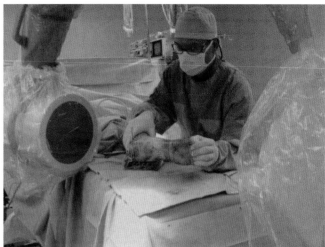

Figure 27-35 I Axial (Harris) view obtained with the distractor in place and corresponding position of C-arm in the clinical setting.

- The pins are cut flush with the capture sleeves of the distractor. This allows for lateral rotation of the limb and fracture repair using a standard lateral approach. Distraction is applied medially allowing for a more mechanically favorable vector, particularly regarding reduction of varus deformity, as well as restoration of height, width, and medialization of the posterior tuberosity.
- The limb is next rotated back into the lateral position for routine fracture repair (Fig. 27-36).

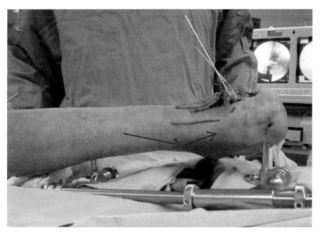
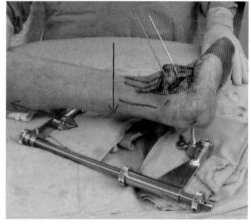

Figure 27-36 I Intraoperative photos showing that the distractor is placed directly on the OR table padding.

- The utility of the distractor is that it can be used for percutaneous, mini-open, or extensile lateral surgical approaches (Fig. 27-37).

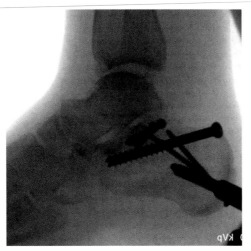 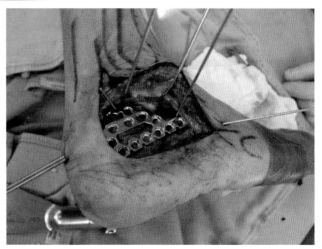

Figure 27-37 I Two different cases, the first showing the distractor being used with percutaneous fixation technique and the second showing the distractor being used with open reduction.

Gastrocnemius Slide (Strayer Procedure)

- The leg is elevated and placed on a triangular pillow.
- An incision is made over the posteromedial aspect of the right calf (approximately halfway between the medial joint line of the knee and the palpable medial malleolus) and carried down through the skin and subcutaneous tissue to the level of the fascia.
- The fascia is then incised longitudinally, and the interval between the gastrocnemius and the soleus muscles is identified and freed from medial to lateral.
  - Take care to identify and cauterize any perforating vessels.
- The plantaris tendon is identified and a 5-cm section is excised.
- The dorsal aspect of the gastrocnemius is then freed from medial to lateral with care being taken to identify and free up all of the dorsal soft tissues including the sural nerve.
- With retraction of all these soft tissues posteriorly and retraction of soleus anteriorly, the gastrocnemius aponeurosis is divided where it blends into the soleus fascia.

References

1. Benirschke SK, Sangeorzan BJ. Extensive intraarticular fractures of the foot. Surgical management of calcaneal fractures. *Clin Orthop Relat Res.* 1993;292:128–134.
2. Gardner MJ, Nork SE, Barei DP, et al. Secondary soft tissue compromise in tongue-type calcaneus fractures. *J Orthop Trauma.* 2008;22(7):439–445.

Chapter 28
Navicular and Cuboid Fractures

MICHAEL F. GITHENS

NICHOLAS M. ROMEO

Sterile Instruments/Equipment

- Tourniquet if desired
- Headlight
- Dental picks and Freer elevators
- Shoulder/bone hook
- Small pointed bone reduction clamps (Weber clamps)
- Small distractor or external fixator
- Kirschner wires and wire driver/drill
- Implants
  - Locking and conventional mini- and small-fragment plates and screws (2.0/2.4/2.7)
  - Precontoured anatomic navicular and cuboid plates
- Allograft cancellous bone chips
- Structural allograft (fibula or tricortical iliac crest)

Navicular Fractures

Positioning and Imaging

- Radiolucent cantilever table.
- Supine with foot at the end of the bed.
- Small bolster under the ipsilateral hip.
- AP, lateral, and oblique radiographic views are evaluated throughout the procedure.
- Comparison contralateral radiographs are often helpful in assessing the patient's native anatomy and alignment.

Surgical Approaches

- Dictated largely by fracture morphology and soft tissue condition.
- Typically, an anteromedial incision is used, with frequent addition of a lateral incision.
- Addition of the lateral approach when lateral column comminution exists or for implant placement.
- For fractures with significant shortening of the columns, distraction through both medial and lateral column external fixators is applied prior to skin incision (Fig. 28-1).
  - Application of fixator allows both for adequate visualization and for obtaining/maintaining reduction.
- Anteromedial approach
  - Incision is created within the interval between the tibialis anterior and tibialis posterior tendons.
  - Deep dissection is performed after deep peroneal nerve and dorsal pedal artery are identified, mobilized, and protected.
  - Capsular incision is repaired at the conclusion of the procedure.

675

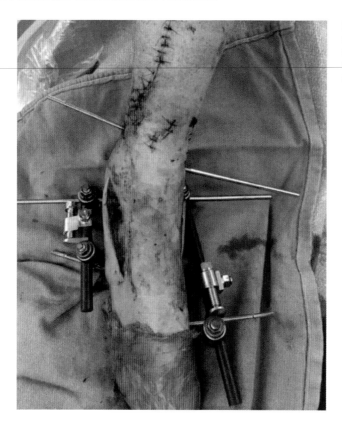

Figure 28-1 ▮ Clinical photo demonstrating medial and lateral external fixators with open compressor-distractor devices to restore midfoot morphology through controlled distraction.

- Lateral approach
  - An incision is marked radiographically at the dorsolateral aspect of the navicular.
  - Deep dissection carried out, mobilizing the EDB.
  - Capsule is incised and later repaired.

Reduction and Fixation Tips

- Gastrocnemius recession (Strayer procedure) should be considered in patients with midfoot fractures and fracture dislocations to unload the mid- and forefoot.
- High-energy injuries with associated tarsal dislocation(s) may be best treated in staged fashion with external fixation assisted reduction/disimpaction followed by definitive ORIF.
- Stress fractures or simple fractures (Fig. 28-2).
  - Dual incisions may be used to access the fracture and for dorsal plate placement.
  - Avoid soft tissue stripping/devascularization via disruption of dorsal blood supply.
  - For displaced fractures, a combination of dental picks and small pointed reduction clamps is used to reduce the fracture after fracture lines are identified and cleansed of any intervening debris.

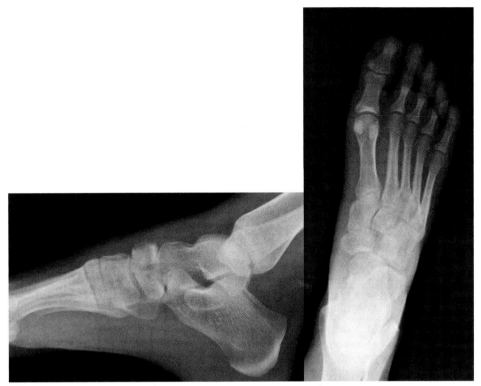

Figure 28-2 I Lateral and AP radiographs demonstrating an isolated navicular fracture without significant comminution.

- Kirschner wires are used for provisional stabilization (Fig. 28-3).
- Dorsal mini-fragment plate applied in compression (Fig. 28-4).
- The plate is placed across the anterior surface of the navicular using both incisions.
- The most medial screw is placed as a lag screw if its trajectory allows or as a position screw.
- The lateral screws are placed sequentially, progressively tensioning the plate as applying compression to the fracture as the screws are tightened.

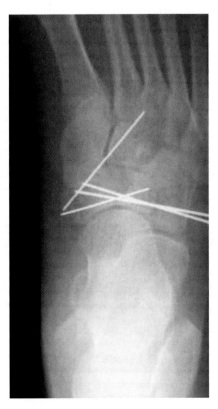

Figure 28-3 I After reduction, K-wires are used for provisional fixation.

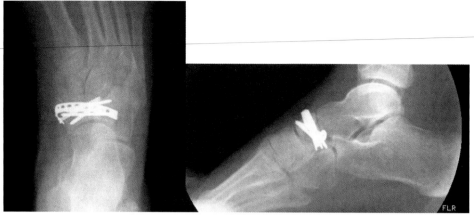

Figure 28-4 I AP and lateral radiographs showing dorsal tension plating of the navicular.

- Fractures with a single large plantar component can be stabilized with independent screw fixation.
  - A single incision is created (typically anteromedial).
  - Any debris is removed from the fracture.
  - Dental picks or small pointed reduction clamps are used to reduce and compress the fracture.
  - Two Kirschner wires are used to temporarily maintain the reduction, and a single screw is placed to compress the fracture.
- Fracture dislocations or fractures with significant comminution.
  - Frequently, the foot lies in a foreshortened position with the lateral aspect of the navicular demonstrating the majority of the comminution and impaction, while the talar head falls into this defect (Fig. 28-5).

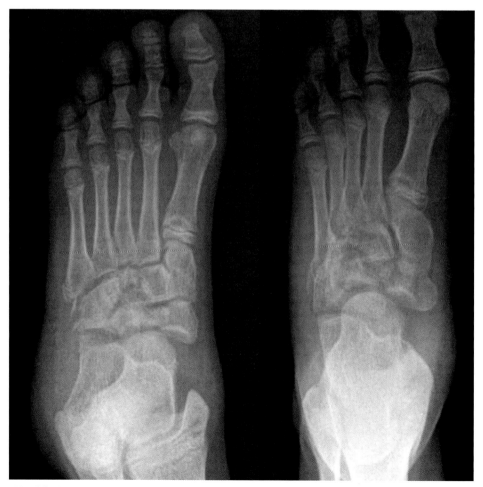

Figure 28-5 I Oblique and AP radiographs of the foot demonstrating a comminuted navicular fracture with significant shortening of the midfoot and medial subluxation of the medial navicular fracture fragment.

- In this setting, where the talar head occupies the navicular's normal location, application of an external fixator is recommended to restore midfoot length and prevent recurrence of the deformity.
- In order to correct shortening, distraction is applied by medial and lateral column distractors.
- The midfoot must be translated laterally to provide talonavicular coverage.
- Reduction is achieved by the following:
  - Lengthening of the column through distractor.
  - Disimpaction of any articular impaction using small osteotomes or elevators.
  - Use of dental picks to manipulate fragments into position.
  - Pointed reduction clamps may be used to compress larger fragments or compress the medial to lateral plane either before or after the plate is provisionally applied.
  - Small (0.045/0.035/0.028) Kirschner wires are used to hold fragments in place.
  - Impaction bone grafting of any defects is performed.
- Spanning fixation via the use of a "T-plate" with expansion onto the cuneiforms provides sufficient stability and maintenance of column length (Fig. 28-6).

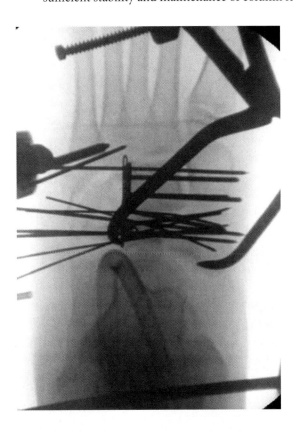

Figure 28-6 I Bridging fixation of the lateral navicular to cuneiform. Note use of medial and lateral distraction to restore midfoot length, thereby allowing restoration of navicular morphology.

- The "T" portion of the plate is applied to the lateral aspect of the navicular, while the long portion of the plate is secured to the lateral cuneiform.
- The plate is held in place temporarily with small Kirschner wires, which can later be replaced by screws.
- To avoid drill bit breakage, Kirschner wires can be used to drill for screws.
- Lateral to medial compression of fracture lines is achieved by placing lag screws through the plate.

- Supplemental independent screws can be applied to provide additional compression.
- A straight plate may be applied plantar to the T-plate to provide an additional buttress (Fig. 28-7).

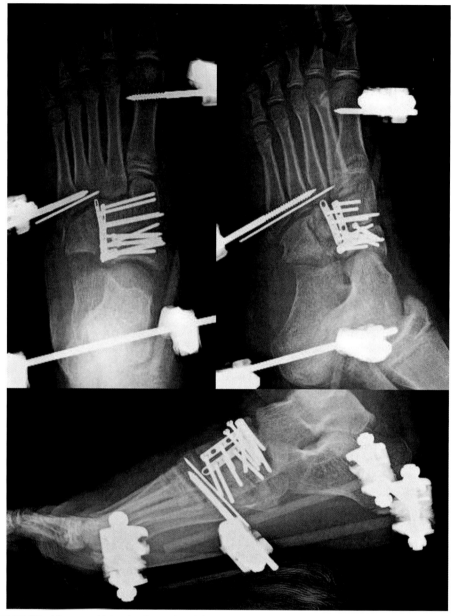

Figure 28-7 | AP, oblique, and lateral radiographs of the foot displaying laterally applied T and straight plates spanning from the navicular to the lateral cuneiform. A bicolumnar external fixator was applied to aid in reduction and was maintained for 6 weeks after fixation.

- In the face of medial comminution or when there is dislocation of the medial fragment, spanning fixation from the navicular to the medial cuneiform can then be similarly applied through a medial approach (Fig. 28-8).
- Alternatively, the external fixator may be left in place for 6 weeks to protect fixation and prevent early recurrence of the injury/deformity.

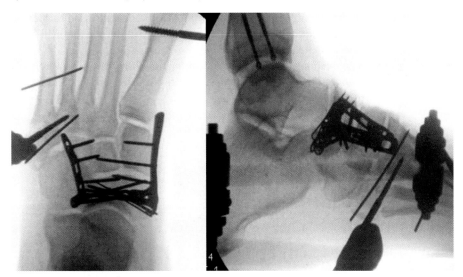

Figure 28-8 I AP and lateral radiographs demonstrating medial and lateral spanning plates for a length-stable construct.

Cuboid Fractures

Positioning and Imaging

- Radiolucent table
- Supine with foot at the end of the bed
- Small bolster ("buttock bump") under the ipsilateral hip
- AP, lateral, and oblique radiographic views

Surgical Approaches

- A skin incision is created directly over the cuboid extending from the anterior calcaneus to the base of the fourth and fifth metatarsals.
- Prior to skin incision, the proximal and distal articulations of the cuboid as well as the dorsal to plantar relationship are identified radiographically to confirm incision placement and length (Fig. 28-9).
- The EBD fascia is elevated and the muscle is elevated dorsally.
- Both the proximal and distal articular surfaces of the cuboid are exposed in their entirety, without compromising stability of the cuboid.
- The medial aspect of the cuboid must be fully visualized to properly reduce intra-articular extension.

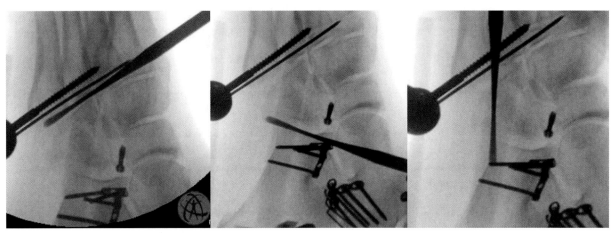

Figure 28-9 I Fluoroscopic images demonstrating the use of a Freer elevator to mark out the planned incision overlying the cuboid.

Reduction and Fixation Strategies

- Cuboid fractures rarely occur in isolation, and other midfoot pathology should be assessed for prior to stabilization.
- High-energy injuries with associated tarsal dislocation(s) may be best treated in staged fashion with external fixation followed by definitive ORIF.
- Any shortening of the lateral column should be addressed surgically.
- If the lateral column heals in a shortened position, the foot will assume an abducted and hyperpronated foot.
- Plate fixation is the usual means of fixation; however, for severely comminuted fractures, temporary bridge plate fixation from the anterior process of the calcaneus onto the fourth metatarsal can be applied (Fig. 28-10).

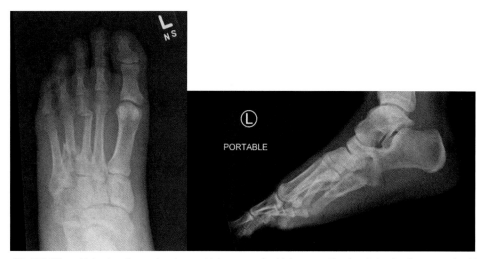

Figure 28-10 | AP and lateral radiographs show a high-energy foot injury resulting in a lateral column crush with a trans-Chopart joint dislocation. Given the severe cuboid comminution, a bridging plate from the calcaneus to the fourth metatarsal shaft is planned.

- Frequently, a large portion of the body is displaced medially (Fig. 28-11).

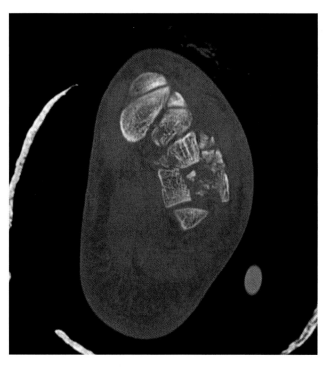

Figure 28-11 | Axial CT scan of the foot demonstrating medial displacement of the medial cuboid body.

- This displacement is largely corrected by distraction of the lateral column.
- Prior to skin incision, place a lateral distractor, with one pin in the calcaneus and one in the fourth and fifth metatarsal bases.
- Initial distraction is applied until the normal lateral column length is restored.
- Typically, both the proximal and distal articular surfaces of the cuboid are impacted and should be elevated using a small osteotome or Freer elevator.
- A dental pick or shoulder hook is used to pull any medially displaced articular fragments laterally.
- The reduction of the articular surfaces is then maintained with the use of small Kirschner wires.
- Impaction bone grafting with cancellous bone chips is performed to maintain articular reduction.
- Massively comminuted segments may be supported with a structural allograft.
- A precontoured cuboid plate or a "T"-plate is then applied to the lateral aspect of the cuboid and held in position with Kirschner wires (Fig. 28-12).

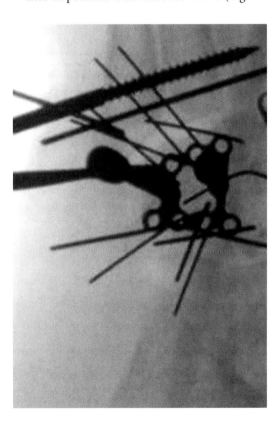

Figure 28-12 I Reduction of the cuboid articular surfaces, as well as the body, is maintained with small Kirschner wires. A precontoured anatomic cuboid plate is applied and position is confirmed radiographically.

- The central screw at each joint surface should be applied first, as a lag screw, if appropriate, in order to prevent any gapping at either the dorsal or plantar articular surfaces (Fig. 28-13).

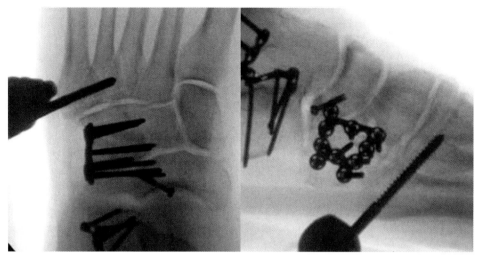

Figure 28-13 I Medial displacement of the medial cuboid body has been corrected with the use of a lateral distractor. Interfragmentary compression through the plate begins with the central screws and then sequentially with the peripheral screws.

- Cortical screws may be later exchanged for locking screws if bone quality is poor or significant comminution exists.
- In cases where definitive cuboid fixation is tenuous, either a bridge plate from the calcaneus to the base of the fourth metatarsal is applied or a lateral column external fixator is left in place.
- Patients are placed in a well-padded short leg splint for 2 to 3 weeks.
- Once sutures are removed, patients are placed into a removable posterior splint, and an early motion protocol is initiated.
- The patient is made non–weight bearing for 3 months.
- External fixator, if left in place, is removed at 6 weeks.
- Bridging plate, if used, is removed between 6 and 8 months.

Chapter 29
Lisfranc Injuries

ANDREW R. EVANS

RANDALL E. MARCUS

Sterile Instruments/Equipment

- Dental picks
- Freer and AO elevators
- Spiked pusher
- Kirschner wires (0.35, 0.45, 0.54, and 0.62 mm)
- Small point-to-point bone clamps
- 2.0- and 2.4-mm screws
- 3.5- and 4.0-mm cortical screws
- 2.4- and 2.7-mm plate/screw sets (straight and T-shaped)

Surgical Approaches

Dorsal Approach to the Midfoot

- Patient positioning
  - Supine.
  - Radiolucent table of cantilever type.
  - Bring the patient to cantilever (foot) end of the table.
  - Place a bump beneath the ipsilateral buttock and flank to neutralize limb rotation.
  - Prep and drape the affected lower extremity to the ipsilateral groin.
  - Place the appropriately sized sterile radiolucent triangle under the knee.
- Fluoroscopically, locate the first intermetatarsal space on the AP view.
- Incise the skin and subcutaneous tissue longitudinally directly over the first intermetatarsal space.
  - Take care to preserve the branches of the superficial and deep peroneal nerves and the dorsalis pedis artery.
    - Retract medially or laterally depending upon their position.
- Dissect the capsules overlying the first and second metatarsocuneiform joints.
  - Typically, these capsules will have been disrupted traumatically.
- Incise the joint capsule along the articular borders of the first metatarsocuneiform articulation to visualize the articular surfaces dorsally, medially, and plantarly.
- Incise the joint capsule along the articular borders of the second metatarsocuneiform articulation to visualize the articular surface dorsally, dorsomedially, and dorsolaterally.
- When the third, fourth, and/or fifth metatarsocuneiform joints are subluxated, dislocated, or fractured, a second incision should be made over the interspace between the third and fourth metatarsals.
  - Adequate visualization of the third metatarsocuneiform joint is difficult through an incision placed over the first intermetatarsal space, requiring the use of this second incision.
  - Determine the location of this incision by identifying the metatarsocuneiform joints and the interspace between the third and fourth metatarsals fluoroscopically.
  - Incise the skin longitudinally directly over the interspace between the third and fourth metatarsals and extend this incision proximally, dissecting through the skin and subcutaneous tissue.
  - Dissect to bone, retracting tendons and neurovascular structures (medially or laterally, as appropriate) to visualize the third and fourth metatarsocuneiform joints.

Crush/Open Injuries

- Consider the use of spanning external fixation to temporize and provisionally stabilize the bony and/or ligamentous midfoot injury.
  - Definitive open reduction and internal fixation should be performed once edema has subsided and the soft tissue injury has healed sufficiently to allow a safe surgical approach.
  - Soft tissues must be followed closely for 1 to 6 weeks in order to determine the time at which incisions for open reduction can be made so as to minimize associated complications.
- Severe crush or open injuries, particularly plantar degloving "slipper foot" injuries and extensive plantar lacerations, should be considered for amputation (Fig. 29-1).

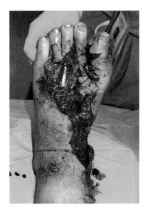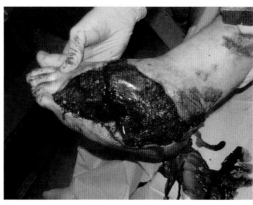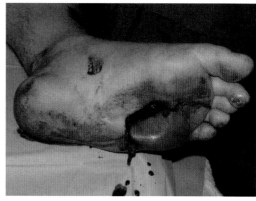

Figure 29-1 I Examples of severe mangled foot injuries that should be considered for amputation.

Reduction and Implant Techniques

External Fixation

- Recommended for initial (provisional) treatment of severe crush or open injuries of the foot, especially in the presence of instability, shortening, dislocation, or deformity.
  - Typically, this first treatment stage is converted to internal fixation when the condition of the soft tissues allows a safe surgical approach.
  - May also be used to supplement internal fixation constructs.
- The objective of this method for provisional stabilization is to restore the foot alignment, especially to restore the length of the medial and/or lateral columns of the foot.
  - Ligamentotaxis assists in the reduction of fractured, impacted, or dislocated tarsal/metatarsal bones.
  - Stabilization of the bones and soft tissues encourages the resolution of inflammation and edema.
- A medial and lateral midfoot external fixation frame typically consists of
  - A 5.0- or 6.0-mm centrally threaded calcaneal transfixion pin (or a medial 5.0-mm half pin for medial column stabilization alone)

- A 4.0-mm first metatarsal Schanz pin
- A 3.0- or 4.0-mm fourth/fifth metatarsal base Schanz pin
- One medial and one lateral bar spanning the medial and lateral columns, respectively (Fig. 29-2)

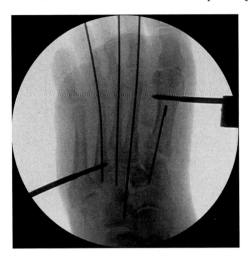

Figure 29-2 | Provisional external fixation of medial and lateral columns using two bars connecting a transcalcaneal pin to a 4.0-mm pin in the bases of the fourth and fifth metatarsals and a 4.0-mm pin in the first metatarsal. Intramedullary K-wires have been placed to provisionally stabilize metatarsal head, neck, shaft fractures (2, 3, and 4), and their TMT articulations. The first TMT dislocation is stabilized temporarily with a transarticular K-wire. The intramedullary K-wires in the third and fourth rays will be withdrawn from the midtarsals to the bases of their respective metatarsals upon definitive fixation of these TMT articulations.

- See Chapter 33 for additional figures.
- Alternatively, a half-pin configuration can be used either medially or laterally for homolateral injuries.
- Manual distraction may be applied to achieve the desired ligamentotaxis.
  - Supplemental distraction may be applied using the open compressor/distractor to facilitate alignment and reduction of fractures/dislocations.
  - Splinting or ankle-spanning external fixator configurations should be considered to maintain neutral ankle dorsiflexion and thereby prevent gastrosoleus equinus contracture.

Open Reduction and Internal Fixation

- Operative fixation of a Lisfranc fracture dislocation should proceed in a medial to lateral direction.
  - Typically, the initial step in the reduction sequence is reduction of the first tarsometatarsal joint followed by provisional K-wire stabilization.
    - Confirmation of an anatomical reduction requires direct visualization and palpation of the dorsal, medial, and plantar-medial aspect of the first TMT joint (to assess any incongruity) and radiographic correlation.
  - This is followed by reduction and provisional K-wire stabilization of the second TMT joint and the lateral TMT joints as necessary (Fig. 29-3).

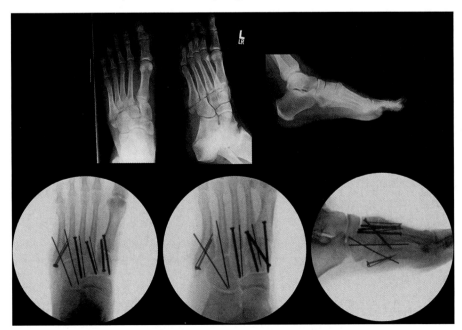

Figure 29-3 | Case example of operative fixation of a complete Lisfranc injury.

- Prior to initiating operative fixation of the Lisfranc injury, evaluate intertarsal joints for the presence of instability.
  - Talonavicular
  - Intercuneiform (Fig. 29-4)

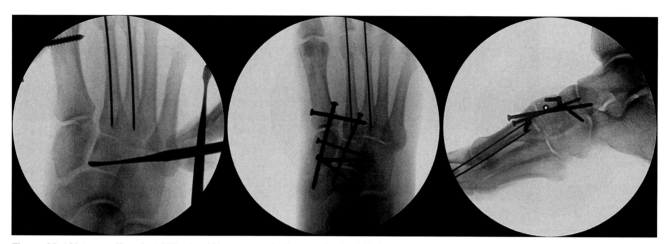

Figure 29-4 | Intercuneiform instability should be assessed prior to reduction initiation to plan the reduction sequence and fixation construct. These intertarsal articulations proved to be unstable and were stabilized in addition to the TMT joints.

- Reduce the first metatarsocuneiform joint, assessing the reduction dorsally, medially, and plantarly to confirm joint congruity.
  - Fracture fragments associated with comminution should be preserved and reduced concomitantly with the TMT dislocations/subluxations.
  - Very small irreducible fracture fragments and hematoma should be irrigated and removed.
  - Given the saucer-like articulation of the first metatarsocuneiform joint, congruity must be confirmed from all sides, especially plantarly.
  - Malreduction of the first metatarsocuneiform joint will likely result in the malreduction of all remaining injured (lateral) metatarsocuneiform joints.
- Once joint congruity and reduction have been established, stabilize it temporarily with K-wires.
  - Subsequently, reduce and stabilize the lateral tarsometatarsal joints with K-wires.
- If dislocated (without fractures), definitively stabilize the first metatarsocuneiform with a 3.5- or 4.0-mm cortical (i.e., "Lisfranc") screw directed dorsal to plantar and distal to proximal, leaving room for a second screw to be placed in the same plane but in the opposite direction, from proximally to distally across this joint.[1]
  - Be sure to countersink these screw heads to distribute their contact pressures over a larger surface area and to avoid prominence of the screw heads.
  - Confirm fluoroscopically on AP, oblique, and lateral views that the screw does not enter the naviculocuneiform joint.

TIP

Lisfranc Screw Path Creation
Randall E. Marcus

Pathoanatomy

When performing internal fixation for a Lisfranc fracture dislocation or fusion of the metatarsal-tarsal articulation, it is important to achieve rigid fixation between each metatarsal and its associated tarsal bone. We recommend using retrograde solid core screws, such as 3.5-mm fully threaded cortical screws (or 4.0-fully threaded cortical screws in the first TMT joint in large individuals). Due to the contour of the metatarsal and the shape of the screw, it can be difficult to perform this procedure without causing an iatrogenic fracture to the proximal metaphyseal portion of the metatarsal as the screws are tightened.

Solution

The peak contact stress between the screw head and bone surface is reduced by increasing the contact area, thereby reducing the force per unit area.

Technique

- Identify the metaphyseal-diaphyseal junction of the proximal metatarsal (usually, the first, second, and third TMT articulations are stabilized with screws in Lisfranc injuries).
- Using a small osteotome placed vertically, 90 degrees to the metaphyseal-diaphyseal junction, a 90-degree "headwall" is developed to be used to buttress each screw's head when seated (Fig. 29-5A).
- A power burr is then used to develop a longitudinal trough over the dorsum of the metatarsal extending distally to the "headwall" at the metaphyseal-diaphyseal junction (Fig. 29-5B).

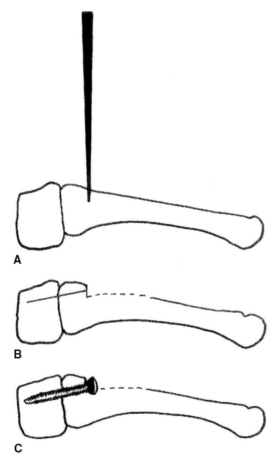

Figure 29-5 **A:** Demonstrates a small osteotome placed vertically at the metaphyseal-diaphyseal junction of the metatarsal to contour a "headwall" at the metatarsal metaphyseal-diaphyseal junction. **B:** A power burr has been utilized to contour a longitudinal trough over the dorsum of the metatarsal extending distally to the "headwall." This trough should be superficial to the medullary canal. **C:** The 3.5-mm fully threaded cortical screw has been inserted in a retrograde direction through the metaphyseal region of the metatarsal crossing the tarsometatarsal articulation into the cuneiform. Note that the peak contact stress between the screw head and the metaphyseal bone surface has been reduced by increasing the contact area.

A

B

C

- The trough should fit the contour of the cortical screw head and approximate half of its diameter (Fig. 29-6).

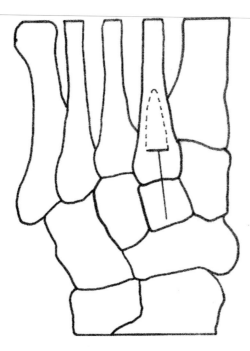

Figure 29-6 I A power burr has been used to contour a longitudinal trough over the dorsum of the metatarsal extending distally to the "headwall." The 2.5-mm drill hole has been placed retrograde extending from the metatarsal metaphysis into the cuneiform.

- The surgeon should be careful not to penetrate the cortex and inadvertently enter the medullary canal of the diaphyseal portion of the metatarsal trough.
- The screw is then inserted retrograde from the proximal metatarsal metaphyseal-diaphyseal junction into the appropriate cuneiform bone with fluoroscopic control. Standard AO technique is used, but if a lag technique is desired, the AO "top hat" will not fit the contour of the metatarsal because of its diameter. Therefore, the 2.5-mm drill bit is used to drill the hole in a retrograde direction, through the metaphyseal region of the metatarsal, across the TMT articulation, and into the cuneiform. If a lag technique is desired for compression, the metaphyseal region of the metatarsal drill hole may be then overdrilled with a 3.5-mm drill bit. Measurements are taken, and the appropriate 3.5-mm fully treaded cortical screw is inserted. As the screw seats, the head of the screw will fill the trough and rest against the metaphyseal headwall of the metatarsal, achieving compression at the fracture site (Figs. 29-5C and 29-7).

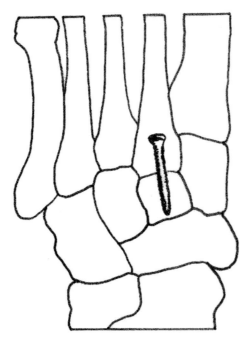

Figure 29-7 I The 3.5-mm fully threaded cortical screw has been inserted retrograde, extending from the metatarsal metaphysis into the cuneiform.

• Solid cortical screws are used instead of cannulated screws because of their increased fatigue strength when compared to cannulated screws. Note that the instruments for placing 3.5-mm cannulated screws may be helpful in aligning each screw's trajectory. However, consider using solid screws rather than cannulated screws due to the cannulated screws reduced strength (Fig. 29-8).

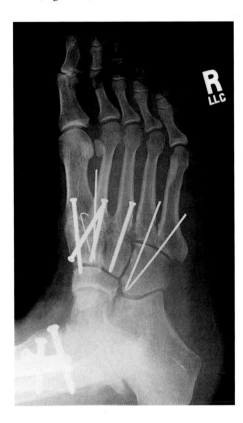

Figure 29-8 | Oblique view of 3.5-mm fully threaded cortical screws inserted in the first, second, and third metatarsal-tarsal articulations for fusion.

• For fusion of the first metatarsal-tarsal articulation, both a retrograde and a second antegrade screw from the medial cuneiform into the first metatarsal metaphysis are inserted for stability.

- Maintain at least two points of fixation in the joint at all times to prevent rotation of the metatarsal and subsequent malreduction.
- Fracture dislocations or fracture comminution of the first metatarsal base, cuneiform, and/or the navicular may necessitate the use of spanning plates/screws from the talus or navicular distally to the first metatarsal.
  - A 2.7-mm compression plate or nonannealed (stiff) 2.7-mm reconstruction plate is generally of adequate strength and low profile for this application (Fig. 29-9).

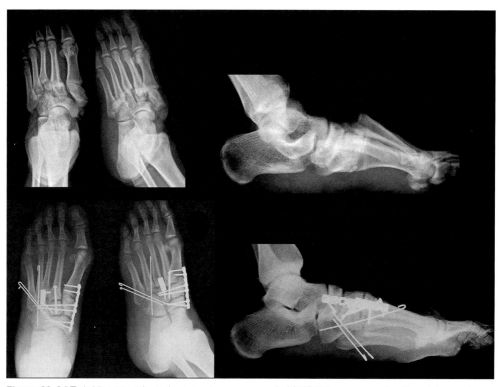

Figure 29-9 I To bridge comminuted segments, a nonannealed (stiff) 2.7-mm reconstruction plate may be used.

  - The use of spanning plates should be avoided in fixation of the fourth/fifth metatarsocuboid joints, the talonavicular, and calcaneocuboid joints due to the significant mobility required for locomotion and function by these articulations.
    - These plates may be placed for initial stabilization, but should be removed by approximately 4 months to restore joint motion.
  - External fixation of either column may also be used instead of, or in combination with, spanning plate fixation.

- Reduce the second metatarsal base so that it fits into its mortise at the first metatarsal and middle cuneiform.
- Small point-to-point clamps are useful to achieve adequate axial compression for anatomic reduction of the second metatarsal base and may also aid in reducing displacement between the second metatarsal base and the first metatarsal/medial cuneiform (Fig. 29-10).

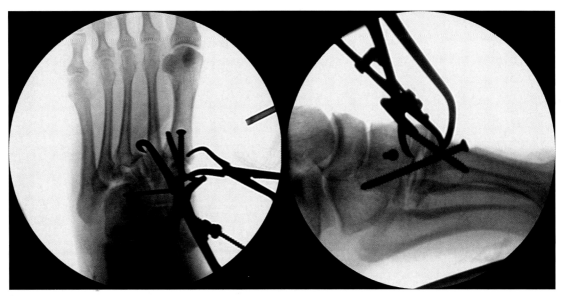

Figure 29-10 | Example of small and large Weber clamps (pointed bone reduction clamps) placed across the first tarsometatarsal joint and between medial cuneiform and base of the second metatarsal.

- Provisionally stabilize the second TMT joint with K-wires.
  - Extensive comminution of the second and/or third metatarsal bases is not uncommon, and if cortical lag screw application is not feasible, then consideration should be given to the use of a spanning 2.4-mm plate and screws from the cuneiform to the respective metatarsal for definitive fixation (Fig. 29-11).

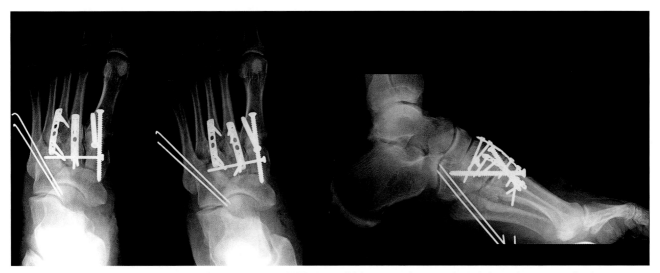

Figure 29-11 | In the presence of comminution of the lesser TMT joints, mini-fragment plates are a good alternative to screw fixation.

- Avoid incorporation of the naviculocuneiform joint, if possible; however, the navicular may be used for supplemental proximal fixation in selected cases with extensive cuneiform comminution or impaction (Figs. 29-12 and 29-13).

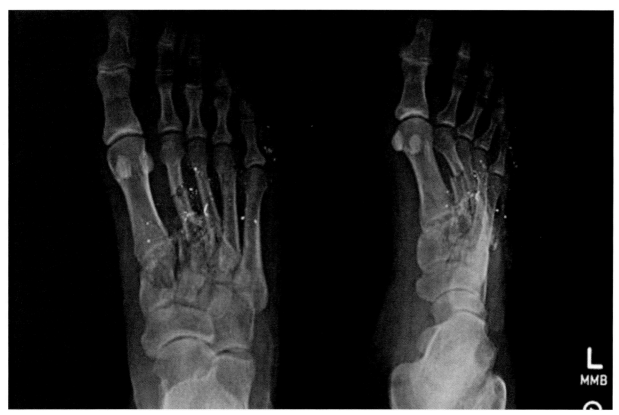

Figure 29-12 I Injury images demonstrating a comminuted Lisfranc injury involving the medial and middle cuneiforms.

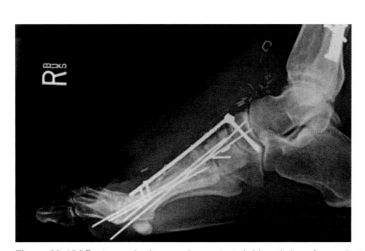
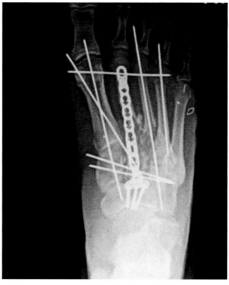

Figure 29-13 I Postoperative images demonstrate bridge plating of comminuted Lisfranc injuries. Because the middle cuneiform comminution prevented stable fixation, the fractures were bridged from the navicular to the distal metatarsal.

- Reduce and provisionally stabilize the third TMT joint with K-wires in a similar fashion to the second metatarsocuneiform joint, and stabilize definitively.
- Perform open reduction and stabilization of the fourth and fifth metatarsocuboid joints with K-wires inserted from the lateral surfaces of the metatarsal bases across the TMT joint into the cuboid.

- This reduction maneuver often requires pushing directly on the fourth metatarsal base in a plantar and medial direction.
- By aiming K-wires toward the proximal-medial corner of the cuboid, the greatest span of cuboid is traversed.
- These K-wires may be inserted percutaneously with their lateral ends left outside the skin, or these ends may be cut short so that they may be buried just underneath the skin.
  - This decision depends on the surgeon's preference, the condition of the skin, and the anticipated length of time required for healing.
- Open reduction and internal fixation of tarsal or hindfoot fractures should also be performed in order to restore articular anatomy, stabilize unstable tarsal segments, and/or reconstruct the medial and lateral column lengths.
- Postoperatively, patients should be maintained in a well-molded splint that maintains the ankle dorsiflexed to neutral.

Midfoot Arthrodesis

- An appropriate treatment option for patients with severe articular comminution and osseous injury, for patients with persistent midfoot instability after fixation, or those with severe posttraumatic arthritis of the midfoot.[2,3]

Associated Gastrosoleus Equinus

- It is the belief of some surgeons that patients with gastrocsoleus equinus have a predilection for Lisfranc injuries, among other fracture patterns.
- In patients who present with this condition (usually bilateral), consideration should be given to performing a Strayer gastrocnemius recession, either at the first stage of provisional treatment (e.g., external fixation) or at the time of definitive stabilization.

References

1. Kuo RS, Tejwani NC, Digiovanni CW, et al. Outcome after open reduction and internal fixation of Lisfranc joint injuries. *J Bone Joint Surg Am.* 2000;82-A:1609–1618.
2. Coetzee JC, Ly TV. Treatment of primarily ligamentous Lisfranc joint injuries: primary arthrodesis compared with open reduction and internal fixation. Surgical technique. *J Bone Joint Surg Am.* 2007;89(Suppl 2 Pt 1):122–127.
3. Ly TV, Coetzee JC. Treatment of primarily ligamentous Lisfranc joint injuries: primary arthrodesis compared with open reduction and internal fixation. A prospective, randomized study. *J Bone Joint Surg Am.* 2006;88(3):514–520.

Chapter 30
Metatarsal Neck Fractures

MICHAEL J. GARDNER

Sterile Instruments/Equipment

- Small pointed bone reduction clamps (Weber clamps)
- Shoulder hook, dental picks, and Freer elevators
- Finger traps and Mastisol for traction
- Implants
  - 0.062 inch K-wires
  - Mini-fragment plates and screws (2.0 and 2.4 mm)
- K-wire driver/drill

Positioning

- Supine on radiolucent table.
- Place a small bump under ipsilateral hip so that the patella faces anteriorly.
- Use tibial nailing triangle turned long-side down to get good AP and oblique views of the midfoot.
- C-arm should enter from opposite side of the table.
- Alternatively, flex knee to 90 degrees over a tibial nailing triangle. With the fluoroscopic beam perpendicular to the floor, five folded towels under the forefoot give a good view and a stable platform for reduction and pin placement (Fig. 30-1).

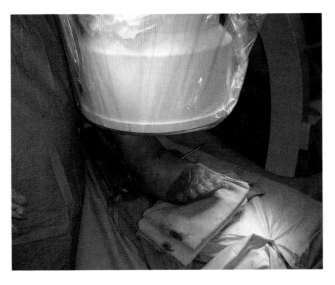

Figure 30-1 ▮ Five folded towels under the forefoot with the fluoroscopic beam perpendicular to the floor give good visualization of the forefoot.

- The C-arm angle is often best determined on a lateral view so that the beam for AP and oblique images is oriented perpendicular to the metatarsal necks and shafts.
- Roll the foot between AP and oblique views to determine both mediolateral and dorsal-plantar K-wire vectors.

Surgical Approaches

- Percutaneous reduction and pinning
  - Strategically placed small incisions for reduction instruments and K-wires.

Reduction and Implant Techniques

- Pull toe axially, and manipulate medially or laterally depending on the fracture obliquity and displacement (Fig. 30-2).

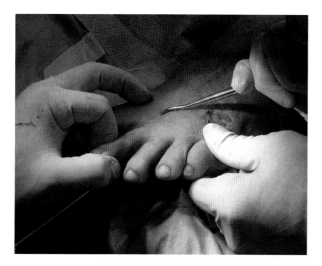

Figure 30-2 | Pulling the toe axially, with medial or lateral translation, assists in fracture reduction.

- If there is difficulty gripping toe, put a finger trap on toes with Mastisol (Fig. 30-3).

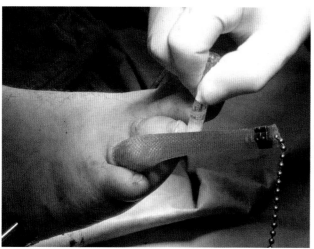
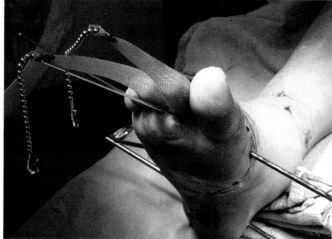

Figure 30-3 | To assist in pulling axial traction on the toes to disimpact the fracture and achieve reduction, Mastisol and finger traps can be a useful technique.

- The starting point is critical and will affect reduction, just as with any intramedullary nailing (Fig. 30-4). A perfectly centered entry site should be confirmed on an AP and 30-degree oblique views in both directions.

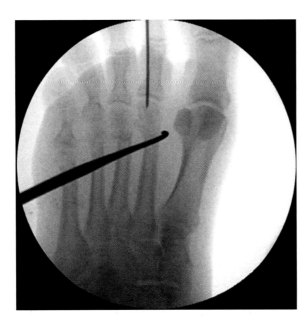

Figure 30-4 ‖ A starting point that is centered on the metatarsal head, regardless of its position relative to the shaft, is critical.

- There are two methods of fixation:
  - In the first method, the K-wire passes under the base of the proximal phalanx.
  - In the second method, the K-wire transfixes the MTP joint.
- Method under base of proximal phalanx
  - Extend and distract the toe slightly for K-wire to enter plantar surface of toe crease.
  - Insert a 0.062-inch K-wire plantarly to clear the base of the proximal phalanx and anchor wire tip on metatarsal head.
  - This technique will result in some extension at the MTP joint, depending on where the K-wire enters the MT head.
  - The K-wire will block MTP flexion, but dorsiflexion will be possible.
- Method of MTP transfixion
  - Start K-wire inferiorly on plantar flare at the base of the proximal phalanx base.
  - Penetrate the base of the proximal phalanx at an acute angle.
  - Advance K-wire through articular surface of proximal phalanx base, but not into head of metatarsal.
  - Position MTP in neutral, and advance K-wire into MT head and either up MT shaft or just out of the plantar surface of MT shaft.

- Reduction aids
  - Percutaneous K-wire: Use a 0.054- or 0.062-inch K-wire as a mini-spiked pusher to translate metatarsal shafts in any direction: medial, lateral, dorsal, or plantar.
  - Control wire by placing in a universal chuck (Fig. 30-5).

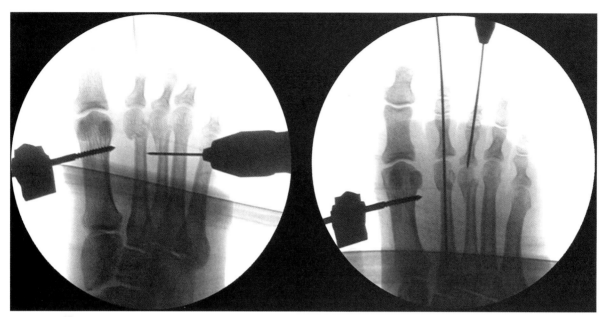

Figure 30-5 ▌ A K-wire on a universal chuck can be a useful reduction tool to manipulate the metatarsal shaft underneath the head. While distal traction is placed on the second phalanx, its MT shaft/neck is translated medially with a chucked K-wire so as to be collinear with the MT head. Then, the K-wire is inserted across the reduced fracture.

- Shoulder hook or dental pick
  - Alternatively, make a stab incision, and place a shoulder hook or dental pick to manipulate shaft relative to metatarsal head (Fig. 30-6).

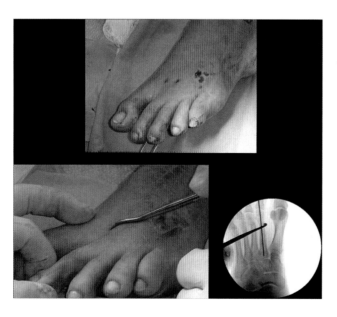

Figure 30-6 ▌ Through small stab incisions on the dorsum of the foot, a shoulder hook can be inserted percutaneously to reduce the metatarsal shaft.

- Anchor pins in the base of the metatarsals, but take care not to perforate the TMT joints (Fig. 30-7).

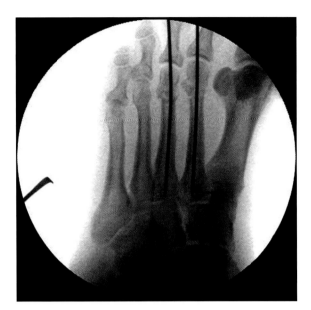

Figure 30-7 | The K-wires are anchored in the bases of the metatarsals.

- After a K-wire is placed, flex or extend MT to bend K-wire and make small corrections.
- Bend K-wires using needle-nose pliers and metal suction tip.
  - Making two 90-degree bends allows the final curve to be approximately 180 degrees and cut short (Fig. 30-8).

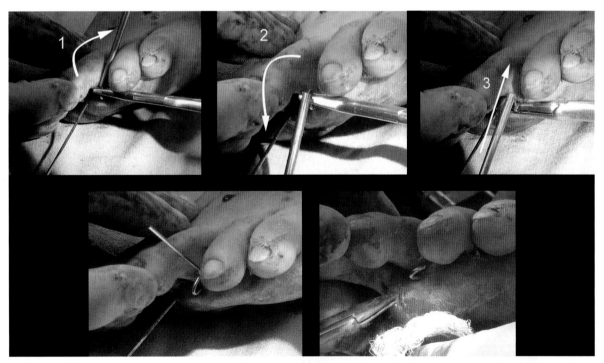

Figure 30-8 | To bend the pins at an acute angle, a three-step technique can be used using a needle-nose pliers and a metal tip suction tip.

- Cover the ends with a protective cap.
- Alternatively, the wires are cut and buried beneath the skin by sliding the wire cutter along the wire, pushing the skin back, and cutting the wire so the skin rebounds over the wire when cut.
  - So that the wires do not migrate proximally and become irretrievable, their insertion depth should be to the subchondral bone at the phalangeal base.
  - A dental pick is used to free the skin and subcutaneous tissue from around the wire.
  - Buried wires may decrease the risk of infection though they are more difficult to remove.

- Standard pinning of a length-unstable metatarsal fracture will likely result in fracture shortening.
  - In this situation, metatarsal length may be maintained by placing a transverse K-wire from a length-stable metatarsal into the length-unstable metatarsal prior to releasing traction (Fig. 30-9).

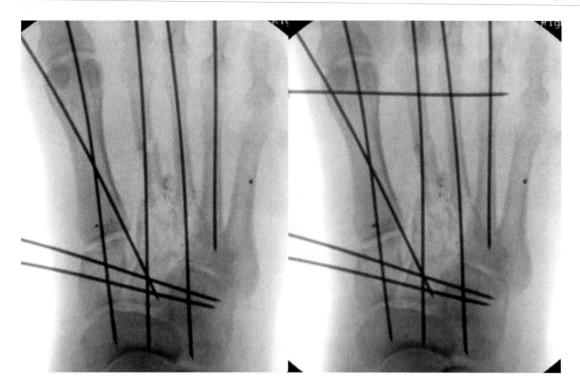

Figure 30-9 I Intraoperative imaging demonstrating pinning of length-unstable metatarsal fractures. The first and fourth metatarsals (length-stable) are used to prevent shortening of the length-unstable second and third metatarsals by transfixing all four with a wire prior to releasing traction.

- Wire is placed through the metatarsal necks, after retrograde wires have been passed.
- Count the cortices while placing the wire to ensure that it is bicortical in each metatarsal.
- Maintaining metatarsal length is important in keeping a normal metatarsal cascade (Fig. 30-10).

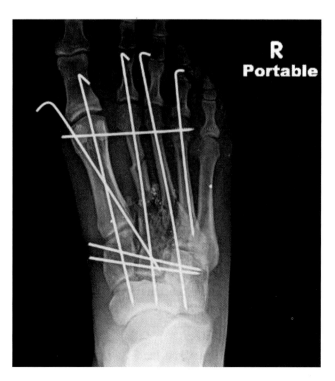

Figure 30-10 I Postoperative AP radiograph demonstrating the pinning technique to prevent shortening of length-unstable metatarsals.

Section 11
External Fixation and Miscellaneous

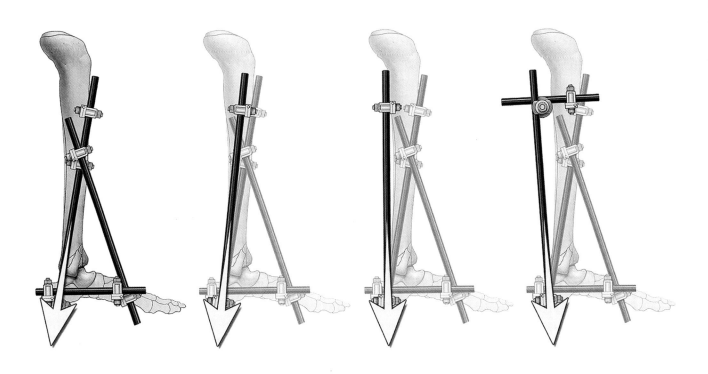

Chapter 31
Knee-Spanning External Fixation

M. BRADFORD HENLEY

MICHAEL J. GARDNER

MICHAEL F. GITHENS

Sterile Instruments/Equipment

- Large external fixation system
- Open compressor-distractor device
- 4.0-mm partially threaded pins for midfoot pin
- Towel bumps

Positioning

- Supine on a cantilever-type table.
- Bring patient to the end of the table.
- Place a small bump under ipsilateral hip and torso.
- Elevate leg on a soft ramp cushion to facilitate lateral radiographs.

Indications

- Staged treatment of complex periarticular fractures about the knee.
- Damage control orthopaedic surgery.
- It is suggested not to obtain CT scans to plan definitive fixation prior to the application of a spanning external fixator, unless the external fixator will be used for definitive fracture management.
- It is best to obtain CT scans after a spanning external fixator is applied.
  - An external fixator can maintain limb length, alignment, and the improvements in fracture reduction achieved through ligamentotaxis.
  - Thus, it is cost-effective and often more efficient to obtain advanced imaging studies, such as CT, prior to definitive fixation, if used as a preoperative tool for planning surgical tactics after external fixation.

Reduction and Implant Techniques

- Assess the fracture pattern on the AP view to determine where the distraction forces will affect the best reduction.
  - Varus deformities will respond to distraction across the joint if the force vector is collinear with the mechanical axis of the limb or just medial to this on an AP image (Fig. 31-1).

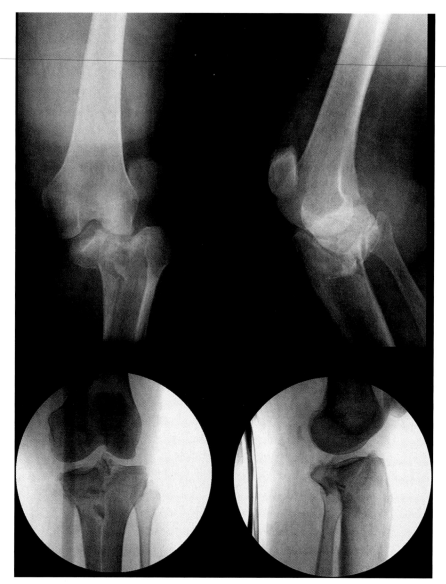

Figure 31-1 I Following fracture-dislocation of the knee, ligamentotaxis through the initial two-pin construct provided accurate length and alignment. Note the initial varus deformity and the position of the external fixator bars medial to the mechanical axis of the extremity.

- Similarly, valgus deformities will respond to distraction across the joint if the force vector is collinear with the mechanical axis of the limb or just lateral to this on an AP image.
- Place pins and pin-bar clamps so as to achieve the above by moving bar to one side of a pin or the other.
- Place one pin in proximal third of femur (5.0 × ~200 mm) and one pin distally in distal tibia (5.0 × ~170 mm) using soft tissue protection sleeves (triple guide) for soft tissue protection.
  - Both pins in the sagittal plane, anterior to posterior.
  - Correct rotational alignment to "near anatomical" before inserting the first two pins in same orientations, orthogonal to proximal femur and distal tibia.
    - If the orientation of these first two pins differs (e.g., the distal tibial pin is not in the same sagittal plane as the proximal femoral pin, but rotationally misaligned) using the external fixator to effect a change in limb length will necessarily effect limb rotation, when the bars are connected to the pins directly.
      - However, if the bars can be aligned so as to be collinear to the axis of the limb (usually requires another connecting bar to offset the longitudinal bar away from the offset pin), using the external fixator to effect a change in limb length should not adversely affect the limb rotation.

- If after distraction, rotation is not anatomical, this should be adjusted using the two pins as joysticks in the femur and tibia.
    - Do not insert a third pin until correct rotation has been achieved, as by doing so, rotation cannot be adjusted by most external fixation systems unless the bar-to-bar clamps have a "ball-joint" connection allowing multiplanar corrections.
  - Ideally, when completed, the first three pins (or even all four pins) will be in the same plane (e.g., sagittal).
- Connect bars to the pins, and connect the two bars with a bar-to-bar clamp in the middle.
  - Ensure the metallic clamps are not overlying joint line to facilitate later imaging.
    - For proximal tibial fractures, place this bar-to-bar connecting clamp over the distal femur.
    - For distal femur fractures, place this bar-to-bar connecting clamp over the proximal tibia.
    - This will facilitate radiographic imaging, intra-operatively during reduction, postoperatively, and during definitive fixation if the fixator is left in place.
    - Such placement will also reduce scanning artifact on the CT scans obtained after provisional fixation.
- The goal is a stabilized lower extremity in a "comfortable" amount of knee flexion, similar to when a long-leg cast is used; approximately 5 to 15 degrees.
  - When the external fixator is placed anteriorly on the lower extremity, distraction will usually increase knee flexion or fracture flexion.
    - Similarly, if the fixator is placed laterally (pins in the coronal plane), it will usually increase the varus.
    - The magnitude of this increase is dependent upon the amount of initial knee flexion/extension (or varus/valgus for coronal pins) and the amount of fixed angulation in the bar-to-bar clamp.
  - To account for this, the limb should be placed in a minimum amount of flexion (−5 to +5 degrees), and the bar-to-bar clamp fixed in a position of minimal angulation (5 to 15 degrees) prior to manual distraction.
    - The final amount of limb angulation will also depend on initial amount of limb shortening and initial position of fracture as it relates to sagittal plane rotation (flexion/extension).
- Distract manually for initial ligamentotaxis and assess reduction on AP and lateral views.
- Correct coronal plane angular deformity (varus/valgus) with manipulation, rotating each fragment around pin axes.
  - Assure that coronal plane translational deformity can also be corrected (this usually requires a minimal amount of manual manipulation).
- Correct sagittal plane translational deformity (anterior/posterior translation) with strategic bumps under the proximal tibia, knee, and/or distal femur.
  - If additional sagittal plane correction is necessary, it may be manually reduced by manipulating the tibia.
- Prior to insertion of the third pin, correct any residual rotational abnormalities.
- Next, use the dynamic compressor-distractor to restore anatomical length to the limb (or minimally overdistract the joint/fracture) before insertion of the third external fixator pin.
- The third pin inserted should be closer to the injury in the nonfractured bone, but not in the surgical field anticipated for definitive fixation.
  - For tibial plateau fractures, this would be the second femoral pin.
  - For supracondylar femoral fractures, this would be the second tibial pin.
  - This pin increases the stability of the reduction and can be used to maintain residual translational or angular deformities corrected just prior to its insertion.

• The final pin, the second tibial pin, should then be inserted. This pin can be used to improve and maintain sagittal reduction in tibial plateau fractures (Fig. 31-2).

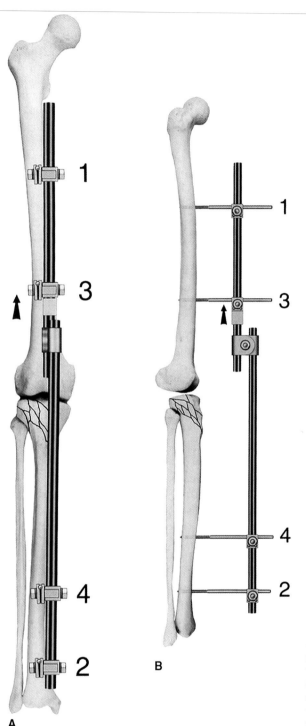

Figure 31-2 I An illustration demonstrating the order of pin placement for knee-spanning external fixation shown in the coronal **(A)** and saggital **(B)** planes. (From Ertl W, Henley MB. Provisional external fixation for periarticular fractures of the tibia. *Tech Orthop.* 2002;17(2):135–144, with permission.)

- An alternative order of pin insertion includes placing the two femoral pins initially, followed by one distal tibial pin. This allows a stable "arm" (e.g., the femur) to reduce the tibia.
  - The disadvantage of this method is that if this "arm" is not collinear with the limb's sagittal plane, the distal bar must be attached to the proximal bar through a bar-to-bar clamp with biplanar angulation.
  - This means that any additional distraction will impart a force vector that affects the fracture reduction in at least two planes and possibly all three (sagittal, coronal, and rotational), in addition to the desired axial distraction.
- After placement of the final pin in the tibia, it can be used to "push" or "pull" the reduction in the sagittal plane, for small additional corrections in translation (Fig. 31-3).

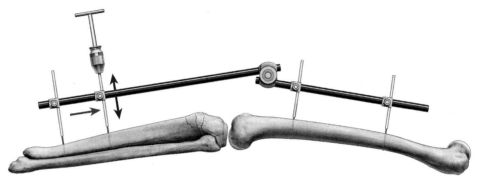

Figure 31-3 I In the case of a tibial plateau fracture, the second (proximal tibial) pin can be inserted last, used as a joystick to fine-tune both the sagittal and coronal planes, and secured to the bar.

  - Larger sagittal plane corrections may require loosening of the clamp-pin fixation (not clamp-bar connection) in this limb segment.
- Using the last pin to adjust the reduction should be planned carefully.
  - This pin position is constrained by the position of the bar and the tibial shaft.
  - The required pin position may result in a pin vector that is not perpendicular to the plane of residual deformity.
- Ensure that the closest pins are away from the planned future incisions.

TIP Adjunct Techniques to Improve Reduction Maintenance During Spanning External Fixation for Floating Knee Injuries, Unstable Tibial Plateau Fractures, and Segmental Lower Extremity Injuries
Michael F. Githens

Pathoanatomy

Knee-spanning external fixators may provide inadequate control of coronal or sagittal plane fracture stability.

Solution

Adjunctive techniques to improve reduction maintenance during spanning external fixation for floating knee injuries, unstable tibial plateau fractures, and segmental lower extremity injuries:

- Improved stability accelerates soft tissue injury resolution and prevents further skin injury.
- Facilitates an easier reduction during the definitive operation.

Techniques

For persistent coronal or sagittal plane instability after external fixation:

- A reduction is obtained using a percutaneously applied Weber clamp, spiked pusher, or shoulder hook (Fig. 31-4).

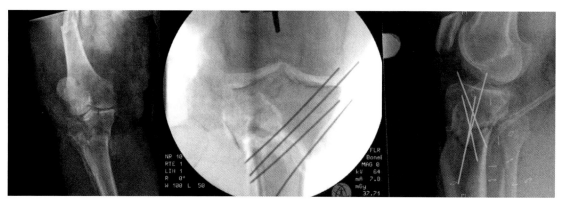

Figure 31-4 I Right injury film of floating knee; after external fixation (center and left), K-wires are placed percutaneously to maintain the relationship of the medial metaphysis and tibial shaft in the setting of severe associated soft tissue injury.

- 0.062-inch or larger diameter K-wires are placed in the obliquity of the clamp.
- Wires are cut below the skin level and buried under the skin using a dental pick to lift the dermis over the cut wire.
- In the setting of an open fracture or fasciotomy wounds, a 2.0-, 2.4-, or 2.7-mm plate may be applied unicortically.
- Ideally, plates should be placed where there is satisfactory soft tissue coverage.
- Plates may be intended as part of the final construct or removed at the time of definitive surgery (Fig. 31-5).

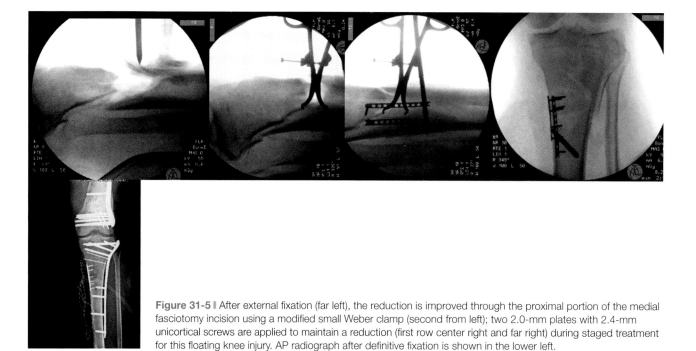

Figure 31-5 I After external fixation (far left), the reduction is improved through the proximal portion of the medial fasciotomy incision using a modified small Weber clamp (second from left); two 2.0-mm plates with 2.4-mm unicortical screws are applied to maintain a reduction (first row center right and far right) during staged treatment for this floating knee injury. AP radiograph after definitive fixation is shown in the lower left.

- Do not apply the plate in a location that interferes with final implant position.

  For displaced tibial tubercle fragments with threatened skin:

- A reduction is obtained using a percutaneously applied shoulder hook (or dental pick).
- 0.062-inch or larger diameter K-wires are placed in the obliquity of the shoulder hook.
- Wires are cut below the skin level and buried under the skin using a dental pick.
- Alternatively, 3.0- or 3.5-mm cannulated or solid screw may be placed if they do not interfere with final construct (Fig. 31-6).

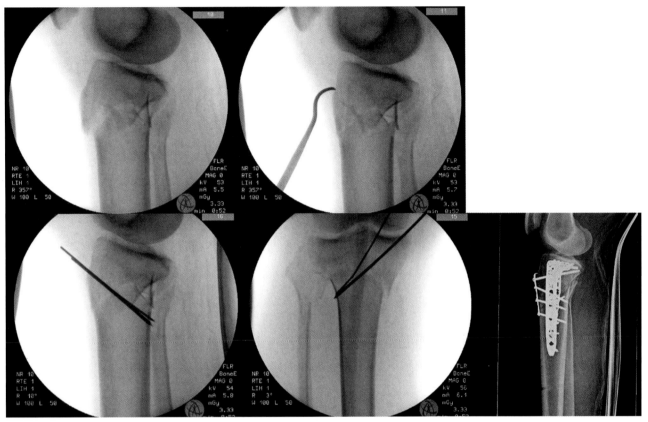

Figure 31-6 I After knee-spanning external fixation, a displaced tibial tuberosity fracture fragment is reduced percutaneously with a shoulder hook. Several 0.062-inch K-wires are used to stabilize the reduced fragment and protect the threatened anterior soft tissue envelope and skin.

- In obese, muscular patients, those with a large body habitus, patients who may be agitated (e.g., traumatic brain injury), or in patients for whom the external fixator will be used for a long period of time, consider augmenting a single bar system with a second bar (e.g., "double-stacked" anterior half-pin unilateral frame) for additional stability (Fig. 31-7).

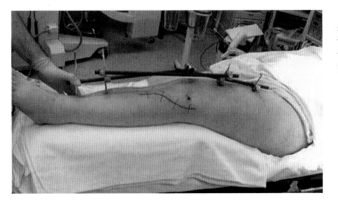

Figure 31-7 I Example of a four-pin knee-spanning external fixator. Note the incision for the definitive fixation of the tibial plateau fracture and the additional augmenting bar between the middle two pins.

- Ensure that there is adequate clearance between the lowest bar and the skin; generally, 2 cm is sufficient.
- At the time of definitive fixation and removal of the external fixator pins, manipulate knee under anesthesia to minimize the potential for quadriceps scarring, adhesions, and heterotopic ossification at the femoral pin sites.
- This technique should only be used for short-term, provisional knee-spanning external fixation.
  - Other pin placement locations and external fixator configurations should be used for external fixators planned for long-term use.

Chapter 32
Ankle-Spanning External Fixation

M. BRADFORD HENLEY

MICHAEL J. GARDNER

Sterile Instruments/Equipment

- Large or medium external fixation system
- Open compressor/distractor device
- 4.0-mm partially threaded pins for midfoot fixation
- Towel bolsters

Positioning

- Supine on a cantilever-type, radiolucent table.
- Bring patient to the cantilever (foot) end of the table.
- Place small bolster (e.g., bump) under ipsilateral hip and torso.
- Elevate the leg on soft ramp cushion to facilitate lateral imaging.

Reduction and Implant Techniques

- Centrally threaded 5.0- or 6.0-mm pin through calcaneus for medial and lateral, "triangular" uniplanar frame.
- Medial 5.0-mm Schanz half pin for medial half-pin frame.
- Calcaneal insertion point is critical to avoid injury to lateral plantar and medial calcaneal nerves, and posterior tibial neurovascular bundle more anteriorly (Fig. 32-1).

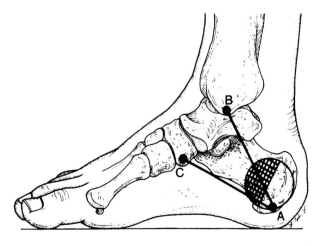

Figure 32-1 ∥ The calcaneal pin should be placed from medial to lateral and in the posterior-inferior half of a circle that approximates the contour of the posterior tuberosity. Avoid inserting the pin into cross-hatched area. Place the pin in coronal plane. It may be inserted as either medial half pin or transcalcaneal pin. Point A (posterior-inferior medial calcaneus), point B (inferior medial malleolus), and point C (navicular tuberosity). (Adapted from Casey D, McConnell T, Parekh S, et al. Percutaneous pin placement in the medial calcaneus: is anywhere safe? *J Orthop Trauma*. 2004;18(8 Suppl):S39–S42, with permission.)

- Place calcaneal pin first, posteriorly and inferiorly in the tuberosity, using a lateral fluoroscopic view (Fig. 32-2).

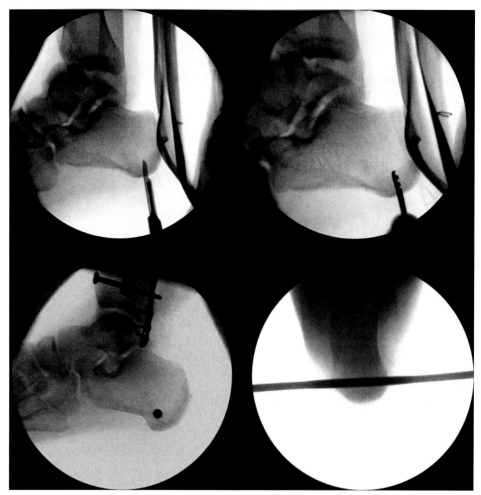

Figure 32-2 For placement of a transcalcaneal pin, the location for the incision should be estimated with a knife under fluoroscopy, and the position of the drill bit and pin should be confirmed. Ideally, the pin should be transverse on the axial view.

- If the fibula is intact or was treated with acute ORIF, the stable lateral column can be used to tension a medial frame (medial calcaneal half pin only) against the lateral fibular plate to restore limb length and angulatory alignment (Fig. 32-3).

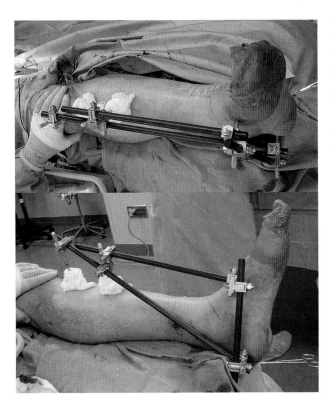

Figure 32-3 I Following fixation of the fibula, a medial frame can be used to tension against the reconstructed lateral column to restore anatomic length. An alternative to a sagittal half pin in the anterior tibia is to place a coronal half pin in the medial aspect of the proximal tibia. This configuration allows for precise control of fracture reduction, as distraction along the tibial-calcaneal bar's axis will result in uniplanar changes. With distraction, in this example, this configuration will result in multiplanar corrections (e.g., distraction and posterior translation with an additional rotational moment).

- Midfoot pin is placed from medial to lateral through the two medial cuneiforms or through all three cuneiforms.
  - Because the midfoot architecture is an arch, it is important to stay in the dorsal half of the medial cuneiform, on the lateral view to avoid exiting plantarly and potentially resulting in a neural or vascular injury (Fig. 32-4).

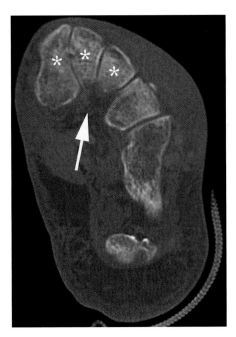

Figure 32-4 I An axial CT scan of the foot demonstrates the arch configuration of the cuneiforms (*asterisks*). A medial to lateral pin should enter the dorsal half of the most medial cuneiform to avoid the structures plantar to the arch (*arrow*).

- Use a 2.5-mm drill bit to drill a pilot hole for a 4.0- × 100-mm partially threaded Schanz half pin (Fig. 32-5).

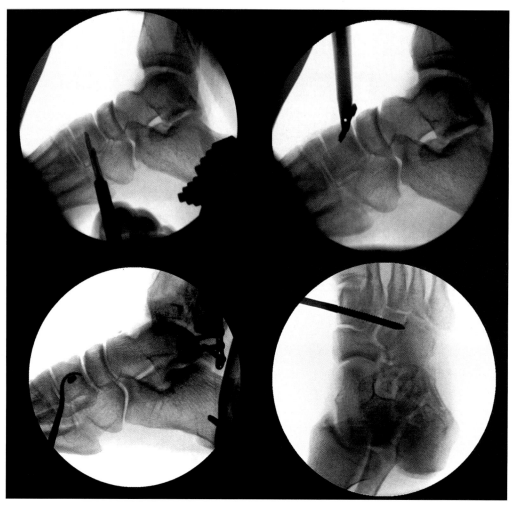

Figure 32-5 I The dorsal starting point is marked with a knife, and the drill entry site and pin position are confirmed on lateral and oblique views.

- In large patients where the osseous pathway allows, a 5.0-mm Schanz pin may be placed in the midfoot.
  - The 5.0-mm pin has longer thread length and may be particularly useful when the external fixator is planned to remain in place for an extended time period.
- It is easier to place the midfoot pin first, prior to distracting across the ankle joint.
  - After distraction across the ankle and subtalar joints, the gastrocsoleus complex tightens, making it more difficult to dorsiflex the foot and obtain an AP fluoroscopic view of the foot.
- To place the midfoot pin, flex the knee to 90 degrees.
  - An assistant can hold the knee flexed, or a tibial triangle can be useful when placed under the knee to assist flexion.

- To obtain a true AP view of the Lisfranc joints, place five folded towels under the forefoot and orient the fluoroscopic beam vertically to the floor (orthogonal to the midfoot and parallel to the TMT joints).
- The cuneiform pin should be placed using this view (Fig. 32-6).

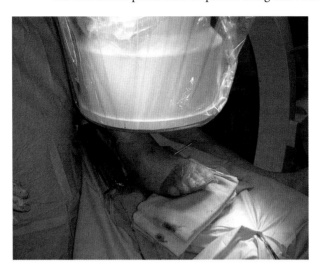

Figure 32-6 | Five folded towels under the forefoot with the fluoroscopic beam perpendicular to the floor gives good visualization of the midfoot for insertion of the medial cuneiform pin.

- Two pins anteriorly, anteromedially, or medially in the tibia.
  - Ensure that these are distal to the knee joint, proximal to the future surgical field, and not through any muscular or fascial compartment (i.e., avoid all lateral tibial diaphyseal pins).
  - In particular, avoid traversing the anterior (or lateral) compartment, as this is associated with an increase in pin drainage, loosening, muscle necrosis, neurovascular injury, and infection.
  - 5.0- × 170-mm pins are generally of appropriate size and should be inserted after predrilling the cortical bone with a 3.5-mm drill bit.
  - Irrigate the drill bit while drilling the pilot hole to prevent thermal necrosis.
- Place bar(s) from proximal tibial pin to calcaneus pin either medially or medially and laterally, depending on the frame configuration desired.
- Tighten both pin-clamp connections and one of the two bar-clamp connections.
- Apply traction manually and tighten pin-bar clamps loosely (Fig. 32-7).

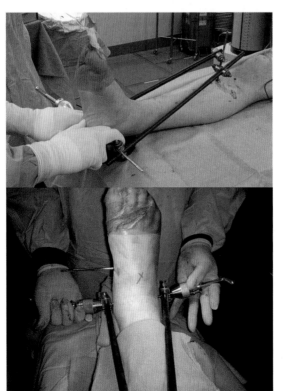

Figure 32-7 | After tightening one end of the pin-bar connections, manual traction will reduce the majority of the limb shortening.

- If a medial frame is used, the first step is restoring the length and tightening the clamps between the proximal tibial pin and the calcaneal pin (Fig. 32-8).

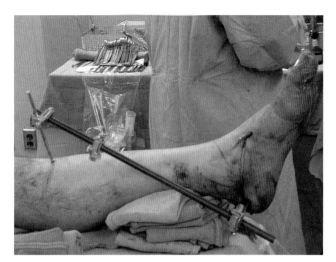

Figure 32-8 | With a medial frame, the first step is establishing the length with a single medial bar between a proximal tibial pin and the calcaneus. If the type of clamps available do not clip on to the open section of the bar, an extra clamp should be placed on the bar between the others pin-bar clamps, for insertion of the second tibial pin.

- When attention is focused on the multiplanar reduction, the clamps and bars may unknowingly slip toward the skin, resting in an undesirable position.
    - These are then in a poor position to tighten once the manipulative reduction is achieved.
    - To prevent this, place several towels or sponges between the bars and skin to maintain the skin-bar distance during manipulation (Fig. 32-9).

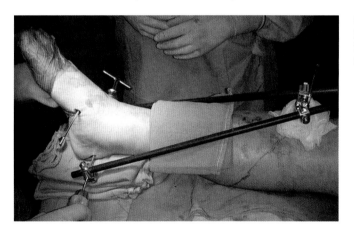

Figure 32-9 | Towels placed under the bars keep them in an acceptable position in which to tighten after a manual reduction is obtained.

- The open compressor/distractor device for the external fixator can be useful for obtaining additional controlled axial distraction.
  - This can also be used to fine-tune the varus/valgus reduction (Fig. 32-10).

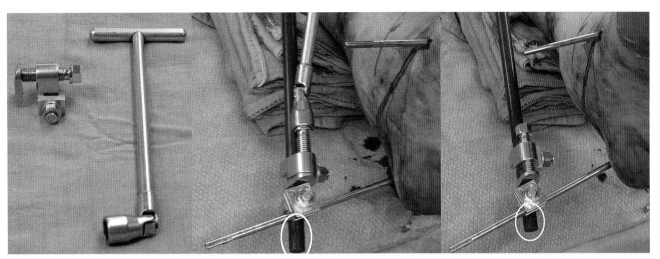

Figure 32-10 | The open compressor-distractor device for external fixation (*left*) can be useful. After the compressor is tightened to the bar, the pin-bar clamp is loosened. The amount of distraction can be tracked by the change in bar excess (*center*, before distraction; *right*, after distraction).

- When using an anterior to posterior sagittal half pin, distraction will create an apex anterior deformity at the fracture site.
  - This can be anticipated and avoided prior to distraction if a bolster is placed under the heel to produce a slight apex posterior deformity.
  - Also the fracture should be placed in slight varus when distracting on the medial bar when using an external fixator in this configuration.
  - Both planes will be corrected with distraction of a medially based frame.
  - These multiplanar deformities (posterior angulation, valgus with rotation) can be avoided by applying a uniplanar (coronal plane only) external fixator, with the tibia pin(s) and the calcaneal pins inserted from medial to lateral in the same plane.
    - If pin-bar clamps are applied to these pins, such that the medial bar is in the exact same coronal plane as the tibial-talar axis, distraction will only create a valgus moment.
    - This is often the preferred configuration (especially if the fibula has been plated so as to create a lateral buttress) as it avoids posterior angulation and rotation.
    - The valgus can be anticipated and counteracted by placing the limb in slight varus, before distraction along the medial bar, between the tibial and calcaneal pins.[1]
- It is important to assess the sagittal plane angular deformity, all translational deformities, and limb rotation prior to the insertion of the third pin.
  - Initially, bumps placed under the heel, Achilles tendon, or calf can partially correct the deformities seen with external fixation of pilon fractures.
  - The position and direction of the initial tibial pin and the position of the pin-bar clamps can be planned strategically to produce variations in the force vector(s) and rotational moments so as to preferentially move a subluxated or dislocated talus anteriorly or posteriorly, medially or laterally, etc.

- If the fracture pattern involves a posterior tibiotalar fracture dislocation, a proximal-posterior to distal-anterior force vector needs to be established "along" the axis of the limb to maintain the talar reduction.
  - The proximal tibial pin can be placed posteromedially to allow for a posterior starting point for the force vector (Fig. 32-11).

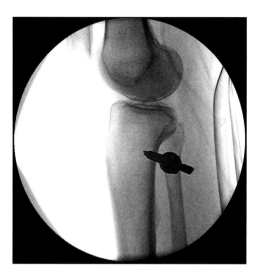

Figure 32-11 | In this case, the proximal tibial pin was placed from posteromedially to anterolaterally to accentuate the posterior to anterior vector across the ankle, when connected to a medial calcaneal half pin.

- The clamps should be rotated such that the bar is angled maximally from proximal-posterior to distal-anterior (Fig. 32-12).

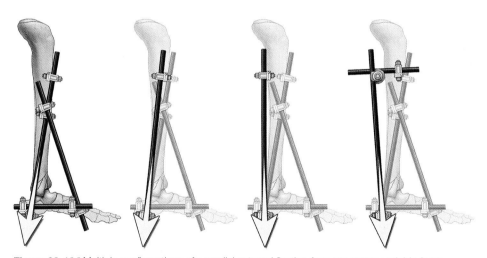

Figure 32-12 | Multiple configurations of a medial external fixation frame to create variable force vectors in the sagittal plane, from anterior to posterior (*left*) to progressively more posterior to anterior (*right*). Standard frame, rotated clamps, posteromedial proximal tibial pin, and posterior extension bar from tibial pin.

- An anterior extension bar is frequently required to connect to the second tibial pin to avoid placing the pin through the posteromedial soft tissue (e.g., gastrocsoleus).
  - If a substantially large posterior to anterior vector is needed, a short bar can be run posteriorly from the anteromedial tibial pin, with the longitudinal bar connecting the posterior extension bar and the calcaneus pin.
- The second and more distal of the two proximal tibial pins is placed proximal to the planned surgical incision.
  - The position is based on the path determined by the line created between the first two pins inserted at each end of the longitudinal bar.
  - As such, its position and vector are relatively constrained.
    - The pin should be inserted once the fracture is reduced to further stabilize the reduction and prevent any rotation around the pins at each end of the bar.

- Pushing along the axis of the pin to improve the reduction is not reliable, because it cannot be placed along the exact vector of the deformity.
- However, if the pin is straight anterior to posterior, and the talus is still translated slightly anteriorly (or posteriorly), or the metaphyseal fracture shows translational displacement, a laminar spreader can be used between a pin-bar clamp and a universal T-chuck to correct a small sagittal plane deformity (Fig. 32-13).
- As the last step of the procedure, the foot is brought to neutral, and a short bar is used to connect the midfoot to the tibial shaft pin(s) (Fig. 32-14).

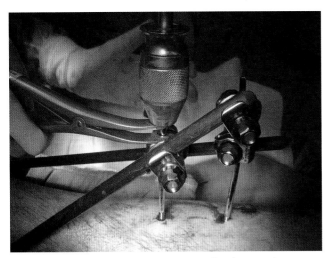

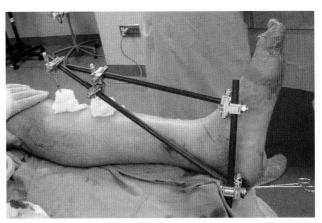

Figure 32-14 I The midfoot pin is connected to the distal of the tibial pins, as the final step to maintain the foot in neutral.

Figure 32-13 I A laminar spreader between the clamp and a universal chuck can be used to pull the tibial fracture fragment anteriorly to correct sagittal plane deformity.

Reference

1. Ertl W, Henley MB. Provisional external fixation for periarticular fractures of the tibia. *Tech Orthop.* 2002;17(2):135–144.

Chapter 33
Foot External Fixation

MICHAEL L. BRENNAN

Sterile Instruments/Equipment

- Large/medium external fixation system
- Open compressor/distractor device
- 4.0-mm partially threaded pins for forefoot fixation
- Towel bolsters/bumps
- Dental pick
- Triangular bolster

Positioning

- Supine on a radiolucent cantilever-type table.
- Bring patient to the radiolucent (foot) end of the table.
- Place small bolster/bump under the ipsilateral hemipelvis and torso.
- Elevate the leg on soft ramp cushion to facilitate lateral imaging.
- Triangular bolster improves imaging of foot (Fig. 33-1).
- With the knee fully flexed, five folded towels under the forefoot allow correct radiographic view of Lisfranc joint with AP fluoroscopy, if necessary.

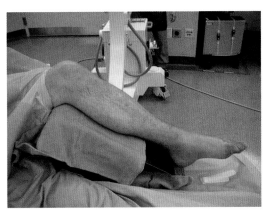 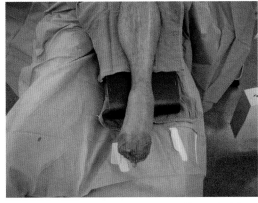

Figure 33-1 ▮ Foot position for external fixation. Note radiolucent triangle flexing hip and knee to facilitate obtaining true AP and oblique views of the foot, when C-arm is in vertical position.

Surgical Approach

- Percutaneous placement of Schanz pins using fluoroscopy

Reduction and Implant Techniques

- Centrally threaded 5.0- or 6.0-mm Schanz pin in calcaneus or medial/lateral 5.0-mm half pins depending on the injury pattern and deformity.
- 4.0 × 100 mm pin in the first and second cuneiforms or in the first metatarsal (Fig. 33-2).

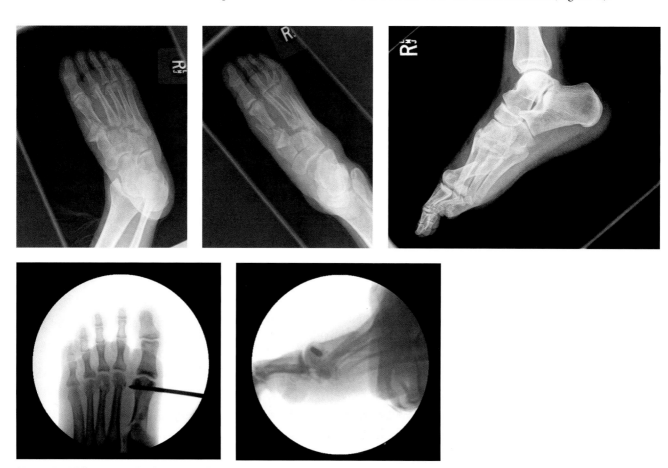

Figure 33-2 I Case example of a severe midfoot crush injury. A 4.0-mm half pin is placed in the distal first metatarsal and connected to the medial side of a calcaneal pin to span the medial column.

- K-wire through base of fourth and fifth metatarsals.
- Use wire hole in drill guide with K-wire to drill; place a 4.0- or 5.0-mm pin.
  - This is used if the lateral column has been disrupted.
- Distraction applied between Schanz pins.
- For Lisfranc injuries, place a medium external fixator frame medially and tighten provisionally.
- Universal T-handle chucks on Schanz pins used as joysticks to manipulate and reduce fracture/dislocations under fluoroscopy (Fig. 33-2).
- Assistant tightens the ex-fix pin-bar clamps.

- Fragment reduction using percutaneous incisions and dental pick (Figs. 33-3–33-4).

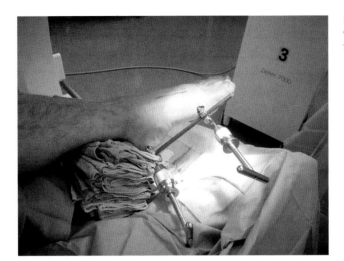

Figure 33-3 | Medial Schanz pins are used with universal chucks to restore length and facilitate realignment of the medial column.

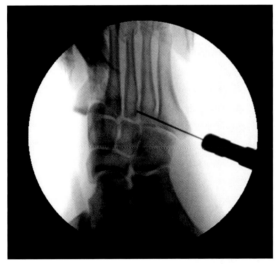 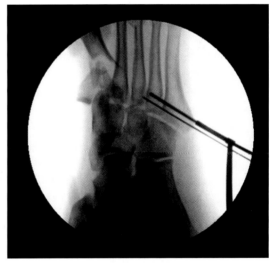

Figure 33-4 | If necessary, a lateral 4.0-mm half pin is placed in the base of the fourth and fifth metatarsals. A K-wire is first inserted through the parallel adjacent hole in the 2.5-mm drill guide to facilitate alignment of the drill bit/drill hole prior to pin insertion.

- Percutaneous K-wire fixation may be used to augment the stability of temporizing external fixation if TMT or tarsal subluxation remains after manipulative reduction and external fixation (Figs. 33-5–33-6).
  - Pins are cut short and buried just beneath the skin.

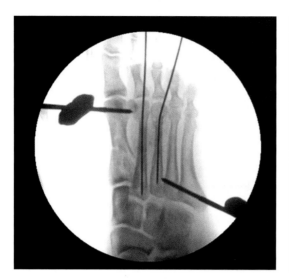
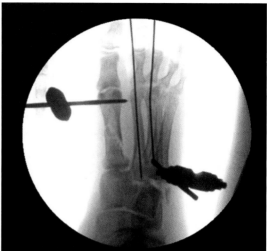
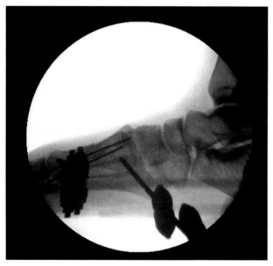

Figure 33-5 I Subsequent to insertion of the 4-mm Schanz pin, the alignment K-wire is removed. Final construct showing ex-fix pins in place.

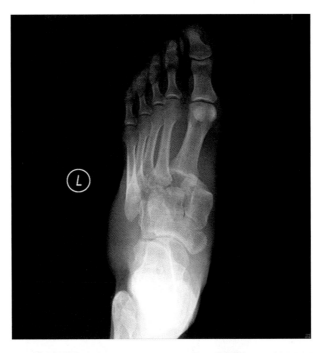

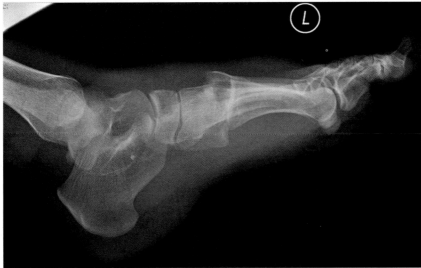

Figure 33-6 ▌ Another clinical example of provisional external fixation applied to a Lisfranc fracture/dislocation. Due to significant lateral soft tissue injury, a medially based frame was selected.

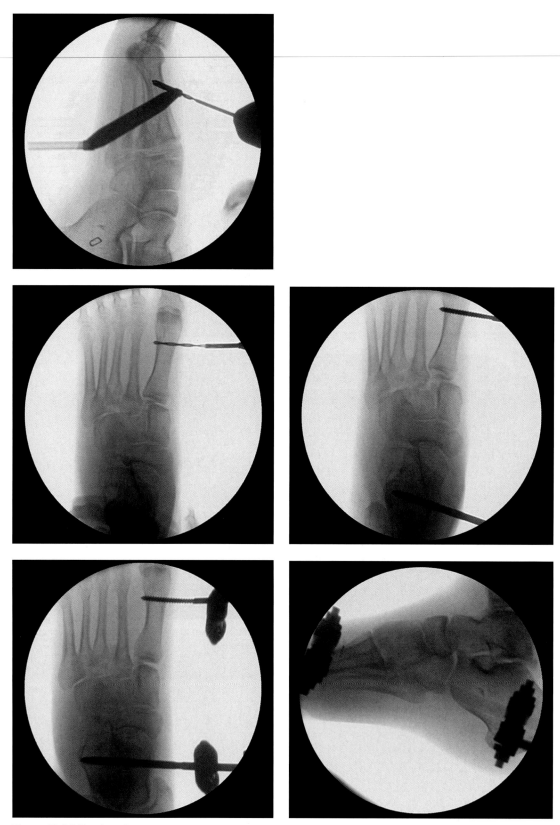

Figure 33-6 | (*Continued*)

Chapter 34
Miscellaneous and Hardware Removal Tips

STEPHEN K. BENIRSCHKE
DAVID BROKAW
CHRISTOPHER DOMES
ERIC D. FARRELL
REZA FIROOZABADI
M. BRADFORD HENLEY
LISA A. TAITSMAN

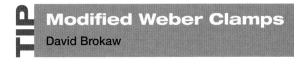

TIP | Modified Weber Clamps
David Brokaw

Pathoanatomy

Osteosynthesis requires reduction of fracture fragments to recreate anatomy and reestablish stability. Maintaining soft tissue attachments is crucial to preserving the vascularity of bone. At times, it is difficult to reduce fracture fragments without disrupting the soft tissue attachments. Unmodified tenaculums (Weber clamps) are not always shaped to apply the needed compression or they may slip off hard cortical bone surfaces. Instruments used to provide compression and reduction can get in the way of definitive hardware positioning. A custom modified tenaculum clamp avoids this.

Solution

Customization of a small and large fracture tenaculum reduction forceps (Weber clamps/"point-to-point" clamps) can assist in compression of fractures and nonunions where the instrument does not obstruct the placement of the fixation hardware (Fig. 34-1).

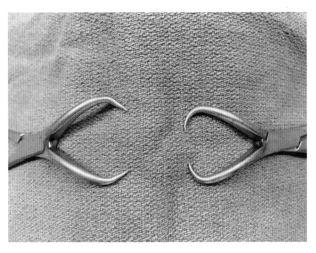

Figure 34-1 ‖ Left, a modified tenaculum bone clamp compared to a nonmodified clamp, right.

Technique

Cortical density may be such that even sharpened tenaculum tines will not engage the bone cortex without slippage. Transverse fracture planes can be compressed using modified tenaculum clamps, but their position may obstruct definitive implant placement. Predrilling colinear, off-plate axis unicortical holes in the cortices adjacent to the fracture line for each clamp tine can assist in fracture reduction and stabilization with compression (Figs. 34-2 and 34-3).

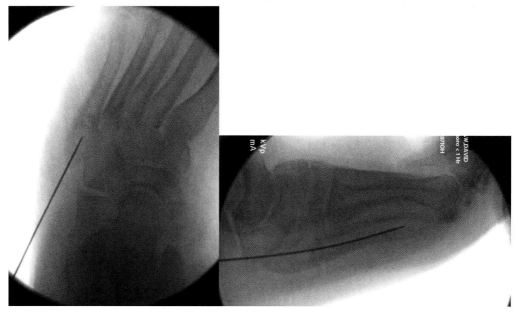

Figure 34-2 I AP and lateral images after starting guide wire inserted for treatment of a fifth metatarsal fracture.

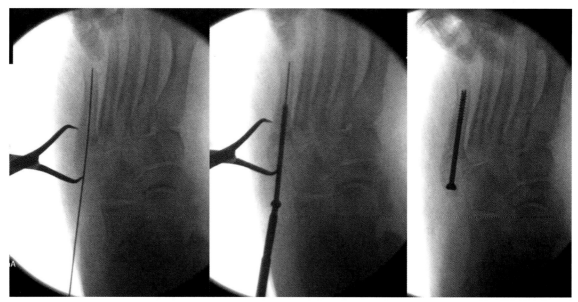

Figure 34-3 I A modified tenaculum (Weber) clamp has been applied to compress the fracture using a drill hole in the diaphysis, and then the guide wire is inserted fully (**left**). A lag screw is inserted to maintain and obtain additional interfragmentary compression (**center**) prior to removing the modified tenaculum clamp (**right**).

- The sharpened tips (tines) of the tenaculum clamp are straightened, by bending them outward leaving a small, varus arc that can engage predrilled unicortical holes on one or both sides of a fracture or nonunion (Fig. 34-1).
  - Alternatively, three different modified clamps may be created by straightening both tines, just the left tine and just the right tine to create a complete set of modifier reduction clamps.

- To stabilize fractures with a large surface area or when bone loss may cause angulation when uniplanar compression is applied, two modified unicortical reduction clamps may be beneficial. This technique can be used with either definitive plate of IM nail fixation (Fig. 34-4).

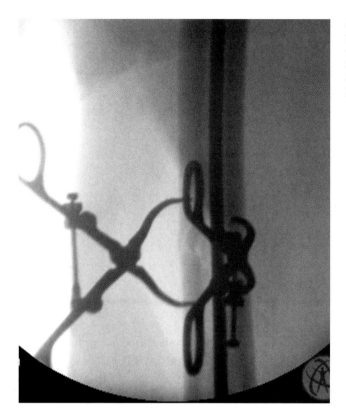

Figure 34-4 ▮ A type 3 A open right femur fracture after debridement, stabilized and compressed with two modified Weber small fragment clamps (one lateral and one anterolateral) during an intramedullary nailing procedure.

- When a fracture pattern is encountered where small vascularized butterfly fragments are necessary to reestablish stability, a very small area of periosteum can be cleared and a small 2.0 unicortical drill hole can be created by directing the drill bit toward the fracture at approximately 30 degrees (Fig. 34-5).

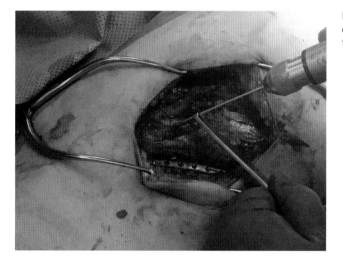

Figure 34-5 ▮ A 2.0 drill bit is used to create an aperture for one tine of a modified tenaculum bone clamp.

- This unicortical hole allows the fragment to be more easily captured by the tenaculum's tine, especially if the adjacent cortex is also predrilled to capture the opposing tenaculum's tine.
  - Using dental picks and the tenaculum bone clamp, the bone fragment(s) can be translated in a controlled manner in all three degrees of freedom before compression is instilled through the clamp's mechanism. This technique allows fracture fragment control and maintains the vascularized muscle attachments (Fig. 34-6).

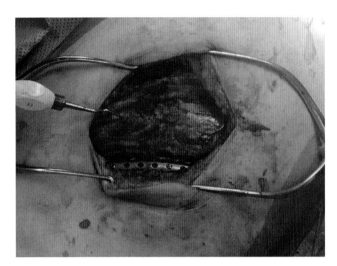

Figure 34-6 I A dental pick can also be used to mobilize fracture fragments in preparation for reduction and tenaculum clamp stabilization.

- These same drill holes can be engaged with a sharp end of a dental pick with one hand, while the opposing fracture fragment is mobilized and secured with the tenaculum clamp. Once these small butterfly fracture fragments are reduced and stabilized with the tenaculum clamp(s), they can be secured with K-wires or minifragment plates. Alternatively, if the modified clamp does not interfere with planned definitive fixation, it can be maintained until appropriate fracture stability has been achieved.
- Considering the optimal position of the plate or final implant construct will direct the surgeon as to the best location of these predrilled, unicortical holes. These small holes are designed to not interfere with the stability of the fracture or cause undo stripping of periosteal and muscular attachments. They also do not interfere with subsequent intrafragmentary screw fixation if necessary for fracture stability.

TIP | Kirschner Wire Bending

Reza Firoozabadi
Stephen K. Benirschke

Pathoanatomy

Kirschner wires are used extensively though their use has led to a number of problems. The two most common problems are protrusion of the wire from the bone surface, which causes soft tissue irritation and wire migration.

Solution

To eliminate these issues, we have developed a technique that introduces a 180-degree bend in the end of the wire that anchors the wire into the bone. This bend allows the wire to present a smooth surface that is flush to the surface of the bone and prevents migration of the wire.[1] Additionally, this bend facilitates easy wire removal if necessary.

Technique

This method is specifically designed for wires that are meant to be impacted into bone, such as is the case for tension band techniques and permanent fracture fixation techniques. It can, however, be used for cases in which the K-wires are placed for temporary measures, allowing for easier retrieval. The recommended instruments are displayed in Figure 34-7.

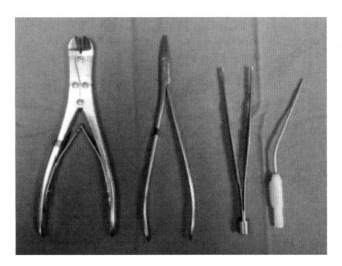

Figure 34-7 | Recommended instruments: wire cutter; needle-nose pliers; impacting forceps; and 7, 10, or 12Fr suction tip depending on gauge of wire to be bent.

The technique consists of seven key steps, which are designed to bend the K-wire 180 degrees. Key steps are as follows:

1. The first step is pull the wire 5 to 10 mm back from its desired final depth using the K-wire driver. This will prevent overpenetration of the second cortex after the wire is bent and impacted into place.
2. A pair of needle-nose pliers is placed flush to bone (Fig. 34-8A) and a 7, 8, 9, or 10 French suction tip is placed over the complete exposed length of the K-wire, that is, from exposed end to the pliers (Fig. 34-8B). Holding the wire firm with the pliers, the suction and wire are rotated 90 degrees perpendicular to the pliers (Fig. 34-8C). This results in a 90-degree bend in the K-wire.

A

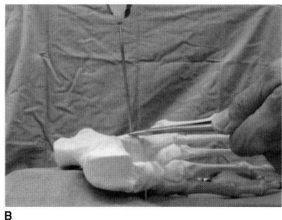

B

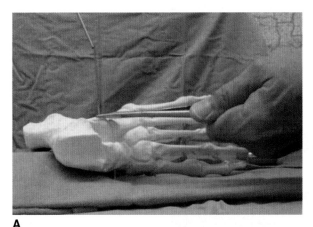

C

Figure 34-8 | A–C: Demonstrate the steps to achieve the first 90-degree bend in the K-wire.

3. The suction tip is slid along the K-wire and the pair of needle-nose pliers is moved so that it grasps the wire in the plane in which it was bent, within 5 mm of the bend that was just created. The sucker with wire within it is then bent 120 degrees back on itself (Fig. 34-9).

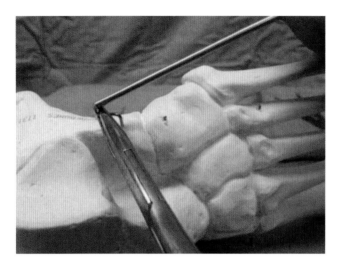

Figure 34-9 I The second bend is placed in the wire, resulting in 120-degree bend.

4. The pliers are moved back at the initial starting point, flush with bone (Fig. 34-10A). The sucker's tip is placed down to the second bend, and the second bend is used as a lever to continue the initial bend (Fig. 34-10B). This results in a 170-degree bend. Note that the first bend cannot be made to 170 degrees initially because the bone is in the way. The second bend is necessary to provide access for the K-wire and sucker.

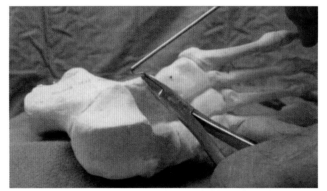

Figure 34-10 I The third bending sequence results in a 170-degree bend.

A

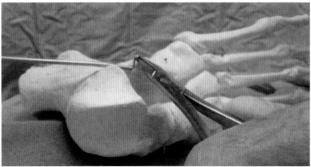
B

5. The wire is then clipped with wire clippers 5mm from the first bend (Fig. 34-11).
6. Using the needle-nose pliers, the bend is increased to 170 to 180 degrees (Fig. 34-12).

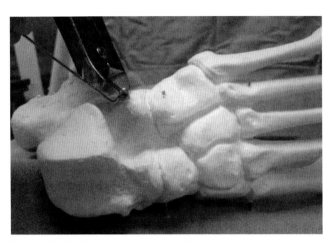

Figure 34-11 | The wire is then clipped in preparation for final bending and tamping.

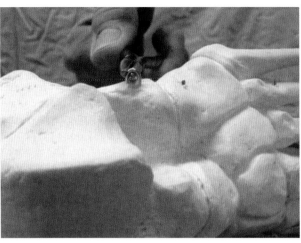

Figure 34-12 | Using the needle-nose pliers, the bend is increased to 170 to 180 degrees.

7. A tamp is then used to push the K-wire into bone (Fig. 34-13A). This results in an impacted hook that is flush with the bone surface (Fig. 34-13B).

Sample X-rays demonstrating the use of K-wire bending (Fig. 34-14):

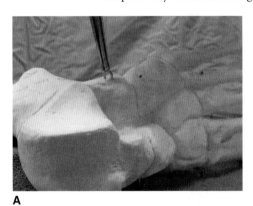

A

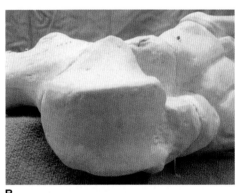

B

Figure 34-13 | The wire is the tamped (A) into the bone so it is flush with the cortex (B).

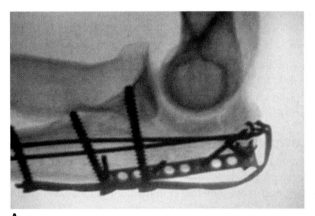

A

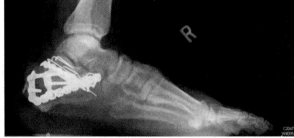

B

Figure 34-14 | X-rays demonstrating the use of K-wire bending.

Reference

1. Firoozabadi R, Kramer PA, Benirschke SK. Kirschner wire bending. *J Orthop Trauma*. 2013;27(11):e260–e263.

Kirschner Wire(s) to Definitive Screw Fixation Technique

Christopher Domes
Lisa Taitsman

Pathoanatomy

Kirschner wires (K-wires) are commonly used to temporarily stabilize fractures, and often, they are inserted in the ideal place for a definitive screw. In small bone fragments, it can be challenging to find space for adequate provisional fixation in addition to the definitive implants. Initial K-wire placement is usually done perpendicular to the fracture pattern to allow for maximal temporary stability of the fracture. The K-wire trajectories are often ideal for screw fixation; however, the wire placement often makes it hard to maneuver a drill and insert a screw in close proximity of the K-wire.

Solution

When fixing small fragments, it can be beneficial to use the K-wire hole/path and replace it with the correctly sized screw for definitive fixation. To use this technique, it is necessary to know the size of the wire and thus which wire matches the proper drill size for a corresponding screw.

Technique

- The fracture to be fixed is exposed and the fracture fragments are identified in the usual manner. Provisional fixation with K-wires is achieved initially (Fig. 34-15).

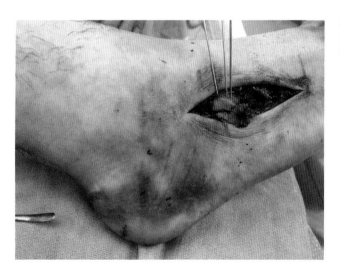

Figure 34-15 | Fracture reduction and provisional fixation with K-wires of a small fracture fragment.

- Depending on the size of the fracture fragment, there may be little or insufficient space to place one or more screws between the K-wires without further comminuting the fracture fragment. In the case depicted, the central K-wire is in an ideal location and direction for a screw. A subtraction method can be used to measure the portion of the K-wire within the bone and hence the anticipated screw length.
  - The provisional wire to be replaced is assessed radiographically to ensure that it is inserted to exactly the depth of the anticipated final screw.
  - A K-wire of the same length is placed directly next to the K-wire that is going to be replaced. The amount of wire that extends past the end of the wire that is in the bone is measured with a ruler and that measurement corresponds to the appropriate length for the screw.
  - Alternatively, the K-wire may be removed and a standard mini-depth gauge can be used.

- Knowing the diameter of the wire, the appropriate size screw is selected as the wire has served functionally as a drill bit (Table 34-1).

Table 34-1 I Kirschner Wire Sizes, with Corresponding Mini- and Small Fragment Screw Sizes and Recommended Drill Bit Diameters for the Screws

K-wire Size (inch)	K-wire Size (mm)	Corresponding Screw	Corresponding Drill Diameter
0.045	1.1 mm	1.5 mm	1.1 mm
0.054	1.4 mm	2.0 mm	1.5 mm
0.062	1.8 mm	2.4 mm	1.8 mm
(5/64) 0.078	2.0 mm	2.7 mm	2.0 mm

Note that this table is also helpful when inserting K-wires into dense cortical bone as a pilot hole may be drilled bicortically for the K-wire (to prevent heat necrosis) with an undersized drill bit. For example, a 1.5 mm bit is ideal for a 0.062-inch K-wire and a 1.1 bit is ideal for a 0.054-inch K-wire.

- Thus, a 0.062-inch K-wire has a diameter of 1.8 mm, which is the same size as the drill bit used for a 2.4-mm screw (1.8 mm core diameter). The screw is inserted in the usual manner (Fig. 34-16).
  - Note that the screw will not be placed in lag fashion unless the near cortex has been overdrilled with a 2.4-mm bit in this example.

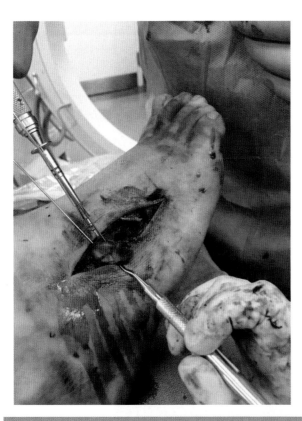

Figure 34-16 I Standard insertion of a 2.4-mm screw following removal of a 0.062-inch K-wire used to create the bone tunnel.

TIP

Screw Lasso Technique
David Brokaw

Pathoanatomy

Advances in plate osteosynthesis have evolved using percutaneous and submuscular techniques. Transcutaneous screw placement can be challenging especially if the screw becomes disengaged from the screwdriver. This can lead to the screw becoming entrapped in the muscular envelope. Screw removal increases surgical time as well as fluoroscopy usage.

Solution

Suture may be used to secure any size screw to the end of a screwdriver using ordinary suture material. This can be used for both cortical or lag screws.

Technique

- A size 0, 1, or larger Vicryl suture is tied around the top of the screw shank adjacent to the screwhead with a simple overhand knot (Fig. 34-17).

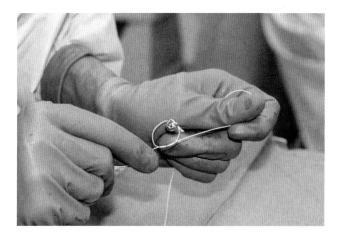

Figure 34-17 ▌The middle of a 1 Vicryl suture that is used to tie an overhand ("simple") knot is tied around the screw just below the screw's head

- Use the midpoint of the suture to tie the simple knot. It is then tightened at the junction between the upper shaft and the screwhead (Fig. 34-18).

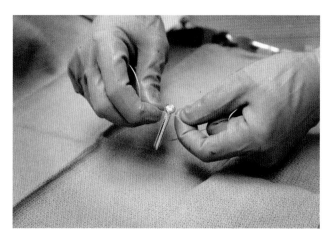

Figure 34-18 ▌The knot is tightened just below the screwhead.

- The surgeon maintains tension on this suture with a nondominant hand while using a power or hand screwdriver to place the screw transcutaneously into the appropriate predrilled screw hole.
  - Sufficient suture length allows the surgeon to pull gentle rearward tension with the nondominant hand while using the dominant hand to direct the screw transcutaneously into the predrilled hole (Figs. 34-19–34-21).

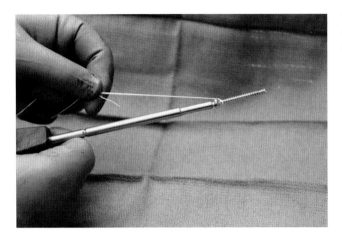

Figure 34-19 I Tension on both free ends of the suture is used to maintain firm engagement of the screw and screwdriver.

- During the insertion, gentle tension applied to both free ends of the suture maintains engagement of the screw onto the screwdriver head (Figs. 34-19–34-21). This prevents disengagement when the screw has to be either withdrawn completely or redirected for repositioning.

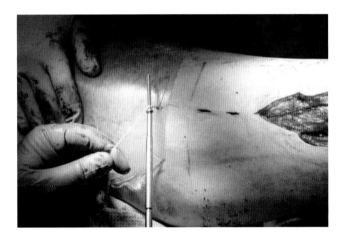

Figure 34-20 I Screw mated to screwdriver prior to percutaneous insertion.

- Many times, adjustments are necessary to reposition the screw into the appropriate slot of the plate by tactile feel or fluoroscopic guidance. Without this rearward tension, the screw may become disengaged from the screwdriver and "lost" within the soft tissue envelope.
  - Maintaining rearward tension with a disposable suture can maximize the accuracy of screw placement and minimize the need for retrieving disengaged screws.
  - This decreases surgical time as well as fluoroscopic exposure to the surgeon or patient.

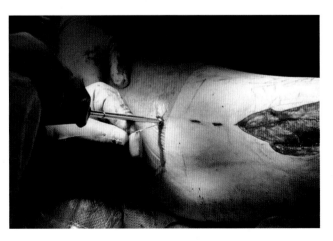

Figure 34-21 I Transcutaneous introduction of the screw is performed while tension is maintained on both free ends of the suture.

- Once the screw is fully seated, the suture can usually be pulled free by releasing one free end and pulling on the other free end.
  - Alternatively, the suture may be abraded and transected as the screw interdigitates and is seated in the plate or both free ends can be cut below the skin (Fig. 34-22).

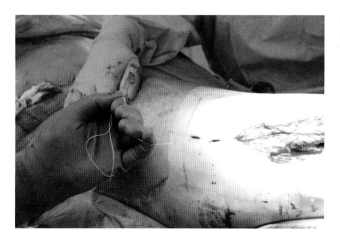

Figure 34-22 | To remove the suture, release one end and pull on the other free end.

- The simple overhand knot allows the screw to spin freely while it is advanced, and not wind up the suture on the screwdriver shaft.
  - However, fully threaded cortical screws may capture and wind up the suture regardless of the knot type. Sufficient length of suture, approximately 10 to 12 inch, will permit this occurrence and provide enough length for seating the screw fully.

TIP | Minimally Invasive Technique for Implant Removal
Eric D. Farrell

Pathophysiology

Internal fixation placed percutaneously or through small incisions increases the complexity of implant removal. Additionally, if an extensile approach was used for ORIF, removal of implants through the original incision may add to morbidity and increase the potential for wound complications.

Solution

A minimally invasive technique for the implant removal can often be used through the original incision(s) or through a new approach.

Technique

- The proximal or distal portion of the plate is marked using fluoroscopy and/or palpation. Ensure that the implant is collinear with the previous incision.
- If implant is not collinear, reopen the previous incision making the incision length sufficient to expose at least the end of the plate and the closest screw hole.
  - If implant is significantly distant from the previous incision, consider making a new incision provided there will be an adequate skin bridge.
- Continue dissection to the fascia, which is then incised and then tagged with suture.

- Elevate soft tissue off the superficial aspect of the plate (Fig. 34-23).

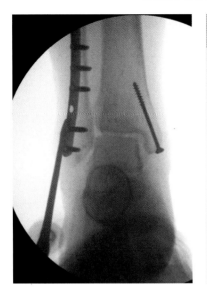 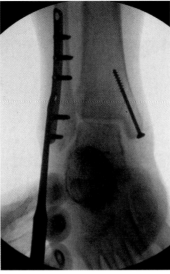

Figure 34-23 An elevator is placed through a small distal incision (in this case, previous incision was used) over the distal two holes. The elevator is used to release soft tissues superficial to plate up to its most proximal extent.

- Fluoroscopy is used to locate the screwheads and area marked.
- A small K-wire can be used to further localize the implant(s) in line with the screw trajectory(ies) (Figs. 34-24 and 34-25).

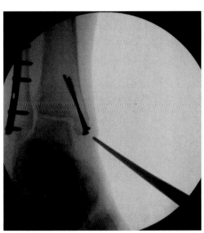 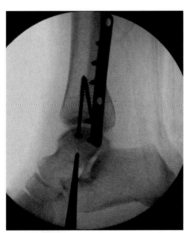

Figure 34-24 Screwheads localized with fluoroscopy on AP and lateral views. In this case, one incision was used to remove both medial screws. An incision is made distal to and between the two screwheads.

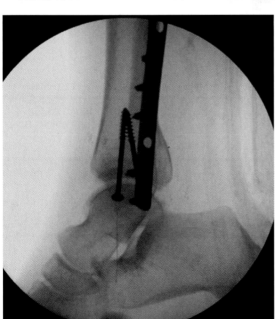

Figure 34-25 A small K-wire is used to percutaneously locate the anterior screwhead and its trajectory.

- A small incision is made over the screwhead and a straight mosquito used to spread to the screwhead. Cannulated screws can be recannulated with a K-wire facilitating removal.
- Screwdriver is inserted onto the screwhead and screw(s) removed (Fig. 34-26).

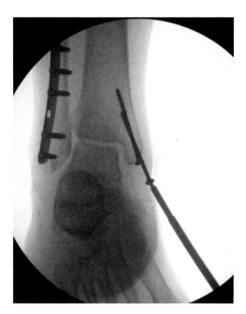

Figure 34-26 I Screw removed through a percutaneous incision.

- For thicker soft tissue envelopes, place a partially opened hemostat over the screwhead and apply pressure to compress the soft tissue, which may facilitate exposure of the screwhead (Fig. 34-27).

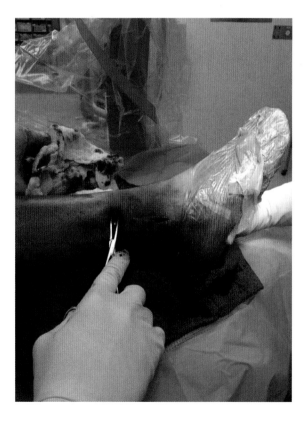

Figure 34-27 I Hemostat may facilitate exposure of screwhead after it is partially removed.

- Following removal of all screws, a freer is then used to elevate the soft tissue off the sides of the plate proximally and continued to the undersurface of the implant.

- A small key elevator is now used to free the soft tissue from underneath the plate (again using tactile and fluoroscopic guidance). This maneuver will facilitate releasing the soft tissues, which have grown over the edges of the plate and through empty screw holes (Fig. 34-28).

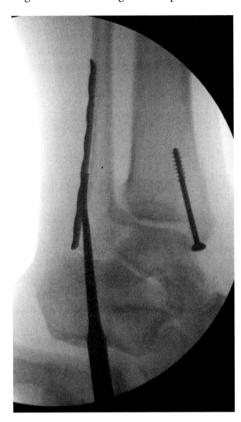

Figure 34-28 | Key elevator freeing underneath the plate through the distal wound.

- Once the plate is free of screws, a small bone hook or similar device is placed through the near end-hole in the plate by inserting its pointed tip adjacent to the plate's terminus. The tip then "exits" the terminal hole so that the tip of the hook is superficial to the plate. The bone hook is now back-slapped with a mallet and plate removed. Note, a pliers, Cobb elevator, or similar instrument can be placed through the bone hook to facilitate mallet strikes (Fig. 34-29).

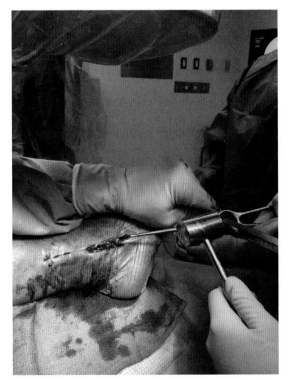

Figure 34-29 | Bone hook placed through the distal hole in the plate (tip is superficial) and mallet used to generate shear forces for plate removal.

- Alternatively, if the soft tissues surrounding the plate are not tenacious, an attempt can be made to remove the plate using mallet strikes alone so as to apply sufficient shear forces without elevating the soft tissues surrounding the plate. This works in the majority of subcutaneous plate locations.
- The wound is irrigated and then fascia closed followed by the skin incision using a nylon suture.

Case Example

- A 30-year-old female s/p ORIF of a lateral tibial plateau fracture at an outside institution. The ORIF was performed through an extensile anterior incision. The patient presented with knee pain and implant-related symptoms (Fig. 34-30).

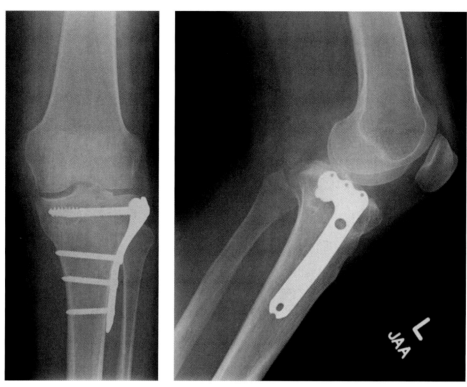

Figure 34-30 ▌ Healed lateral tibial plateau fracture with lateral buttress plate.

- The decision was made to remove implants through new small incisions in order to avoid elevating a large lateral flap, which would be required if the previous incision was used (Fig. 34-31).

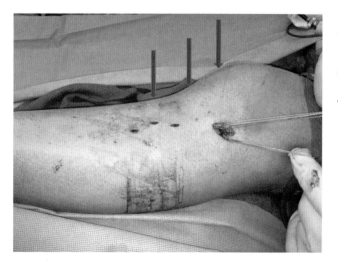

Figure 34-31 ▌ The approach is made and the fascia is tagged with sutures for retraction. The proximal screws were removed though the proximal incision, and distal screws were removed percutaneously. Note the extensile anterior incision (*red arrows*).

- Proximal plate is visualized and plate has been freed from deep and superficial tissue using freer and small Cobb (Figs. 34-32 through 34-36).

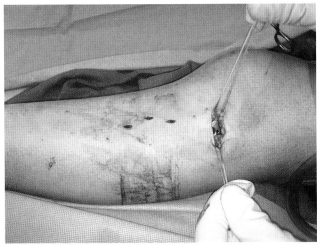

Figure 34-32 I Proximal plate has been elevated with a freer and proximal hole is accessible to bone hook.

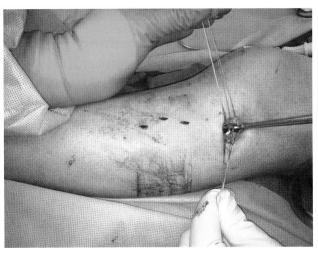

Figure 34-33 I A bone hook inserted so that the pointed tip is superficial preventing injury to the skin and underlying bone.

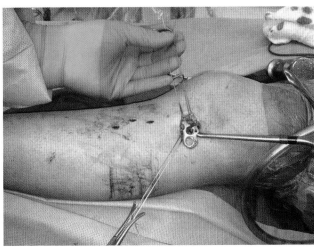

Figure 34-34 I The plate is removed with gentle backslaps from mallet. In this case, bone hook/plate was initially internally rotated and traction placed on posterior fascial tags to expose and clear the posterior corner of the plate.

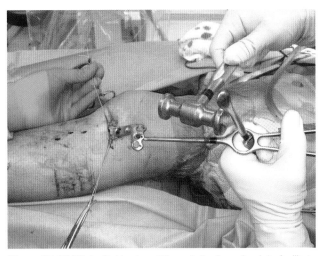

Figure 34-35 I Note Cobb placed through the bone hook to facilitate mallet strikes. Alternate instruments, such as pliers may also be used.

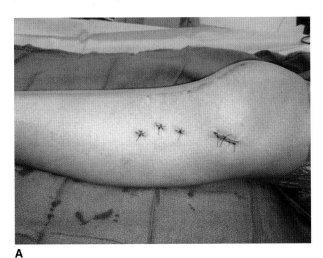

A

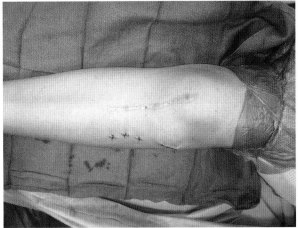

B

Figure 34-36 I **A and B:** Postop incisions and relation to previous incision.

Removal of a Slotted Tibial IM Nail
Eric D. Farrell

Pathoanatomy

Removal of implants can be a difficult task especially when they are well fixed or long lived. Special instruments may be required, and the surgeon may also need to think "outside the box." Despite adequate preoperative planning, special commercially available instrumentation sets designed specifically for IM nail removal may be unavailable or inadequate.

Solution

A 1/3 tubular locking plate and 2.4-mm guide pin can be used as flexible osteotomes to aid in removal of a slotted tibial intramedullary nail.

Technique

This 49-year-old male is approximately 30 years following placement of a slotted IM nail for a midshaft tibial fracture. The patient developed ankle arthritis and has a failed ankle fusion in which cannulated screws were used. The tibial nail requires removal to facilitate a revision ankle fusion (Figs. 34-37 and 34-38).

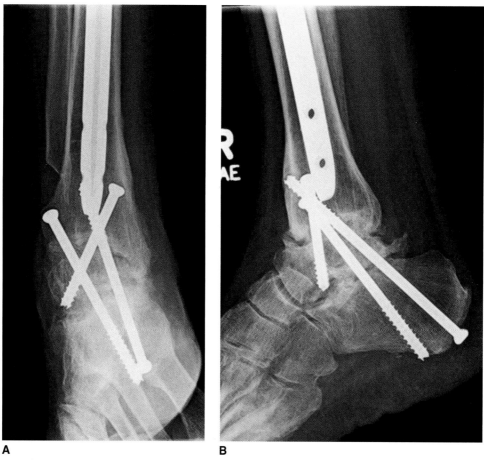

A   **B**

Figure 34-37 I **A and B:** Failed ankle fusion with cannulated screws.

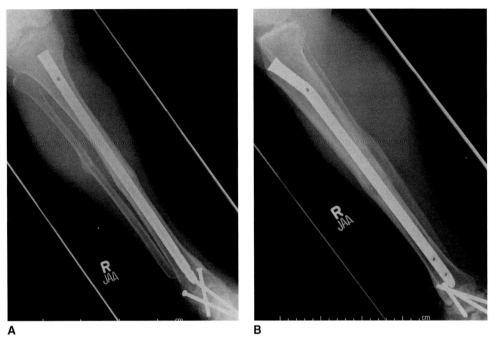

A **B**

Figure 34-38 I **A and B:** Slotted tibial nail. Interlocking screws were removed previously. The fracture is well healed.

- The previous patellar incision/approach is used to expose the proximal tibial insertion site. A 2.4-mm terminally threaded guide pin is inserted into the proximal portion of the nail and confirmed under fluoroscopy (Fig. 34-39A and B).

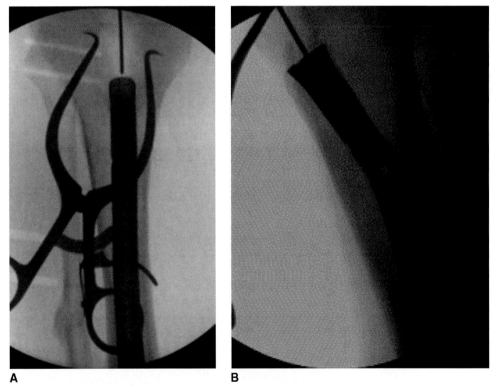

A **B**

Figure 34-39 I **A and B:** Guide pin inserted into the nail confirmed on AP and lateral.

- A cannulated opening drill (~8 to 11 mm) is then inserted over the guide pin and advanced to the top of the nail. Care is taken to protect the patellar tendon and nail threads.

- The remaining bone above the proximal nail is carefully removed using a combination of curettes and small burr. The bone within the threads is also removed without damaging the threads.
- In this case, there is a generous Herzog curve, which can make nail removal more difficult. Attention should be made to freeing up and removing some bone posterior to the nail and cephalad to the curve.
- Flexible osteotomes are ideal for freeing the bone around the nail without removing excess bone. If these are not available, a 1/3 tubular plate can be used as a flexible osteotome.
- Trick: A long 1/3 tubular plate is contoured with a small bend at the 2 to 3 hole. The plate is then placed posterior to the proximal nail, and a mallet is used to advance distally. A pair of vise-grip pliers can be clamped to the plate near the tibia and used to receive mallet blows (Fig. 34-40A–C).

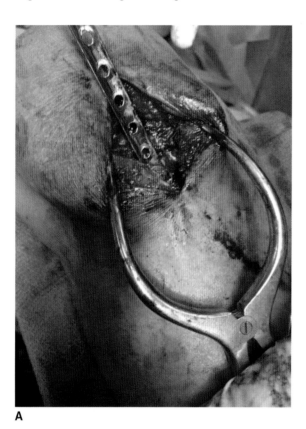

A

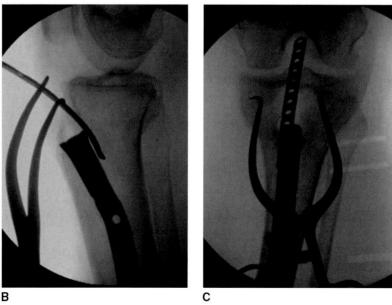

B   **C**

Figure 34-40 | **A–C:** Plate used as flexible osteotome to free proximal nail.

- The plate is advanced distally and posteriorly as far as possible (Fig. 34-41A and B).

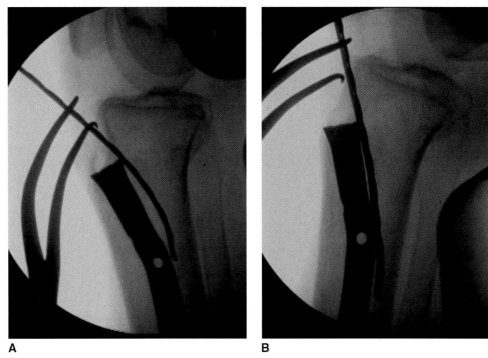

A   **B**

Figure 34-41 ‖ A and B: Plate advanced posteriorly and distally.

- The plate is then used to free anterior to the plate and, if possible, medially and laterally (Fig. 34-42A and B).

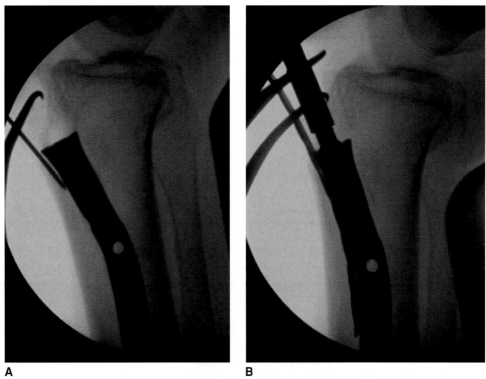

A   **B**

Figure 34-42 ‖ A and B: Anterior freeing.

- Freeing distally on the medial and lateral sides of the nail may be difficult using the plate. A 2.4-mm guide pin can be used in this case. Under fluoroscopic guidance, the threaded tip guide pin is advanced. Placing the drill on oscillate may aid in redirecting the trajectory (Figs. 34-43A and B and 34-44).

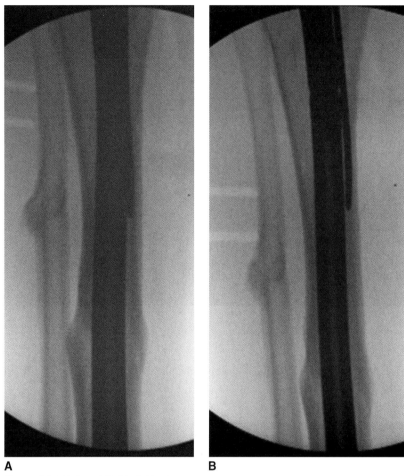

A   **B**

Figure 34-43 I **A and B:** Medial freeing.

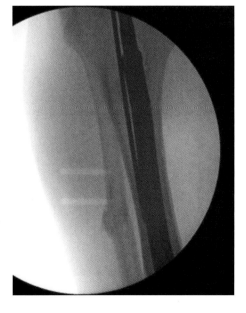

Figure 34-44 I Lateral freeing.

- In the absence of locking screws in long-lived implants, bone tends to grow into the holes. These cylinders of bone "fix" the nail to the metaphyseal bone in the proximal and distal portions of an interlocking nail. These bone cylinders may be released by freeing the nail medially and laterally to the nail.

- Alternatively, the holes can be "drilled out" with an appropriate-sized drill bit (3.2 or 4.3 mm). Use a C-arm–assisted free hand technique similar to placing interlocking screws.
- An implant-appropriate extraction bolt is then affixed to the nail. The guide pin (2.8/3.2/4.3 mm) or drill bit can be placed into one of the interlocking screw holes to prevent the nail from rotating as the extraction bolt is tightened.
- The extractor is then fastened to the bolt, and a large mallet or sliding hammer is used to backslap the nail.
  - CAUTION: Striking the proximal aspect on some nail extraction systems may create excessive bending stresses, and it reduces the mechanical advantage. In addition, repeated offset strikes may cause the extractor to break at the top of the extraction bolt.
- TIP: If the nail removal does not appear to be progressing using the manufacturer's recommended technique, use the mallet to strike the bottom portion of the extraction device.
- In this case, once the extraction handle was struck closer to the bolt, nail removal progressed immediately. The nail was removed without further difficulty (Fig. 34-45A–C).

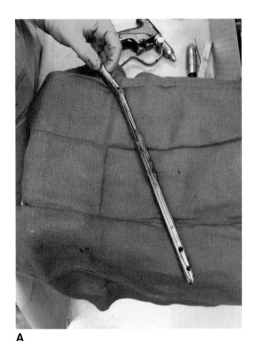

A

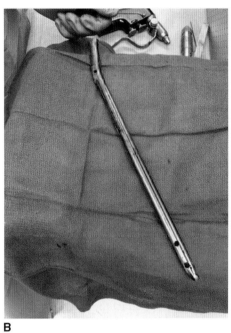

B

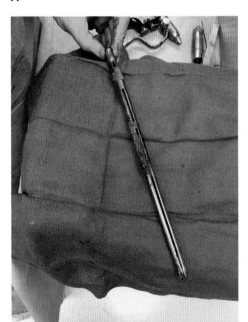

C

Figure 34-45 | A–C: Slotted tibial nail successfully removed. Note the evidence of extensive bony ingrowth.

- Ankle fusion was then performed, and 8-month postop X-rays reveal progressive healing (Fig. 34-46A and B).

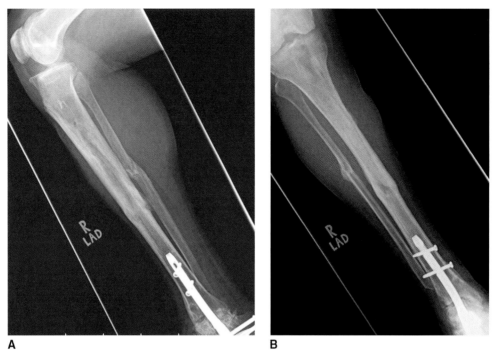

A   B

Figure 34-46 ▮ A and B: Healing ankle fusion and tibia.

- Should all attempts at nail removal be unsuccessful, the next step is to create a lateral cortical "episi-otomy" to increase the medullary diameter and decrease the force required for nail extraction.
  - Make an anterolateral skin incision at the level of the tibial isthmus. This should extend a few centimeter proximal and distal to the tight isthmic contact with the IM nail.
  - Incise the anterior tibialis fascia approximately 5 mm lateral to its insertion on the anterolateral tibial crest.
  - Retract the anterior compartment muscles laterally and make 4.5-mm drill holes in the midportion of the lateral tibial cortex just proximal and distal to the tibial isthmus. The midportion of the lateral cortex should correspond to the middle of the IM canal and a midaxial line of the IM nail on a lateral image.
    - These two 4.5 holes will serve to relieve stress when the diaphysis is expanded.
  - Created a lateral corticotomy with a micro-oscillating saw. Advance the saw to the nail.
  - Insert several thin osteotomes into the corticotomy, thereby enlarging the medullary canal.
  - Make another attempt at nail removal with the osteotomes in situ.
  - If this fails, then increase the width of the corticotomy by inserting slightly thicker osteotomes or chisels until the medullary pressure on the IM nail has been reduced sufficiently to permit IM nail extraction.
  - Alternatively, the corticotomy can be lengthened both proximally and distally by creating two more 4.5-mm stress-relieving holes proximal and distal to the original holes. Connect the two proximal and the two distal holes with the oscillating saw thereby extending the length of the lateral corticotomy. Introduce additional osteotomes or chisels into these corticotomy extensions to allow for further expansion of the medullary canal.

Index

Page numbers in *italics* denote figures.